NOVEL THERAPEUTIC TARGETS FOR ANTIARRHYTHMIC DRUGS

NOVEL THERAPEUTIC TARGETS FOR ANTIARRHYTHMIC DRUGS

Edited by

George Edward Billman
Professor of Physiology and Cell Biology
The Ohio State University

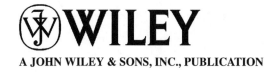

A JOHN WILEY & SONS, INC., PUBLICATION

Published by John Wiley & Sons, Inc., Hoboken, New Jersey
Published simultaneously in Canada

For general information on our other products and services or for technical support, please contact our Customer Care Department within the United States at (800) 762-2974, outside the United States at (317) 572-3993 or fax (317) 572-4002.

Wiley also publishes its books in a variety of electronic formats. Some content that appears in print may not be available in electronic formats. For more information about Wiley products, visit our web site at www.wiley.com

Library of Congress Cataloging-in-Publication Data:

Novel therapeutic targets for antiarrhythmic drugs / [edited by] George E. Billman.
     p. ; cm.
   Includes bibliographical references and index.
   ISBN 978-0-470-26100-2 (cloth)
     1. Myocardial depressants. 2. Arrhythmia–Chemotherapy. I. Billman, George E.
     [DNLM: 1. Antiarrhythmia Agents. 2. Arrhythmias, Cardiac–drug therapy.
   QV 150 N937 2010]
   RM347.N68 2010
   616.1'28061–dc22

                                                    2009020796

Printed in the United States of America

10   9   8   7   6   5   4   3   2   1

To Rosemary, friend, confidante, soul mate, and life partner—semper gaude.

CONTENTS

◼◼◼ ACKNOWLEDGMENTS

As John Donne, the 17th century, British metaphysical poet and Anglican Priest so beautifully stated, "No man is an island, entire in itself. . ." (from Mediation XVII), this book results from the efforts of many. I wish to express my gratitude to many individuals who not only assisted in the preparation of this book but also guided me along my life's journey. First, I wish to thank my parents who nurtured my curiosity as well as my wife and children for their love and support in both the good times and the bad. I also thank the faculty of the Department of Physiology and Biophysics at the University of Kentucky for their support while I earned my doctorate degree. In particular, I wish to acknowledge Dr. James Zolman, who taught me how to analyze research articles critically and interpret statistical results accurately. I am deeply indebted to my mentor, Dr. David C. Randall, who gave me the freedom to fail and the support to succeed. My career development was enhanced even more by my postdoctoral advisor Dr. H. Lowell Stone (deceased) at the University of Oklahoma, who taught me the art of "grantsmanship" and gave me the opportunity to pursue independent research interests that led to my first grant. I also appreciate the help and good humor of Dr. M. Jack Keyl (deceased), whose infectious enthusiasm kept research fun and exciting, even in those all too common times when experiments did not work as planned and funding fell short of expected. I would not be the scientist that I am today without the guidance and support of the individuals mentioned above. Finally, I wish to thank Mr. Jonathan Rose for inviting me to write this book and to the authors of the individual chapters; truly without their contributions, this book would not have been possible.

CONTRIBUTORS

Takeshi Aiba, M.D., Ph.D.
Johns Hopkins University

Gudrun Antoons, Ph.D.
Laboratory of Experimental Cardiology
Catholic University of Leuven (KUL)
Belgium

Charles Antzelevitch, Ph.D., F.A.C.C., F.A.H.A., F.H.R.S.
Executive Director and Director of Research
Gordon K. Moe Scholar
Masonic Medical Research Laboratory

Andrea Barbuti, Ph.D.
Departmento of Biomolecular Sciences and Biotechnology
Università degli Studi di Milano

Mirko Baruscotti, Ph.D.
Departmento of Biomolecular Sciences and Biotechnology
Università degli Studi di Milano, Italy

Andriy E. Belevych, Ph.D.
Davis Heart and Lung Research Institute
The Ohio State University Medical Center

George E. Billman, Ph.D, F.A.H.A.
Department of Physiology and Cell Biology
The Ohio State University

Penelope A. Boyden, Ph.D.
Department of Pharmacology
Center for Molecular Therapeutics
Columbia College of Physicians and Surgeons

Annalisa Bucchi, Ph.D.
Departmento of Biomolecular Sciences and Biotechnology
Università degli Studi di Milano, Italy

Alexander Burashnikov, Ph.D.
Masonic Medical Research Laboratory

Cynthia A. Carnes, Pharm.D., Ph.D., F.A.H.A., F.H.R.S.
College of Pharmacy
The Ohio State University

Hugh Clements-Jewery, Ph.D.
Division of Functional Biology
West Virginia School of Osteopathic Medicine

Ruben Coronel, M.D., Ph.D.
Department of Experimental Cardiology
Academic Medical Center, The Netherlands

Michael Curtis, Ph.D, F.H.E.A., F.B.Pharmcol.S
Cardiovascular Division
Rayne Institute
St. Thomas' Hospital
King's College London
United Kingdom

Jacques M.T. de Bakker, Ph.D.
Department of Experimental Cardiology
Academic Medical Center, The Netherlands

Stefan Dhein, M.D., Ph.D.
Heart Centre Leipzig
University of Leipzig
Germany

Dario DiFrancesco, Ph.D.
Departmento of Biomolecular Sciences and Biotechnology
Università degli Studi di Milano, Italy

Wen Dun, Ph.D.
Department of Pharmacology
Center for Molecular Therapeutics
Columbia College of Physicians and Surgeons

J. Michael Frangiskakis, M.D., Ph.D
UPMC Cardiovascular Institute
University of Pittsburgh

Gary Gintant, Ph.D.
Department of Integrative Pharmacology
Abbot Laboratories

Sandor Györke, Ph.D.
Davis Heart and Lung Research Institute
The Ohio State University Medical Center

Anja Hagen, Ph.D.
University of Leipzig
University Hospital for Children and Adolescents
Germany

Armando Lagrutta, Ph.D.
Senior Investigator, Safety and Exploratory Pharmacology
Merck Research Laboratories

Barry London, M.D., Ph.D.
UPMC Cardiovascular Institute
University of Pittsburgh

Lars S. Maier, M.D.
Department of Cardiology and Pneumology / Heart Center
Georg-August-University Göttingen
Germany

Jeanne Nerbonne, Ph.D.
Department of Molecular Biology and Pharmacology
Washington University
School of Medicine

Noriko Niwa, Ph.D.
Department of Molecular Biology and Pharmacology
Washington University
School of Medicine

Brian O'Rourke, Ph.D.
Division of Cardiology
Department of Medicine
Johns Hopkins University

Peter J. Schwartz, M.D.
Professor and Chairman
Department of Cardiology
Fondazione IRCCS Policlinico S. Matteo
Italy

Joseph J. Salata, Ph.D.
Director, Safety and Exploratory Pharmacology
Safety Assessment
Merck Research Laboratories

Arun Sridhar, Ph.D.
Safety Pharmacology GlaxoSmithKline United Kingdom

Karin R. Sipido, M.D., Ph.D.
Laboratory of Experimental Cardiology
Catholic University of Leuven (KUL)
Belgium

Zhi Su, Ph.D.
Department of Integrative Pharmacology
Abbot Laboratories

Dmitry Terentyev, Ph.D.
Davis Heart and Lung Research Institute
The Ohio State University Medical Center

Gordon F. Tomaselli, M.D.
Michel Mirowski MD Professor of Cardiology
Chair of Cardiology
Johns Hopkins University

András Varró, M.D., Ph.D., Sc.D.
Department of Pharmacology and Pharmacotherapy
University of Szeged
Albert Szent-Györgyi Medical Center, Hungary

Rik Willems, M.D.
Department of Cardiology
University Hospital of Leuven
Belgium

CHAPTER 1

Introduction

GEORGE E. BILLMAN

"... ignorance more frequently begets confidence than does knowledge: it is those who know little, and not those who know much, who so positively assert that this or that problem will never be solved by science." Charles Darwin [1]

"The greatest failure – not trying in the first place. *The best angle to approach problems is the try-angle.*" Jean Shirer Ingold [2]

The effective management of cardiac arrhythmias, either of atrial or ventricular origin, remains a major challenge for the cardiologist. Sudden cardiac death (defined as unexpected death from cardiac causes that occurs within 1 hour of the onset of symptoms [3]) remains the leading cause of death in industrially developed countries, and it accounts for between 300,000 and 500,000 deaths each year in the United States [4–6]. Holter monitoring studies reveal that these sudden deaths most frequently (up to 93%) resulted from ventricular tachyarrhythmias [7–9]. In a similar manner, atrial fibrillation is the most common rhythm disorder contributing to a substantial mortality, as well as a reduction in the quality of life, among these patients [10, 11]. Atrial fibrillation currently accounts for about 2.3 million cases in the United States and has been projected to increase by 2.5 fold over the next half century [12]. Indeed, the prevalence of this arrhythmia increases with each decade of life (0.5% patient population between the ages of 50 to 59 years climbing to almost 9% at age 80–89 years) and contributes to approximately one quarter of ischemic strokes in the elderly population [10, 11]. The economic impact associated with the morbidity and mortality resulting from cardiac arrhythmias is enormous (incremental cost per quality-adjusted life-year as much as U.S. $558,000 [13]).

Despite the enormity of this problem, the development of safe and effective antiarrhythmic agents remains elusive. In fact, several initially promising antiarrhythmic drugs have actually been shown to increase, rather than to decrease, the risk

Novel Therapeutic Targets for Antiarrhythmic Drugs, Edited by George Edward Billman
Copyright © 2010 John Wiley & Sons, Inc.

for arrhythmic death in patients recovering from myocardial infarction. For example, the Cardiac Arrhythmia Suppression Trial (CAST study [14]) demonstrated that, although class I antiarrhythmic drugs (i.e., drugs that block sodium channels) effectively suppressed premature ventricular contractions, some of these compounds (flecainide and encainide) increased the risk for arrhythmic cardiac death. In a similar manner, many class III antiarrhythmic drugs (drugs that prolong refractory period, most likely via modulation of potassium channels) have been shown to prolong QT interval, to promote the life-threatening tachyarrhythmia torsades de pointes (i.e., polymorphic ventricular tachycardia in which the QRS waves seem to "twist" around the baseline), and to increase cardiac mortality in some patient populations [15, 16]. Unfortunately, only a few drugs have been clinically proven to reduce cardiac mortality in high-risk patients, such as patients recovering from myocardial infarction. To date, only β-adrenergic receptor antagonists and amiodarone, which is a class III antiarrhythmic drug that also blocks β-adrenergic receptors, have been shown to reduce sudden cardiac death [5, 17–21]. However, even optimal pharmacological therapy does not completely suppress malignant ventricular arrhythmias. For example, mortality after myocardial infarction remains high among patients with substantial ventricular dysfunction, even when placed on β-adrenergic receptor antagonist therapy [21]. The 1-year mortality is 10% or higher, with sudden death accounting for approximately one third of the deaths in these high-risk patients [21]. Furthermore, the long-term use of amiodarone is limited because of adverse side effects that include pulmonary fibrous, hepatotoxicity, and thyroid toxicity [22]. Given the adverse actions of many antiarrhythmic medications, as well as the partial protection afforded by even the best agents (e.g., β-adrenergic receptor antagonists), it is obvious that more effective antiarrrhythmic therapies must be developed.

Old ideas never truly die, just the people who hold them. Eventually, newer ideas gain acceptance as the younger generation replaces the older generation. The major obstacle to progress often results from the inertia of conventional thinking [23]. This book attempts to overcome this inertia by describing some novel approaches for the management of arrhythmias. The primary focus of the book will be on ventricular arrhythmias, but a few chapters will also address aspects of atrial arrhythmias (see Chapters 3, 17, and 18). The book is divided into four sections. The first section opens with a comprehensive review of basic cardiac electrophysiology (Chapters 2 and 3) and mechanisms responsible for arrhythmias in the setting of ischemia (Chapter 4) and closes with a review of basic pharmacology, focusing on the classification of antiarrhythmic drugs (Chapter 5). Section two addresses safety pharmacology: the concept of "repolarization reserve" (Chapter 6), safety challenges (Chapter 7), and regulatory issues (Chapter 8) for the development of novel antiarrhythmic drugs. Section three describes several novel pharmacological targets for antiarrhythmic drugs (Chapters 9–18). Finally, section four describes a few promising nonpharmacological antiarrhythmic interventions, including selective cardiac neural disruption or nerve stimulation (Chapter 19), endurance exercise training (Chapter 20), and dietary supplements (omega-3 polyunsaturated fatty acids, Chapter 21). The reader is encouraged to approach each chapter with an open mind, for the prejudice of conventional wisdom can blind. Sometimes to be a visionary, one simply has to open one's eyes.

REFERENCES

1. Hayden, T. (2009). What Darwin didn't know. Smithsonian Magazine, 39, 40–49.
2. Heat-Moon, W.L. Roads to Quoz: An American Mossey. Little, Brown and Co., New York, 2008, pp. 314.
3. Torp-Pedersen, C., Kober, L., Elming, H., Burchart, H. (1997). Classification of sudden and arrhythmic death. PACE—Pacing and Clinical Electrophysiology, 20, 2545–2552.
4. Abildstrom, S.Z., Kobler, L., Torp-Pedersen, C. (1999) Epidemiology of arrhythmic and sudden death in the chronic phase of ischemic heart disease. Cardiac Electrophysiology Reviews, 3, 177–179.
5. Zipes, D.P., Wellens, H.J. (1998). Sudden cardiac death. Circulation, 98, 2334–2351.
6. Zheng, Z.-J., Croft, J.B., Giles, W.H., Mensah, G.A. (2001) Sudden cardiac death in the United States, 1989 to 1998. Circulation, 104, 2158–2163.
7. Bayes de Luna, A., Coumel, P., LeClercq, J.F. (1989). Ambulatory sudden cardiac death: Mechanisms of production of fatal arrhythmia on the basis of data from 157 cases. American Heart Journal, 117, 151–159.
8. Hinkle, L.E.J., Thaler, H.T. (1982) Clinical classification of cardiac deaths. Circulation, 65, 457–464.
9. Greene, H.L. (1990). Sudden arrhythmic cardiac death: Mechanisms, resuscitation and classification: The Seattle perspective. American Journal of Cardiology, 65, 4B–12.
10. Kannel, W.B., Wolf, P.A., Levy, D. (1998). Prevalence, incidence, prognosis, and predisposing conditions for atrial fibrillation: Population-based estimates. American Journal of Cardiology, 82, 2N–9N.
11. Lakshminarayan, K., Solid, C.A., Collins, A.J., Anderson, D.C., Herzog, C.A. (2006). Atrial Fibrillation and stroke in the general Medicare population: A 10-year perspective (1992 to 2002). Stroke, 37, 1969–1974.
12. (1998). Risk Factors for stroke and efficacy of antithrombotic therapy in atrial fibrillation. Analysis of pooled data from five randomized controlled trials. Archives of Internal Medicine, 154, 1449–1457.
13. Byrant, J., Brodin, H., Loveman, E., Clegg, A. (2005). The clinical and cost-effectiveness of implantable cardioverter defibrillators: A systemic review. Health Technology Assessment, 9, 1–150.
14. Echt, D.S., Liebson, P.R., Mitchell, L.B., Peters, R.W., Obiasmanno, D., Barker, A.H., Arensberg, D., Baker, A., Freedman, L., Greene, H.L., Hunter, M.L., Richardson, D.W. (1991). Mortality and morbidity in patients receiving encainide, flecainide, or placebo. New England Journal of Medicine, 324, 782–788.
15. Sager, P.T. (1999). New advances in class III antiarrhythmic drug therapy. Current Opinions in Cardiology, 14, 15–23.
16. Waldo, A.L., Camm, A.J., de Ruyter, H., Friedman, P.L., MacNeil, D.J., Pauls, J.F., Pitt, B., Pratt, C.M., Schwartz, P.J., Veltri, E.P. for the SWORD Investigators. (1996). Effect of d-sotalol on mortality in patients with left ventricular dysfunction after recent and remote myocardial infarction. Lancet, 348, 7–12.

17. Amiodarone trials meta-analysis investigators. (1997). Effects of Prophylactic amiodarone on mortality after acute myocardial infarction and in congestive heart failure: Meta-analysis of individual data from 6500 patients in randomized trials. Lancet, 350, 1417–1424.

18. Held, P., Yusuf, S. (1989). Early intravenous beta-blockade in acute myocardial infarction. Cardiology, 76, 132–143.

19. Held, P.H., Yusuf, S. (1993) Effects of beta-blockers and Ca^{2+} channel blockers in acute myocardial infarction. European Heart Journal, 14, 18–25.

20. Kendall, M.J., Lynch, K.P., Hjalmarson, A., Kjekshus, J. (1995). β-Blockers and sudden cardiac death. Annals of Internal Medicine, 123, 353–367.

21. Buxton, A.E., Lee, K.L., Fisher, J.D., Josephson, M.E., Prystowsky, E.N., Hafley, G. (1999) A randomized study of the prevention of sudden death in patients with coronary artery disease. New England Journal of Medicine, 341, 1882–1890.

22. Nattel, S. Class III drugs: Amiodarone, Bertylium, Ibutilide, and sotalol. In: Zipes, D.P. and Jalife, J. Eds. Cardiac Electrophysiology from Cell to Bedside, 3rd Edition. W. B. Saunders Co., Philadelphia, PA, 2000, pp. 921–932.

23. Wainer, H. (2008) Why is a raven like a writing desk? American Scientist, 96, 446–449.

CHAPTER 2

Myocardial K$^+$ Channels: Primary Determinants of Action Potential Repolarization

NORIKO NIWA and JEANNE NERBONNE

2.1 INTRODUCTION

The heart beats automatically at regular intervals, and this rhythmic contractile activity is driven by myocardial electrical activity: the generation of action potentials in individual cardiomyocytes and the propagation of activity through the myocardium [1, 2]. The normal cardiac cycle begins with action potential generation in the sinoatrial node and propagates through the atria to the atrioventricular node. Activity then spreads through the His-Purkinje system to the apex of the ventricles and into the working, ventricular myocardium. The propagation of activity triggers dynamic changes in the membrane potentials of individual cardiomyocytes, and action potentials are generated [1, 2]. Electrical coupling, mediated by gap junctions, underlies the spread of activity in the myocardium, ensuring that ventricular excitation proceeds in an orderly manner and that pump function is maintained [3]. Importantly, perturbations of myocardial electrical functioning can lead to rhythm disturbances and to changes in pump function [3–6].

Myocardial action potentials reflect the coordinated functioning of voltage-gated ion channels carrying depolarizing (Na$^+$ and Ca^{2+}) and repolarizing (K$^+$) currents [1, 2]. Of these, the K$^+$ channels are the most numerous and diverse, and these channels play essential roles in controlling resting membrane potentials, determining the shapes and durations of action potentials and influencing refractory periods [7]. Multiple voltage-gated K$^+$ (Kv) channels, as well as non-voltage-gated, inwardly rectifying K$^+$ (Kir) currents, have been identified (Table 2.1), and have

Novel Therapeutic Targets for Antiarrhythmic Drugs, Edited by George Edward Billman
Copyright © 2010 John Wiley & Sons, Inc.

Table 2.1. Cardiac K$^+$ Currents Contributing to Action Potential Repolarization

Channel Type	Current Name	Activation	Inactivation	Recovery	Tissue[1]
Kv (I$_{to}$)					
	I$_{to,f}$	fast	fast	fast	A, P, V
	I$_{to,s}$	fast	moderate	slow	V(A, AVN, SAN)[2]
Kv (I$_k$)					
	I$_{Kr}$	moderate	fast	slow	A, P, V, SAN, AVN
	I$_{Ks}$	very slow	no	—	A, P, V, SAN
	I$_{Kur}$	very fast	very slow	slow	A (V??)
	I$_{K,slow1}$	very fast	slow	slow	A, V[3]
	I$_{Kp}$	fast	no	—	V[3]
	I$_{K,slow2}$	fast	very slow	slow	A, V[3]
	I$_K$	slow	slow	slow	V[3]
	I$_{SS}$	slow	no	—	A, V, AVN
Kir					
	I$_{KI}$	—	—	—	A, P, V

[1]A = atrial; P = Purkinje; V = ventricular; SAN = sinoatrial node; AVN = atrioventricular node. The dashed boxes are placed around currents given different names in different species that likely are encoded by the same channel subunits.
[2]Only identified in nonventricular cells in the rabbit, to date.
[3]Currents identified in rodents.

been shown to contribute to myocardial action potential repolarization [2, 7]. The various K$^+$ channels display distinct time- and voltage-dependent properties and pharmacological sensitivities [7, 8]. Kv channels, for example, open in response to membrane depolarization and are primary determinants of action potential repolarization [2, 7, 9]. Cardiac Kv currents are classified into two broad groups based on characteristic differences in time- and voltage-dependent properties: transient outward Kv (I$_{to}$, I$_{to,f}$, and I$_{to,s}$) and delayed rectifying Kv (I$_{Kr}$, I$_{Ks}$, and I$_{Kur}$) currents (Table 2.1). Heterogeneities in the expression levels and/or the biophysical properties of the various K$^+$ currents contribute to regional differences in action potential waveforms [7, 9, 10]. In addition, changes in the densities and/or the properties of myocardial K$^+$ channels are evident in a number of inherited and acquired cardiac diseases, and these changes can have profound electrical consequences, including the initiation or maintenance of potentially life-threatening cardiac arrhythmias [4, 6].

It is now also clear that the functional diversity of myocardial K$^+$ channels reflects the expression of a large number of K$^+$ channel pore-forming (α) and accessory (β) subunits [2, 7, 9]. Although less well understood, more diversity is possible through the heteromeric assembly of K$^+$ channel α subunits and the multiplicity of β subunit actions, as well as the coexpression of a variety of additional regulatory proteins that modulate myocardial K$^+$ channel stability, trafficking, and/or functioning [11–13].

2.2　ACTION POTENTIAL WAVEFORMS AND REPOLARIZING K$^+$ CURRENTS

The activity of cardiac ion channels is evident in the profiles of action potentials (Figure 2.1). In human ventricular myocytes, for example, the fast action potential upstroke (phase 0), because of the activation of voltage-gated Na$^+$ channels, is followed by a rapid repolarization phase (phase 1) attributed to Na$^+$ channel inactivation and the activation of the fast component of I_{to}, $I_{to,f}$, channels. During the plateau (phase 2), the membrane potential is maintained at a positive level, reflecting the balance of inward Na$^+$/Ca^{2+} currents and outward K$^+$ currents. With the increased activation of the rapid (I_{Kr}) and the slow (I_{Ks}) components of delayed rectification, the outward K$^+$ currents dominate and the membrane repolarizes (phase 3). The Kir current, I_{K1}, also participates in the final phase of repolarization. In addition, I_{K1} plays an important role in the maintenance of ventricular (and atrial) resting membrane potentials (phase 4).

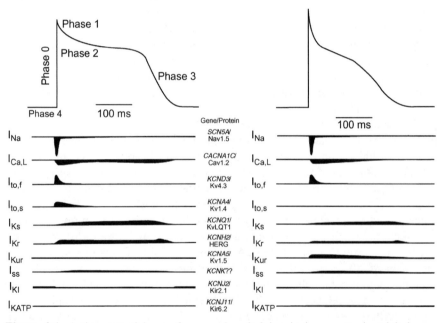

Figure 2.1. Action potential waveforms and underlying ionic currents in adult human ventricular (**left**) and atrial (**right**) myocytes. The time- and voltage-dependent properties of the voltage-gated inward Na$^+$ (Nav) and Ca^{2+} (Cav) currents expressed in human atrial and ventricular myocytes are similar. In contrast, there are multiple types of K$^+$ currents, particularly Kv currents, contributing to atrial and ventricular action potential repolarization. The time- and voltage-dependent properties of the various Kv currents are distinct. Differences in the expression and/or the densities of repolarizing Kv and Kir channels contribute to atrial-ventricular differences in action potential waveforms. The genes encoding the pore-forming (α) subunits underlying the various cardiac ion channels are indicated (**center**).

There are marked differences in the waveforms of action potentials in different regions of the myocardium [7, 10]. Compared with ventricular cells, for example, resting membrane potentials are less negative in atrial myocytes, and atrial action potentials display less positive plateau potentials, slower phase 3 repolarization, and shorter durations (Figure 2.1). These atrioventricular differences reflect variations in the expression of ion channels, particularly K$^+$ channels. The atrial-specific expression of ultra-rapid component delayed rectification, I_{Kur} [14–16], for example, together with the high density of $I_{to,f}$ in atrial [17], compared with ventricular [18], myocytes increases the rate of early repolarization, which results in lower plateau potentials and shorter action potential durations. In most species, acetylcholine-sensitive inwardly rectifying K$^+$ (I_{KACh}) channels are more abundant in atrial, than in ventricular, myocytes [19–21]. These (I_{KACh}) channels play a role in action potential shortening and in the hyperpolarization of resting membrane potentials in response to parasympathetic stimulation. The lower density of I_{K1} accounts for the slower final phase (phase 3) of repolarization and the less negative resting potentials in atrial (compared with ventricular) myocytes [10].

Even within the ventricles, action potential waveforms are variable [7, 10]. Myocytes in the epicardium, for example, typically display a more prominent phase 1 and notch, often described as a "spike and dome" morphology, and action potential durations are shorter than in cells in the endocardium [22]. These epicardial-endocardial differences are also attributed to heterogeneities in the expression of ion channels, particularly K$^+$ channels. The density of $I_{to,f}$, for example, is higher in epicardial, compared with endocardial, myocytes and underlies the prominent phase 1 "notch" in epicardial action potentials [23]. In guinea pig [24] and feline [25] ventricles, delayed rectifier K$^+$ current densities are lower in the endocardium than in the epicardium, which contributes to the longer duration of endocardial action potentials. The M cells, which are observed in the deep subepicardial layers of canine [26] and human [27] ventricles, also display unique electrophysiological properties. Action potentials in canine M cells, for example, display a prominent phase 1 and notch similar to those in epicardial myocytes, although action potentials are much longer in M cells [26]. Action potential durations in M cells are prolonged as pacing rates are slowed [26], which are attributed to lower I_{Ks} densities [28]. Action potential waveforms are also distinct in the right and left ventricles. In canine right ventricular epicardial and M cells, for example, action potentials display a more prominent phase 1 and notch and are shorter than in the left ventricle [29, 30]. Observed interventricular and apical-basal regionaldifferences in differences in $I_{to,f}$ and I_{Ks} densities underlie ventricular action potential deviations [29–31].

Efforts focused on understanding arrhythmia mechanisms and on exploring underlying mechanisms and/or possible antiarrhythmic therapies have been facilitated by developing model systems. These can be animal, cellular, and/or mathematical models to allow mechanisms to be probed and mechanistic insights to be revealed. Although many experimental models have been and are currently used, mice have been used extensively, largely because of the ease with which genetic manipulations can be made and molecular/cellular mechanisms can be probed [32–35]. Action potentials in adult mouse atrial and ventricular myocytes, however, are really different from those recorded in humans; in particular, repolarization is rapid and there is no clear plateau phase [32, 34, 36]. The characteristic waveforms and the short durations of mouse (ventricular and atrial) action potentials are attributed primarily to the rapid activation and the high density of repolarizing K^+ currents [32, 34, 36]. The high density of $I_{to,f}$, for example, dominates the early repolarization phase and contributes to the shorter action potential durations in the murine myocardium [34, 36]. In contrast, I_{to} in human ventricular myocytes partially repolarizes the membrane potential and sets the early plateau potential but only indirectly influences action potential durations [37]. The marked differences in ventricular repolarization in mice and humans is clearly reflected in electrocardiographic (ECG) recordings, particularly in repolarization parameters; in the mouse, the T-wave is not well defined and the QT interval is short ($\sim$50 ms) compared with the human ($\sim$400 ms) [32].

2.3 FUNCTIONAL DIVERSITY OF REPOLARIZING MYOCARDIAL K^+ CHANNELS

Electrophysiological studies have revealed that multiple types of K^+ channels are coexpressed in the myocardium (Table 2.1) and that differences in the relative expression levels of these channels contribute to regional, chamber, and species specific differences in action potential waveforms [7, 10, 36, 38]. On membrane depolarization, I_{to} activates (and inactivates) rapidly (Figure 2.1), which contributes to rapid phase 1 of repolarization and to the plateau [39, 40]. Thus, I_{to} indirectly influences the activation of L-type Ca^{2+} channels, Na^+/Ca^{2+} exchange currents, and delayed rectifying Kv channels during the plateau phase, and it modulates action potential durations. Two components of I_{to} with different rates of inactivation and recovery from inactivation have been distinguished, $I_{to,fast}$ ($I_{to,f}$) and $I_{to,slow}$ ($I_{to,s}$) [41, 42]. The fast component $I_{to,f}$ is characterized by time constants of inactivation and recovery of $\sim$30 to 100 ms and $\sim$60 to 100 ms, respectively [41, 42]. In contrast, the slow component $I_{to,s}$ inactivates with time constants of several hundreds of milliseconds and recovers with time constants on the order of seconds [42, 43]. Millimolar concentrations of 4-aminopyridine (4-AP) block both $I_{to,f}$ and $I_{to,s}$, albeit by different mechanisms: closed-state block for $I_{to,f}$ and open-state block for $I_{to,s}$ [40, 42]. Several spider toxins, *Heteropoda* toxin-2 and toxin-3 and phrixotoxins, however, selectively block $I_{to,f}$ and do not affect other Kv channels, including $I_{to,s}$ channels [40, 43, 44].

In ferret left ventricles, $I_{to,f}$ is prominently expressed in epicardial cells, whereas $I_{to,s}$ predominates in endocardial myocytes [41]. In human left ventricles, I_{to} in epicardial myocytes recovers from inactivation quickly (time constants < 50 ms), whereas a slowly recovering I_{to} component predominates in endocardial myocytes, which suggests that $I_{to,f}$ and $I_{to,s}$ also are differentially expressed in human ventricles [18, 23]. In both human and ferret, I_{to} densities are $\sim$4-to 5-fold higher in epicardial, than in endocardial, left ventricular myocytes [18, 41]. In canine left ventricle, only $I_{to,f}$ has been reported and $I_{to,f}$ densities are ~5-to 6-fold higher in epicardial, than in endocardial, cells [38]. In mice, $I_{to,f}$ densities are higher in the right, than in left, ventricles and are low in the intraventricular septum, whereas $I_{to,s}$ is expressed only in septum cells [42, 43, 45]. Human atrial I_{to} displays very fast recovery from inactivation [17], which suggests that only $I_{to,f}$ is expressed.

Although it is clear that I_{to} affects early repolarization and the plateau potential in large mammals, the influence of I_{to} on action potential durations is complex. The inhibition of I_{to} by 4-AP, for example, prolongs human ventricular action potential durations [46, 47]. In addition, reduced I_{to} density in failing ventricles is accompanied by marked action potential prolongation [46–48]. Mathematical simulations and dynamic clamp experiments, however, suggest that reduced I_{to} densities can prolong or shorten (or leave unaffected) action potential durations in human and canine ventricular myocytes [49–51], which reflects the complex interactions between I_{to} and other depolarizing and repolarizing currents [37, 39]. The application of 4-AP also prolongs action potentials in human atrial myocytes [52, 53] through effects on I_{Kur} [16], as well as I_{to}, and modeling studies suggest that attenuation of I_{to} has more dramatic effects on the phase 1 notch and on the plateau potential [54, 55].

Multiple components of delayed rectification (I_K) are coexpressed in cardiac myocytes, and these are distinguished based on differences in time- and voltage-dependent properties and/or pharmacological sensitivities (Table 2.1). Two prominent I_K components, for example, I_{Kr} and I_{Ks}, were first distinguished in guinea pig atrial [56, 57] and ventricular [58] myocytes: I_{Kr} activates rapidly, inactivates rapidly, and displays marked inward rectification, whereas I_{Ks} activates slowly [57, 58]. The marked inward rectification of I_{Kr} is caused by rapid voltage-dependent inactivation [57], and I_{Kr} amplitudes decrease as the membrane depolarizes [2]. Thus, I_{Kr} is small during the action potential plateau [59]. In addition, however, I_{Kr} displays relatively slow deactivation and rapid recovery from inactivation [2, 59]. As the membrane begins to repolarize, I_{Kr} channels recover from inactivation, which produces large outward currents and contributes to phase 3 repolarization [59]. In contrast, the contribution of I_{Ks} increases gradually on depolarization [59]. In addition, because these channels deactivate slowly and do not inactivate [60, 61], I_{Ks} contributes importantly to the plateau and to phase 3 repolarization [59]. The slow deactivation and absence of inactivation of I_{Ks} channels are physiologically important in rate-dependent adaptation of action potential durations. As heart rate increases, I_{Ks} channels do not have sufficient time to deactivate prior to the next action potential, and channels accumulate in the open state. The accumulation of open channels generates a large I_{Ks} at times late during the plateau phase, which leads to rate-dependent action potential shortening [59, 61]. Notably, I_{Ks} is increased in response to β-adrenergic stimulation, whereas I_{Kr} is unaffected [62, 63]. The augmentation of I_{Ks} contributes to ventricular action potential shortening in response to sympathetic activation [64]. In addition, I_{Kr} is selectively blocked by lanthanum and by methanesulfonanilide class III antiarrhythmics (dofetilide, E4031), whereas I_{Ks} is selectively blocked by chromanols (293B, HMR-1556) [8]. Both I_{Kr} and I_{Ks} are expressed in human [65, 66] and canine [28, 67] atrial and ventricular myocytes and in rabbit ventricular myocytes [68], albeit with heterogeneous distributions [24, 28, 69, 70]. In rodent ventricular and atrial myocytes, however, I_{Ks} and I_{Kr} are negligible [71, 72], and distinct components of delayed rectification have been identified, including $I_{K,slow}$, $I_{K,slow1}$, and $I_{K,slow2}$ [42, 43, 73–75] (Table 2.1).

In human [14, 16, 66], rat [76], and canine [77] atrial myocytes, a rapidly activating and slowly inactivating outward Kv current, referred to as $I_{Kultrarapid}$ (I_{Kur}), has been identified. I_{Kur} channels are selectively blocked by micromolar concentration of 4-AP [14, 66, 77], prolonging atrial action potential durations markedly [14, 77]. Importantly, I_{Kur} is not detected in human ventricular myocytes [16, 66], and one of the selective rate-dependent I_{Kur} channel blockers, diphenyl phosphine oxide (DPO), reportedly prolongs human atrial action potential durations and is without effects on ventricular cells [78]. Because it has been suggested to be an atrial specific repolarizing current [14, 16, 66, 76, 77], I_{Kur} is considered a promising therapeutic target for the treatment of atrial arrhythmias [78, 79]. It was reported recently, however, that a 4-AP-sensitive I_{Kur}-like current is expressed in canine left ventricular midmyocardial myocytes [80]; this observation suggests that more studies focused on detailing the properties and the expression levels of Kv channels in human ventricular myocytes are needed.

The other subfamily of K$^+$ channels, which includes the inwardly rectifying K$^+$ (Kir) channels that are prominently expressed in the myocardium, also contribute to shaping the resting and active membrane properties of cardiac cells. Although preferentially carrying inward K$^+$ currents, Kir channels only carry outward K$^+$ currents under physiological conditions because cell membrane potentials are always more positive than the K$^+$ equilibrium potential ($\sim$ -90 mV) [81]. Several types of Kir channels are expressed in the mammalian heart, including I_{K1}, acetylcholine-sensitive I_{KACh}, and adenosine triphosphate (ATP)-inhibited I_{KATP} channels. The I_{K1} channels display strong inward rectification, attributed to voltage-dependent channel block by cytoplasmic Mg^{2+} and polyamines [82, 83]. The block of I_{K1} channels is relieved on membrane repolarization, which contributes to outward K$^+$ currents during the terminal phase of repolarization [59]. Around the resting membrane potential, the total conductance contributed by I_{K1} channels is much larger than that of any other currents, clamping the resting membrane potential close to the K$^+$ equilibrium potential [8, 84].

Binding of acetylcholine to muscarinic M2 receptors activates I_{KACh} channels through direct coupling to G-protein $\beta\gamma$ subunits [85, 86]. The activation of I_{KACh} channels hyperpolarizes pacemaker cells and slows spontaneous pacemaking activity [9, 86]. In the atria and sinoatrial node, I_{KACh} channels play a role in heart rate regulation in response to parasympathetic activation [9, 86]. Sarcolemmal I_{KATP} channels, in contrast, are predominantly expressed in the ventricles. These channels are inhibited by physiological levels of intracellular ATP and are activated by decreased ATP levels and by MgADP [87]. Thus, cardiac I_{KATP} channels are predominantly closed under normal physiological conditions and are opened under metabolic stress, such as during ischemia or hypoxia [87]. Reduced intracellular ATP and the opening of I_{KATP} channels shorten action potential durations, thereby reducing Ca^{2+} entry and inhibiting myocardial contractility [87].

By blocking I_{KATP} channels, sulfonylureas inhibit the action potential shortening induced by hypoxia or ischemia [88]. In contrast, the I_{KATP} channel opener, pinacidil, shortens ventricular action potential durations, and interestingly, this (shortening) effect is more prominent during ischemia [89]. Pinacidil also improves myocardial contractile function after ischemia [89], which suggests cardioprotective effects of I_{KATP} channels [90].

2.4 MOLECULAR DIVERSITY OF K$^+$ CHANNEL SUBUNITS

Accumulating evidence suggests that functional K$^+$ channels are integral membrane protein complexes composed of pore-forming (α) subunits and several accessory (β) and regulatory proteins [2, 7, 9]. Each Kv channel α subunit contains six transmembrane-spanning segments (S1 to S6), a pore region, and cytoplasmic N- and C-terminal domains (Figure 2.2). The pore region is formed by the S5 and S6 transmembrane segments, along with the linker region containing the amino acid sequence TxGYG as the K$^+$ selectivity signature motif [9]. The S4 segment serves as the voltage sensor with positively charged basic residues at approximately every third position [9]. In the Kv1-Kv4 subfamilies (Table 2.2), the assembly of Kv α subunits (Figure 2.2) is mediated by N-terminal tetramerization (T1) domains immediately preceding the S1 segment [91]. A large number of Kv α subunit genes (Table 2.2), as well as alternatively spliced variants, have been identified [92–97]. Heterologous expression of the various Kv α subunits produces Kv currents with distinct biophysical properties [7, 9, 98]. In heterologous cells, Kv α subunits in the same subfamily can also form heteromeric channels, which is a potential mechanism for generating further K$^+$ channel diversity [98, 99].

In addition, K$^+$ channel diversity seems to be enhanced even more through interactions with K$^+$ channel accessory (β) subunits, which modulate channel biophysical properties as well as cell surface expression [11, 12]. A variety of cytoplasmic K$^+$ channel accessory subunits (Table 2.2), which include the Kvβ subunits, the K$^+$ channel-interacting proteins (KChIPs), and the K$^+$ channel-associated protein (KChAP), and transmembrane accessory subunits, which include the minimal K$^+$ channel protein (minK), the minK-related peptides (MiRPs) and the diaminopeptidy transferase-like (DPPX-like) proteins, have been identified [7, 11, 12]. There are three homologous Kvβ subunits, Kvβ1, Kvβ2, and Kvβ3 [100–102], each with multiple splice variants [103, 104]. Structural analyses suggest that the conserved C-terminal domains of Kvβ subunits interact with the N-terminal T1 domains of Kv1 α subunits in a 1 : 1 stoichiometry [105]. The N-terminal domains of Kvβ subunits are unique, and the long N-termini in the Kvβ1 and Kvβ3 subunits are thought to function as inactivating ball peptides and to produce rapid, N-type inactivation of Kv1α-subunit encoded channels [104, 106–108]. The Kvβ1 and Kvβ2 subunits reportedly modulate the surface expression of Kv1 and Kv4 channels [109, 110].

The intracellular KChIP proteins belong to the neuronal Ca^{2+} sensor (NCS) subfamily of Ca^{2+} binding proteins, each of which contains four Ca^{2+}-binding

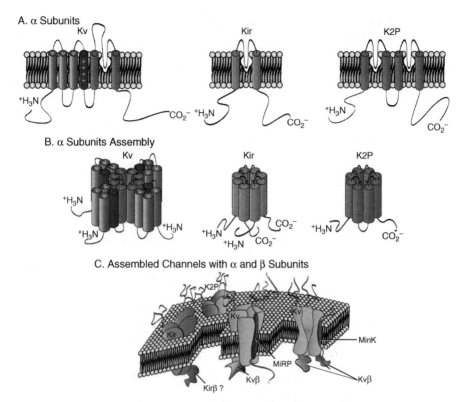

Figure 2.2. Pore-forming subunits and assembly of cardiac Kv, Kir, and K2P channels. Membrane topologies of individual Kv, Kir, and K2P pore-forming (α) subunits (**A**) and the tetrameric assembly of Kv and Kir subunits and the dimeric assembly of K2P subunits (**B**) are illustrated. (**C**) Schematic of assembled Kv, Kir, and K2P α subunits with associated transmembrane and cytoplasmic accessory subunits. See color insert.

EF-hand motifs [111, 112]. The KChIPs bind to a distal N-terminal domain of Kv4 α subunits in a 1 : 1 stoichiometry [113]. Co-expression with KChIPs increases the surface expression of Kv4 channels [111, 114] and modulates channel gating [111, 114, 115]. KChAP, which also interacts with the N-termini of Kv α subunits [116, 117], seems to function as a chaperone protein, facilitating the cell surface expression, without influencing the time- and/or voltage-dependent properties of Kv2- and Kv4-encoded channels [116, 117]. The minK/MiRP subunits are (single) transmembrane spanning domain proteins with extracellular N-termini and cytoplasmic C-termini [118]. Studies in heterologous cells revealed that minK associates with *KCNQ1* and reconstitutes the slow activation properties of native I$_{Ks}$ channels [119, 120]. It has also been suggested that minK functions as a binding partner of ERG1 [121] and, in addition, that another member of this subfamily, MiRP1 (*KCNE2*), modulates the properties of *KCNQ1*-encoded currents [122].

Table 2.2. Diversity of Voltage-Gated K$^+$ (Kv) Channel Pore-Forming (α) and Assessory (β) Subunits

Subfamily	Protein	Gene	Human	Mouse	Cardiac Current
			Locus		
Kv1					
	Kv1.1	KCNA1	12p13.32	6F3	
	Kv1.2	KCNA2	1p13.3	3F2.3	$I_{K,slow}, (I_{K,DTX})$
	Kv1.3	KCNA3	1p13.3	3F2.3	
	Kv1.4	KCNA4	11p14.1	2E3	$I_{to,s}$
	Kv1.5	KCNA5	12p13.32	6F3	$I_{kur}, I_{K,slow1}$
	Kv1.6	KCNA6	12p13.32	6F3	
	Kv1.7	KCNA7	12p13.33	7B4	
	Kv1.8	KCNA8	1p13.3	2F2.3	
Kv2					
	Kv2.1	KCNB1	20q13.13	2H3	$I_{K,slow2}$
	Kv2.2	KCNB2	8q13.3	1A3	??
Kv3					
	Kv3.1	KCNC1	11p15.1	7B4	
	Kv3.2	KCNC2	12q21.1	10D2	
	Kv3.3	KCNC3	19q13.33	7B4	
	Kv3.4	KCNC4	1p13.3	3F2.3	
Kv4					
	Kv4.1	KCND1	Xp11.23	XA1.1	??
	Kv4.2	KCND2	7q31.31	6A2	$I_{to,f}$
	Kv4.3	KCND3	1p13.2	3F2.2	$I_{to,f}$
Kv5					
	Kv5.1	KCNF1	2p25.1	12A1.1	??
Kv6					
	Kv6.1	KCNG1	20q13.13	2H3	
	Kv6.2	KCNG2	18q23	18E3	
	Kv6.3	KCNG3	2p21	17E4	
	Kv6.4	KCNG4	16q24.1	8E1	

Table 2.2 (*Continued*)

Subfamily	Protein	Gene	Locus Human	Locus Mouse	Cardiac Current
Kv7					
	KvLQT1	*KCNQ1*	11p15.5	7F5	i_{ks}
	KCNQ2	*KCNQ2*	20q13.33	2H4	
	KCNQ3	*KCNQ3*	8q24.22	15D1	
	KCNQ4	*KCNQ4*	1p34.2	4D2.2	
	KCNQ5	*KCNQ5*	6q13	1A4	
Kv8					
	Kv8.1	*KCNV1*	8q23.2	15B3.3	
	Kv8.2	*KCNV2*	9p24.2	19C1	
Kv9					
	Kv9.1	*KCNS1*	20q13.12	2H3	
	Kv9.2	*KCNS2*	8q22.2	15B3.1	
	Kv9.3	*KCNS3*	2q24.2	12A1.1	
Kv11					
	eag	*KCNH1*	1q32.2	1H6	
	erg1	*KCNH2*	7q36.1	5A3	I_{kr}
	erg2	*KCNH3*	12q13.12	15F1	
	erg3	*KCNH4*	17q21.2	11D	
	erg4	*KCNH5*	14q23.2	12C3	
	erg5	*KCNH6*	17q23.3	11E1	
	erg6	*KCNH7*	2q24.2	2C1.3	
	erg7	*KCNH8*	3p24.3	17C	
Kvβ					
	Kvβ1	*KCNAB1*	3q25.31	3E1	??
	Kvβ2	*KCNAB2*	1p36.31	4E2	??
	Kvβ3	*KCNAB3*	17p13.1	11B3	
KCNE					
	Mink	*KCNE1*	21q22.12	16C4	I_{Ks}
	MiRP1	*KCNE2*	21q22.11	16C4	I_{Kr}??, $I_{to,f}$??
	MiRP2	*KCNE3*	11q13.4	7E2	$I_{to,f}$??
	MiRP3	*KCNE4*	2q36.1	1C4	
	MiRP4	*KCNE5*	Xq22.3	XF2	

(*continued*)

Table 2.2 (*Continued*)

Subfamily	Protein	Gene	Locus Human	Locus Mouse	Cardiac Current
KchAP					
	KChAP	*PIAS3*	1q21.1	3F2.1	$I_{to,f}$, I_K??
KChIP					
	KChIP1	*KCNIP1*	5q35.1	11A4	
	KChIP2	*KCNIP2*	10q24.32	19C3	$I_{to,f}$, I_{Kur}??
	KChIP3	*KCNIP3*	2q11.1	2F1	
	KChIP4	*KCNIP4*	4p15.3	5B3	
NCS					
	NCS-1	*FREQ*	9q34.11	2B	$I_{to,f}$

☐ Expressed in Mammalian Heart

2.5   MOLECULAR DETERMINANTS OF FUNCTIONAL CARDIAC I_{to} CHANNELS

Consistent with differences in biophysical properties, myocardial $I_{to,f}$ and $I_{to,s}$ channels are encoded by distinct Kv α subunits. Tetrameric assembly of Kv4.2 and/ or Kv4.3 α subunits, for example, underlies $I_{to,f}$ channels [7]. In human and canine ventricles, only Kv4.3 is expressed [95, 123, 124], whereas both Kv4.2 and Kv4.3 are expressed in rodent ventricles [125–127]. The expression of Kv4.3 seems to be uniform in human and canine ventricles [128], whereas there is a transmural Kv4.2 expression gradient in rodent ventricles that parallels the transmural gradient in $I_{to,f}$ density [125, 126, 129]. There are two isoforms of human Kv4.3, and the long variant contains a 19 amino acid insertion in the C-terminus [95, 130]. This insert also contains additional consensus protein kinase C (PKC) phosphorylation sites [95, 130], which seem to be targets of α-adrenergic modulation [131].

Considerable evidence suggests that KChIP2 plays a critical role in regulating the functional cell surface expression of $I_{to,f}$ channels. KChIP2, for example, coimmunoprecipitates with Kv4.2 (and Kv4.3) from adult mouse ventricles [129] and modifies the gating properties of Kv4 channels [111, 114]. In addition, the targeted disruption of *KCNIP2* (KChIP2) results in complete loss of $I_{to,f}$ [132]. Although the mechanisms involved in increased membrane targeting of Kv4 channels by KChIP2 have not been clarified, it has been reported that palmitoylation of KChIP2 is important [133]. It has also been suggested that binding of KChIP2 to an endoplasmic reticulum (ER) retention signal in the N terminus of Kv4 masks the ER retention signal, which allows Kv4 channels to traffic to the cell surface [114, 134], although retention signals that prevent export from the ER have not been identified [134, 135].

It has also been suggested that the KChIPs are mainly involved in forward trafficking from the ER to the Golgi via a pathway different from coat protein II (COPII)-coated vesicles and Sar1 activity [135]. In human and canine hearts, there is a marked transmural gradient of KChIP2 transcript expression across the ventricular wall [128, 136], correlated with the gradient in $I_{to,f}$ [128]. An epicardial-endocardial gradient in KChIP2 mRNA expression in adult mouse ventricles has also been reported [137]. Another EF-hand motif-containing Ca^{2+} binding protein, neuronal calcium sensor-1 (NCS-1), coimmunoprecipitates with Kv4 α subunits from adult mouse ventricles [138]. Coexpression of NCS-1 increases Kv4 current densities and affects rates of inactivation [138, 139]. Biochemical studies have revealed that Kv4.2 also coimmunoprecipitates with Kvβ1.1 and Kvβ1.2 from mouse ventricles and that the loss of Kvβ1 reduces the functional expression of mouse ventricular $I_{to,f}$ channels [140]. In heterologous cells, both Kvβ1 and Kvβ2 increase the cell surface expression of Kv4.3 and Kv4.3 current densities, without altering channel gating [109]. Coexpression with Kvβ1.2 has also been shown to confer sensitivity to redox modulation and hypoxia to Kv4.2 channels without affecting gating kinetics [141].

Dipeptidyl-aminopeptidase-like protein 6 (DPP6) is a transmembrane protein that coimmunoprecipitates with Kv4 α subunits from the brain [142]. Coexpression of DPP6 with Kv4 α subunits increases Kv4 channel surface expression and accelerates channel inactivation and recovery [142]. It has been reported that DPP6 is expressed in human heart and that the coexpression with KChIP2 exerts additive effects on the rates of Kv4 channel inactivation and recovery, reconstituting properties similar to native cardiac $I_{to,f}$ [143]. Another DPP protein, DPP10, also interacts with Kv4.2 α subunits in rat brain [144] and has similar effects on heterologously expressed Kv4 channels [145–147].

Studies in heterologous cells also suggest functional roles for minK/MiRP subunits in the generation of cardiac I_{to} channels. It has been demonstrated, for example, that coexpression of MiRP1 modulates the time- and voltage-dependent properties of Kv4 channels [148, 149]. It has also been reported that the targeted deletion of *kcne2* (MiRP1) in mice resulted in reduced (~25%) ventricular $I_{to,f}$ densities with no measurable changes in the total or the surface expression of the Kv4.2 protein [150]. In addition, MiRP1 and Kv4.2 (but not Kv4.3) coimmunoprecipitate from adult mouse heart [150]. Augmentation of heterologously expressed Kv4.3 currents by MiRP1, however, has been observed in HEK293 cells, and MiRP1 coexpression slowed inactivation [148]. It has also been reported, however, that coexpression of MiRP1 with Kv4.3 and KChIP2 accelerated activation without affecting current densities [151]. Interestingly, a missense mutation (R99H) in *KCNE3* (MiRP2) was recently identified in an individual with Brugada syndrome [152]. This same mutation was also identified in four (of four) phenotypically positive family members but not in three (of three) phenotypically negative family members. Experiments in CHO cells revealed that coexpression of wild type and mutant *KCNE3* markedly affected Kv4.3 current densities, whereas KvLQT1 currents were unaffected [152]. It was also reported that MiRP3 and Kv4.3 can be coimmunoprecipitated from human left atrial appendages; these observations were interpreted as suggesting a physiological role for *KCNE3* in the generation of Kv4-encoded cardiac $I_{to,f}$ channels [152]. Clearly, more studies are needed to define the *in vivo* functional roles of the minK/MiRP subfamily of Kv accessory subunits in the human heart.

Accumulating evidence suggests that the slow component of I_{to}, $I_{to,s}$, is encoded by Kv1.4 [7]. Targeted disruption in the *KCNA4* (Kv1.4) locus in mice [153], for example, eliminates $I_{to,s}$, whereas $I_{to,f}$ is unaffected [45, 153]. In human ventricles, Kv1.4 transcripts are more abundant in the endocardium than epicardium [124], which is consistent with the observation that $I_{to,s}$ is preferentially expressed in the endocardium [18, 23]. Although Kv1.4 transcripts are also expressed in human atrium [124], the Kv1.4 protein is undetectable and exposure to specific antisense oligodeoxynucleotides targeting Kv1.4 has no effect on human atrial I_{to} [154]. In addition, oxidizing treatments, such as H_2O_2, have no effect on human atrial I_{to} inactivation, although oxidative stress slows the inactivation of heterologously expressed Kv1.4 (but not Kv4) channels [155–157]. It seems, therefore, that Kv1.4-encoded channels ($I_{to,s}$) do not contribute to human atrial repolarization.

Studies in heterologous expression systems have revealed that the gating properties of Kv1.4-encoded channels are modified by coexpression of accessory Kvβ subunits. Coexpression with Kvβ1 or Kvβ3, for example, markedly accelerates fast Kv1.4 channel inactivation, which is suggested to be mediated by the N-terminal "ball" peptides in the N-termini of Kvβ1 and Kvβ3 [100, 106, 158]. Interestingly, however, Kvβ2 also increases Kv1.4 current densities and accelerates inactivation despite lacking an N-terminal "ball" peptide domain [159–161]. Although Kvβ1.2 reportedly coimmunoprecipitates with Kv1.4 from (rat) brain [159], no role for Kvβ subunits in the generation of cardiac Kv1.4 ($I_{to,s}$) channels has been demonstrated directly to date.

2.6   MOLECULAR DETERMINANTS OF FUNCTIONAL CARDIAC I_K CHANNELS

Considerable evidence suggests that human atrial I_{Kur} channels are encoded by the Kv1.5 α subunit [162]. Heterologously expressed *KCNA5* (Kv1.5) generates delayed rectifier currents with biophysical and pharmacological (4-AP sensitivity) properties similar to native I_{Kur}, and antisense oligodeoxynucleotides targeted against Kv1.5 selectively attenuate I_{Kur} in human atrial myocytes [162]. A non-sense mutation in *KCNA5* has been identified in a family presenting with a history of atrial fibrillation [163]. The mutation results in the production of a truncated Kv1.5 protein that exerts a dominant negative effect, which results in the prolongation of atrial action potential duration and in increasing susceptibility to atrial fibrillation [163]. Although also present in human ventricles, the expression levels of Kv1.5 transcripts are ~25–30 fold lower than in the atria [124, 164], and I_{Kur} has not been described in human ventricular myocytes [16, 66]. Immunohistochemical studies suggest membrane expression of the Kv1.5 protein with high densities at intercalated disks in human and canine atria [165, 166]. Kv1.5 immunoreactivity has also been reported in human ventricular tissue, although strictly localized at the intercalated disks [165]. One component of delayed rectification in mice, I$_{K,slow1}$, is found in both atrial and ventricular myocytes and is indistinguishable from human atrial I$_{Kur}$ in terms of biophysical and pharmacological properties [42, 43, 167–169]. Indeed, it has been demonstrated that mouse I$_{K,slow1}$ channels are also encoded by Kv1.5 [170].

Previous studies suggested that canine atrial I$_{Kur}$ channels are encoded by Kv3.1 (rather than Kv1.5) based on the robust expression of the Kv3.1 message and protein (with low expression of Kv1.5) in canine atria [171]. In addition, canine atrial I$_{Kur}$ channels reportedly display sensitivity to tetraethylammonium (TEA) comparable with that observed for heterologously expressed Kv3.1 channels [171]. It was subsequently reported, however, that Kv1.5, not Kv3.1, is expressed in canine atria [166]. This latter study also reported that the TEA sensitivity of canine atrial I$_{Kur}$ is really different from Kv3.1 but that the currents are blocked by the Kv1.5 channel specific blocker, C9356 [166], which suggests that Kv1.5 likely also encodes canine atrial I$_{Kur}$. Although not viewed in earlier studies [171], it has also been reported that Kv1.5 is expressed in canine ventricles [166]. In addition, I$_{Kur}$-like currents in canine ventricular myocytes are blocked by the Kv1.5 specific blocker, DPO-1 [80].

Heterologous coexpression of Kvβ subunits, such as Kvβ1.1 [107], Kvβ1.2 [172], Kvβ3 [102, 173], and Kvβ3.1 [108], modifies the kinetics of Kv1.5 current inactivation, effects attributed to N-terminal inactivation domains [106] and to phosphorylation by protein kinase C or a related kinase [174]. Coexpression of Kvβ1–3 subunits also produces hyperpolarizing shifts in the voltage dependence of Kv1.5 current activation [102, 107, 172, 175]. In addition, Kvβ1.2 coimmunoprecipitates with Kv1.5 from human atria [159], although not from mouse ventricles [140], and heterologously expressed Kvβ2 and Kv1.5 also coimmunoprecipitate [175]. Exploiting a glutathione-S-transferase (GST)-Kv1.5 C-terminal fusion protein and mass spectrometry, one of the cytoskeletal-associater LIM domain proteins, FHL1, was identified as a potential Kv1.5 binding protein [176]. The LIM proteins, which include FHL1, contain multiple (four and a half in the case of the FHL proteins) highly conserved double zinc-finger (LIM) motifs [177]. The LIM proteins shuttle between cellular compartments and subserve multiple roles, which contribute to the control of gene expression and to the regulation of protein localization and functioning [177]. The heterologous coexpression of FHL1 increases Kv1.5 current densities and modulates the kinetics and voltage dependences of current activation and inactivation [176].

It was reported recently that targeted disruption of the *KCNE2* (MiRP1) locus results in a marked (50%) reduction in mouse ventricular I$_{K,slow}$ densities [150]. In addition, MiRP1 was shown to co-immunoprecipitate with Kv1.5 from adult mouse ventricles, and the attenuation of I$_{K,slow}$ was accompanied by reduced membrane expression of Kv1.5 [150]. Taken together, these results suggest that MiRP1 may play an important role in the generation of Kv1.5-encoded Kv channels *in vivo*. The cytoplasmic Kv accessory subunit, KChIP2, has also been shown to associate with Kv1.5 in adult mouse ventricles and to reduce the cell surface expression of Kv1.5 channels in HEK-293 cells; these observations are interpreted as reflecting an inhibitory effect of KChIP2 on the trafficking of Kv1.5 channels [178]. These observations suggest that more studies are needed to identify the molecular composition of functional cardiac I_{Kur} channels and to define the mechanisms that control the assembly, trafficking, and cell surface expression of these channels.

The *KCNQ1* locus, which is linked to inherited long QT syndrome 1 (LQTS1) [179], encodes the KvLQT1 protein that, when expressed alone, generates rapidly activating and slowly deactivating Kv currents [119, 120]. The coexpression of minK with KvLQT1, however, produces slowly activating Kv currents that closely resemble native I_{Ks} [60, 119, 120]. Loss-of-function mutations in *KCNE1* (minK) result in reduced I_{Ks} current densities and have been linked to LQTS5 [180] and atrial fibrillation [181, 182]. Homozygous mutations in *KCNQ1* or *KCNE1* have been identified in autosomal recessive long QT syndrome (Jervelle and Lange-Nielsen syndrome) with severe phenotypes, including congenital deafness [183–185]. In contrast, gain-of-function mutations in *KCNQ1* are associated with short QT syndrome (SQTS2) [186–188]. Although *in vitro* expressed minK was shown to coimmunoprecipitate with KvLQT1 [119], neither the molecular determinants of this interaction nor the stoichiometry of minK:KvLQT1 interactions have been determined [11]. It has been suggested that 2 [189, 190], 14 [191], or variable numbers [192] of minK subunits coassemble with KvLQT1 α subunits to generate functional I_{Ks} channels. It has also been suggested that minK interacts (directly) with the pore-loop of KvLQT1 [193, 194], perhaps lining the pore [195, 196], and that minK-dependent modulation of KvLQT1 activation kinetics reflects direct interaction(s) between the KvLQT1 C-terminus and the transmembrane domain of minK [197, 198]. An alternatively spliced valiant of KvLQT1 with a truncated N-terminus (isoform 2) that exerts a dominant negative effect on KvLQT1 isoform 1 has been identified in the human heart [96, 199, 200]. Interestingly, isoform 2 is preferentially expressed in the midmyocardium [96] and may contribute to transmural differences in the expression of I_{Ks} (i.e., the lower densities of I_{Ks} in the midmyocardium), compared with the epicardium and endocardium [28]. Although *KCNQ1* (KvLQT1) message is expressed in neonatal and adult mouse heart [201], I_{Ks} is readily detected in neonatal myocytes but is small or undetectectable in adult cells [71, 72]. It has been suggested that developmental changes in minK expression [201, 202] are responsible for the loss of functional I_{Ks} channels in adult mouse ventricles [42, 43]. In the adult mouse heart, the expression of minK messenger RNA (mRNA) is limited to the conduction system [203] and transgenic mice overexpressing dominant negative human KvLQT1 exhibit abnormalities in sinus node function and atrio-venticular conduction, as well as prolonged QT intervals [204], which suggests important contributions of I_{Ks} to cardiac automaticity and electrical conduction in adult mouse heart.

In addition to minK/MiRPs, two cytoplasmic proteins, Yotiao and fh12, seem to play important roles in the regulation of cardiac I_{Ks} channels. Yotiao (AKAP9) is an A-kinase anchoring protein (AKAP), which tethers cyclic adenosine $3',5'$-monophosphate (cAMP) dependent protein kinase A (PKA) in the vicinity of target substrates and mediates PKA-dependent phosphorylation [205]. In humans, Yotiao links PKA and protein phosphatase 1 to the C-terminus of KvLQT1, forming a macromolecular signaling complex [206]. The interaction between Yotiao and KvLQT1 is mediated by a leucine/isoleucine zipper (LIZ) motif in the C-terminus of KvLQT1 [206]; Yotiao and this LIZ motif are required for cAMP (PKA)-dependent upregulation of KvLQT1-minK channels [206]. Although it was reported that PKA targets serine-27 in the N-terminus of KvLQT1 and upregulates KvLQT1-minK channels [64, 207], subsequent work revealed that minK is required for the functional consequences of KvLQT phosphorylation [64]. In addition, it is also now clear that Yotiao is phosphorylated by PKA and independently regulates KvLQT1-minK channels *in vitro* [207]. Interestingly, missense mutations in the KvLQT1 LIZ domain [206, 208], the C-terminus of minK [64, 209], or in Yotiao [210] identified in individuals with LQT1, LQT5, and LQT11 lack cAMP/PKA-mediated current upregulation [64, 206, 210, 211]. The enhancement of I_{Ks} by β-adrenergic receptor activation [62, 63] mediated by the cAMP/PKA pathway [64, 206, 211] contributes, in part, to action potential shortening during sympathetic stimulation [211]. The loss of cAMP/PKA-mediated regulation of I_{Ks} in LQT mutant channels may account, at least in part, for the increased risk of arrhythmic events in response to increased sympathetic tone in LQT1 and LQT5 patients [212, 213].

As noted, *KCNH2* has been identified as the locus of mutations in familial LQTS2 [214]. The heterologous expression of ERG1 (*KCNH2*) reveals voltage-gated, inwardly rectifying K^+-selective channels with properties similar to cardiac I_{Kr} channels [215, 216]. Inherited short QT syndrome is also linked to mutations in *KCNH2* (SQTS1) [217]. The full length, cell-surface ERG1 protein (ERG1a) in heterologous expression systems and in the heart seems to be heavily glycosylated [218, 219]. In addition to the full-length ERG1a, N- and C-terminal variants have been identified [93, 94, 97], and several lines of evidence suggest that the N-terminal ERG1 variant, ERG1b, coassembles with full length ERG1a to form heteromeric I_{Kr} channels [220–222]. Biochemical studies suggest that ERG1a:ERG1b subunit assembly proceeds cotranslationally [223, 224], although the stoichiometry of functional cell surface ERG1a:ERG1b channels has not been determined [221, 222]. Additional support for a physiological role for ERG1b was provided with the identification of an ERG1b-specific missense mutation that results in an arginine to valine conversion in amino acid position 8 (A8V) in a LQT patient that was absent in 400 controls [221]. Interestingly, it has been reported that ERG1b reflects translation through an alternate start site compared with ERG1a [225], rather than an alternatively spliced variant, as had been suggested previously. In contrast with ERG1b, no physiological role has yet to be assigned to the C-terminal variant of ERG1, ERG1-USO [97], and the role (if any) of this variant in the generation of functional cardiac I_{Kr} channels is presently unclear.

The role(s) of accessory subunits in the generation of functional *KCNH2*-encoded cardiac I_{Kr} channels is not well understood [12, 121, 226–229]. It has been reported that heterologously expressed ERG1 and minK coimmunoprecipitate [227] and that antisense oligodeoxynucleotides targeted against minK attenuate I_{Kr} amplitudes in an atrial tumor (AT-1) cell line [230]. It has also been reported, however, that heterologous coexpression of another member of the *KCNE* subfamily of accessory subunits, MiRP1 (*KCNE2*), modifies the properties of ERG1 currents [226]. Mutations in *KCNE2* have been identified in inherited long QT syndrome (LQTS6) [226, 228] and familial atrial fibrillation [231], and it has been suggested that these mutations affect the functional expression of I$_{Kr}$ channels. Although biochemical experiments in heterologous cells suggested that HERG1 is more likely to associate with minK than with MiRP1 [229], it is not known currently whether the minK or MiRP1 (or both) accessory subunits associate with ERG1a and/or ERG1b in the myocardium and contribute to the generation of functional cardiac I$_{Kr}$ channels [12]. Clearly, additional experiments focused on defining the roles of the *KCNE* subfamily of Kv channel accessory subunits in the generation of myocardial I$_{Kr}$ (and other Kv) channels are needed to address this important point.

Accumulating evidence also suggests roles for several additional accessory/regulatory proteins in the generation of functional, cell surface cardiac I$_{Kr}$ channels. A yeast two hybrid screen using the C terminus of human ERG1, HERG1, as the bait, for example, identified the Golgi-associated protein GM130, shown to be involved in vesicular transport, as an HERG1 binding protein [232]. The GM130 interaction mapped to two non-contiguous regions of HERG1 and to a region just upstream of the GRASP-65 domain in GM130 [232]. Additional biochemical studies revealed that the heat shock proteins, Hsp70 and Hsp90, co-immunoprecipitate with heterologously expressed HERG1 and that geldanamycin, a specific inhibitor of Hsp90, prevents the maturation (post-translational processing) and increases the proteosomal degradation of the ERG1 protein [233]. Interestingly, the interaction between the ERG1 protein and Hsp70/Hsp90 are increased in LQT2 trafficking deficient *KCNH2* mutants, such as HERG1G601S [234]. In addition, the mutant HERG1G601S protein is retained in the endoplasmic reticulum [233]. It was also reported that inhibition of Hsp90 decreased I$_{Kr}$ densities in isolated ventricular myocytes [233]. Taken together, these results suggest that GM-130, Hsp70, and Hsp90 function as chaperone proteins, facilitating the trafficking of ERG1-encoded I$_{Kr}$ channels to the cell surface [233]. Additional potential ERG1-I$_{Kr}$ channel regulatory proteins, including FKBP38 [235] and FHL2 [236], have also been identified and are suggested to play roles in the regulation of channel trafficking and targeting. Considerable evidence now indicates that many LQT2 mutations, as well as many I$_{Kr}$ channel "blocking" drugs, affect ERG1-I$_{Kr}$ channel assembly, trafficking and targeting, in addition to influencing the properties of assembled cell-surface channels [235, 237]. It has also been reported that the PKA-specific AKAP inhibitory peptide AKAP-IS reduces PKA-dependent phosphorylation of HERG1 [238]. In addition, PKA activity was found to coimmunoprecipitate with heterologously expressed (in HEK-293 cells) HERG1, which is consistent with AKAP-IS-mediated interactions between PKA and HERG1 [238]. The recent development of a rabbit model of LQT2, in which the LQT2 G628S mutant HERG1 protein is overexpressed [230], should provide a model system to begin to dissect the molecular mechanisms regulating the assembly, trafficking, targeting, and functioning of cardiac HERG1-I$_{Kr}$ channels in isolated cardiac cells and in the intact heart. The development of rabbit models of KvLQT1- (KCNQ1-) linked LQT1 [230, 239, 240] is expected to have a major impact on the field.

2.7 MOLECULAR DETERMINANTS OF FUNCTIONAL CARDIAC Kir CHANNELS

Distinct types of inwardly rectifying K^+ (Kir) channels are expressed in the myocardium [241, 242], encoded by different Kir α subunits [243]. Several Kir subunit subfamilies, Kir1 through Kir6, most with several members, have been identified (Table 2.3). The Kir α subunits have two (not six) transmembrane domains (Figure 2.2A), although like Kv α subunits, Kir α subunits also assemble as tetramers to form functional K^+ selective channels (Figure 2.2B). The strongly inwardly rectifying Kir channels, I_{K1}, in cardiac cells [242, 243] reflect the expression of α subunits of the Kir2 subfamily, and all (three) members of the Kir 2 subfamily (Table 2.3) are expressed in the myocardium [244, 245]. Interestingly, KCNJ2, which encodes Kir2.1, is the locus of mutations in Andersen's syndrome [246, 247], an inherited, multisystem disorder that can be life threatening because of QT prolongation and increased (ventricular) arrhythmia risk [248]. Most Andersen syndrome mutations produce mutant Kir2.1 proteins that function as dominant negatives to suppress Kir2.x-encoded I_{K1} currents [249–251]. These mutations, therefore, result in reduced I_{K1} density and action potential prolongation [252, 253]. Individuals carrying Andersen's syndrome mutations in KCNJ2 can display QT prolongation (LQTS7) and periodic paralysis, as well as craniofacial malformations [248, 250, 254, 255], alone or in combination. Because only KCNJ2 is involved, the fact that many organ systems are affected suggests that Kir2.x-encoded channels are expressed and are functional in a variety of cells/tissues. Myocardial I_{K1} channels are regulated directly by phosphatidyl inositide bisphosphate, PIP2 [256–259], and many of the Andersen's mutations are in the PIP2 binding region [260], observations that suggest that PIP2-mediated regulation is also altered in Andersen's syndrome mutant I_{K1} channels.

The first direct molecular evidence that Kir 2 α subunits encode cardiac I_{K1} channels was provided in studies completed on myocytes isolated from (Kir2.1$^{-/-}$ and Kir2.2$^{-/-}$) mice bearing targeted disruptions in *KCNJ2* (Kir2.1) or *KCNJ12* (Kir 2.2) [261]. The Kir2.1$^{-/-}$ mice have cleft palate and die shortly after birth, precluding electrophysiological studies on adult cells [261]. Experiments conducted on isolated neonatal Kir2.1$^{-/-}$ ventricular myocytes, however, revealed that I_{K1} is absent [261]. An inwardly rectifying current, with properties distinct from wild type I_{K1}, was observed in Kir2.1$^{-/-}$ myocytes [262], suggesting either that an additional Kir current component is present but is difficult to resolve in wild-type cells or, alternatively, that a novel I_{K1} is upregulated in Kir2.1$^{-/-}$ hearts. In contrast, voltage-clamp recordings from adult Kir2.2$^{-/-}$ ventricular myocytes revealed that, although I_{K1} densities are reduced, the properties of the residual I_{K1} are indistinguishable from I_{K1} in wild-type cells [262]. These observations suggest that both Kir2.1 and Kir2.2

Table 2.3. Diversity of Inwardly Rectifying K$^+$ (Kir) and Two Pore Domain K$^+$ (K2P) Channel Subunits

Family	Subfamily	Protein	Gene	Location Human	Location Mouse	Cardiac Current
Kir						
	Kir1					
		Kir1.1	KCNJ1	11q24.3	9A4	??
	Kir2					
		Kir2.1	*KCNJ2*	17q24.3	11E2	I_{K1}
		Kir2.2	*KCNJ12*	17p11.2	11B2	I_{K1}
		Kir2.3	*KCNJ4*	22q13.1	15E1	??
		Kir2.4	*KCNJ14*	19q13.32	7B4	??
	Kir3					
		Kir3.1	KCNJ3	2q24.1	2C1.1	I_{KACh}
		Kir3.2	KCNJ6	21q22.13	16C4	
		Kir3.3	KCNJ9	1q23.2	1H3	
		Kir3.4	KCNJ5	11q24.3	9A4	I_{KACh}
	Kir4					
		Kir4.1	KCNJ10	1q23.2	1H3	
		Kir4.2	KCNJ15	21q22.13	16C4	
	Kir5					
		Kir5.1	KCNJ16	17q24.3	11E2	
	Kir6					
		Kir6.1	KCNJ8	12p12.1	6G2	I_{KATP}??
		Kir6.2	KCNJ11	11p15.1	7B4	I_{KATP}
SUR						
	SUR	SUR1	KBCC8	11p15.1	7B4	I_{KATP}
		SUR2	ABCC9	12p12.1	6G2	I_{KATP}
K2P						
	TWIK					
		TWIK-1	KCNK1	1q42.2	8E2	??
		TWIK-2	KCNK6	19q13.2	7B1	??
		TWIK-3	KCNK7	11q13.1	19A	
	TREK					
		TREK-1	KCNK2	1q41	1H6	I_{ss} ??
		TREK-2	KCNK10	14q31.3	12E	

Table 2.3 (*Continued*)

Family	Subfamily	Protein	Gene	Location Human	Location Mouse	Cardiac Current
	TASK					
		TASK-1	KCNK3	2p23.3		I_{ss} ??
		TASK-2	KCNK5	6p21.2	14A3	
		TASK-3	*KCNK9*	8q24.3	15D3	
		TASK-4	*KCNK15*	20q13.12	2H3	
	TRAAK					
		TRAAK-1	KCNK4	11q13.1	19A	
	THIK					
		THIK-1	KCNK13	14q32.11	12E	
		THIK-2	KCNK12	2p16.3	17E4	??
	TALK					
		TALK-1	KCNK16	6p21.2	14A3	??
		TALK-2	KCNK17	6p21.2		

☐ Expressed in Mammalian Heart

contribute to (mouse) ventricular I_{K1} channels, a hypothesis supported by subsequent biochemical and molecular analyses [263, 264]. The finding that the inwardly rectifying channels identified in the absence of Kir2.1 have properties distinct from wild-type I_{K1} channels further suggests that functional cardiac I_{K1} channels are heteromeric. Consistent with this hypothesis, detailed comparisons of the properties of heterologously expressed Kir2.1, Kir2.2, and Kir 2.3 α subunits and endogenous guinea pig, sheep, and mouse myocytes suggest marked regional differences in the molecular composition of I_{K1} channels [264–266].

Transgenic overexpression of *KCNJ2* (Kir2.1) results in ventricular action potential shortening [267] and increased arrhythmogenesis [268, 269] consistent with the view that I_{K1} plays a critical role in the regulation of normal cardiac rhythms [81]. Interestingly, these observations led directly to the identification of mutations in *KCNJ2* linked to congenital short QT syndrome, SQTS3 [270]. Importantly, hypoxia has also now been shown to result in the functional upregulation of ventricular I_{K1} densities, leading to action potential shortening, an acquired short QT phenotype, and increased arrhythmia risk [271, 272].

Although the weakly inwardly rectifying I_{KATP} channels are thought to play a role in ischemia and preconditioning [233, 273, 274], these channels do not seem to function in the regulation of resting membrane potentials or action potential waveforms under normal physiological conditions [87, 274]. In heterologous cells, coexpression of Kir6.x subunits (Table 2.3) with one of the ATP-binding cassette proteins that encode the sulfonylurea receptors (SURx) can generate I_{KATP} channels with properties similar to those described in native channels, including sensitivities to ATP, ADP, and sulfonylureas [87, 275, 276]. Functional I_{KATP} channels are formed by four Kir6 subunits, each of which associated with one SUR subunit [277, 278]. In addition to playing a regulatory role, SUR subunits bind to the C-terminus of Kir6.2, masking a C-terminal ER retention signal [279]. Deletion of the Kir6.2 C-terminus enables the Kir6.2 homomeric channels to reach the cell surface without SUR [280]. Kir6.2 channels (without SUR) can be inhibited by ATP, indicating that Kir6 subunits determine ATP-dependent channel regulation [280]. In contrast, SUR subunits are responsible for MgADP-dependent channel activation [281, 282], and a missense mutation in *ABCC9* which encodes SUR2A predisposes individuals to adrenergic induced atrial fibrillation originating from the vein of Marshall [283].

Pharmacological and molecular studies suggest that cardiac sarcolemmal I_{KATP} channels reflect the heteromeric assembly of Kir6.2 and SUR2A subunits, although Kir6.1 is also expressed [284]. In addition, antisense oligodeoxynucleotides against SUR1 reduce I_{KATP} channel densities in neonatal rat ventricular myocytes [285], suggesting that I_{KATP} channels are molecularly heterogeneous. Electrophysiological recordings from myocytes isolated from mice (Kir $6.2^{-/-}$) harboring a targeted disruption of the *KCNJ11* (Kir 6.2) locus [276, 286, 287], however, revealed no detectable I_{KATP} channel activity [286, 287], suggesting an absolute requirement for Kir6.2. Although these findings suggest that Kir6.1 cannot form functional cardiac I_{KATP} channels in the absence of Kir6.2, it is possible that Kir6.1 coassembles with Kir6.2 to form Kir6.1/Kir 6.2 heteromeric cardiac I_{KATP} channels.

The suggestion that SUR2 plays a pivotal role in the generation of cardiac I_{KATP} channels is supported by the finding that ventricular I_{KATP} channel density is reduced in myocytes from animals (SUR2$^{-/-}$) in which SUR2 has been deleted [288]. In contrast, it has also been reported that there are no measurable cardiac effects of the targeted disruption of SUR1 [276, 289]. Nevertheless, it is clear that I_{KATP} channel density is not eliminated in SUR2$^{-/-}$ ventricular myocytes [288] and that the properties of the residual I_{KATP} channels are similar to those produced on heterologous coexpression of Kir6.2 and SUR1 [288], suggesting that SUR1 also coassembles with Kir 6.2 in ventricular myocytes to produce functional I_{KATP} channels, at least in the absence of SUR2. Importantly, it was recently reported that SUR1 is required for the generation of (mouse) atrial I_{KATP} channels, suggesting that the molecular determinants of atrial and ventricular I_{KATP} channels are distinct [290]. The results of immunohistochemical studies have been interpreted as suggesting that Kir6.2 and SUR2A assemble to form plasmalemmal cardiac I_{KATP} channels [291]. In contrast, both Kir6.1 and Kir6.2 (and SUR2A) are expressed in mitochondria, observations interpreted as suggesting that the molecular compositions of functional I_{Kr} channels in different cellular compartments are distinct [291]. Similar to I_{K1} channels, myocardial I_{KATP} channels are also modulated by the binding of PIP2 and other membrane lipids [254, 256].

Action potentials recorded from isolated Kir6.2$^{-/-}$ ventricular myocytes are indistinguishable from those recorded from wild-type cells [287], which is consistent with suggestions that I_{KATP} channels do not play a role in shaping action potential waveforms under normal physiological conditions [87]. The characteristic ventricular action potential shortening observed during ischemia or metabolic blockade, however, is abolished in Kir 6.2$^{-/-}$ ventricular cells [287]. In addition, the protective effect of ischemic preconditioning is abolished in Kir6.2$^{-/-}$ hearts [276, 292] and infarct size in Kir6.2$^{-/-}$ animals, with and without preconditioning, is the same [292]. These observations are consistent with suggestions that cardiac I_{KATP} channels play an important role under pathophysiological conditions, particularly those involving metabolic stress [87, 90]. Unexpectedly, it has also been reported that ventricular action potential durations are largely unaffected in animals expressing mutant I_{KATP} channels with markedly (40-fold) reduced ATP sensitivity [293]. The mutant I_{KATP} channels would be expected to be open at rest (because of the reduced ATP sensitivity) and to affect cardiac membrane excitability. The fact that action potentials are unaffected in ventricular myocytes expressing the mutant I_{KATP} channels suggests that regulatory mechanisms (in addition to ATP) play a role in the physiological control of cardiac I_{KATP} channel activity *in vivo* [293].

2.8 OTHER POTASSIUM CURRENTS CONTRIBUTING TO ACTION POTENTIAL REPOLARIZATION

Background or leak K^+ conductances play an important role in stabilizing resting membrane potentials close to the K^+ equilibrium potential [294]. Cardiac background K^+ currents were first described in guinea pig ventricular myocytes and referred to as I_{Kp} [295, 296]. In neonatal and adult rat atrial [297, 298] and ventricular [299] myocytes, background K^+ currents that are sensitive to membrane stretch, unsaturated fatty acids, and intracellular acidification have also been identified and termed I_{KAA} [297]. Guinea pig ventricular I_{Kp} activates rapidly on depolarization and is noninactivating [296]. Although I_{K1} channels are major determinants of ventricular and atrial resting membrane potentials, the properties of I_{K1} channels [241, 242, 300] are distinct from those of background K^+ currents. Rather, accumulating evidence suggests that these channels reflect the expression of two pore domain K^+ (K2P) channels [301–303].

Distinct from the Kv and Kir subunit families, each K2P channel α subunit contains four transmembrane segments and two pore loops (Figure 2.2A). There are, however, several K2P subfamilies, as well as multiple members of each subfamily (Table 2.3). Functional K2P channels reflect the dimeric assembly (Figure 2.2B) of two identical subunits [304, 305] or of two different α subunits in the same subfamily [306–308]. The heterologous expression of K2P channel subunits reveals K^+ selective currents that display Goldman–Hodgkin–Katz (GHK) rectification and modest time- and voltage-dependent properties [301]. Of the many K2P channel subunits, the TWIK-related acid-sensitive K^+ channel 1 (TASK-1, *KCNK3*) and TWIK-related K^+ channel 1 (TREK-1, *KCNK2*) are expressed at the mRNA and protein levels in the mammalian heart [309–317], where they are thought to play roles in the generation of background K^+ currents.

Heterologously expressed TASK-1 channels display properties similar to myocardial background K^+ channels: TASK 1 channels activate rapidly, are active over the physiological range of membrane potentials, and do not inactivate [313]. In addition, TASK1 channels are characterized by high sensitivity to changes in extracellular pH, such that the channels are inhibited by acidosis in a narrow physiological range [318]. TASK-1 channels are insensitive to classic K$^+$ channel blockers, such as 4-AP [319], but are blocked selectively by cannabinoids, anandamide, and methananamide [320]. Inhalational anesthetics, such as halothane, augment TASK-1 currents [321], whereas local anesthetics, including lidocaine and bupicaine, inhibit TASK-1 currents [319]. In rat ventricular and atrial myocytes, TASK-1-like-channels/currents have been identified based on similarities with heterologously expressed TASK-1 channels [322] and sensitivity to the novel TASK-1 blocker, A293 [310]. In addition, TASK-1 immunoreactivity has been detected at the intercalated discs in rat atrial and ventricular tissue [314]. To date, however, no TASK-1-like currents have been described in the human heart.

Heterologously expressed TREK-1 channels have low basal activity and are activated by a variety of stimuli, including membrane stretch [323], arachidonic acid, and other polyunsaturated fatty acids [323, 324], and by intracellular acidification [323]. Like other K2P channels, TREK-1 channels display instantaneous activation, no inactivation, and little voltage-dependence [324], which is consistent with the properties of background conductances. Like TASK-1 channels, TREK-1 channels are also resistant to classical K$^+$ channel blockers [324], but, similar to other stretch activated channels, are inhibited by micromolar concentrations of gadolinium (Ga^{3+}), and by the neuroprotective agent, riluzole [325]. Although many inhalational anesthetics affect K2P channels, chloroform specifically potentates TREK-1 channels [321]. The properties of heterologously expressed TREK-1 channels are similar to those previously reported for I$_{KAA}$ in rat cardiac myocytes [297–299]. The pharmacological properties and the single-channel conductances of I$_{KAA}$ channels in rat ventricular and atrial myocytes, for example, are similar to heterologously expressed TREK-1 channels [315, 317, 326]. Immunofluorescence imaging suggests that the TREK-1 protein is arranged in longitudinal stripes at the surface of (rat) cardiomyocytes [327]. Similar to the TASK-1 channels, however, the functional expression of TREK-1 channels has not been demonstrated to date in human cardiomyocytes.

2.8.1   Myocardial K$^+$ Channel Functioning in Macromolecular Protein Complexes

Accumulating evidence suggests that myocardial Kv and Kir channels function as components of macromolecular protein complexes, comprising channel pore-forming α subunits and a variety of accessory subunits and regulatory proteins that are linked to the intracellular actin cytoskeleton and to the extracellular matrix. As with accessory and regulatory proteins, interactions with the cytoskeleton are expected to influence channel stability, trafficking, localization, and/or biophysical properties. Consistent with this suggestion, the properties of sarcolemmal I$_{KATP}$ channels are affected by pharmacological disruption of actin microfilaments. Exposure to deoxyribonuclease (DNase) I or cytochalasin B, for example, attenuated the ATP sensitivity of I$_{KATP}$ channels in guinea pig ventricular myocytes [328, 329]. In addition, I$_{KATP}$ channel rundown was accelerated by cytochalasin B and DNase I, and it was inhibited by agents that stabilize actin microfilaments, including phosphatidylinositol biphosphate (PIP$_2$) and phalloidin [330]. The inhibitory effects of sulfonylureas on (guinea pig and rat) ventricular I$_{KATP}$ channels were also attenuated by DNase I [329]. Similarly, rectification of guinea pig ventricular I$_{K1}$ channels is modified by cytochalasin D [331].

The properties of rat ventricular I$_{to,f}$ channels have also been reported to be regulated by the actin cytoskeleton under pathological conditions, specifically in left ventricular hypertrophy [332]. Although neither phalloidin nor cytochalasin D seems to affect I$_{to,f}$ densities in wild-type (nonhypertrophied) rat ventricular myocytes, phalloidin increased and cytochalasin-D decreased I$_{to,f}$ densities in hypertrophied cells [332]. In addition, phalloidin treatment shortened, whereas cytochalasin D lengthened, action potential durations in hypertrophied rat ventricular myocytes [332]. Interestingly, heterologously expressed (in HEK-293 cells) Kv4.2 channel densities were shown to be augmented after treatment with cytochalasin D [333]. These disparate observations suggest possible roles for Kv4.2 channel accessory/regulatory proteins in mediating interactions between Kv4 channels and the actin cytoskeleton and that these subunits likely are differentially expressed in different cell types [333, 334]. Several actin-binding proteins and other scaffolding proteins have been suggested to mediate the interactions between Kv channels and the actin cytoskeleton. Filamin, for example, has been shown to interact directly with a small (four amino acid) domain in the C-termini of Kv4 α subunits *in vitro* and to increase heterologously expressed Kv4 current densities [335]. In brain, filamin colocalizes with Kv4.2 [335]. Another actin binding protein, α-actinin-2, has also been shown to interact directly with the N termini of several Kv α subunits, including Kv1.4 and Kv1.5 [336, 337]. In HEK-293 cells, Kv1.5 co-localizes with α-actinin-2 at the cell periphery, and this co-localization is disrupted by cytochalasin D [336]. In addition, exposure to cytochalasin D or antisense oligodeoxynucleotides targeted against α-actinin-2 increased Kv1.5 current densities in HEK-293 cells, and the upregulation of Kv1.5 currents was antagonized by phalloidin [336]. It has also been reported that the phosphorylation of Kv1.5 (expressed in *Xenopus* oocytes) requires α-actinin-2 [338]. Kv channel accessory subunits also seem to interact with components of the actin cytoskeleton [339, 340]. The acceleration of Kv1.1 channel inactivation observed with coexpression of Kvβ1.1, for example, seems to be mediated by the actin cytoskeleton [339, 340].

Additional scaffolding proteins, including PDZ-domain-containing membrane-associated guanylate kinases (MAGUKs), have been implicated in the clustering and localization of neurotransmitter receptors and ion channels [341]. The 95 kDa post-synaptic density protein (PSD-95) and synapse-associated protein 97 (SAP97), both PDZ-domain-containing proteins, for example, interact directly with Kv α subunits. PSD-95 binds directly to PDZ-binding domains in the C-termini of Kv1 α subunits, and PSD-95 coimmunoprecipitates with Kv1.4 from the rat brain [342]. Interactions with PSD-95 also increase the clustering and cell-surface expression of heterologously expressed Kv1 channels [342–344]. It has also been reported that coexpression with PSD-95 localizes Kv1.4 channels to specific membrane microdomains known as "lipid rafts" [345–347]. In heterologous cells, Kv1.5 channels also localize to lipid rafts and, more specifically, to a subpopulation of lipid rafts called caveolae [348].

Caveolin, which is a scaffold protein found in caveolae, seems to play a role in targeting Kv1.5 channels to lipid raft microdomains [349] and in mediating interactions with SAP97 [350]. To date, however, there is no evidence of association between Kv1.5 and caveolin-3 in (rat or canine) atrial myocytes [351].

The binding of PSD-95 to Kv1.4 stabilizes Kv1.4-encoded channels in the membrane [352], presumably by suppressing internalization [353]. PSD-95 also reportedly binds to both the N- and C-termini of Kv1.5, exerting distinct effects on Kv1.5-encoded current amplitudes [354]. It has also been reported that PSD-95 binds to C-terminal PDZ-binding motifs in Kv4 α subunits [355], although the functional impact of this binding on Kv4 channel surface expression and clustering is not clear [342, 355]. PSD-95 has been reported to be expressed in human atria [356], although not in adult rat hearts [357, 358]. PDZ-binding motifs in the C-termini of Kv1 α subunits also interact directly with another MAGUK protein, SAP97 [343]. In contrast with the results obtained with PSD-95, however, interaction with SAP97 causes retention of Kv channels in the endoplasmic reticulum [343, 344, 359]. It has also been reported, however, that SAP97 immobilizes and retains Kv1.5 channels on the cell surface in neonatal rat cardiomyocytes and increases heterologously expressed Kv1.5 current amplitudes [356, 359]. In addition, in both human atria and rat ventricles, SAP97 and Kv1.5 seem to be colocalized at the intercalated disks [165, 356], and the two proteins can be co-immunoprecipitated [356, 359]. The observations suggest an indirect association between SAP97 and the N-terminus of Kv1.5, perhaps mediated by α-actinin [360]. Interestingly, the interaction between Kv1.5 and SAP97 is affected by phosphorylation of either protein [360, 361]. The functional roles of PSD-95 and SAP-97 in the regulation Kv1.5-encoded I_{Kur} channels in human atrial myocytes, however, remain to be determined.

The MAGUK proteins also interact with Kir channels, and Kir2 α subunits reportedly complex with multiple MAGUK proteins, including CASK, SAP-97, Veli-3, and Mint-1, in adult rat hearts [362]. Interestingly, in polarized epithelial cells, CASK plays a role in targeting Kir2.2 channels to specific membrane specializations, effects thought to be mediated through direct interactions between the C-terminal PDZ-binding motif of Kir 2.2 and SAP-97 or Veli-1/Veli-3 [363]. The role(s) of CASK and/or of other MAGUK proteins in the targeting, localization, and/or functioning of myocardial Kir channels, however, remain to be determined.

The actin cytoskeleton also likely plays important roles in Kir and Kv channel transport (trafficking), internalization, recycling, and degradation, although little is presently known about the underlying mechanisms in cardiac cells. Motor proteins, such as the kinesins, however, are know to carry vesicles along microtubules and actin filaments [364], and the kinesins have been suggested to function in the forward trafficking of K$^+$ channels in neurons. One kinesin isoform, Kif17, for example, plays a role in the trafficking of Kv4.2 [365], and another isoform, Kif5B, seems to be essential for membrane localization of Kv1 channels [366]. It has also been demonstrated that SAP97 interacts with an actin filament-based motor protein, myosin VI, in rat brains [367]. Interestingly, another motor protein, dynamin, has been suggested to play a role in the endocytosis of Kv1.5 [368]. In addition, in HL-1 (an atrial tumor cell line) cells, retrograde trafficking of channel proteins in early

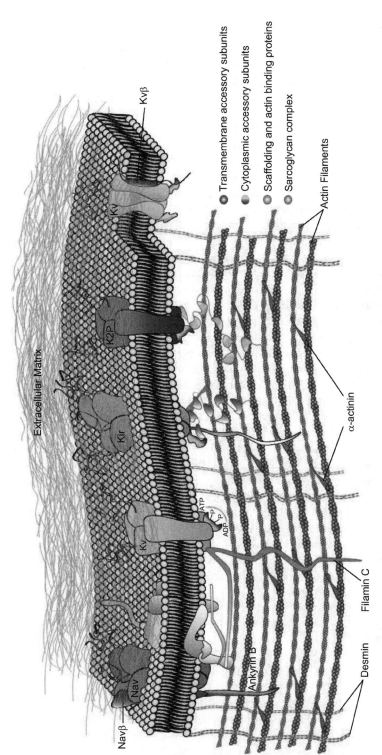

Figure 2.3. Cardiac Kv, Kir, and K2P channels function as components of macromolecular protein complexes. Schematic illustrating functional cardiac K^+ channels, composed of pore-forming α subunits and both transmembrane and cytosolic K^+ channel accessory subunits. Interactions between cardiac K^+ channels and the actin cytoskeleton are mediated through actin-binding proteins, such as filamin and α-actinin, and PDZ domain-containing scaffolding proteins. See color insert.

endosomes is mediated by the microtubule-based motor protein, dynein [369]. Recent studies have also revealed that small GTPases of the Rab family [370] determine the fate of internalized Kv1.5 channels (i.e. whether channels are recycled or degraded) in both HL-1 [369] and HEK-293 [371] cells. It seems certain that a major focus of future research will be on delineating the molecular mechanisms involved in the trafficking, turnover, and recycling of myocardial K$^+$ channels.

Considerable evidence also suggests that ion channels are functionally modulated by cell-cell and cell-extracellular matrix interactions [372]. In cultured rat ventricular myocytes, for example, cell-cell contact results in upregulation of Kv1.5 mRNA expression, whereas Kv4.2 transcripts is downregulated [373]. Neuronal cadherin (N-cadherin), a cell adhesion molecule, reportedly colocalizes with Kv1.5 at intercalated disks in human cardiomyocytes [165] and, in heterologous cells, coexpression of N-cadherin increases Kv1.5 current amplitudes [374]. Interestingly, overexpression of SAP97 in neonatal rat ventricular myocytes *in vitro* results in increased Kv1.5 expression at cell-cell contacts [375]. In addition, membrane expression of Kv1.5 is increased when the cells (neonatal myocytes) reach confluence [375]. These observations suggest that targeting of Kv1.5 to membrane microdomains in cardiac myocytes is mediated by the organized association of N-cadherin, SAP-97, and possibly the actin cytoskeleton, as observed in epithelial cells and fibroblasts [376]. Studies focused on exploring this hypothesis even more are needed to delineate the physiological roles of these interactions and the underlying molecular mechanisms.

Functional links between extracellular matrix adhesion molecules, integrin receptors and K$^+$ channels have also been demonstrated [372]. It was shown, for example, that the integrin β1 subunit binds directly to Kir3 α subunits and regulates Kir3 channel expression in heterologous cells [377]. In neurons, vitronectin-mediated integrin receptor stimulation increases the functional cell surface expression of Kv4.2 channels [378]. In both neuronal and hemopoietic tumor cells, integrin β1 subunit stimulation results in activation of hERG channels [379, 380] and it appears that hERG channels, integrin receptors, and other signaling molecules function specifically in these macromolecular signaling complexes [381, 382]. It seems certain that there will be increased emphasis on studies focused on defining the physiological role(s) of extracellular matrix components, as well as components of the intracellular actin cytoskeleton in the regulation of myocardial Kv and Kir (and K2P), and on delineating the underlying molecular mechanisms controlling these pathways under normal and pathophysiological conditions.

REFERENCES

1. Shin, H.-T. (1994). Anatomy of the action potential in the heart. Texas Heart Institute Journal, 21, 30–41.

2. Roden, D.M., Balser, J.R., George, A.L., Jr., Anderson, M.E. (2002). Cardiac ion channels. Annual Review of Physiology, 64, 431–475.

3. Desplantez, T., Dupont, E., Severs, N.J., Weingart, R. (2007). Gap junction channels and cardiac impulse propagation. Journal of Membrane Biology, 218, 13–28.

4. Wilde, A.A. (2008). Channelopathies in children and adults. Pacing and Clinical Electrophysiology, 31, S41–S45.

5. Raschi, E., Vasina, V., Poluzzi, E., De Ponti, F. (2008). The hERG K^+ channel: Target and antitarget strategies in drug development. Pharmacological Research, 57, 181–195.

6. Nattel, S., Maguy, A., Le Bouter, S., Yeh, Y.H. (2007). Arrhythmogenic ion-channel remodeling in the heart: Heart failure, myocardial infarction, and atrial fibrillation. Physiological Reviews, 87, 425–456.

7. Nerbonne, J.M., Kass, R.S. (2005). Molecular physiology of cardiac repolarization. Physiological Reviews, 85, 1205–1253.

8. Tamargo, J., Caballero, R., Gomez, R., Valenzuela, C., Delpon, E. (2004). Pharmacology of cardiac potassium channels. Cardiovascular Research, 62, 9–33.

9. Snyders, D.J. (1999). Structure and function of cardiac potassium channels. Cardiovascular Research, 42, 377–390.

10. Schram, G., Pourrier, M., Melnyk, P., Nattel, S. (2002). Differential distribution of cardiac ion channel expression as a basis for regional specialization in electrical function. Circulation Research, 90, 939–950.

11. Li, Y., Um, S.Y., McDonald, T.V. (2006). Voltage-gated potassium channels: Regulation by accessory subunits. Neuroscientist, 12, 199–210.

12. Abbott, G.W., Xu, X., Roepke, T.K. (2007). Impact of ancillary subunits on ventricular repolarization. Journal of Electrocardiology, 40, S42–S46.

13. Steele, D.F., Eldstrom, J., Fedida, D. (2007). Mechanisms of cardiac potassium channel trafficking. Journal of Physiology, 582, 17–26.

14. Wang, Z., Fermini, B., Nattel, S. (1993). Sustained depolarization-induced outward current in human atrial myocytes. Evidence for a novel delayed rectifier K^+ current similar to Kv1.5 cloned channel currents. Circulation Research, 73, 1061–1076.

15. Fedida, D., Wible, B., Wang, Z., Fermini, B., Faust, F., Nattel, S., Brown, A.M. (1993). Identity of a novel delayed rectifier current from human heart with a cloned K^+ channel current. Circulation Research, 73, 210–216.

16. Amos, G.J., Wettwer, E., Metzger, F., Li, Q., Himmel, H.M., Ravens, U. (1996). Differences between outward currents of human atrial and subepicardial ventricular myocytes. Journal of Physiology, 491, 31–50.

17. Fermini, B., Wang, Z., Duan, D., Nattel, S. (1992). Differences in rate dependence of transient outward current in rabbit and human atrium. American Journal of Physiology Heart Circulatory Physiology, 263, H1747–H1754.

18. Nabauer, M., Beuckelmann, D.J., Uberfuhr, P., Steinbeck, G. (1996). Regional differences in current density and rate-dependent properties of the transient outward current in subepicardial and subendocardial myocytes of human left ventricle. Circulation, 93, 168–177.

19. McMorn, S.O., Harrison, S.M., Zang, W.J., Yu, X.J., Boyett, M.R. (1993). A direct negative inotropic effect of acetylcholine on rat ventricular myocytes. American Journal of Physiology Heart Circulatory Physiology, 265, H1393–H1400.

20. Koumi, S., Wasserstrom, J.A. (1994). Acetylcholine-sensitive muscarinic K^+ channels in mammalian ventricular myocytes. American Journal of Physiology Heart Circulatory Physiology, 266, H1812–H1821.

21. Boyett, M.R., Kirby, M.S., Orchard, C.H., Roberts, A. (1988). The negative inotropic effect of acetylcholine on ferret ventricular myocardium. Journal of Physiology, 404, 613–635.

22. Litovsky, S.H., Antzelevitch, C. (1988). Transient outward current prominent in canine ventricular epicardium but not endocardium. Circulation Research, 62, 116–126.

23. Wettwer, E., Amos, G.J., Posival, H., Ravens, U. (1994). Transient outward current in human ventricular myocytes of subepicardial and subendocardial origin. Circulation Research, 75, 473–482.

24. Bryant, S.M., Wan, X., Shipsey, S.J., Hart, G. (1998). Regional differences in the delayed rectifier current (I_{Kr} and I_{Ks}) contribute to the differences in action potential duration in basal left ventricular myocytes in guinea-pig. Cardiovascular Research, 40, 322–331.

25. Furukawa, T., Kimura, S., Furukawa, N., Bassett, A.L., Myerburg, R.J. (1992). Potassium rectifier currents differ in myocytes of endocardial and epicardial origin. Circulation Research, 70, 91–103.

26. Sicouri, S., Antzelevitch, C. (1991). A subpopulation of cells with unique electrophysiological properties in the deep subepicardium of the canine ventricle. The M cell. Circulation Research, 68, 1729–1741.

27. Drouin, E., Charpentier, F., Gauthier, C., Laurent, K., Le Marec, H. (1995). Electrophysiologic characteristics of cells spanning the left ventricular wall of human heart: Evidence for presence of M cells. Journal of American Collage of Cardiology, 26, 185–192.

28. Liu, D.W., Antzelevitch, C. (1995). Characteristics of the delayed rectifier current (I_{Kr} and I_{Ks}) in canine ventricular epicardial, midmyocardial, and endocardial myocytes. A weaker I_{Ks} contributes to the longer action potential of the M cell. Circulation Research, 76, 351–365.

29. Di Diego, J.M., Sun, Z.Q., Antzelevitch, C. (1996). I_{to} and action potential notch are smaller in left vs. right canine ventricular epicardium. American Journal of Physiology Heart Circulatory Physiology, 271, H548–H561.

30. Volders, P.G., Sipido, K.R., Carmeliet, E., Spatjens, R.L., Wellens, H.J., Vos, M.A. (1999). Repolarizing K$^+$ currents I_{TO1} and I_{Ks} are larger in right than left canine ventricular midmyocardium. Circulation, 99, 206–210.

31. Szentadrassy, N., Banyasz, T., Biro, T., Szabo, G., Toth, B.I., Magyar, J., Lazar, J., Varro, A., Kovacs, L., Nanasi, P.P. (2005). Apico-basal inhomogeneity in distribution of ion channels in canine and human ventricular myocardium. Cardiovascular Research, 65, 851–860.

32. London, B. (2001). Cardiac arrhythmias: From (transgenic) mice to men. Journal of Cardiovascular Electrophysiology, 12, 1089–1091.

33. Charpentier, F., Demolombe, S., Escande, D. (2004). Cardiac channelopathies: From men to mice. Annals of Internal Medicine, 36, 28–34.

34. Nerbonne, J.M. (2004). Studying cardiac arrhythmias in the mouse–a reasonable model for probing mechanisms? Trends in Cardiovascular Medicine, 14, 83–93.

35. Salama, G., London, B. (2007). Mouse models of long QT syndrome. Journal of Physiology, 578, 43–53.

36. Gussak, I., Chaitman, B.R., Kopecky, S.L., Nerbonne, J.M. (2000). Rapid ventricular repolarization in rodents: Electrocardiographic manifestations, molecular mechanisms, and clinical insights. Journal of Electrocardiology, 33, 159–170.

37. van der Heyden, M.A., Wijnhoven, T.J., Opthof, T. (2006). Molecular aspects of adrenergic modulation of the transient outward current. Cardiovascular Research, 71, 430–442.

38. Liu, D.W., Gintant, G.A., Antzelevitch, C. (1993). Ionic bases for electrophysiological distinctions among epicardial, midmyocardial, and endocardial myocytes from the free wall of the canine left ventricle. Circulation Research, 72, 671–687.

39. Oudit, G.Y., Kassiri, Z., Sah, R., Ramirez, R.J., Zobel, C., Backx, P.H. (2001). The molecular physiology of the cardiac transient outward potassium current (I_{to}) in normal and diseased myocardium. Journal of Molecular and Cellular Cardiology, 33, 851–872.

40. Patel, S.P., Campbell, D.L. (2005). Transient outward potassium current, 'Ito', phenotypes in the mammalian left ventricle: Underlying molecular, cellular and biophysical mechanisms. Journal of Physiology, 569, 7–39.

41. Brahmajothi, M.V., Campbell, D.L., Rasmusson, R.L., Morales, M.J., Trimmer, J.S., Nerbonne, J.M., Strauss, H.C. (1999). Distinct transient outward potassium current (I_{to}) phenotypes and distribution of fast-inactivating potassium channel α subunits in ferret left ventricular myocytes. Journal of General Physiology, 113, 581–600.

42. Xu, H., Guo, W., Nerbonne, J.M. (1999). Four kinetically distinct depolarization-activated K^+ currents in adult mouse ventricular myocytes. Journal of General Physiology, 113, 661–678.

43. Brunet, S., Aimond, F., Li, H., Guo, W., Eldstrom, J., Fedida, D., Yamada, K.A., Nerbonne, J.M. (2004). Heterogeneous expression of repolarizing, voltage-gated K^+ currents in adult mouse ventricles. Journal of Physiology, 559, 103–120.

44. Brahmajothi, M.V., Campbell, D.L., Rasmusson, R.L., Morales, M.J., Trimmer, J.S., Nerbonne, J.M., Strauss, H.C. (1999). Distinct transient outward potassium current (I_{to}) phenotypes and distribution of fast-inactivating potassium channel alpha subunits in ferret left ventricular myocytes. Journal of General Physiology, 113, 581–600.

45. Guo, W., Xu, H., London, B., Nerbonne, J.M. (1999). Molecular basis of transient outward K^+ current diversity in mouse ventricular myocytes. Journal of Physiology, 521, 587–599.

46. Beuckelmann, D.J., Nabauer, M., Erdmann, E. (1993). Alterations of K^+ currents in isolated human ventricular myocytes from patients with terminal heart failure. Circulation Research, 73, 379–385.

47. Mubagwa, K., Flameng, W., Carmeliet, E. (1994). Resting and action potentials of nonischemic and chronically ischemic human ventricular muscle. Journal of Cardiovascular Electrophysiology, 5, 659–671.

48. Kääb, S., Nuss, H.B., Chiamvimonvat, N., O'Rourke, B., Pak, P.H., Kass, D.A., Marban, E., Tomaselli, G.F. (1996). Ionic mechanism of action potential prolongation in ventricular myocytes from dogs with pacing-induced heart failure. Circulation Research, 78, 262–273.

49. Priebe, L., Beuckelmann, D.J. (1998). Simulation study of cellular electric properties in heart failure. Circulation Research, 82, 1206–1223.

50. Greenstein, J.L., Wu, R., Po, S., Tomaselli, G.F., Winslow, R.L. (2000). Role of the calcium-independent transient outward current I_{to1} in shaping action potential morphology and duration. Circulation Research, 87, 1026–1033.

51. Sun, X., Wang, H.S. (2005). Role of the transient outward current (I_{to}) in shaping canine ventricular action potential—a dynamic clamp study. Journal of Physiology, 564, 411–419.

52. Shibata, E.F., Drury, T., Refsum, H., Aldrete, V., Giles, W. (1989). Contributions of a transient outward current to repolarization in human atrium. American Journal of Physiology Heart Circulatory Physiology, 257, H1773–H1781.

53. Firek, L., Giles, W.R. (1995). Outward currents underlying repolarization in human atrial myocytes. Cardiovascular Research, 30, 31–38.

54. Courtemanche, M., Ramirez, R.J., Nattel, S. (1998). Ionic mechanisms underlying human atrial action potential properties: Insights from a mathematical model. American Journal of Physiology Heart Circulatory Physiology, 275, H301–H321.

55. Nygren, A., Fiset, C., Firek, L., Clark, J.W., Lindblad, D.S., Clark, R.B., Giles, W.R. (1998). Mathematical model of an adult human atrial cell: The role of K^+ currents in repolarization. Circulation Research, 82, 63–81.

56. Horie, M., Hayashi, S., Kawai, C. (1990). Two types of delayed rectifying K + channels in atrial cells of guinea pig heart. Japanese Journal of Physiology, 40, 479–490.

57. Sanguinetti, M.C., Jurkiewicz, N.K. (1991). Delayed rectifier outward K^+ current is composed of two currents in guinea pig atrial cells. American Journal of Physiology Heart Circulatory Physiology, 260, H393–H399.

58. Sanguinetti, M.C., Jurkiewicz, N.K. (1992). Role of external Ca^{2+} and K^+ in gating of cardiac delayed rectifier K^+ currents. Pflügers Archives European Journal of Physiology, 420, 180–186.

59. Oudit, G.Y., Ramirez, R.F., Backx, P.H. Cardiac Electrophysiology: From Cell to Bedside, 4th edition. Saunders, Philadelphia, PA, 2004, pp. 19–32.

60. Tristani-Firouzi, M., Sanguinetti, M.C. (1998). Voltage-dependent inactivation of the human K^+ channel KvLQT1 is eliminated by association with minimal K^+ channel (minK) subunits. Journal of Physiology, 510, 37–45.

61. Ravens, U., Wettwer, E. (1998). Electrophysiological aspects of changes in heart rate. Basic Research in Cardiology, 93, 60–65.

62. Sanguinetti, M., Jurkiewicz, N., Scott, A., Siegl, P. (1991). Isoproterenol antagonizes prolongation of refractory period by the class III antiarrhythmic agent E-4031 in guinea pig myocytes. Mechanism of action. Circulation Research, 68, 77–84.

63. Han, W., Wang, Z., Nattel, S. (2001). Slow delayed rectifier current and repolarization in canine cardiac purkinje cells. American Journal of Physiology Heart Circulatory Physiology, 280, H1075–H1080.

64. Kurokawa, J., Chen, L., Kass, R.S. (2003). Requirement of subunit expression for cAMP-mediated regulation of a heart potassium channel. Proceedings of the National Academy of Sciences USA, 100, 2122–2127.

65. Wang, Z., Fermini, B., Nattel, S. (1994). Rapid and slow components of delayed rectifier current in human atrial myocytes. Cardiovascular Research, 28, 1540–1546.

66. Li, G.R., Feng, J., Yue, L., Carrier, M., Nattel, S. (1996). Evidence for two components of delayed rectifier K^+ current in human ventricular myocytes. Circulation Research, 78, 689–696.

67. Yue, L., Feng, J., Li, G.R., Nattel, S. (1996). Transient outward and delayed rectifier currents in canine atrium: Properties and role of isolation methods. American Journal of Physiology Heart Circulatory Physiology, 270, H2157–H2168.

68. Veldkamp, M.W., van Ginneken, A.C., Bouman, L.N. (1993). Single delayed rectifier channels in the membrane of rabbit ventricular myocytes. Circulation Research, 72, 865–878.

69. Li, D., Zhang, L., Kneller, J., Nattel, S. (2001). Potential ionic mechanism for repolarization differences between canine right and left atrium. Circulation Research, 88, 1168–1175.

70. Cheng, J., Kamiya, K., Liu, W., Tsuji, Y., Toyama, J., Kodama, I. (1999). Heterogeneous distribution of the two components of delayed rectifier K^+ current: A potential mechanism of the proarrhythmic effects of methanesulfonanilideclass III agents. Cardiovascular Research, 43, 135–147.

71. Wang, L., Feng, Z.P., Kondo, C.S., Sheldon, R.S., Duff, H.J. (1996). Developmental changes in the delayed rectifier K^+ channels in mouse heart. Circulation Research, 79, 79–85.

72. Babij, P., Askew, G.R., Nieuwenhuijsen, B., Su, C.M., Bridal, T.R., Jow, B., Argentieri, T. M., Kulik, J., DeGennaro, L.J., Spinelli, W., Colatsky, T.J. (1998). Inhibition of cardiac delayed rectifier K^+ current by overexpression of the long-QT syndrome HERG G628S mutation in transgenic mice. Circulation Research, 83, 668–678.

73. Zhou, J., Jeron, A., London, B., Han, X., Koren, G. (1998). Characterization of a slowly inactivating outward current in adult mouse ventricular myocytes. Circulation Research, 83, 806–814.

74. Apkon, M., Nerbonne, J.M. (1991). Characterization of two distinct depolarization-activated K^+ currents in isolated adult rat ventricular myocytes. Journal of General Physiology, 97, 973–1011.

75. Fiset, C., Clark, R.B., Larsen, T.S., Giles, W.R. (1997). A rapidly activating sustained K^+ current modulates repolarization and excitation-contraction coupling in adult mouse ventricle. Journal of Physiology, 504, 557–563.

76. Boyle, W.A., Nerbonne, J.M. (1992). Two functionally distinct 4-aminopyridine-sensitive outward K^+ currents in rat atrial myocytes. Journal of General Physiology, 100, 1041–1067.

77. Yue, L., Feng, J., Li, G.R., Nattel, S. (1996). Characterization of an ultrarapid delayed rectifier potassium channel involved in canine atrial repolarization. Journal of Physiology, 496, 647–662.

78. Lagrutta, A., Wang, J., Fermini, B., Salata, J.J. (2006). Novel, potent inhibitors of human Kv1.5 K^+ channels and ultrarapidly activating delayed rectifier potassium current. Journal of Pharmacology and Experimental Therapeutics, 317, 1054–1063.

79. Brendel, J., Peukert, S. (2003). Blockers of the Kv1.5 channel for the treatment of atrial arrhythmias. Cardiovascular & Hematological Agents in Medicinal Chemistry, 1, 273–287.

80. Sridhar, A., da Cunha, D.N.Q., Lacombe, V.A., Zhou, Q., Fox, J.J., Hamlin, R.L., Carnes, C.A. (2007). The plateau outward current in canine ventricle, sensitive to 4-aminopyridine, is a constitutive contributor to ventricular repolarization. British Journal of Pharmacology, 152, 870–879.

81. Dhamoon, A.S., Jalife, J. (2005). The inward rectifier current (I_{K1}) controls cardiac excitability and is involved in arrhythmogenesis. Heart Rhythm, 2, 316–324.

82. Lopatin, A.N., Makhina, E.N., Nichols, C.G. (1994). Potassium channel block by cytoplasmic polyamines as the mechanism of intrinsic rectification. Nature, 372, 366–369.

83. Stanfield, P.R., Davies, N.W., Shelton, P.A., Khan, I.A., Brammar, W.J., Standen, N.B., Conley, E.C. (1994). The intrinsic gating of inward rectifier K^+ channels expressed

from the murine IRK1 gene depends on voltage, K$^+$ and Mg^{2+}. Journal of Physiology, 475, 1–7.

84. Lopatin, A.N., Nichols, C.G. (2001). Inward rectifiers in the heart: An update on I$_{K1}$. Journal of Molecular and Cellular Cardiology, 33, 625–638.

85. Logothetis, D.E., Kurachi, Y., Galper, J., Neer, E.J., Clapham, D.E. (1987). The βγ subunits of GTP-binding proteins activate the muscarinic K$^+$ channel in heart. Nature, 325, 321–326.

86. Pfaffinger, P.J., Martin, J.M., Hunter, D.D., Nathanson, N.M., Hille, B. (1985). GTP-binding proteins couple cardiac muscarinic receptors to a K$^+$ channel. Nature, 317, 536–538.

87. Flagg, T.P., Nichols, C.G. (2005). Sarcolemmal K$_{ATP}$ channels: What do we really know? Journal of Molecular and Cellular Cardiology, 39, 61–70.

88. Gogelein, H. (2001). Inhibition of cardiac ATP-dependent potassium channels by sulfonylurea drugs. Current Opinion in Investigational Drugs, 2, 72–80.

89. Cole, W.C., McPherson, C.D., Sontag, D. (1991). ATP-regulated K$^+$ channels protect the myocardium against ischemia/reperfusion damage. Circulation Research, 69, 571–581.

90. Grover, G.J., Garlid, K.D. (2000). ATP-sensitive potassium channels: A review of their cardioprotective pharmacology. Journal of Molecular and Cellular Cardiology, 32, 677–695.

91. Shen, N.V., Pfaffinger, P.J. (1995). Molecular recognition and assembly sequences involved in the subfamily-specific assembly of voltage-gated K$^+$ channel subunit proteins. Neuron, 14, 625–633.

92. Attali, B., Lesage, F., Ziliani, P., Guillemare, E., Honore, E., Waldmann, R., Hugnot, J.P., Mattei, M.G., Lazdunski, M., Barhanin, J. (1993). Multiple mRNA isoforms encoding the mouse cardiac Kv1-5 delayed rectifier K$^+$ channel. Journal of Biological Chemistry, 268, 24283–24289.

93. Lees-Miller, J.P., Kondo, C., Wang, L., Duff, H.J. (1997). Electrophysiological characterization of an alternatively processed ERG K$^+$ channel in mouse and human hearts. Circulation Research, 81, 719–726.

94. London, B., Trudeau, M.C., Newton, K.P., Beyer, A.K., Copeland, N.G., Gilbert, D.J., Jenkins, N.A., Satler, C.A., Robertson, G.A. (1997). Two isoforms of the mouse ether-a-go-go-related gene coassemble to form channels with properties similar to the rapidly activating component of the cardiac delayed rectifier K$^+$ current. Circulation Research, 81, 870–878.

95. Kong, W., Po, S., Yamagishi, T., Ashen, M.D., Stetten, G., Tomaselli, G.F. (1998). Isolation and characterization of the human gene encoding I$_{to}$: Further diversity by alternative mRNA splicing. 275, H1963–H1970.

96. Pereon, Y., Demolombe, S., Baro, I., Drouin, E., Charpentier, F., Escande, D. (2000). Differential expression of KvLQT1 isoforms across the human ventricular wall. American Journal of Physiology Heart Circulatory Physiologyl, 278, H1908–H1915.

97. Kupershmidt, S., Snyders, D.J., Raes, A., Roden, D.M. (1998). A K$^+$ channel splice variant common in human heart lacks a C-terminal domain required for expression of rapidly activating delayed rectifier current. Journal of Biological Chemistry, 273, 27231–27235.

98. Po, S., Roberds, S., Snyders, D.J., Tamkun, M.M., Bennett, P.B. (1993). Heteromultimeric assembly of human potassium channels. Molecular basis of a transient outward current? Circulation Research, 72, 1326–1336.

99. Covarrubias, M., Wei, A.A., Salkoff, L. (1991). *Shaker, shal, shab*, and *shaw* express independent K^+ current systems. Neuron, 7, 763–773.

100. Morales, M.J., Castellino, R.C., Crews, A.L., Rasmusson, R.L., Strauss, H.C. (1995). A novel β subunit increases rate of inactivation of specific voltage-gated potassium channel α subunits. Journal of Biological Chemistry, 270, 6272–6277.

101. England, S.K., Uebele, V.N., Kodali, J., Bennett, P.B., Tamkun, M.M. (1995). A novel K^+ channel β-subunit (hkvβ1.3) is produced via alternative mRNA splicing. Journal of Biological Chemistry, 270, 28531–28534.

102. England, S.K., Uebele, V.N., Shear, H., Kodali, J., Bennett, P.B., Tamkun, M.M. (1995). Characterization of a voltage-gated K^+ channel β subunit expressed in human heart. Proceedings of the National Academy of Sciences USA, 92, 6309–6913.

103. Pongs, O., Leicher, T., Berger, M., Roeper, J., Bahring, R., Wray, D., Giese, K.P., Silva, A.J., Storm, J.F. (1999). Functional and molecular aspects of voltage-gated K^+ channel beta subunits. Annals of the New York Academy of Sciences, 868, 344–355.

104. Martens, J.R., Kwak, Y.-G., Tamkun, M.M. (1999). Modulation of Kv Channel α/β subunit interactions. Trends in Cardiovascular Medicine, 9, 253–258.

105. Gulbis, J.M., Zhou, M., Mann, S., MacKinnon, R. (2000). Structure of the cytoplasmic β subunit—T1 assembly of voltage-dependent K^+ channels. Science, 289, 123–127.

106. Rettig, J., Heinemann, S.H., Wunder, F., Lorra, C., Parcej, D.N., Dolly, J.O., Pongs, O. (1994). Inactivation properties of voltage-gated K^+ channels altered by presence of β-subunit. Nature, 369, 289–294.

107. Heinemann, S.H., Rettig, J., Wunder, F., Pongs, O. (1995). Molecular and functional characterization of a rat brain Kvβ3 potassium channel subunit. FEBS Letters, 377, 383–389.

108. Leicher, T., Bahring, R., Isbrandt, D., Pongs, O. (1998). Coexpression of the KCNA3B gene product with Kv1.5 leads to a novel A-type potassium channel. Journal of Biological Chemistry, 273, 35095–35101.

109. Yang, E.K., Alvira, M.R., Levitan, E.S., Takimoto, K. (2001). Kvβ subunits increase expression of Kv4.3 channels by interacting with their C termini. Journal of Biological Chemistry, 276, 4839–4844.

110. Shi, G., Nakahira, K., Hammond, S., Rhodes, K.J., Schechter, L.E., Trimmer, J.S. (1996). Beta subunits promote K^+ channel surface expression through effects early in biosynthesis. Neuron, 16, 843–852.

111. An, W.F., Bowlby, M.R., Betty, M., Cao, J., Ling, H.P., Mendoza, G., Hinson, J.W., Mattsson, K.I., Strassle, B.W., Trimmer, J.S., Rhodes, K.J. (2000). Modulation of A-type potassium channels by a family of calcium sensors. Nature, 403, 553–556.

112. Burgoyne, R.D. (2004). The neuronal calcium-sensor proteins. Biochimica et Biophysica Acta-Molecular Cell Research, 1742, 59–68.

113. Kim, L.A., Furst, J., Gutierrez, D., Butler, M.H., Xu, S., Goldstein, S.A., Grigorieff, N. (2004). Three-dimensional structure of I_{to};Kv4.2-KChIP2 ion channels by electron microscopy at 21 angstrom resolution. Neuron, 41, 513–519.

114. Bahring, R., Dannenberg, J., Peters, H.C., Leicher, T., Pongs, O., Isbrandt, D. (2001). Conserved Kv4 N-terminal domain critical for effects of Kv channel-interacting protein 2.2 on channel expression and gating. Journal of Biological Chemistry, 276, 23888–23894.

115. Beck, E.J., Bowlby, M., An, W.F., Rhodes, K.J., Covarrubias, M. (2002). Remodelling inactivation gating of Kv4 channels by KChIP1, a small-molecular-weight calcium-binding protein. Journal of Physiology, 538, 691–706.

116. Wible, B.A., Yang, Q., Kuryshev, Y.A., Accili, E.A., Brown, A.M. (1998). Cloning and expression of a novel K$^+$ channel regulatory protein, KChAP. Journal of Biological Chemistry, 273, 11745–11751.

117. Kuryshev, Y.A., Gudz, T.I., Brown, A.M., Wible, B.A. (2000). KChAP as a chaperone for specific K$^+$ channels. American Journal of Physiology Cell Physiology, 278, C931–C941.

118. McCrossan, Z.A., Abbott, G.W. (2004). The MinK-related peptides. Neuropharmacology, 47, 787–821.

119. Barhanin, J., Lesage, F., Guillemare, E., Fink, M., Lazdunski, M., Romey, G. (1996). KvLQT1 and IsK (minK) proteins associate to form the I$_{Ks}$ cardiac potassium current. Nature, 384, 78–80.

120. Sanguinetti, M.C., Curran, M.E., Zou, A., Shen, J., Spector, P.S., Atkinson, D.L., Keating, M.T. (1996). Coassembly of KvLQT1 and minK (IsK) proteins to form cardiac I$_{Ks}$ potassium channel. Nature, 384, 80–83.

121. McDonald, T.V., Yu, Z., Ming, Z., Palma, E., Meyers, M.B., Wang, K.W., Goldstein, S.A., Fishman, G.I. (1997). A minK-HERG complex regulates the cardiac potassium current I$_{Kr}$. Nature, 388, 289–292.

122. Tinel, N., Diochot, S., Borsotto, M., Lazdunski, M., Barhanin, J. (2000). KCNE2 confers background current characteristics to the cardiac KCNQ1 potassium channel. EMBO Journal, 19, 6326–6330.

123. Dixon, J.E., Shi, W., Wang, H.S., McDonald, C., Yu, H., Wymore, R.S., Cohen, I.S., McKinnon, D. (1996). Role of the Kv4.3 K$^+$ channel in ventricular muscle. A molecular correlate for the transient outward current. Circulation Research, 79, 659–668.

124. Gaborit, N., Le Bouter, S., Szuts, V., Varro, A., Escande, D., Nattel, S., Demolombe, S. (2007). Regional and tissue specific transcript signatures of ion channel genes in the non-diseased human heart. Journal of Physiology, 582, 675–693.

125. Dixon, J.E., McKinnon, D. (1994). Quantitative analysis of potassium channel mRNA expression in atrial and ventricular muscle of rats. Circulation Research, 75, 252–260.

126. Wickenden, A.D., Jegla, T.J., Kaprielian, R., Backx, P.H. (1999). Regional contributions of Kv1.4, Kv4.2, and Kv4.3 to transient outward K$^+$ current in rat ventricle. American Journal of Physiology Heart Circulatory Physiology, 276, H1599–H1607.

127. Marionneau, C., Brunet, S., Flagg, T.P., Pilgram, T.K., Demolombe, S., Nerbonne, J.M. (2008). Distinct cellular and molecular mechanisms underlie functional remodeling of repolarizing K + currents with left ventricular hypertrophy. Circulation Research, 102, 1406–1415.

128. Rosati, B., Pan, Z., Lypen, S., Wang, H.S., Cohen, I., Dixon, J.E., McKinnon, D. (2001). Regulation of KChIP2 potassium channel β subunit gene expression underlies the gradient of transient outward current in canine and human ventricle. Journal of Physiology, 533, 119–125.

129. Guo, W., Li, H., Aimond, F., Johns, D.C., Rhodes, K.J., Trimmer, J.S., Nerbonne, J.M. (2002). Role of heteromultimers in the generation of myocardial transient outward K^+ currents. Circulation Research, 90, 586–593.

130. Dilks, D., Ling, H.P., Cockett, M., Sokol, P., Numann, R. (1999). Cloning and expression of the human Kv4.3 potassium channel. Journal of Neurophysiology, 81, 1974–1977.

131. Po, S.S., Wu, R.C., Juang, G.J., Kong, W., Tomaselli, G.F. (2001). Mechanism of α-adrenergic regulation of expressed hKv4.3 currents. American Journal of Physiology Heart Circulatory Physiology, 281, H2518–H2527.

132. Kuo, H.C., Cheng, C.F., Clark, R.B., Lin, J.J., Lin, J.L., Hoshijima, M., Nguyen-Tran, V. T., Gu, Y., Ikeda, Y., Chu, P.H., Ross, J., Giles, W.R., Chien, K.R. (2001). A defect in the Kv channel-interacting protein 2 (KChIP2) gene leads to a complete loss of I_{to} and confers susceptibility to ventricular tachycardia. Cell, 107, 801–813.

133. Takimoto, K., Yang, E.K., Conforti, L. (2002). Palmitoylation of KChIP splicing variants is required for efficient cell surface expression of Kv4.3 channels. Journal of Biological Chemistry, 277, 26904–26911.

134. Shibata, R., Misonou, H., Campomanes, C.R., Anderson, A.E., Schrader, L.A., Doliveira, L.C., Carroll, K.I., Sweatt, J.D., Rhodes, K.J., Trimmer, J.S. (2003). A fundamental role for kchips in determining the molecular properties and trafficking of Kv4.2 potassium channels. Journal of Biological Chemistry, 278, 36445–36454.

135. Hasdemir, B., Fitzgerald, D.J., Prior, I.A., Tepikin, A.V., Burgoyne, R.D. (2005). Traffic of Kv4 K^+ channels mediated by KChIP1 is via a novel post-er vesicular pathway. Journal of Cell Biology, 171, 459–469.

136. Rosati, B., Grau, F., Rodriguez, S., Li, H., Nerbonne, J.M., McKinnon, D. (2003). Concordant expression of KChIP2 mRNA, protein and transient outward current throughout the canine ventricle. Journal of Physiology, 548, 815–822.

137. Teutsch, C., Kondo, R.P., Dederko, D.A., Chrast, J., Chien, K.R., Giles, W.R. (2007). Spatial distributions of Kv4 channels and KChip2 isoforms in the murine heart based on laser capture microdissection. Cardiovascular Research, 73, 739–749.

138. Guo, W., Malin, S.A., Johns, D.C., Jeromin, A., Nerbonne, J.M. (2002). Modulation of Kv4-encoded K^+ currents in the mammalian myocardium by neuronal calcium sensor-1. Journal of Biological Chemistry, 277, 26436–26443.

139. Nakamura, T.Y., Pountney, D.J., Ozaita, A., Nandi, S., Ueda, S., Rudy, B., Coetzee, W.A. (2001). A role for frequenin, a Ca^{2+}-binding protein, as a regulator of Kv4 K^+-currents. Proceedings of the National Academy of Sciences USA, 98, 12808–12813.

140. Aimond, F., Kwak, S.P., Rhodes, K.J., Nerbonne, J.M. (2005). Accessory Kvβ1 subunits differentially modulate the functional expression of voltage-gated K^+ channels in mouse ventricular myocytes. Circulation Research, 96, 451–458.

141. Perez-Garcia, M.T., Lopez-Lopez, J.R., Gonzalez, C. (1999). Kvβ1.2 subunit coexpression in HEK293 cells confers O_2 sensitivity to Kv4.2 but not to *shaker* channels. Journal of General Physiology, 113, 897–907.

142. Nadal, M.S., Ozaita, A., Amarillo, Y., Vega-Saenz de Miera, E., Ma, Y., Mo, W., Goldberg, E.M., Misumi, Y., Ikehara, Y., Neubert, T.A., Rudy, B. (2003). The CD26-related dipeptidyl aminopeptidase-like protein DPPX is a critical component of neuronal A-type K^+ channels. Neuron, 37, 449–461.

143. Radicke, S., Cotella, D., Graf, E.M., Ravens, U., Wettwer, E. (2005). Expression and function of dipeptidyl-aminopeptidase-like protein 6 as a putative β-subunit of human

cardiac transient outward current encoded by Kv4.3. Journal of Physiology, 565, 751–756.

144. Zagha, E., Ozaita, A., Chang, S.Y., Nadal, M.S., Lin, U., Saganich, M.J., McCormack, T., Akinsanya, K.O., Qi, S.Y., Rudy, B. (2005). DPP10 modulates Kv4-mediated A-type potassium channels. Journal of Biological Chemistry, 280, 18853–18861.

145. Jerng, H.H., Qian, Y., Pfaffinger, P.J. (2004). Modulation of Kv4.2 channel expression and gating by dipeptidyl peptidase 10 (DPP10). Biophysical Journal, 87, 2380–2396.

146. Jerng, H.H., Kunjilwar, K., Pfaffinger, P.J. (2005). Multiprotein assembly of Kv4.2, KChIP3 and DPP10 produces ternary channel complexes with I$_{SA}$-like properties. Journal of Physiology, 568, 767–788.

147. Li, H.L., Qu, Y.J., Lu, Y.C., Bondarenko, V.E., Wang, S., Skerrett, I.M., Morales, M.J. (2006). DPP10 is an inactivation modulatory protein of Kv4.3 and Kv1.4. American Journal of Physiology Cell Physiology, 291, C966–C976.

148. Deschênes, I., Tomaselli, G.F. (2002). Modulation of Kv4.3 current by accessory subunits. FEBS Letters, 528, 183–188.

149. Zhang, M., Jiang, M., Tseng, G.N. (2001). minK-related peptide 1 associates with Kv4.2 and modulates its gating function: Potential role as beta subunit of cardiac transient outward channel? Circulation Research, 88, 1012–1019.

150. Roepke, T.K., Kontogeorgis, A., Ovanez, C., Xu, X., Young, J.B., Purtell, K., Goldstein, P. A., Christini, D.J., Peters, N.S., Akar, F.G., Gutstein, D.E., Lerner, D.J., Abbott, G.W. (2008). Targeted deletion of *kcne2* impairs ventricular repolarization via disruption of I$_{K,slow1}$ and I$_{to,f}$. FASEB Journal, 22, 3648–3660.

151. Radicke, S., Cotella, D., Graf, E.M., Banse, U., Jost, N., Varro, A., Tseng, G.N., Ravens, U., Wettwer, E. (2006). Functional modulation of the transient outward current I$_{to}$ by KCNE β-subunits and regional distribution in human non-failing and failing hearts. Cardiovascular Research, 71, 695–703.

152. Delpón, E., Cordeiro, J.M., Nunez, L., Thomsen, P.E.B., Guerchicoff, A., Pollevick, G.D., Wu, Y., Kanters, J.K., Larsen, C.T., Burashnikov, E., Christiansen, M., Antzelevitch, C. (2008). Functional effects of KCNE3 mutation and its role in the development of Brugada syndrome. Circulation: Arrhythmia and Electrophysiology, 1, 209–218.

153. London, B., Wang, D.W., Hill, J.A., Bennett, P.B. (1998). The transient outward current in mice lacking the potassium channel gene Kv1.4. Journal of Physiology, 509, 171–182.

154. Wang, Z., Feng, J., Shi, H., Pond, A., Nerbonne, J.M., Nattel, S. (1999). Potential molecular basis of different physiological properties of the transient outward K$^+$ current in rabbit and human atrial myocytes. Circulation Research, 84, 551–561.

155. Vega-Saenz de Miera, E., Rudy, B. (1992). Modulation of K$^+$ channels by hydrogen peroxide. Biochemical and Biophysical Research Communications, 186, 1681–1687.

156. Serodio, P., Kentros, C., Rudy, B. (1994). Identification of molecular components of A-type channels activating at subthreshold potentials. Journal of Neurophysiology, 72, 1516–1529.

157. Duprat, F., Guillemare, E., Romey, G., Fink, M., Lesage, F., Lazdunski, M., Honore, E. (1995). Susceptibility of cloned K$^+$ channels to reactive oxygen species. Proceedings of the National Academy of Sciences USA, 92, 11796–11800.

158. Castellino, R.C., Morales, M.J., Strauss, H.C., Rasmusson, R.L. (1995). Time- and voltage-dependent modulation of a Kv1.4 channel by a β-subunit (Kvβ3) cloned from ferret ventricle. American Journal of Physiology Heart Circulatory Physiology, 269, H385–H391.

159. Kuryshev, Y.A., Wible, B.A., Gudz, T.I., Ramirez, A.N., Brown, A.M. (2001). KChAP/ Kvβ1.2 interactions and their effects on cardiac Kv channel expression. American Journal of Physiology Cell Physiology, 281, C290–C299.

160. Accili, E.A., Kuryshev, Y.A., Wible, B.A., Brown, A.M. (1998). Separable effects of human Kvβ1.2 N- and C-termini on inactivation and expression of human Kv1.4. Journal of Physiology, 512, 325–336.

161. Peri, R., Wible, B.A., Brown, A.M. (2001). Mutations in the Kvβ2 binding site for NADPH and their effects on Kv1.4. Journal of Biological Chemistry, 276, 738–741.

162. Feng, J., Wible, B., Li, G.R., Wang, Z., Nattel, S. (1997). Antisense oligodeoxynucleotides directed against Kv1.5 mRNA specifically inhibit ultrarapid delayed rectifier K^+ current in cultured adult human atrial myocytes. Circulation Research, 80, 572–579.

163. Olson, T.M., Alekseev, A.E., Liu, X.K., Park, S., Zingman, L.V., Bienengraeber, M., Sattiraju, S., Ballew, J.D., Jahangir, A., Terzic, A. (2006). Kv1.5 channelopathy due to KCNA5 loss-of-function mutation causes human atrial fibrillation. Human Molecular Genetics, 15, 2185–2191.

164. rdög, B., Brutyó, E., Puskás, L.G., Papp, J.G., Varró, A., Szabad, J., Boldogkoi, Z. (2006). Gene expression profiling of human cardiac potassium and sodium channels. International Journal of Cardiology, 111, 386–393.

165. Mays, D.J., Foose, J.M., Philipson, L.H., Tamkun, M.M. (1995). Localization of the Kv1.5 K^+ channel protein in explanted cardiac tissue. Journal of Clinical Investigation, 96, 282–292.

166. Fedida, D., Eldstrom, J., Hesketh, J.C., Lamorgese, M., Castel, L., Steele, D.F., Van Wagoner, D.R. (2003). Kv1.5 is an important component of repolarizing K^+ current in canine atrial myocytes. Circulation Research, 93, 744–751.

167. Bou-Abboud, E., Li, H., Nerbonne, J.M. (2000). Molecular diversity of the repolarizing voltage-gated K^+ currents in mouse atrial cells. Journal of Physiology, 529, 345–358.

168. Trepanier-Boulay, V., Lupien, M.A., St-Michel, C., Fiset, C. (2004). Postnatal development of atrial repolarization in the mouse. Cardiovascular Research, 64, 84–93.

169. Brouillette, J., Clark, R.B., Giles, W.R., Fiset, C. (2004). Functional properties of K^+ currents in adult mouse ventricular myocytes. Journal of Physiology, 559, 777–798.

170. London, B., Guo, W., Pan, X., Lee, J.S., Shusterman, V., Rocco, C.J., Logothetis, D.A., Nerbonne, J.M., Hill, J.A. (2001). Targeted replacement of Kv1.5 in the mouse leads to loss of the 4-aminopyridine-sensitive component of $I_{K,slow}$ and resistance to drug-induced QT prolongation. Circulation Research, 88, 940–946.

171. Yue, L., Wang, Z., Rindt, H., Nattel, S. (2000). Molecular evidence for a role of shaw (kv3) potassium channel subunits in potassium currents of dog atrium. Journal of Physiology, 527, 467–478.

172. De Biasi, M., Wang, Z., Accili, E., Wible, B., Fedida, D. (1997). Open channel block of human heart hKv1.5 by the β-subunit hKv β1.2. American Journal of Physiology Heart Circulatory Physiology, 272, H2932–H2941.

173. Majumder, K., De Biasi, M., Wang, Z., Wible, B.A. (1995). Molecular cloning and functional expression of a novel potassium channel β-subunit from human atrium. FEBS Letters, 361, 13–16.

174. Kwak, Y.-G., Navarro-Polanco, R.A., Grobaski, T., Gallagher, D.J., Tamkun, M.M. (1999). Phosphorylation is required for alteration of Kv1.5 K^+ channel function by the Kvβ1.3 subunit. Journal of Biological Chemistry, 274, 25355–25361.

175. Uebele, V.N., England, S.K., Chaudhary, A., Tamkun, M.M., Snyders, D.J. (1996). Functional differences in Kv1.5 currents expressed in mammalian cell lines are due to the presence of endogenous Kvβ2.1 subunits. Journal of Biological Chemistry, 271, 2406–2412.

176. Yang, Z., Browning, C.F., Hallaq, H., Yermalitskaya, L., Esker, J., Hall, M.R., Link, A.J., Ham, A.-J.L., McGrath, M.J., Mitchell, C.A., Murray, K.T. (2008). Four and a half LIM protein 1: A partner for KCNA5 in human atrium. Cardiovascular Research, 78, 449–457.

177. Kadrmas, J.L., Beckerle, M.C. (2004). The LIM domain: From the cytoskeleton to the nucleus. Nature Reviews Molecular Cell Biology, 5, 920–931.

178. Li, H., Guo, W., Mellor, R.L., Nerbonne, J.M. (2005). KChIP2 modulates the cell surface expression of Kv1.5-encoded K⁺ channels. Journal of Molecular and Cellular Cardiology, 39, 121–132.

179. Wang, Q., Curran, M.E., Splawski, I., Burn, T.C., Millholland, J.M., VanRaay, T.J., Shen, J., Timothy, K.W., Vincent, G.M., de Jager, T., Schwartz, P.J., Toubin, J.A., Moss, A.J., Atkinson, D.L., Landes, G.M., Connors, T.D., Keating, M.T. (1996). Positional cloning of a novel potassium channel gene: KvLQT1 mutations cause cardiac arrhythmias. Nature Genetics, 12, 17–23.

180. Splawski, I., Tristani-Firouzi, M., Lehmann, M.H., Sanguinetti, M.C., Keating, M.T. (1997). Mutations in the hmink gene cause long QT syndrome and suppress I_{Ks} function. Nature Genetics, 17, 338–340.

181. Lai, L.P., Su, M.J., Yeh, H.M., Lin, J.L., Chiang, F.T., Hwang, J.J., Hsu, K.L., Tseng, C.D., Lien, W.P., Tseng, Y.Z., Huang, S.K. (2002). Association of the human minK gene 38G allele with atrial fibrillation: Evidence of possible genetic control on the pathogenesis of atrial fibrillation. American Heart Journal, 144, 485–490.

182. Ehrlich, J.R., Zicha, S., Coutu, P., Hebert, T.E., Nattel, S. (2005). Atrial fibrillation-associated minK38G/S polymorphism modulates delayed rectifier current and membrane localization. Cardiovascular Research, 67, 520–528.

183. Splawski, I., Timothy, K.W., Vincent, G.M., Atkinson, D.L., Keating, M.T. (1997). Molecular basis of the long-QT syndrome associated with deafness. New England Journal of Medicine, 336, 1562–1567.

184. Neyroud, N., Tesson, F., Denjoy, I., Leibovici, M., Donger, C., Barhanin, J., Faure, S., Gary, F., Coumel, P., Petit, C., Schwartz, K., Guicheney, P. (1997). A novel mutation in the potassium channel gene KvLQT1 causes the Jervell and Lange-Nielsen cardioauditory syndrome. Nature Genetics, 15, 186–189.

185. Schulze-Bahr, E., Wang, Q., Wedekind, H., Haverkamp, W., Chen, Q., Sun, Y., Rubie, C., Hordt, M., Towbin, J.A., Borggrefe, M., Assmann, G., Qu, X., Somberg, J.C., Breithardt, G., Oberti, C., Funke, H. (1997). KCNE1 mutations cause Jervell and Lange-Nielsen syndrome. Nature Genetics, 17, 267–268.

186. Chen, Y.H., Xu, S.J., Bendahhou, S., Wang, X.L., Wang, Y., Xu, W.Y., Jin, H.W., Sun, H., Su, X.Y., Zhuang, Q.N., Yang, Y.Q., Li, Y.B., Liu, Y., Xu, H.J., Li, X.F., Ma, N., Mou, C.P., Chen, Z., Barhanin, J., Huang, W. (2003). KCNQ1 gain-of-function mutation in familial atrial fibrillation. Science, 299, 251–254.

187. Bellocq, C., van Ginneken, A.C., Bezzina, C.R., Alders, M., Escande, D., Mannens, M.M., Baro, I., Wilde, A.A. (2004). Mutation in the KCNQ1 gene leading to the short QT-interval syndrome. Circulation, 109, 2394–2397.

188. Hong, K., Piper, D.R., Diaz-Valdecantos, A., Brugada, J., Oliva, A., Burashnikov, E., Santos-de-Soto, J., Grueso-Montero, J., Diaz-Enfante, E., Brugada, P., Sachse, F., Sanguinetti, M.C., Brugada, R. (2005). De novo KCNQ1 mutation responsible for atrial fibrillation and short QT syndrome in utero. Cardiovascular Research, 68, 433–440.

189. Wang, K.W., Goldstein, S.A. (1995). Subunit composition of minK potassium channels. Neuron, 14, 1303–1309.

190. Chen, H., Kim, L.A., Rajan, S., Xu, S., Goldstein, S.A. (2003). Charybdotoxin binding in the I_{Ks} pore demonstrates two MinK subunits in each channel complex. Neuron, 40, 15–23.

191. Tzounopoulos, T., Guy, H.R., Durell, S., Adelman, J.P., Maylie, J. (1995). Min k channels form by assembly of at least 14 subunits. Proceedings of the National Academy of Sciences USA, 92, 9593–9597.

192. Wang, W., Xia, J., Kass, R.S. (1998). MinK-KvLQT1 fusion proteins, evidence for multiple stoichiometries of the assembled IsK channel. Journal of Biological Chemistry, 273, 34069–34074.

193. Tai, K.K., Goldstein, S.A. (1998). The conduction pore of a cardiac potassium channel. Nature, 391, 605–658.

194. Melman, Y.F., Um, S.Y., Krumerman, A., Kagan, A., McDonald, T.V. (2004). KCNE1 binds to the KCNQ1 pore to regulate potassium channel activity. Neuron, 42, 927–937.

195. Wang, K.W., Tai, K.K., Goldstein, S.A. (1996). MinK residues line a potassium channel pore. Neuron, 16, 571–577.

196. Goldstein, S.A., Miller, C. (1991). Site-specific mutations in a minimal voltage-dependent K^+ channel alter ion selectivity and open-channel block. Neuron, 7, 403–408.

197. Tapper, A.R., George, A.L., Jr. (2000). MinK subdomains that mediate modulation of and association with KvLQT1. Journal of General Physiology, 116, 379–390.

198. Gage, S.D., Kobertz, W.R. (2004). KCNE3 truncation mutants reveal a bipartite modulation of KCNQ1 K^+ channels. Journal of General Physiology, 124, 759–771.

199. Demolombe, S., Baro, I., Pereon, Y., Bliek, J., Mohammad-Panah, R., Pollard, H., Morid, S., Mannens, M., Wilde, A., Barhanin, J., Charpentier, F., Escande, D. (1998). A dominant negative isoform of the long QT syndrome 1 gene product. Journal of Biological Chemistry, 273, 6837–6843.

200. Jiang, M., Tseng-Crank, J., Tseng, G.N. (1997). Suppression of slow delayed rectifier current by a truncated isoform of KvLQT1 cloned from normal human heart. Journal of Biological Chemistry, 272, 24109–24112.

201. Drici, M.-D., Arrighi, I., Chouabe, C., Mann, J.R., Lazdunski, M., Romey, G., Barhanin, J. (1998). Involvement of IsK-associated K^+ channel in heart rate control of repolarization in a murine engineered model of Jervell and Lange-Nielsen syndrome. Circulation Research, 83, 95–102.

202. Honore, E., Attali, B., Romey, G., Heurteaux, C., Ricard, P., Lesage, F., Lazdunski, M., Barhanin, J. (1991). Cloning, expression, pharmacology and regulation of a delayed rectifier K^+ channel in mouse heart. EMBO Journal, 10, 2805–2811.

203. Kupershmidt, S., Yang, T., Anderson, M.E., Wessels, A., Niswender, K.D., Magnuson, M. A., Roden, D.M. (1999). Replacement by homologous recombination of the minK gene with lacz reveals restriction of minK expression to the mouse cardiac conduction system. Circulation Research, 84, 146–152.

204. Demolombe, S., Lande, G., Charpentier, F., van Roon, M.A., van den Hoff, M.J., Toumaniantz, G., Baro, I., Guihard, G., Le Berre, N., Corbier, A., de Bakker, J., Opthof,

T., Wilde, A., Moorman, A.F., Escande, D. (2001). Transgenic mice overexpressing human KvLQT1 dominant-negative isoform. Part I: Phenotypic characterisation. Cardiovascular Research, 50, 314–327.

205. Diviani, D. (2008). Modulation of cardiac function by A-kinase anchoring proteins. Current Opinion in Pharmacology Cardiovascular and Renal, 8, 166–173.

206. Marx, S.O., Kurokawa, J., Reiken, S., Motoike, H., D'Armiento, J., Marks, A.R., Kass, R.S. (2002). Requirement of a macromolecular signaling complex for β adrenergic receptor modulation of the KCNQ1-KCNE1 potassium channel. Science, 295, 496–499.

207. Chen, L., Kurokawa, J., Kass, R.S. (2005). Phosphorylation of the A-kinase-anchoring protein Yotiao contributes to Protein Kinase A regulation of a heart potassium channel. Journal of Biological Chemistry, 280, 31347–31352.

208. Piippo, K., Swan, H., Pasternack, M., Chapman, H., Paavonen, K., Viitasalo, M., Toivonen, L., Kontula, K. (2001). A founder mutation of the potassium channel KCNQ1 in long QT syndrome: Implications for estimation of disease prevalence and molecular diagnostics. Journal of American College of Cardiology, 37, 562–568.

209. Bianchi, L., Shen, Z., Dennis, A.T., Priori, S.G., Napolitano, C., Ronchetti, E., Bryskin, R., Schwartz, P.J., Brown, A.M. (1999). Cellular dysfunction of LQT5-minK mutants: Abnormalities of I_{Ks}, I_{Kr} and trafficking in long QT syndrome. Human Molecular Genetics, 8, 1499–1507.

210. Chen, L., Marquardt, M.L., Tester, D.J., Sampson, K.J., Ackerman, M.J., Kass, R.S. (2007). Mutation of an A-kinase-anchoring protein causes long-QT syndrome. Proceedings of the National Academy of Sciences USA, 104, 20990–20995.

211. Terrenoire, C., Clancy, C.E., Cormier, J.W., Sampson, K.J., Kass, R.S. (2005). Autonomic control of cardiac action potentials: Role of potassium channel kinetics in response to sympathetic stimulation. Circulation Research, 96, e25–e34.

212. Chiang, C.E. (2004). Congenital and acquired long QT syndrome. Current concepts and management. Cardiology in Review, 12, 222–234.

213. Schwartz, P.J., Priori, S.G., Spazzolini, C., Moss, A.J., Vincent, G.M., Napolitano, C., Denjoy, I., Guicheney, P., Breithardt, G., Keating, M.T., Towbin, J.A., Beggs, A.H., Brink, P., Wilde, A.A., Toivonen, L., Zareba, W., Robinson, J.L., Timothy, K.W., Corfield, V., Wattanasirichaigoon, D., Corbett, C., Haverkamp, W., Schulze-Bahr, E., Lehmann, M.H., Schwartz, K., Coumel, P., Bloise, R. (2001). Genotype-phenotype correlation in the long-QT syndrome: Gene-specific triggers for life-threatening arrhythmias. Circulation, 103, 89–95.

214. Curran, M.E., Splawski, I., Timothy, K.W., Vincent, G.M., Green, E.D., Keating, M.T. (1995). A molecular basis for cardiac arrhythmia: HERG mutations cause long QT syndrome. Cell, 80, 795–803.

215. Sanguinetti, M.C., Jiang, C., Curran, M.E., Keating, M.T. (1995). A mechanistic link between an inherited and an acquired cardiac arrhythmia: HERG encodes the I_{Kr} potassium channel. Cell, 81, 299–307.

216. Trudeau, M.C., Warmke, J.W., Ganetzky, B., Robertson, G.A. (1995). HERG, a human inward rectifier in the voltage-gated potassium channel family. Science, 269, 92–95.

217. Brugada, R., Hong, K., Dumaine, R., Cordeiro, J., Gaita, F., Borggrefe, M., Menendez, T. M., Brugada, J., Pollevick, G.D., Wolpert, C., Burashnikov, E., Matsuo, K., Wu, Y.S., Guerchicoff, A., Bianchi, F., Giustetto, C., Schimpf, R., Brugada, P., Antzelevitch, C.

(2004). Sudden death associated with short-QT syndrome linked to mutations in HERG. Circulation, 109, 30–35.

218. Zhou, Z., Gong, Q., Ye, B., Fan, Z., Makielski, J.C., Robertson, G.A., January, C.T. (1998). Properties of HERG channels stably expressed in HEK293 cells studied at physiological temperature. Biophysical Journal, 74, 230–241.

219. Pond, A.L., Scheve, B.K., Benedict, A.T., Petrecca, K., Van Wagoner, D.R., Shrier, A., Nerbonne, J.M. (2000). Expression of distinct ERG proteins in rat, mouse, and human heart. Relation to functional I_{Kr} channels. Journal of Biological Chemistry, 275, 5997–6006.

220. Jones, E.M., Roti Roti, E.C., Wang, J., Delfosse, S.A., Robertson, G.A. (2004). Cardiac I_{Kr} channels minimally comprise hERG 1a and 1b subunits. Journal of Biological Chemistry, 279, 44690–44694.

221. Sale, H., Wang, J., O'Hara, T.J., Tester, D.J., Phartiyal, P., He, J.Q., Rudy, Y., Ackerman, M.J., Robertson, G.A. (2008). Physiological properties of hERG 1a/1b heteromeric currents and a hERG 1b-specific mutation associated with long-QT syndrome. Circulation Research, 103, e81–e95.

222. Larsen, A.P., Olesen, S.P., Grunnet, M., Jespersen, T. (2008). Characterization of hERG1a and hERG1b potassium channels-a possible role for hERG1b in the I_{Kr} current. Pflugers Archiv—European Journal of Physiology, 456, 1137–1148.

223. Phartiyal, P., Jones, E.M., Robertson, G.A. (2007). Heteromeric assembly of human ether-a-go-go-related gene (hERG) 1a/1b channels occurs cotranslationally via N-terminal interactions. Journal of Biological Chemistry, 282, 9874–9882.

224. Phartiyal, P., Sale, H., Jones, E.M., Robertson, G.A. (2008). Endoplasmic reticulum retention and rescue by heteromeric assembly regulate human ERG 1a/1b surface channel composition. Journal of Biological Chemistry, 283, 3702–3207.

225. Luo, X., Xiao, J., Lin, H., Lu, Y., Yang, B., Wang, Z. (2008). Genomic structure, transcriptional control, and tissue distribution of HERG1 and KCNQ1 genes. American Journal of Physiology Heart Circulatory Physiology, 294, H1371–H1380.

226. Abbott, G.W., Sesti, F., Splawski, I., Buck, M.E., Lehmann, M.H., Timothy, K.W., Keating, M.T., Goldstein, S.A. (1999). MiRP1 forms I_{Kr} potassium channels with HERG and is associated with cardiac arrhythmia. Cell, 97, 175–187.

227. Yang, T., Kupershmidt, S., Roden, D.M. (1995). Anti-minK antisense decreases the amplitude of the rapidly activating cardiac delayed rectifier K^+ current. Circulation Research, 77, 1246–1253.

228. Gordon, E., Panaghie, G., Deng, L., Bee, K.J., Roepke, T.K., Krogh-Madsen, T., Christini, D.J., Ostrer, H., Basson, C.T., Chung, W., Abbott, G.W. (2008). A KCNE2 mutation in a patient with cardiac arrhythmia induced by auditory stimuli and serum electrolyte imbalance. Cardiovascular Research, 77, 98–106.

229. Um, S.Y., McDonald, T.V. (2007). Differential association between HERG and KCNE1 or KCNE2. PLoS one, 2, 1–10.

230. Brunner, M., Peng, X., Liu, G.X., Ren, X.Q., Ziv, O., Choi, B.R., Mathur, R., Hajjiri, M., Odening, K.E., Steinberg, E., Folco, E.J., Pringa, E., Centracchio, J., Macharzina, R.R., Donahay, T., Schofield, L., Rana, N., Kirk, M., Mitchell, G.F., Poppas, A., Zehender, M., Koren, G. (2008). Mechanisms of cardiac arrhythmias and sudden death in transgenic rabbits with long QT syndrome. Journal of Clinical Investigation, 118, 2246–2259.

231. Yang, Y., Xia, M., Jin, Q., Bendahhou, S., Shi, J., Chen, Y., Liang, B., Lin, J., Liu, Y., Liu, B., Zhou, Q., Zhang, D., Wang, R., Ma, N., Su, X., Niu, K., Pei, Y., Xu, W., Chen, Z., Wan, H., Cui, J., Barhanin, J. (2004). Identification of a KCNE2 gain-of-function mutation in patients with familial atrial fibrillation. American Journal of Human Genetics, 75, 899–905.

232. Roti, E.C., Myers, C.D., Ayers, R.A., Boatman, D.E., Delfosse, S.A., Chan, E.K., Ackerman, M.J., January, C.T., Robertson, G.A. (2002). Interaction with GM130 during HERG ion channel trafficking. Disruption by type 2 congenital long QT syndrome mutations. Human ether-a-go-go-related gene. J Biol Chem, 277, 47779–47785.

233. Ficker, E., Dennis, A.T., Wang, L., Brown, A.M. (2003). Role of the cytosolic chaperones Hsp70 and Hsp90 in maturation of the cardiac potassium channel HERG. Circulation Research, 92, e87–e100.

234. Furutani, M., Trudeau, M.C., Hagiwara, N., Seki, A., Gong, Q., Zhou, Z., Imamura, S., Nagashima, H., Kasanuki, H., Takao, A., Momma, K., January, C.T., Robertson, G.A., Matsuoka, R. (1999). Novel mechanism associated with an inherited cardiac arrhythmia: Defective protein trafficking by the mutant HERG (G601S) potassium channel. Circulation, 99, 2290–2294.

235. Walker, V.E., Atanasiu, R., Lam, H., Shrier, A. (2007). Co-chaperone FKBP38 promotes HERG trafficking. Journal of Biological Chemistry, 282, 23509–23516.

236. Lin, J., Lin, S., Yu, X., Choy, P.C., Shen, X., Deng, C., Kuang, S., Wu, J. (2008). The four and a half LIM domain protein 2 interacts with and regulates the HERG channel. FEBS Journal, 275, 4531–4539.

237. Eckhardt, L.L., Rajamani, S., January, C.T. (2005). Protein trafficking abnormalities: A new mechanism in drug-induced long QT syndrome. British Journal of Pharmacology, 145, 3–4.

238. Li, Y., Sroubek, J., Krishnan, Y., McDonald, T.V. (2008). A-kinase anchoring protein targeting of protein kinase a and regulation of HERG channels. Journal of Membrane Biology, 223, 107–116.

239. Odening, K.E., Kirk, M., Lorvidhaya, P., Brunner, M., Hyder, O., Centracchio, J., Schofield, L., Donahay, T., Chaves, L., Peng, X., Zehender, M., Koren, G. (2008). Transgenic LQT1 and LQT2 rabbits provide a new model for safety screening for I_{Kr} or I_{Ks} blocking propensity of drugs. Journal of Pharmacological Toxicological Methods, 58, 148–149.

240. Odening, K.E., Hyder, O., Chaves, L., Schofield, L., Brunner, M., Kirk, M., Zehender, M., Peng, X., Koren, G. (2008). Pharmacogenomics of anesthetic drugs in transgenic LQT1 and LQT2 rabbits reveal genotype-specific differential effects on cardiac repolarization. American Journal of Physiology Heart Circulatory Physiology, 295, H2264–H2272.

241. Nichols, C.G., Makhina, E.N., Pearson, W.L., Sha, Q., Lopatin, A.N. (1996). Inward rectification and implications for cardiac excitability. Circulation Research, 78, 1–7.

242. Nichols, C.G., Lopatin, A.N. (1997). Inward rectifier potassium channels. Annual Review of Physiology, 59, 171–191.

243. Doupnik, C.A., Davidson, N., Lester, H.A. (1995). The inward rectifier potassium channel family. Current Opinion in Neurobiology, 5, 268–277.

244. Liu, G.X., Derst, C., Schlichthorl, G., Heinen, S., Seebohm, G., Bruggemann, A., Kummer, W., Veh, R.W., Daut, J., Preisig-Muller, R. (2001). Comparison of cloned Kir2 channels with native inward rectifier K⁺ channels from guinea-pig cardiomyocytes. Journal of Physiology, 532, 115–126.

245. Takahashi, N., Morishige, K., Jahangir, A., Yamada, M., Findlay, I., Koyama, H., Kurachi, Y. (1994). Molecular cloning and functional expression of cDNA encoding a second class of inward rectifier potassium channels in the mouse brain. Journal of Biological Chemistry, 269, 23274–23279.

246. Jongsma, H.J., Wilders, R. (2001). Channelopathies: Kir2.1 mutations jeopardize many cell functions. Current Biology, 11, R747–R750.

247. Plaster, N.M., Tawil, R., Tristani-Firouzi, M., Canun, S., Bendahhou, S., Tsunoda, A., Donaldson, M.R., Iannaccone, S.T., Brunt, E., Barohn, R., Clark, J., Deymeer, F., George, A.L., Jr., Fish, F.A., Hahn, A., Nitu, A., Ozdemir, C., Serdaroglu, P., Subramony, S.H., Wolfe, G., Fu, Y.H., Ptacek, L.J. (2001). Mutations in Kir2.1 cause the developmental and episodic electrical phenotypes of Andersen's syndrome. Cell, 105, 511–519.

248. Tawil, R., Ptacek, L.J., Pavlakis, S.G., DeVivo, D.C., Penn, A.S., Ozdemir, C., Griggs, R. C. (1994). Andersen's syndrome: Potassium-sensitive periodic paralysis, ventricular ectopy, and dysmorphic features. Annals of Neurology, 35, 326–330.

249. Ai, T., Fujiwara, Y., Tsuji, K., Otani, H., Nakano, S., Kubo, Y., Horie, M. (2002). Novel KCNJ2 mutation in familial periodic paralysis with ventricular dysrhythmia. Circulation, 105, 2592–2594.

250. Lange, P.S., Er, F., Gassanov, N., Hoppe, U.C. (2003). Andersen mutations of KCNJ2 suppress the native inward rectifier current I_{K1} in a dominant-negative fashion. Cardiovascular Research, 59, 321–327.

251. Preisig-Muller, R., Schlichthorl, G., Goerge, T., Heinen, S., Bruggemann, A., Rajan, S., Derst, C., Veh, R.W., Daut, J. (2002). Heteromerization of Kir2.X potassium channels contributes to the phenotype of Andersen's syndrome. Proceedings of the National Academy of Sciences USA, 99, 7774–7779.

252. Sung, R.J., Wu, S.N., Wu, J.S., Chang, H.D., Luo, C.H. (2006). Electrophysiological mechanisms of ventricular arrhythmias in relation to Andersen-tawil syndrome under conditions of reduced I_{K1}: A simulation study. American Journal of Physiology Heart Circulatory Physiology, 291, H2597–H2605.

253. Seemann, G., Sachse, F.B., Weiss, D.L., Ptacek, L.J., Tristani-Firouzi, M. (2007). Modeling of I_{K1} mutations in human left ventricular myocytes and tissue. American Journal of Physiology Heart Circulatory Physiology, 292, H549–H559.

254. Andelfinger, G., Tapper, A.R., Welch, R.C., Vanoye, C.G., George, A.L., Jr., Benson, D. W. (2002). KCNJ2 mutation results in Andersen syndrome with sex-specific cardiac and skeletal muscle phenotypes. American Journal of Human Genetics, 71, 663–668.

255. Tristani-Firouzi, M., Jensen, J.L., Donaldson, M.R., Sansone, V., Meola, G., Hahn, A., Bendahhou, S., Kwiecinski, H., Fidzianska, A., Plaster, N., Fu, Y.H., Ptacek, L.J., Tawil, R. (2002). Functional and clinical characterization of KCNJ2 mutations associated with LQT7 (Andersen syndrome). Journal of Clinical Investigation, 110, 381–388.

256. Hilgemann, D.W., Feng, S., Nasuhoglu, C. (2001). The complex and intriguing lives of PIP2 with ion channels and transporters. Science Signaling: Signal Transduction Knowledge Environment, 2001, RE19.

257. Huang, C.L., Feng, S., Hilgemann, D.W. (1998). Direct activation of inward rectifier potassium channels by PIP2 and its stabilization by Gβγ. Nature, 391, 803–806.

258. Shyng, S.L., Cukras, C.A., Harwood, J., Nichols, C.G. (2000). Structural determinants of PIP_2 regulation of inward rectifier K_{ATP} channels. Journal of General Physiology, 116, 599–608.

259. Takano, M., Kuratomi, S. (2003). Regulation of cardiac inwardly rectifying potassium channels by membrane lipid metabolism. Progress in Biophysics and Molecular Biology, 81, 67–79.

260. Donaldson, M.R., Jensen, J.L., Tristani-Firouzi, M., Tawil, R., Bendahhou, S., Suarez, W. A., Cobo, A.M., Poza, J.J., Behr, E., Wagstaff, J., Szepetowski, P., Pereira, S., Mozaffar, T., Escolar, D.M., Fu, Y.H., Ptacek, L.J. (2003). PIP2 binding residues of Kir2.1 are common targets of mutations causing Andersen syndrome. Neurology, 60, 1811–1816.

261. Zaritsky, J.J., Eckman, D.M., Wellman, G.C., Nelson, M.T., Schwarz, T.L. (2000). Targeted disruption of Kir2.1 and Kir2.2 genes reveals the essential role of the inwardly rectifying K⁺ current in K⁺-mediated vasodilation. Circulation Research, 87, 160–166.

262. Zaritsky, J.J., Redell, J.B., Tempel, B.L., Schwarz, T.L. (2001). The consequences of disrupting cardiac inwardly rectifying K⁺ current I_{K1} as revealed by the targeted deletion of the murine Kir2.1 and Kir2.2 genes. Journal of Physiology, 533, 697–710.

263. McLerie, M., Lopatin, A.N. (2003). Dominant-negative suppression of I_{K1} in the mouse heart leads to altered cardiac excitability. Journal of Molecular and Cellular Cardiology, 35, 367–378.

264. Zobel, C., Cho, H.C., Nguyen, T.T., Pekhletski, R., Diaz, R.J., Wilson, G.J., Backx, P.H. (2003). Molecular dissection of the inward rectifier potassium current I_{K1} in rabbit cardiomyocytes: Evidence for heteromeric co-assembly of Kir2.1 and Kir2.2. Journal of Physiology, 550, 365–372.

265. Dhamoon, A.S., Pandit, S.V., Sarmast, F., Parisian, K.R., Guha, P., Li, Y., Bagwe, S., Taffet, S.M., Anumonwo, J.M.B. (2004). Unique Kir2.X properties determine regional and species differences in the cardiac inward rectifier K⁺ current. Circulation Research, 94, 1332–1339.

266. Panama, B.K., McLerie, M., Lopatin, A.N. (2007). Heterogeneity of I_{K1} in the mouse heart. American Journal of Physiology Heart Circulatory Physiology, 293, H3558–H3567.

267. Li, J., McLerie, M., Lopatin, A.N. (2004). Transgenic upregulation of I_{K1} in the mouse heart leads to multiple abnormalities of cardiac excitability. American Journal of Physiology Heart Circulatory Physiology, 287, H2790–H2802.

268. Piao, L., Li, J., McLerie, M., Lopatin, A.N. (2007). Transgenic upregulation of I_{K1} in the mouse heart is proarrhythmic. Basic Research in Cardiology, 102, 416–428.

269. Noujaim, S.F., Pandit, S.V., Berenfeld, O., Vikstrom, K., Cerrone, M., Mironov, S., Zugermayr, M., Lopatin, A.N., Jalife, J. (2007). Up-regulation of the inward rectifier K⁺ current (I_{K1}) in the mouse heart accelerates and stabilizes rotors. Journal of Physiology, 578, 315–326.

270. Priori, S.G., Pandit, S.V., Rivolta, I., Berenfeld, O., Ronchetti, E., Dhamoon, A., Napolitano, C., Anumonwo, J., di Barletta, M.R., Gudapakkam, S., Bosi, G., Stramba-Badiale, M., Jalife, J. (2005). A novel form of short QT syndrome (SQT3) is caused by a mutation in the KCNJ2 gene. Circulation Research, 96, 800–807.

271. Piao, L., Li, J., McLerie, M., Lopatin, A.N. (2007). Cardiac I_{K1} underlies early action potential shortening during hypoxia in the mouse heart. Journal of Molecular and Cellular Cardiology, 43, 27–38.

272. Xu, Y., Zhang, Q., Chiamvimonvat, N. (2007). I_{K1} and cardiac hypoxia: After the long and short QT syndromes, what else can go wrong with the inward rectifier K⁺ currents? Journal of Molecular and Cellular Cardiology, 43, 15–17.

273. Isomoto, S., Kurachi, Y. (1997). Function, regulation, pharmacology, and molecular structure of ATP-sensitive K^+ channels in the cardiovascular system. Journal of Cardiovascular Electrophysiology, 8, 1431–1446.

274. Noma, A. (1983). ATP-regulated K^+ channels in cardiac muscle. Nature, 305, 147–148.

275. Babenko, A.P., Aguilar-Bryan, L., Bryan, J. (1998). A view of sur/KIR6.X, K_{ATP} channels. Annual Review of Physiology, 60, 667–687.

276. Seino, S., Miki, T. (2004). Gene targeting approach to clarification of ion channel function: Studies of Kir6.x null mice. Journal of Physiology, 554, 295–300.

277. Clement, J.P.t., Kunjilwar, K., Gonzalez, G., Schwanstecher, M., Panten, U., Aguilar-Bryan, L., Bryan, J. (1997). Association and stoichiometry of K_{ATP} channel subunits. Neuron, 18, 827–838.

278. Shyng, S., Nichols, C.G. (1997). Octameric stoichiometry of the K_{ATP} channel complex. Journal of General Physiology, 110, 655–664.

279. Zerangue, N., Schwappach, B., Jan, Y.N., Jan, L.Y. (1999). A new er trafficking signal regulates the subunit stoichiometry of plasma membrane K_{ATP} channels. Neuron, 22, 537–548.

280. Tucker, S.J., Gribble, F.M., Zhao, C., Trapp, S., Ashcroft, F.M. (1997). Truncation of Kir6.2 produces ATP-sensitive K^+ channels in the absence of the sulphonylurea receptor. Nature, 387, 179–183.

281. Nichols, C.G., Shyng, S.L., Nestorowicz, A., Glaser, B., Clement, J.P.t., Gonzalez, G., Aguilar-Bryan, L., Permutt, M.A., Bryan, J. (1996). Adenosine diphosphate as an intracellular regulator of insulin secretion. Science, 272, 1785–1787.

282. Shyng, S.L., Ferrigni, T., Shepard, J.B., Nestorowicz, A., Glaser, B., Permutt, M.A., Nichols, C.G. (1998). Functional analyses of novel mutations in the sulfonylurea receptor 1 associated with persistent hyperinsulinemic hypoglycemia of infancy. Diabetes, 47, 1145–1151.

283. Olson, T.M., Alekseev, A.E., Moreau, C., Liu, X.K., Zingman, L.V., Miki, T., Seino, S., Asirvatham, S.J., Jahangir, A., Terzic, A. (2007). K_{ATP} channel mutation confers risk for vein of marshall adrenergic atrial fibrillation. Nature Clinical Practice Cardiovascular Medicine, 4, 110–116.

284. Pountney, D.J., Sun, Z.Q., Porter, L.M., Nitabach, M.N., Nakamura, T.Y., Holmes, D., Rosner, E., Kaneko, M., Manaris, T., Holmes, T.C., Coetzee, W.A. (2001). Is the molecular composition of K_{ATP} channels more complex than originally thought? Journal of Molecular and Cellular Cardiology, 33, 1541–1546.

285. Yokoshiki, H., Sunagawa, M., Seki, T., Sperelakis, N. (1999). Antisense oligodeoxynucleotides of sulfonylurea receptors inhibit ATP-sensitive K^+ channels in cultured neonatal rat ventricular cells. Pflügers Archives European Journal of Physiology, 437, 400–408.

286. Li, R.A., Leppo, M., Miki, T., Seino, S., Marban, E. (2000). Molecular basis of electrocardiographic ST-segment elevation. Circulation Research, 87, 837–839.

287. Suzuki, M., Li, R.A., Miki, T., Uemura, H., Sakamoto, N., Ohmoto-Sekine, Y., Tamagawa, M., Ogura, T., Seino, S., Marban, E., Nakaya, H. (2001). Functional roles of cardiac and vascular ATP-sensitive potassium channels clarified by Kir6.2-knockout mice. Circulation Research, 88, 570–577.

288. Pu, J., Wada, T., Valdivia, C., Chutkow, W., Burant, C., Makielski, J. (2001). Evidence of K_{ATP} channels in native cardiac cells without SUR. Biophysical Journal (Annual Meeting Abstracts), 80, 625e–626.

289. Seghers, V., Nakazaki, M., DeMayo, F., Aguilar-Bryan, L., Bryan, J. (2000). SUR1 knockout mice. A model for K_{ATP} channel-independent regulation of insulin secretion. Journal of Biological Chemistry, 275, 9270–9277.

290. Flagg, T.P., Kurata, H.T., Masia, R., Caputa, G., Magnuson, M.A., Lefer, D.J., Coetzee, W. A., Nichols, C.G. (2008). Differential structure of atrial and ventricular K_{ATP} atrial K_{ATP} channels require SUR1. Circulation Research, 103, 1458–1465.

291. Singh, H., Hudman, D., Lawrence, C.L., Rainbow, R.D., Lodwick, D., Norman, R.I. (2003). Distribution of Kir6.0 and SUR2 ATP-sensitive potassium channel subunits in isolated ventricular myocytes. Journal of Molecular and Cellular Cardiology, 35, 445–459.

292. Suzuki, M., Sasaki, N., Miki, T., Sakamoto, N., Ohmoto-Sekine, Y., Tamagawa, M., Seino, S., Marban, E., Nakaya, H. (2002). Role of sarcolemmal K_{ATP} channels in cardioprotection against ischemia/reperfusion injury in mice. Journal of Clinical Investigation, 109, 509–516.

293. Koster, J.C., Knopp, A., Flagg, T.P., Markova, K.P., Sha, Q., Enkvetchakul, D., Betsuyaku, T., Yamada, K.A., Nichols, C.G. (2001). Tolerance for ATP-insensitive K_{ATP} channels in transgenic mice. Circulation Research, 89, 1022–1029.

294. Hodgkin, A.L., Huxley, A.F. (1952). A quantitative description of membrane current and its application to conduction and excitation in nerve. Journal of Physiology, 117, 500–544.

295. Yue, D.T., Marban, E. (1988). A novel cardiac potassium channel that is active and conductive at depolarized potentials. Pflügers Archives European Journal of Physiology, 413, 127–133.

296. Backx, P.H., Marban, E. (1993). Background potassium current active during the plateau of the action potential in guinea pig ventricular myocytes. Circulation Research, 72, 890–900.

297. Kim, D., Clapham, D.E. (1989). Potassium channels in cardiac cells activated by arachidonic acid and phospholipids. Science, 244, 1174–1176.

298. Kim, D. (1992). A mechanosensitive K⁺ channel in heart cells. Activation by arachidonic acid. Journal of General Physiology, 100, 1021–1040.

299. Kim, D., Duff, R.A. (1990). Regulation of K⁺ channels in cardiac myocytes by free fatty acids. Circulation Research, 67, 1040–1046.

300. Noma, A., Nakayama, T., Kurachi, Y., Irisawa, H. (1984). Resting K⁺ conductances in pacemaker and non-pacemaker heart cells of the rabbit. Japanese Journal of Physiology, 34, 245–254.

301. Goldstein, S.A., Bockenhauer, D., O'Kelly, I., Zilberberg, N. (2001). Potassium leak channels and the KCNK family of two-p-domain subunits. Nature Reviews Neuroscience, 2, 175–184.

302. Kim, D. (2005). Physiology and pharmacology of two-pore domain potassium channels. Current Pharmaceutical Design, 11, 2717–2736.

303. Gurney, A., Manoury, B. (2008). Two-pore potassium channels in the cardiovascular system. Europian Biophysics Journal, 38, 305–318.

304. Lesage, F., Lauritzen, I., Duprat, F., Reyes, R., Fink, M., Heurteaux, C., Lazdunski, M. (1997). The structure, function and distribution of the mouse TWIK-1 K⁺ channel. FEBS Letters, 402, 28–32.

305. Maingret, F., Lauritzen, I., Patel, A.J., Heurteaux, C., Reyes, R., Lesage, F., Lazdunski, M., Honore, E. (2000). TREK-1 is a heat-activated background K⁺ channel. EMBO Journal, 19, 2483–2491.

306. Kang, D., Han, J., Talley, E.M., Bayliss, D.A., Kim, D. (2004). Functional expression of TASK-1/TASK-3 heteromers in cerebellar granule cells. Journal of Physiology, 554, 64–77.

307. Larkman, P.M., Perkins, E.M. (2005). A TASK-like pH- and amine-sensitive 'leak' K^+ conductance regulates neonatal rat facial motoneuron excitability *in vitro*. European Journal of Neuroscience, 21, 679–691.

308. Czirjak, G., Enyedi, P. (2002). Formation of functional heterodimers between the TASK-1 and TASK-3 two-pore domain potassium channel subunits. Journal of Biological Chemistry, 277, 5426–5432.

309. Kim, D., Fujita, A., Horio, Y., Kurachi, Y. (1998). Cloning and functional expression of a novel cardiac two-pore background K^+ channel (cTBAK-1). Circulation Research, 82, 513–518.

310. Putzke, C., Wemhoner, K., Sachse, F.B., Rinne, S., Schlichthorl, G., Li, X.T., Jae, L., Eckhardt, I., Wischmeyer, E., Wulf, H., Preisig-Muller, R., Daut, J., Decher, N. (2007). The acid-sensitive potassium channel TASK-1 in rat cardiac muscle. Cardiovascular Research, 75, 59–68.

311. Medhurst, A.D., Rennie, G., Chapman, C.G., Meadows, H., Duckworth, M.D., Kelsell, R.E., Gloger, I.I., Pangalos, M.N. (2001). Distribution analysis of human two pore domain potassium channels in tissues of the central nervous system and periphery. Molecular. Brain Research, 86, 101–114.

312. Liu, W., Saint, D.A. (2004). Heterogeneous expression of tandem-pore K^+ channel genes in adult and embryonic rat heart quantified by real-time polymerase chain reaction. Clinical and Experimental Pharmacology and Physiology, 31, 174–178.

313. Lopes, C.M., Gallagher, P.G., Buck, M.E., Butler, M.H., Goldstein, S.A. (2000). Proton block and voltage gating are potassium-dependent in the cardiac leak channel kcnk3. Journal of Biological Chemistry, 275, 16969–16978.

314. Jones, S.A., Morton, M.J., Hunter, M., Boyett, M.R. (2002). Expression of TASK-1, a pH-sensitive twin-pore domain K^+ channel, in rat myocytes. American Journal of Physiology Heart Circulatory Physiology, 283, H181–H185.

315. Aimond, F., Rauzier, J.M., Bony, C., Vassort, G. (2000). Simultaneous activation of p38 MAPK and p42/44 MAPK by ATP stimulates the K^+ current I_{TREK} in cardiomyocytes. Journal of Biological Chemistry, 275, 39110–39116.

316. Tan, J.H., Liu, W., Saint, D.A. (2004). Differential expression of the mechanosensitive potassium channel TREK-1 in epicardial and endocardial myocytes in rat ventricle. Experimental Physiology, 89, 237–242.

317. Terrenoire, C., Lauritzen, I., Lesage, F., Romey, G., Lazdunski, M. (2001). A TREK-1-like potassium channel in atrial cells inhibited by β-adrenergic stimulation and activated by volatile anesthetics. Circulation Research, 89, 336–342.

318. Duprat, F., Lesage, F., Fink, M., Reyes, R., Heurteaux, C., Lazdunski, M. (1997). TASK, a human background K^+ channel to sense external pH variations near physiological pH. EMBO Journal, 16, 5464–5471.

319. Leonoudakis, D., Gray, A.T., Winegar, B.D., Kindler, C.H., Harada, M., Taylor, D.M., Chavez, R.A., Forsayeth, J.R., Yost, C.S. (1998). An open rectifier potassium channel with two pore domains in tandem cloned from rat cerebellum. Journal of Neuroscience, 18, 868–877.

320. Maingret, F., Patel, A.J., Lazdunski, M., Honore, E. (2001). The endocannabinoid anandamide is a direct and selective blocker of the background K$^+$ channel TASK-1. EMBO Journal, 20, 47–54.

321. Patel, A.J., Honore, E., Lesage, F., Fink, M., Romey, G., Lazdunski, M. (1999). Inhalational anesthetics activate two-pore-domain background K$^+$ channels. Nature Neuroscience, 2, 422–426.

322. Kim, Y., Bang, H., Kim, D. (1999). TBAK-1 and TASK-1, two-pore K$^+$ channel subunits: Kinetic properties and expression in rat heart. American Journal of Physiology Heart Circulatory Physiology, 277, H1669–H1678.

323. Maingret, F., Patel, A.J., Lesage, F., Lazdunski, M., Honore, E. (1999). Mechano- or acid stimulation, two interactive modes of activation of the TREK-1 potassium channel. Journal of Biological Chemistry, 274, 26691–26696.

324. Fink, M., Lesage, F., Duprat, F., Heurteaux, C., Reyes, R., Fosset, M., Lazdunski, M. (1998). A neuronal two P domain K$^+$ channel stimulated by arachidonic acid and polyunsaturated fatty acids. EMBO Journal, 17, 3297–3308.

325. Duprat, F., Lesage, F., Patel, A.J., Fink, M., Romey, G., Lazdunski, M. (2000). The neuroprotective agent riluzole activates the two p domain K$^+$ channels TREK-1 and TRAAK. Molecular Pharmacology, 57, 906–912.

326. Tan, J.H., Liu, W., Saint, D.A. (2002). Trek-like potassium channels in rat cardiac ventricular myocytes are activated by intracellular ATP. Journal of Membrane Biology, 185, 201–207.

327. Li, X.T., Dyachenko, V., Zuzarte, M., Putzke, C., Preisig-Muller, R., Isenberg, G., Daut, J. (2006). The stretch-activated potassium channel TREK-1 in rat cardiac ventricular muscle. Cardiovascular Research, 69, 86–97.

328. Terzic, A., Kurachi, Y. (1996). Actin microfilament disrupters enhance K$_{ATP}$ channel opening in patches from guinea-pig cardiomyocytes. Journal of Physiology, 492, 395–404.

329. Brady, P.A., Alekseev, A.E., Aleksandrova, L.A., Gomez, L.A., Terzic, A. (1996). A disrupter of actin microfilaments impairs sulfonylurea-inhibitory gating of cardiac K$_{ATP}$ channels. American Journal of Physiology Heart Circulatory Physiology, 271, H2710–H2716.

330. Furukawa, T., Yamane, T., Terai, T., Katayama, Y., Hiraoka, M. (1996). Functional linkage of the cardiac ATP-sensitive K$^+$ channel to the actin cytoskeleton. Pflügers Archives European Journal of Physiology, 431, 504–512.

331. Mazzanti, M., Assandri, R., Ferroni, A., DiFrancesco, D. (1996). Cytoskeletal control of rectification and expression of four substates in cardiac inward rectifier K$^+$ channels. FASEB Journal, 10, 357–361.

332. Yang, X., Salas, P.J.I., Pham, T.V., Wasserlauf, B.J., Smets, M.J.D., Myerburg, R.J., Gelband, H., Hoffman, B.F., Bassett, A.L. (2002). Cytoskeletal actin microfilaments and the transient outward potassium current in hypertrophied rat ventriculocytes. Journal of Physiology, 541, 411–421.

333. Wang, Z., Eldstrom, J.R., Jantzi, J., Moore, E.D., Fedida, D. (2004). Increased focal Kv4.2 channel expression at the plasma membrane is the result of actin depolymerization. American Journal of Physiology Heart Circulatory Physiology, 286, H749–H759.

334. Choi, B.H., Park, J.-A., Kim, K.-R., Lee, G.-I., Lee, Y.-T., Choe, H., Ko, S.-H., Kim, M.-H., Seo, Y.-H., Kwak, Y.-G. (2005). Direct block of cloned hKv1.5 channel by

cytochalasins, actin-disrupting agents. American Journal of Physiology Cell Physiology, 289, C425–C436.

335. Petrecca, K., Miller, D.M., Shrier, A. (2000). Localization and enhanced current density of the Kv4.2 potassium channel by interaction with the actin-binding protein filamin. Journal of Neuroscience, 20, 8736–8744.

336. Maruoka, N.D., Steele, D.F., Au, B.P.-Y., Dan, P., Zhang, X., Moore, E.D.W., Fedida, D. (2000). Alpha-actinin-2 couples to cardiac Kv1.5 channels, regulating current density and channel localization in HEK cells. FEBS Letters, 473, 188–194.

337. Cukovic, D., Lu, G.W., Wible, B., Steele, D.F., Fedida, D. (2001). A discrete amino terminal domain of Kv1.5 and Kv1.4 potassium channels interacts with the spectrin repeats of α-actinin-2. FEBS Letters, 498, 87–92.

338. Mason, H.S., Latten, M.J., Godoy, L.D., Horowitz, B., Kenyon, J.L. (2002). Modulation of Kv1.5 currents by protein kinase a, tyrosine kinase, and protein tyrosine phosphatase requires an intact cytoskeleton. Molecular Pharmacology, 61, 285–293.

339. Levin, G., Chikvashvili, D., Singer-Lahat, D., Peretz, T., Thornhill, W.B., Lotan, I. (1996). Phosphorylation of a K^+ channel α subunit modulates the inactivation conferred by a β subunit. Involvement of cytoskeleton. Journal of Biological Chemistry, 271, 29321–29328.

340. Nakahira, K., Matos, M.F., Trimmer, J.S. (1998). Differential interaction of voltage-gated K^+ channel β-subunits with cytoskeleton is mediated by unique amino terminal domains. Journal of Molecular Neuroscience, 11, 199–208.

341. Elias, G.M., Nicoll, R.A. (2007). Synaptic trafficking of glutamate receptors by MAGUK scaffolding proteins. Trends in Cell Biology, 17, 343–352.

342. Kim, E., Niethammer, M., Rothschild, A., Nung Jan, Y., Sheng, M. (1995). Clustering of *shaker*-type K^+ channels by interaction with a family of membrane-associated guanylate kinases. Nature, 378, 85–88.

343. Kim, E., Sheng, M. (1996). Differential K^+ channel clustering activity of PSD-95 and SAP97, two related membrane-associated putative guanylate kinases. Neuropharmacology, 35, 993–1000.

344. Tiffany, A.M., Manganas, L.N., Kim, E., Hsueh, Y.P., Sheng, M., Trimmer, J.S. (2000). PSD-95 and SAP97 exhibit distinct mechanisms for regulating K^+ channel surface expression and clustering. Journal of Cell Biology, 148, 147–158.

345. Wong, W., Schlichter, L.C. (2004). Differential recruitment of Kv1.4 and Kv4.2 to lipid rafts by PSD-95. Journal of Biological Chemistry, 279, 444–452.

346. Martens, J.R., O'Connell, K., Tamkun, M. (2004). Targeting of ion channels to membrane microdomains: Localization of Kv channels to lipid rafts. Trends in Pharmacological Sciences, 25, 16–21.

347. Maguy, A., Hebert, T.E., Nattel, S. (2006). Involvement of lipid rafts and caveolae in cardiac ion channel function. Cardiovascular Research, 69, 798–807.

348. Martens, J.R., Sakamoto, N., Sullivan, S.A., Grobaski, T.D., Tamkun, M.M. (2001). Isoform-specific localization of voltage-gated K^+ channels to distinct lipid raft populations. Targeting of Kv1.5 to caveolae. Journal of Biological Chemistry, 276, 8409–8414.

349. McEwen, D.P., Li, Q., Jackson, S., Jenkins, P.M., Martens, J.R. (2008). Caveolin regulates Kv1.5 trafficking to cholesterol-rich membrane microdomains. Molecular Pharmacology, 73, 678–685.

350. Folco, E.J., Liu, G.-X., Koren, G. (2004). Caveolin-3 and SAP97 form a scaffolding protein complex that regulates the voltage-gated potassium channel Kv1.5. American Journal of Physiology Heart Circulatory Physiology, 287, H681–H690.

351. Eldstrom, J., Van Wagoner, D.R., Moore, E.D., Fedida, D. (2006). Localization of Kv1.5 channels in rat and canine myocyte sarcolemma. FEBS Letters, 580, 6039–6046.

352. Burke, N.A., Takimoto, K., Li, D., Han, W., Watkins, S.C., Levitan, E.S. (1999). Distinct structural requirements for clustering and immobilization of K$^+$ channels by PSD-95. Journal of General Physiology, 113, 71–80.

353. Jugloff, D.G., Khanna, R., Schlichter, L.C., Jones, O.T. (2000). Internalization of the Kv1.4 potassium channel is suppressed by clustering interactions with PSD-95. Journal of Biological Chemistry, 275, 1357–1364.

354. Eldstrom, J., Doerksen, K.W., Steele, D.F., Fedida, D. (2002). N-terminal PDZ-binding domain in Kv1 potassium channels. FEBS Letters, 531, 529–537.

355. Wong, W., Newell, E.W., Jugloff, D.G., Jones, O.T., Schlichter, L.C. (2002). Cell surface targeting and clustering interactions between heterologously expressed PSD-95 and the *shal* voltage-gated potassium channel, Kv4.2. Journal of Biological Chemistry, 277, 20423–20430.

356. Godreau, D., Vranckx, R., Maguy, A., Rucker-Martin, C., Goyenvalle, C., Abdelshafy, S., Tessier, S., Couetil, J.P., Hatem, S.N. (2002). Expression, regulation and role of the MAGUK protein SAP-97 in human atrial myocardium. Cardiovascular Research, 56, 433–442.

357. Seeber, S., Becker, K., Rau, T., Eschenhagen, T., Becker, C.M., Herkert, M. (2000). Transient expression of NMDA receptor subunit NR2B in the developing rat heart. Journal of Neurochemistry, 75, 2472–2477.

358. Kistner, U., Wenzel, B.M., Veh, R.W., Cases-Langhoff, C., Garner, A.M., Appeltauer, U., Voss, B., Gundelfinger, E.D., Garner, C.C. (1993). SAP90, a rat presynaptic protein related to the product of the drosophila tumor suppressor gene dlg-A. Journal of Biological Chemistry, 268, 4580–4583.

359. Murata, M., Buckett, P.D., Zhou, J., Brunner, M., Folco, E., Koren, G. (2001). SAP97 interacts with Kv1.5 in heterologous expression systems. American Journal of Physiology Heart Circulatory Physiology, 281, H2575–H2584.

360. Eldstrom, J., Choi, W.S., Steele, D.F., Fedida, D. (2003). SAP97 increases Kv1.5 currents through an indirect N-terminal mechanism. FEBS Letters, 547, 205–211.

361. Mathur, R., Choi, W.-S., Eldstrom, J., Wang, Z., Kim, J., Steele, D.F., Fedida, D. (2006). A specific N-terminal residue in Kv1.5 is required for upregulation of the channel by SAP97. Biochemical and Biophysical Research Communications, 342, 1–8.

362. Leonoudakis, D., Conti, L.R., Anderson, S., Radeke, C.M., McGuire, L.M., Adams, M.E., Froehner, S.C., Yates, J.R., 3rd, Vandenberg, C.A. (2004). Protein trafficking and anchoring complexes revealed by proteomic analysis of inward rectifier potassium channel (Kir2.X)-associated proteins. Journal of Biological Chemistry, 279, 22331–22346.

363. Leonoudakis, D., Conti, L.R., Radeke, C.M., McGuire, L.M., Vandenberg, C.A. (2004). A multiprotein trafficking complex composed of SAP97, CASK, Veli, and Mint1 is associated with inward rectifier Kir2 potassium channels. Journal of Biological Chemistry, 279, 19051–19063.

364. Karcher, R.L., Deacon, S.W., Gelfand, V.I. (2002). Motor-cargo interactions: The key to transport specificity. Trends in Cell Biology, 12, 21–27.

365. Chu, P.J., Rivera, J.F., Arnold, D.B. (2006). A role for kif17 in transport of Kv4.2. Journal of Biological Chemistry, 281, 365–373.

366. Rivera, J., Chu, P.J., Lewis, T.L., Jr., Arnold, D.B. (2007). The role of kif5b in axonal localization of Kv1 K^+ channels. Eurorean Journal of Neuroscience, 25, 136–146.

367. Wu, H., Nash, J.E., Zamorano, P., Garner, C.C. (2002). Interaction of SAP97 with minus-end-directed actin motor myosin VI. Implications for ampa receptor trafficking. Journal of Biological Chemistry, 277, 30928–30934.

368. Choi, W.S., Khurana, A., Mathur, R., Viswanathan, V., Steele, D.F., Fedida, D. (2005). Kv1.5 surface expression is modulated by retrograde trafficking of newly endocytosed channels by the dynein motor. Circulation Research, 97, 363–371.

369. McEwen, D.P., Schumacher, S.M., Li, Q., Benson, M.D., Iniguez-Lluhi, J.A., Van Genderen, K.M., Martens, J.R. (2007). Rab-GTPase-dependent endocytic recycling of Kv1.5 in atrial myocytes. Journal of Biological Chemistry, 282, 29612–29620.

370. Jordens, I., Marsman, M., Kuijl, C., Neefjes, J. (2005). Rab proteins, connecting transport and vesicle fusion. Traffic, 6, 1070–1077.

371. Zadeh, A.D., Xu, H., Loewen, M.E., Noble, G.P., Steele, D.F., Fedida, D. (2008). Internalized Kv1.5 traffics via Rab-dependent pathways. Journal of Physiology, 586, 4793–7813.

372. Arcangeli, A., Becchetti, A. (2006). Complex functional interaction between integrin receptors and ion channels. Trends in Cell Biology, 16, 631–639.

373. Hershman, K.M., Levitan, E.S. (1998). Cell-cell contact between adult rat cardiac myocytes regulates Kv1.5 and Kv4.2 K^+ channel mRNA expression. American Journal of Physiology Cell Physiology, 275, C1473–C1480.

374. Koutsouki, E., Lam, R.S., Seebohm, G., Ureche, O.N., Ureche, L., Baltaev, R., Lang, F. (2007). Modulation of human Kv1.5 channel kinetics by N-cadherin. Biochemical and Biophysical Research Communications, 363, 18–23.

375. Abi-Char, J., El-Haou, S., Balse, E., Neyroud, N., Vranckx, R., Coulombe, A., Hatem, S.N. (2008). The anchoring protein SAP97 retains Kv1.5 channels in the plasma membrane of cardiac myocytes. American Journal of Physiology Heart Circulatory Physiology, 294, H1851–H1861.

376. Reuver, S.M., Garner, C.C. (1998). E-cadherin mediated cell adhesion recruits SAP97 into the cortical cytoskeleton. Journal of Cell Science, 111, 1071–1080.

377. McPhee, J.C., Dang, Y.L., Davidson, N., Lester, H.A. (1998). Evidence for a functional interaction between integrins and G protein-activated inward rectifier K^+ channels. Journal of Biological Chemistry, 273, 34696–34702.

378. Vasilyev, D.V., Barish, M.E. (2003). Regulation of an inactivating potassium current (I_A) by the extracellular matrix protein vitronectin in embryonic mouse hippocampal neurones. Journal of Physiology, 547, 859–871.

379. Arcangeli, A., Becchetti, A., Mannini, A., Mugnai, G., De Filippi, P., Tarone, G., Del Bene, M.R., Barletta, E., Wanke, E., Olivotto, M. (1993). Integrin-mediated neurite outgrowth in neuroblastoma cells depends on the activation of potassium channels. Journal of Cellular Biology, 122, 1131–1143.

380. Hofmann, G., Bernabei, P.A., Crociani, O., Cherubini, A., Guasti, L., Pillozzi, S., Lastraioli, E., Polvani, S., Bartolozzi, B., Solazzo, V., Gragnani, L., Defilippi, P., Rosati, B., Wanke, E.,

Olivotto, M., Arcangeli, A. (2001). HERG K^+ channels activation during β_1 integrin-mediated adhesion to fibronectin induces an up-regulation of $\alpha_v\beta_3$integrin in the pre-osteoclastic leukemia cell line FLG 29.1. Journal of Biological Chemistry, 276, 4923–4931.

381. Cherubini, A., Hofmann, G., Pillozzi, S., Guasti, L., Crociani, O., Cilia, E., Di Stefano, P., Degani, S., Balzi, M., Olivotto, M., Wanke, E., Becchetti, A., Defilippi, P., Wymore, R., Arcangeli, A. (2005). Human ether-a-go-go-related gene 1 channels are physically linked to β1 integrins and modulate adhesion-dependent signaling. Molecular Biology of the Cell, 16, 2972–2983.

382. Pillozzi, S., Brizzi, M.F., Bernabei, P.A., Bartolozzi, B., Caporale, R., Basile, V., Boddi, V., Pegoraro, L., Becchetti, A., Arcangeli, A. (2007). Vegfr-1 (flt-1), β_1 integrin, and hERG K^+ channel for a macromolecular signaling complex in acute myeloid leukemia: Role in cell migration and clinical outcome. Blood, 110, 1238–1250.

CHAPTER 3

The "Funny" Pacemaker Current

ANDREA BARBUTI, ANNALISA BUCCHI, MIRKO BARUSCOTTI, and
DARIO DIFRANCESCO

3.1 INTRODUCTION: THE MECHANISM OF CARDIAC PACEMAKING

The ordered sequence of repetitive contractions and relaxations of the healthy heart is determined in the first place by the oscillatory electrical properties of the sinoatrial node (SAN), which acts both as a biological cardiac metronome and as a driving stimulus for the whole heart (pacemaker). The understanding of the cellular and molecular mechanisms responsible for the intrinsic automaticity of SAN tissue is clearly fundamental to cardiac physiology. Decades of intense investigation have been devoted to collect evidence elucidating the key points of this process. Electrophysiological studies have shown that the most specific aspect of the action potential of pacemaker cells of the SAN is the lack of a stable resting level during diastole.

In SAN myocytes, the interval between consecutive action potentials (APs) is characterized by a slow transition from the maximum diastolic potential (MDP, around $-60\,mV$) to the threshold (around $-40\,mV$) for the initiation of a new AP. This fraction of the AP is commonly known as pacemaker phase (or slow diastolic depolarization or phase 4). The diastolic depolarization (DD) represents the "heart rate controller," because changes of cardiac rate, caused, for example, by the modulatory actions exerted by the autonomic nervous system, are determined largely by changes of its duration. Several ionic currents, pumps, and exchange mechanisms are at work in pacemaker cells to build up the set of conditions suitable for automatic activity to ensue. Among them, one special mechanism, the activation at the end of repolarization of the "funny" (I_f), current has the specific role of initiating the slow DD and of controlling its rate of development, by means of which cardiac rate is in turn controlled. The properties of the funny current, termed "pacemaker" current, to highlight its role are described below.

Novel Therapeutic Targets for Antiarrhythmic Drugs, Edited by George Edward Billman
Copyright © 2010 John Wiley & Sons, Inc.

3.2 THE "FUNNY" CURRENT

3.2.1 Historical Background

Early electrophysiological experiments investigating pacemaking were carried out in Purkinje fibers, and they indicated a decline in membrane conductance during the DD [1, 2]. This, and the observation that the current flowing during the pacemaker phase appeared to reverse near the K^+ equilibrium potential [3], suggested that pacemaking could result from the decay of a K^+ conductance during diastole. The "K^+-conductance decay" hypothesis was strengthened by two reports describing the presence in Purkinje fibers of an outward current deactivating during hyperpolarization to the diastolic range of potentials, with a reversal similar to that of a pure K^+ component, and termed I_{K2} [4, 5]. The relevance to pacemaking was also supported by evidence that I_{K2} was modified by catecholamines in a way compatible with rate acceleration [6].

The "K^+-conductance decay" hypothesis in Purkinje fibers held for over 10 years, and I_{K2} was considered the best described K^+ current in the heart, although some unexplained features of its behavior called for a more complex scenario; for example, the current disappeared in low external Na^+ solutions [7], and its reversal potential was clearly far too negative for a pure K^+ current [8].

This universally accepted hypothesis was seriously challenged only with the description in 1979 of the funny current in SAN cells [9]. I_f, which is an inward current activated on hyperpolarization to pacemaker voltages, had properties suitable for generation of the DD phase in the true pacemaker region of the heart as well as for the control of spontaneous rate by sympathetic stimulation, given its sensitivity to catecholamines [9, 10]. The description of I_f in the SAN represented a provocative new proposal in the theory of pacemaking, because it is explained as the result of activation of an inward, rather than deactivation of an outward, current, and at the same time, it represented a disturbing, clashing contrast with pacemaking in Purkinje fibers. Was it really possible that pacemaking in two distinct, but connected regions of the heart was so dramatically different, based on two perfectly symmetrical mechanisms? It seemed paradoxical, and the puzzle was solved only with a careful reinvestigation of the I_{K2} current in Purkinje fibers. DiFrancesco, Ohba, and Ojeda [11] realized that the reversal potential of I_{K2} could be strongly affected by depletion of K^+ ions in the extracellular spaces (clefts); DiFrancesco and Ojeda [12] noted that I_{K2} and I_f had similar features, despite their apparently different ionic nature. Starting from these observations, DiFrancesco [13, 14] solved the puzzle by reinterpreting the ionic nature of I_{K2} and showed that I_{K2} had been incorrectly assumed to be a K^+ current based on a fake reversal potential; in fact it was the same as I_f in the SAN (Figure 3.1).

The discovery of I_f in the SAN and the identification with I_{K2} in Purkinje fibers set the stage, in the early 1980s, for a comprehensive and conceptually new interpretation of cardiac pacemaking. According to this interpretation, a specific ionic mechanism, the activation during diastole of I_f, a slowly developing inward current, was in charge of generating the DD and of determining its slope, and hence, cardiac rate.

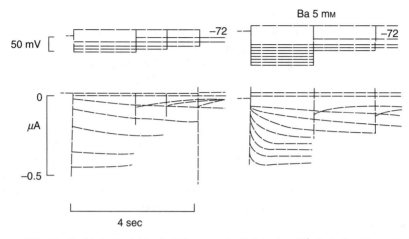

Figure 3.1. The Purkinje fiber's I_{K2} (left) becomes I_f (right) when K^+ depletion (due to I_{K1}) is blocked by barium. The fake reversal at about -127 mV on the left disappears when depletion is removed, and no reversal is observed any more, revealing the true inward nature of the pacemaker current in Purkinje fibers on the right. From ref. 14 with permission.

3.2.2 Biophysical Properties of the I_f Current

After the discovery of the I_f current, extensive biophysical investigation was carried out to describe the details of its ionic, kinetic, and modulatory properties [15, 16]. These studies were essential for the newly found current to more accurately characterize and to verify the causal relationship between current properties and ability to generate and control pacemaker activity.

3.2.2.1 Voltage Dependence of Activation. Published data reporting the voltage range of activation of I_f in the SAN reveal a high variability, with threshold values in the range $-32/-70$ mV and half-activation voltages in the range $-50/-120$ mV (Table 1 in Baruscotti et al. [17]). Such variability is even greater when considering the I_f current expressed in other cardiac regions [17]. Although some variability is expected to derive from different experimental conditions, it is now clear that the large scattering of data reflects a specific property of f-channels, whose voltage dependence of activation shifts widely under varying environmental conditions. A cyclic adenosine 3′,5′-monophosphate (cAMP)-dependent shift of the f-channel activation curve is the main mechanism of channel modulation by the autonomic nervous system (see below), but several other mechanisms affect f-channel kinetics, such as phosphorylation [18, 19], interaction with auxiliary subunits [20], or structural proteins [21]. These mechanisms may act synergistically to fine tune the current activation range and kinetics and thus set the amount of current that can be recruited at appropriate times during cell activity.

More recently, experiments on rabbit SAN cells showed modulation of the f-channels by phosphoinositides [22, 23]. Under normal conditions, the I_f activation curve recorded by whole-cell experiments is known to shift negatively with time; this phenomenon is known as run-down [24]. Recent experiments have shown that run-down can be partially due to depletion of PI(4,5)P2 ([22]; see Section 3.3). This process can clearly lead to substantial underestimation of the I_f contribution [25]; thus, in the presence of run-down, the most depolarized threshold/half-activation voltage data reported in the literature are most likely to be close to real values.

The position of the f-channel activation curve in SAN cells is also strongly modified by disruption of caveolae, indicating that channel kinetics are modulated by specific membrane localization [21]. A novel mechanism proposed to explain the wide range of voltage-dependent activation in various cardiac regions involves a regulation of the I_f current by Src-mediated tyrosine phosphorylation [19, 26, 27] (see Section 3.3). The observation that in other cells of the cardiac conduction system such as Purkinje fibers [28] and cells of the working myocardium [29] the I_f activation threshold is more negative than in the SAN supports the role of I_f in primary pacemaking.

3.2.2.2 Kinetics. The pacemaker current slowly activates during hyperpolarization and deactivates during depolarization with time constants that change steeply with voltage. The I_f activation process typically proceeds with sigmoidal time course, which can be described as a proper channel opening preceded by a brief delay that can be removed by conditioning pre-hyperpolarizing steps [30]. Whereas the proper channel opening can be accurately described by a single- [31, 32] or double-exponential Hodgkin-Huxley kinetics [33–35], the presence of the delay requires complex, multistate, non-Hodgkin-Huxley kinetic models based on the existence of distinct "delaying" and proper "gating" processes [36]. A similar approach has been used to describe kinetics of clonal pacemaker currents [37].

3.2.2.3 Ionic Nature. The earliest data on the ionic permeability of f-channels derive from experiments in Purkinje fibers, later confirmed in SAN cells [13,14, 24]. Values of about $-10/-20$ mV were recorded when he I_f reversal potential was measured; these values are consistent with a mixed ionic composition. Ionic substitution experiments identified Na^+ and K^+ ions as the physiological carriers of I_f [13], the Na/K permeability ratio being about 0.27–0.33 [38, 39]. Although Na^+ ions permeate the channel according to the expected ohmic behavior, K^+ ions at physiological concentrations induce outward rectification of the current [13], similar to what observed in other K^+-permeable channels [40], and influence channel conductance. In particular, an increase in external K^+ concentration determines an increase in the channels conductance. This effect is physiologically relevant because a higher external K^+ concentration tends to decrease, by depolarization, the fraction of f-channels activated at the termination of an action potential, and thus decrease substantially the slope of DD and heart rate; an increase in the I_f conductance may thus compensate at least partially for the bradycardic effect of hyperkalemia.

In a recent work, Bucchi et al. [41] reported that SAN f-channels can be described as multi-ion, single-file pores. It is thus reasonable that pore residues involved in ion coordination during the crossing of the channel have less energetically favored bonds for Na^+ than for K^+, which would explain the different permeability ratio.

3.2.3   Autonomic Modulation

3.2.3.1 I_f-Mediated Autonomic Modulation of Cardiac Rate. The cardiac conduction system, and more specifically the SAN region, is extensively innervated by the autonomic nervous system, which exerts a tonic control of pacemaker activity. Fine modulation of heart rate is achieved by accurate control of the steepness of the slow DD operated by autonomic neurotransmitters. Sympathetic stimulation accelerates the heart rate and parasympathetic stimulation slows the heart rate, through the activation of β-adrenergic receptors (β-ARs) and muscarinic M2 receptors, which controls the cytosolic concentration of cAMP. The voltage dependence of activation of the pacemaker I_f current is controlled by the cytosolic cAMP concentration: an increase of cAMP shifts the opening probability of f-channels toward more positive potentials, via direct binding to the channel [42]. Thus, sympathetic/parasympathetic-stimulated changes of intracellular cAMP induce, through cAMP-dependent f-channel modulation, an increase/decrease of the net inward current during the DD, leading to a consequent increase/decrease of the steepness of DD, hence of heart rate [43, 44]. In cardiac cells, the physiological response to sympathetic stimulation is mediated by both β_1 and β_2 subtypes of β-ARs. In the whole heart, both β_1-ARs and β_2-ARs receptors are present, and β_1-ARs are the most abundant and widely distributed; it is worth mentioning that in the SAN β_2-ARs are highly expressed, although not as much as β_1-ARs.

Recent data have shown that in the SAN, β_2-ARs are confined to specific membrane microdomains (e.g., caveolae; see also Section 3.3) together with pacemaker channels, whereas β_1-ARs are largely excluded from these domains. Specific stimulation of β_2-ARs gives rise to a larger shift of the I_f activation curve and stronger rate acceleration than β_1-AR stimulation [45].

3.2.4   Cardiac Distribution of I_f

After its original discovery in the SAN and Purkinje fibers, I_f was also identified in adult ventricular and atrial myocytes. The current density is, however, too low, and the activation threshold is too negative for I_f to play a significant role in the working cardiac muscle under physiological conditions [46, 47], which suggests that the amount of current detected represents a remnant of embryonic expression (see below). Interestingly, pathological conditions such as cardiac hypertrophy lead to upregulation of I_f [48, 49], although the underlying mechanisms are not yet clear.

During development, I_f is functionally expressed in newborn myocytes committed to atrial and ventricular phenotypes [48, 50–53], which correlates with the ability of newborn myocytes to beat spontaneously. Interestingly, f-channel messenger RNA (mRNA) can also be detected in undifferentiated embryonic stem cells [54, 55].

The widespread presence of a functional I_f current in embryonic/neonatal heart, together with the known mechanisms of reexpression of fetal genes during pathology-induced cardiac remodeling [48, 49, 56, 57], lends support to the view that I_f may become an important trigger to induce arrhythmias in conditions such as chronic hypertension and cardiac failure.

Spontaneously beating cardiac cells are found not only throughout the conduction system but also in other regions such as the tissue surrounding atrioventricular valves [58, 59] and the tissue surrounding pulmonary veins [60–63]. In the rabbit, spontaneously beating cells isolated from the region surrounding the mitral valve were shown to express a large I_f, again in agreement with an association between the presence of spontaneous activity and the expression of the pacemaker current [64]. More recently, I_f was also recorded from spontaneously beating cells isolated from canine and human pulmonary veins [60, 61, 63].

The observation that atrial fibrillation is often triggered by the electrical activity of regions surrounding the pulmonary veins and that fast atrial pacing upregulates I_f and increases the arrhythmogenic potential of cardiomyocytes of this region suggests a possible arrhythmogenic contribution of I_f of pulmonary vein myocytes to atrial fibrillation [60–63].

3.3 MOLECULAR DETERMINANTS OF THE I_f CURRENT

The advent of the cloning era in the last few decades has substantially advanced our understanding of the biology of ion channels. Whereas cloning of the first voltage-dependent Na^+, Ca^{2+}, and K^+ channels was accomplished in the 1980s, cloning of funny channels had to wait until the late 1990s, some 20 years after their discovery, partly because the commonly used homology cloning was unsuccessful in SAN tissue (although it did provide evidence for an isoform of cyclic nucleotide-gated [CNG], channels [65]). Funny channels were eventually cloned by chance in 1997 while searching for proteins interacting with the SH3 domain of the neural N-src with a yeast-two-hybrid system, which yielded a protein sequence with high homology with Eag, hERG, and CNG channels [66].

An analysis of the primary sequence of these newly identified protein suggested six transmembrane domains, a highly charged S4 segment, a pore region, and a putative cyclic nucleotide binding domain (CNBD); all these features strongly suggested that this protein, which was named brain CNG1 (BCNG1), was the first member of a new family of ionic channels. The final functional proof came a year later when the heterologous expression of the protein yielded a channel with all the functional hallmarks of the pacemaker current [67, 68]. These channels were later renamed hyperpolarization-activated cyclic nucleotide (HCN) gated channels. A homologous sequence was also found in sea urchin sperm [69]. The identification of the first member of HCN family paved the way for additional cloning by sequence homology of additional members across different phyla [70]. To date, four different HCN gene isoforms have been identified in mammals (HCN1-4, [71]), and in humans, the genes have been localized in different chromosomes (HCN1: 5p12; HCN2: 19p13.3; HCN3: 1q22; HCN4: 15q24-25 [72, 73]).

3.3.1 HCN Clones and Pacemaker Channels

HCN channels belong to the six transmembrane (TM)-domain family of pore-loop channels and are formed by a relatively short intracellular N-terminal region, the six

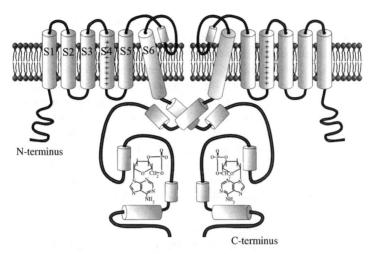

Figure 3.2. Schematic topology of HCN channels. Channels are tetramers, and two subunits only are depicted here. Each subunit is composed of six transmembrane domains (S1-S6); the S4 domain is the putative voltage sensor, and the S5, S6, and S5-S6 linker domains represented the pore-forming region. The domains involved in CNBD in the C-terminus and the cAMP molecules are also represented.

TM segments S1-S6 (with a highly basic S4 segment), a pore (P) region comprised between the S5 and S6, a C-linker that extends from the end of S6 to the beginning of the CNBD, and a relatively long intracellular C-terminus (Figure 3.2). This basic molecular structure confers to all HCN isoforms specific functional properties, including activation during hyperpolarization, time-dependent activation and deactivation, mixed Na^+ and K^+ permeability, and modulation by the second messenger cAMP. Data also indicate that functional HCN channels, like the Kv and CNG channels of the same superfamily, are tetramers [74–77].

The properties of the four HCN isoforms differ quantitatively. For example, reported values of the half activation voltage ($V^1/_2$) of the activation curves of human HCN1 through 4 are −69.5, −95.6, −77, and −92 mV, respectively [78]. The rates of activation are also different; the typical values of time constant of activation at −95 mV are 0.11 s, 1.13 s, 1.24 s (at −100 mV), and 2.52 s for HCN1 through 4, respectively [37, 78]. Furthermore, the sensitivity to cAMP (a positively directed shift of the activation curve, see below) varies considerably, with the HCN1 isoform poorly affected (4.3–5.8 mV shift), whereas HCN2 and HCN4 display a much more substantial cAMP-dependence, with shifts of 16.9–19.2 (HCN2) and 11–23 mV (HCN4). Interestingly, cAMP stimulation of HCN3 induces a negative shift of the activation curve (2.9–5 mV) [17, 78, 79].

The presence of several HCN isoforms with quantitatively different properties poses the problem of the isoform distribution in f-channel expressing tissues and of the subunit composition of native channels. Surprisingly, when expressed heterologously, none of the homomeric channels display properties overlapping those of native pacemaker channels [74, 75, 80]. Several possible explanations for this behavior are given here. First, homomeric assembly is not the only possible functional tetrameric organization because *in vitro* and *in vivo* expression studies have shown that heteromeric channel assembly can occur (with the notable exception of HCN3 and HCN2 channels, which do not co-assemble [77]), and the resulting channels often display characteristics intermediate between those of their individual components [74, 75, 77, 80–82]. Second, the properties of HCN channels are affected by accessory subunits such as MIRP1, by phosphorylation, and by membrane phospholipids such as phosphatidylinositol 4,5-bisphosphate (PI(4,5)P2) [20, 22, 83–86], as well as by environmental conditions such as the membrane lipid composition [21] and possibly by other yet unidentified mechanisms. Altogether, these modulatory influences are referred to as "context dependence" of f-channels [87].

Additional information on the molecular composition of funny channels comes from investigation of SAN tissue. Two lines of evidence indicate that the HCN4 isoform represents by far the largest component of HCN proteins expressed in the SAN. One involves mRNA measurements in rabbit SAN cells by RNase protection assays; according to these experiments, the HCN4 and HCN1 mRNAs are distributed with a 4:1 ratio, whereas the HCN2 mRNA signal is present only in traces [88]. A second one involving immunolabeling experiments later confirmed these early findings at the protein level in mice, rats, and rabbits; these experiments clearly showed that HCN4 is by far the most highly expressed isoform in the SAN region [45, 84–92]. Even though a faint mRNA signal of HCN3 was found in mouse ventricle (but not human hearts), an HCN3 protein signal was never detected [78, 79].

3.3.2 Identification of Structural Elements Involved in Channel Gating

Several studies have attempted to identify the structural domains responsible for the biophysical properties of HCN channels. These attempts have involved investigation of the ionic selectivity and permeability pathway, the voltage dependence of gating, the cAMP-dependent modulation, and the interaction with cytoskeletal elements.

3.3.2.1 *Ionic Selectivity and Permeability Pathway.* Permeable pores of HCN channels derive from a reentrant loop of the regions connecting transmembrane segments 5 and 6. A more precise identification of the pore recognizes three distinct parts named S5-P, P loop, and P-S6 (see Figure 3.2). The selectivity filter is represented by the triplet GYG that is common to all HCN isoforms and K^+ channels. An intriguing question is how the marked differences between K^+ channels (highly selective for K^+ ions) and HCN channels (also permeable to Na^+ ions) are generated. A possible explanation proposed by a theoretical approach is that the inner pore of HCN channels should be less rigid than that of K^+ channels, and thus, it can accommodate partially hydrated Na^+ as well as K^+ ions [93].

An investigation on the mechanism of block of HCN1 channels by the drug ZD7288 has also provided hints on the structural organization of the permeability pathway [94]. This study showed that ZD7288 interacts with specific residues in the S6 domain and that the drug can be trapped into the pore when the channel closes. A possible explanation of these data, also confirmed by the homology model with the

KcsA K^+ channel crystal [95], is that the S6 segments line the inner wall of HCN1 pores and that access to the S6 residues involved in ZD7288 binding is guarded by a gating structure likely to comprise the last part of the S6 segment.

3.3.2.2 Voltage Dependence of Gating. The voltage-dependent gating of ion channels is provided by the combined contribution of at least two functional domains: a voltage-sensing module that first responds to membrane voltage changes and a coupling domain that transfers this movement to the "proper" gating structure, which finally completes the electromechanical coupling by opening/closing the permeability pathway of the channel. In six TM channels, the module responsible for voltage sensing resides within the S1-S4 domain region, and it involves specifically the positively charged S4 TM segment [96–100]. Membrane voltage changes and the corresponding change of the electrical field induce rotational and/or translocational movements of the S4 segment [101]. Since all HCN isoforms have a fully conserved sequence in the S4 segment, it cannot be considered the structural site, giving rise to the differences in the voltage dependence ($V^1/_2$) or in the opening/closing kinetics observed among the HCN channel isoforms. It is also interesting to observe that although the S4 segment is positively charged in both HCN and in Kv channels, the voltage dependence of the opening is opposite, with HCN channels opening on hyperpolarization and Kv channels opening on depolarization. Recent data have shown that the S4 segments of Kv and HCN channels move in the same direction when similar voltage changes are applied, which demonstrates that the voltage dependence of kinetics is determined by the coupling mechanism, not by S4 segments [102].

After the identification of S4 as the voltage sensor, an important point that needed to be addressed was how the movement of S4 can ultimately result in channel gating. A first explanation was based on the hypothesis that voltage-dependent ion channels act as rigid structures, such that any movement of the voltage sensor immediately drives a general rearrangement of the protein leading to the opening of the pore [101]. This idea proved to be wrong, and the search for a potential coupling element focused on the cytoplasmic prolongation of the S4 TM domain, the S4-S5 linker. Given its direct connection to the S4, any S4 movement originated in response to voltage changes will likely also pull/rotate the S4-S5 linker. This hypothesis was confirmed experimentally in both Kv and HCN channels [98, 101]. In particular, an Ala scanning mutagenesis of this region in HCN2 channels has allowed the identification of several amino acids whose change alters profoundly channel kinetics [98]. Single substitutions of three of these amino acids (E324, Y331, and R339) yield channels unable to close. Although these experiments highlighted the relevance of the S4-S5 linker, they did not provide specific clues on the molecular nature of the interacting elements of the gating domain. This important aspect was investigated later, and the evidence in HCN channels suggests that the S4-S5 linker functionally interacts with the C-linker region. For example, an electrostatic interaction between the Arg-339 of the S4-S5 linker and the Asp-443 of the C-linker has been shown to stabilize the closed state of HCN2 channels [99].

More support to the coupling role of the S4-S5 linker comes from evidence in spHCN channels showing that the S4-S5 linker and the C-linker come in close proximity during gating, and cross-linking of these two domains profoundly alters channel gating [103].

At the same time, it is worth noting that the C-linker is not essential to confer voltage-dependence to channel gating, because at least in HCN2 channels, a partial deletion of this structure leaves unaltered this biophysical property [99]. Clear evidence for the coupling role of the S4-S5 domain has also been shown in Kv potassium channels [101, 104, 105].

An additional relevant aspect that has been investigated is the role of pore residues as structural elements involved in channel gating. An analysis of accessibility from the external medium of the C318 residue positioned in the pore region of HCN1 channel has shown that sulfhydryl modification of this residue profoundly influences channel kinetic parameters [106]. Also, investigation of nearby residues in the descending portion of the P-loop further supports an active role of this region in gating [107]. A gating hypothesis that directly derives from these experiments is that the pore and gate of mammalian HCN channels undergo concerted allosteric movements defined as "pore-to-gate coupling."

3.3.2.3 cAMP-Dependent Modulation.

The ability of the second messenger cAMP to interact functionally with native pacemaker channels was discovered several years before the cloning of the genes coding for pacemaker channels [42]. Thus, the unique characteristic of pacemaker channels of being dually gated by voltage and by a direct interaction with the second messenger cAMP was established before the primary sequence of the cloned HCN isoforms and the presence of a CNBD in the C-terminus were known.

In short, changes in cytoplasmic cAMP levels induced by metabolic cell requirements (whether as a consequence of autonomic stimulation and/or of hormonal stimuli) cause a shift of the activation curve of the pacemaker current [42, 108]. Depolarizing/hyperpolarizing shifts lead to an increased/decreased contribution of the I_f current during diastole, hence an increased/decreased steepness of the DD, thus allowing fine regulation of heart rate.

The observation that cAMP and voltage operate jointly to control the probability of channel opening (Po), with cAMP acting in a way equivalent to voltage hyperpolarization, was incorporated into an allosteric model of channel gating able to explain several aspects of channel kinetics [37, 109].

This model describes the dependence of Po on voltage and cAMP according to the following modified Boltzmann equation:

$$Po = 1/(1 + \exp((V - V_{1/2} - s)/v))$$

where V is voltage, $V_{1/2}$ is the half activation voltage, and v is the inverse slope factor. The factor s, which is not normally present in the Boltzmann equation, expresses a shift in millivolts that depends on the cAMP concentration (for details, see [109]). This model provides an interpretation of the effects of cAMP and voltage in terms of concerted actions controlling the open probability of channels, and by simply assuming higher affinity of cAMP for the open than for the closed channel configuration, it explains why cAMP acts exactly like a voltage hyperpolarization [109].

Several studies have investigated the structural rearrangements of HCN channels mediating cAMP-induced modulation. cAMP exerts its action on gating by interacting with the CNBD, the binding pocket located in the C-terminus region.

A first insight into the mechanism operating in cAMP-dependent activation was gained with the experimental observation originally made by Barbuti et al. [110] on native f-channels in SAN cells. Those intracellular portions of the channel exert a basal inhibitory action on channel opening, and channel activation by cAMP binding involves removal of this inhibition.

This observation was confirmed at a molecular level by the demonstration that the C-terminal of HCN channels in the absence of bound cAMP exerts a basal inhibitory action on channel gating [111]. This study showed that deletion of the whole CNBD shifts the activation curves of both HCN1 and HCN2 to more depolarized voltage, and that the voltage dependence of activation of CNBD-deleted HCN1 and HCN2 channels are similar ($V^1/_2$ of -103.5 and $-105.8\,\mathrm{mV}$, respectively). The different voltage dependence of intact HCN1 and HCN2 channels can therefore be accounted for by the different extent of inhibition exerted by the two C-termini.

Progress in the understanding of the structural domains involved in cAMP modulation came from the crystallization of part of the C-terminus of the HCN2 isoform [76], and specifically of the region delimited by Asp443 and His 645. This region comprises the C-linker and the CNBD. The crystallization was carried out in the presence of cAMP. Results indicate that the C-termini assemble in a tetrameric structure with a 4-fold axis of rotational symmetry; the N-termini of the four subunits are spatially organized close to each other and linked to the four S6 domains where the gating region of HCN channels is located. The regions of contact between the four subunits are large and include the C-linker domains, which are composed by six α-helices, A' to F'. Helices A' and B' of each subunit assemble in a helix-turn-helix structure and interact with the C' and D' helices of the adjacent subunit. Such a tetrameric assembly occurs in the presence of cAMP, whereas in its absence, assembly of the subunits is less likely.

Data from crystallization and previously evidence [110–112] agree to suggest a structure in which the cAMP-unbound C termini, arranged as monomeric or dimeric structures, exert a basal inhibition. cAMP binding removes this inhibition by inducing the rearrangement of the structure of these domains and particularly of the C-linker regions, which can now assemble into a 4-fold-symmetry gating ring.

A comparison among C-linker regions of CNG and HCN channels allows for identification of the three amino acidic residues (QEK) that are necessary to couple cyclic nucleotide binding to channel gating [113]. Analyzing which residues of the CNBD are relevant for cAMP-induced-response of HCN2 channels through molecular dynamics simulations supports the view that R632 in the C-helix of the CNBD is the residue providing selective stabilization of the cyclic nucleotide binding to the open state of the channel [114]. Additional analysis supports the view that binding of cAMP induces a local movement in the CNBD that is then transferred to the

C-linker region. Because C-linker regions represent the boundaries between subunits, the movement of the CNBDs associated with cAMP binding induces the complete rearrangement of the four C-termini [114].

3.3.3   Regulation of Pacemaker Channel Activity: "Context" Dependence and Protein-Protein Interactions

The differences in kinetics and cAMP sensitivity of the various HCN subunits together with their heterogeneous distribution throughout the heart [88] could be the basis for the changing properties of I_f in different cardiac regions. However, heterologous expression of various HCN isoforms either alone or in combination fails to recapitulate fully the properties of the native pacemaker current. It is known, for example, that SAN myocytes of different species express predominantly the HCN4 and to a much lesser extent the HCN1 and/or HCN2 subunits [88, 90–92, 115], but neither the coexpression of these isoforms nor the expression of covalently linked tandem constructs can reproduce native f-channel properties [80]. These data indicate that HCN subunit assembling cannot be the only determinant of the properties of native I_f.

Furthermore, heterologous expression of HCN2 or HCN4 in HEK 293 cells generates currents activating at voltages significantly more positive than currents generated by overexpression of the same isoforms in neonatal ventricular myocytes, indicating that a "context dependence" plays an important role in defining f-channel characteristics [116]. This "context" dependence could, for example, arise from specific cellular environments, in which channels are located that may favor/disfavor efficient interaction with ancillary proteins and signaling molecules.

HCN channels do indeed interact with several proteins. It is known, for example, that MiRP-1, which is a single TM-domain β-subunit of hERG channels, encoded by the KCNE2 gene, interacts with and modifies the conductance and activation kinetics of HCN1, HCN2, and HCN4 channels [20, 83, 84]. It has also been shown that HCN4 channels interact with caveolin 3 and thus localize in caveolin-rich membrane microdomains (caveolae), which are specialized membrane compartments that normally group proteins involved in specific signal transduction pathways. Disorganization of caveolae strongly affects channel properties [21]. Also, the confinement of pacemaker channels within membrane caveolae plays an important role in their modulation by β-adrenergic receptors, as indicated by the fact that I_f and rate of SAN myocytes are modulated more efficiently by stimulation of β_2 –adrenergic receptors than β_1-adrenergic receptors, because of colocalization of β_2-adrenergic receptors and f-channels within caveolae [45].

HCN channels are also regulated by local pools of phospholipids (PI(4,5)P2 and PI(3,4,5)P3), which are normally produced by activation of PLC mediated by stimulation of receptors such as the bradykinin BK2 receptor and the muscarinic M1 receptor [22, 23, 117]. It has been shown that PI(4,5)P2 acts as a ligand that allosterically opens HCN channels by a phosphatidylinositol (PI) kinase-dependent, cAMP-independent mechanism. Specifically, an increase in PI(4,5)P2 level induces a depolarizing shift of the voltage-dependence of HCN channels activation (about

+ 20 mV for HCN2 and about + 6 mV for HCN1), a faster channel activation, and a slower channels deactivation; furthermore, activation of BK2 also inhibited the peak tail current amplitude in a protein kinase C (PKC)-independent-way [23].

The pacemaker current is modulated by phosphorylation-dependent processes that are controlled by various cellular kinases and phosphatases; because these processes may be isoform and tissue specific, Scr-mediated tyrosine phosphorylation of HCN has been suggested as a novel mechanism that could partially explain the wide range of voltage-dependent activation observed in various cardiac regions and at different developmental stages [29, 85, 86, 118, 119]. In *Xenopus oocytes,* for example, the tyrosine kinase inhibitor genistein has no effect on HCN1, decreases the HCN4 current amplitude, and reduces the HCN2 current by decreasing its amplitude and by shifting its activation curve to more negative potentials [120].

A recent work has shown that tyrosine phosphorylation of HCN4 channel protein expressed in HEK293 cells shifts the channel activation curve to more positive potentials, speeds the activation time constant, and reduces the initial delay, which makes HCN4 properties more similar to those of native sinoatrial f-channels [86]. Coimmunoprecipitation experiments revealed that Src forms a complex with HCN2 and HCN4 channels as well as phosphorylates HCN4 in at least two different highly conserved tyrosine residues in the C-linker: Tyr 531, which is responsible for most of Src's actions, and Tyr 554, which is associated only with kinetic changes [86, 118].

In addition, receptor-like protein tyrosine phosphatase alpha (RPTPα) has been shown to significantly inhibit or eliminate HCN2 channel expression in HEK293 cells through reduction of tyrosine phosphorylation of the channel protein [121]. Interestingly, Src proteins expression seems to be higher in neonatal than in adult rat ventricle myocytes [122], whereas the total RPTPα protein expression is higher in adult than in neonatal ventricles [121]; these findings are in agreement with the physiological activation of neonatal ventricular I_f and nonphysiological activation of adult ventricular I_f.

3.3.4 HCN Gene Regulation

HCN transcriptional regulation plays an important role during cardiac development. HCN mRNA is expressed at much higher levels in the embryonic stage than after birth, and in general, HCN expression decreases with additional development [51, 123]. This trend is reversed under pathological conditions, such as cardiac hypertrophy and heart failure [56, 124]. It has been shown that the use of mineralo-corticoid receptor antagonists in patients affected by heart failure decreases the incidence of sudden cardiac death [125, 126] and that activation of mineralcorticoid receptors stimulates transcription of both HCN2 and HCN4, which results in an increase of protein synthesis and thus an increase of I_f current [127]. These findings suggest a possible role of HCN channel upregulation in an increased susceptibility to arrhythmias during cardiac hypertrophy and heart failure. The full regulatory mechanisms responsible for HCN gene upregulation or downregulation are still largely unknown. Starting from the observation that transgenic mice expressing a dominant negative form of the transcription silencer NRSF (Neuron-Restrictive

Silencer Factor) show an increased propensity to arrhythmias and upregulation of the HCN4 channel, Kuratomi et al. [129] have recently found two sequences in the noncoding region of the HCN4 gene, which regulate its transcription. The first is a highly conserved 846-bp sequence, located at the 5′ of the ATG, which functions as a basal promoter; the second sequence is a NRSE (Neuron-Restrictive Silencer Element), a sequence recognized by the NRSF silencer, located in the intronic region between exon 1 and 2, which represses promoter activity [128, 129].

3.4 BLOCKERS OF FUNNY CHANNELS

Ion channel blockers inhibit the flow of ions through channel pores. When their action is specific for a given type of channel, they allow pharmacological dissection of the contribution of this channel to cellular electrical activity. The importance of ion channel blockers is that they are tools potentially useful in both basic research and clinical therapy.

Ion channel dysfunctions are responsible for several types of diseases known as channelopathies, and the development of drugs targeting specific ion channels has, as a consequence, become a rapidly growing field of pharmacological research. The relevance of I_f in the generation of the DD phase of the action potential in pacemaker cells makes it an important pharmacological target in the search of tools able to reduce heart rate without interfering with other currents that may affect the duration of the action potential (typically K^+ channels) and/or the inotropic state of the heart (typically Ca^{2+} channels). Drugs able to block f-channels are indeed expected to control the cardiac chronotropic state via modification of the DD phase, and they should have a potential for treatment of heart diseases, such as for example angina pectoris, heart failure, and ischemic heart disease.

All these pathologies greatly benefit from a slowing of heart rate, because this condition reduces cardiac oxygen consumption and improves oxygen supply to cardiomyocytes by increasing the duration of diastole and the consequent increase in the time of perfusion through coronary circulation. Conventional pharmacological interventions aimed to reduce heart rate (β-adrenergic receptor blockers, calcium channels blockers, and nitrates) have potentially adverse side effects and are not well tolerated by all affected individuals; heart rate reduction induced by these drugs is often associated with mild to severe vascular side effects and with a decrease in cardiac inotropism. Consequently, interest in the development of specific heart-rate-reducing agents has grown significantly in recent years.

In the last few years, several substances, termed "specific heart rate-reducing agents," have become available that indeed can slow rate with essentially no other cardiovascular effects. Their action has been extensively characterized both *in vitro* and *in vivo* studies [17]. The specific negative chronotropic action is caused by the highly specific block of funny channels exerted by these substances, which show little or no interaction with other channels (such as K^+ or Ca^{2+} channels) and β-adrenergic receptors. This family includes alinidine (ST567), zatebradine (UL-FS49), cilobradine (DK-AH26), ZD-7288, and ivabradine (S16257) [41, 130–133].

3.4.1 Alinidine (ST567)

Alinidine, the first specific bradycardic agent reported in the literature, is an imidazoline derivative of the antihypertensive drug clonidine, which was however found to have a pharmacological profile different from the parent drug because its properties included analgesic [134] and bradycardic effects [135–138]. Alinidine reduced sinus rate by about 30% in isolated guinea-pig atria ($\sim$8 μM [137]) and by about 20% in rabbit SAN cells ($\sim$1 μM [139]). An analysis of action potential parameters showed an $\sim$10% decrease of the DD slope accompanied by a prolongation of the action potential duration, but no effects on MDP, maximal dV/dt, and action potential amplitude were observed [139]. Voltage-clamp experiments showed that the action of the drug was caused by an interaction with ion channels, but the drug specificity was partial: 100 μg/mL ($\sim$300 μM) alinidine reduced K^+ currents by $\sim$52%, Ca^{2+} currents by $\sim$57%, and the pacemaker I_f current by $\sim$80% [139]. The effects of alinidine on DD slope and action potential duration were confirmed by experiments in sheep Purkinje fibers and rabbit SAN cells [140, 141]. According to these data, alinidine (28 μM) was reported to inhibit I_f by shifting its activation curve to more negative voltages (by 7.8 mV) and by reducing its fully activated conductance (by 27.0%); no use or frequency dependence were observed, thus suggesting that the drug binds equally well to open and closed channel states.

Studies on intact animal models and humans confirmed the prominent bradycardic properties of alinidine [136, 138, 142]. In normal healthy subjects, the heart rate was significantly reduced by a single oral administration of alinidine (80 mg) by $\sim$4% and 14% in resting conditions and after exercise, respectively [143]. Although alinidine displayed a new pharmacodynamic profile when compared with contemporary drugs used in clinical therapy, its development was discontinued because of a lack of specificity and the presence of central side effects in the shape of visual disturbances, which were found in some healthy volunteers and occasionally in patients [142]. Among the adverse effects induced by alinidine were also vertigo, psychoreactive disorders, drowsiness, dry mouth, hypototonia, and negative inotropism [142, 144].

3.4.2 Falipamil (AQ-A39), Zatebradine (UL-FS 49), and Cilobradine (DK-AH269)

Other molecules were subsequently developed with the aim of improving the specificity for the I_f current and thus for the rate-slowing action versus side effects. A second group of molecules with bradycardic action, derived from the calcium channel inhibitor verapamil, included falipamil (AQ-A39), zatebradine (UL-FS49), and cilobradine (DK-AH269). Like alinidine, these drugs were shown to induce bradycardia mainly by a decrease of the DD slope, and their efficacies were tested in a variety of cardiac cell/tissue preparations, in intact animals and, in the case of zatebradine and falipamil, also in humans [130, 132, 145–152]. Experiments investigating the mode of I_f block showed that, in contrast to alinidine, these molecules do not modify the voltage dependence of the current but reduce the I_f maximal conductance [130, 132, 153].

3.4.2.1   Falipamil (AQ-A39). Falipamil reduces sinus frequency in isolated guinea-pig heart (by $\sim$50% at 21.5 μM) mainly by reducing DD slope in various cardiac preparations and in intact animals [137, 145, 154]. In addition to the bradycardic effect, a marked prolongation of the action potential duration (APD_{90} $\sim +60\%$) and a reduction of the contractile tension ($\sim -30\%$) in papillary muscles were also observed [145]. These undesired proarrhythmic effects, probably caused by a block of calcium and potassium channels [130, 141, 155, 156], likely caused termination of development of this drug.

3.4.2.2   Zatebradine (UL-FS49). When compared with alinidine and falipamil, zatebradine was more potent in rate slowing and had greater selectivity for I_f. Investigation in rabbit SAN cells showed that zatebradine (1 μM) induces a $\sim$65% use-dependent block of I_f and acts from the intracellular side; minor effects on delayed K^+ currents and no changes of Ca^{2+} current amplitude were also reported [153, 157]. Similar data were also obtained in several other cardiac preparations [150, 158–160]. In a detailed study carried out in rabbit SAN myocytes, DiFrancesco [153] showed that the I_f block by UL-FS49 develops with time constants in the order of several tens of seconds and that it can only occur when channels are in the open state; the site of block is positioned within the pore, at a distance of about 39% of the electrical field from the intracellular side. Block is also strongly influenced by the electrical gradient across the membrane and negative voltages induce partial drug unbinding [153].

In rabbit SAN tissue, zatebradine (3 μM) reduced spontaneous rate by $\sim$28%, and an analysis of AP parameters showed that the bradycardic action was predominantly induced by a decrease of the rate of the DD; however, a prolongation of the AP duration ($\sim$30%) was also observed [150]. In intact animal models, zatebradine was shown to reduce heart rate with little or no effects on other cardiovascular parameters and to prevent exercise-induced myocardial dysfunction [149, 161–163]. Despite the promising results in animal studies, a phase 3 clinical trial concluded that zatebradine does not provide any greater exercise tolerance benefit in *angina* patients treated with extended-release nifedipine [164]. In addition, undesired visual effects that included persistence of images and flashes were observed in patients treated with the drug [164, 165]. Evaluation of the effects of zatebradine on photoreceptors showed that these effects are caused by the inhibition of the I_h current, the neuronal equivalent of I_f, which is also expressed in the retina [166, 167].

3.4.2.3   Cilobradine. Cilobradine is a congener of zatebradine developed more recently. Experiments carried out in isolated single SAN cells [132] showed that cilobradine (1 μM) induces a use-dependent block (82%) of the I_f current. The drug needs open channels to reach the binding site and acts intracellularly; also, block is voltage-dependent and is relieved by strong hyperpolarization. However, despite its high affinity for f-channels and associated rate-slowing effect, cilobradine (1 μM) also increases action potential duration (APD) in single murine SAN cells ($\sim$60%; [168]) by block of outward K^+ currents, and this APD prolongation confers potentially proarrhythmic properties. Interestingly, cilobradine (0.25 mg/kg) was reported to reduce heart rate ($\sim$20%) without negative inotropic effects in a rabbit model of myocardial infarction [169]. A study carried out in rodents showed that contrary to zatebradine, cilobradine does not modify the visual response at doses able to elicit bradycardia [170]; whether this difference is caused by differences in the affinities of cilobradine and zatebradine for cardiac SAN and retinal channels is a possibility that needs more investigations. Similarly, comparison of data obtained in Purkinje and SAN cells revealed that cilobradine blocks I_f more effectively in sheep Purkinje fibers (IC_{50}, 66 nM) than in rabbit SAN cells (IC_{50}, 480 nM) [132]; whether this difference, too, arises from a different heteromeric composition of f-channels in the two tissues remains an open question.

3.4.3   ZD7288

The compound ZD7288, which is a lipophilic quaternary cation, was developed after alinidine and UL-FS49, and its bradycardic action was first investigated in isolated beating atria and intact SAN tissue of guinea-pig [171, 172] and in anaesthetized dogs [173]. In intact atria ZD7288 (0.1–100 μM) reduced spontaneous rate (maximal slowing of 50%) without modifying the contractile force of electrically stimulated left atria [171]; similar effects were observed in intact SAN tissue (60% rate reduction at 0.3 μM), although a moderate but measurable prolongation of the APD ($+10\%$) was also observed [131]. In anaesthetized dogs, ZD7288 (1.0 mg/kg) lowered heart rate from 152 to 77 bpm. Myocardial contractile function decreased along with rate while the stroke volume increased [173].

The selectivity of ZD7288 was verified by testing in guinea-pig SAN cells its inhibitory action on I_f and on Ca^{2+} and K^+ currents [131]. At the concentration of 0.1 μM, ZD7288 was shown to induce a 7% decrease of the spontaneous frequency and a robust block of I_f (-44%), while blocking poorly K^+ (-1%) and Ca^{2+} currents (-18%). The mechanism of action of I_f block by 0.3 μM ZD7288, evaluated in isolated guinea pig SAN cells, consisted of both a negative shift of the activation curve (-16 mV) and a decrease of the maximal conductance (-52%; [131]). Furthermore, ZD7288, like alinidine and unlike UL-FS49, induced a block that did not depend on use or frequency, suggesting that ZD7288 interacts with its binding site independently from the channel state. The slow kinetics of block onset (several minutes) suggested that the drug must first cross the membrane before it can act [131, 174].

When the effects of ZD7288 were evaluated on the funny current in different types of neurons, a substantial block was observed [166, 174–176]; this property represents a limit in the potential use of this drug as a specific I_f blocker in cardiac tissue. Gasparini and DiFrancesco [175] observed that block of the funny current in the hippocampus requires higher doses of the drug than in the SAN, leading to the suggestion of a possible difference in the cardiac versus hippocampal HCN-isoform channel composition.

3.4.4   Ivabradine (S16257)

Ivabradine is the only heart-rate-reducing agent having passed all clinical tests for therapeutic application. Based on its selective action on the funny current and heart rate in the absence of side effects, ivabradine is used today for pharmacological treatment of chronic stable angina in patients with normal sinus rhythm who have a contraindication or intolerance to β-adrenergic receptor blockers. Ivabradine is a phenylalkylamine that at physiological pH has a net positive charge of about $+1$.

In rabbit SAN, ivabradine ($3\,\mu M$) induces a slowing of spontaneous rate comparable with those elicited by the same concentration of zatebradine (24% versus 28%), but a less pronounced prolongation of APD (9% versus 29%; [150]). Bois et al. [159] showed that, in agreement with its specific action on the DD rate, ivabradine ($3\,\mu M$) reduces the pacemaker current amplitude ($\sim -60\%$) without significantly modifying T- and L-type Ca^{2+} currents and delayed K^+ currents.

The main features of an ivabradine-induced block of f-channels can be summarized as follows: 1) the block can only occur from the intracellular side, 2) drug binding and unbinding reactions are limited to the open channel configuration; and 3) the block is use and current dependent [41, 159]. The current dependence suggests that f-channels are multi-ion single file pores and that ivabradine blocks ion flow by accessing the intracellular vestibule of the channel and by directly interacting with the permeation pathway Figure 3.3. In other words, block can be viewed as a process where ivabradine molecules, which bear a positive charge at physiological pH, are "kicked into" the pore from the intracellular side of the channel by the transient outward flow that occurs during depolarization, and they are "kicked out" when ions flow in the inward direction during cell hyperpolarization. The current-dependence is a property specific of f-channel block by ivabradine, not found in the f-channel block by other molecules such as ZD7288 and zatebradine, which are instead pure voltage-dependent blockers [41].

f-channel block by ivabradine thus depends on the following two separate features: the state of the channel and the direction of the current flow. Channels open on hyperpolarization when the driving force is inward; in this case, although the binding site is accessible, the direction of the current tends to displace ivabradine molecules from the binding site within the pore. The reverse situation occurs on depolarization: In this case, f-channels deactivate, but for a brief time channels meet the condition of being open with the current flowing in the outward direction, and this is when block occurs. Channels therefore undergo repetitive cycling between conditions favoring block and conditions favoring block removal. This is the basis for a marked "use-dependence" of block, a condition under which block accumulates during repetitive channel opening-closing cycles.

The selective action of ivabradine on heart rate has been confirmed in both preclinical and clinical tests. Several studies performed in animals and humans have shown that ivabradine reduces heart rate at rest and during exercise without significantly affecting the QT interval or myocardial contractility [177–184]. Trials in patients with stable *angina pectoris* showed the efficacy of ivabradine as an anti-anginal and anti-ischemic compound, and they showed that this efficacy is maintained over 12 months without development of acquired tolerance [185–187]. The anti-anginal effects of ivabradine and β-blockers have been shown to be comparable, but unlike β-adrenergic receptor blockers (the most common current treatment for angina), ivabradine treatment is free of side effects such as sexual disturbances,

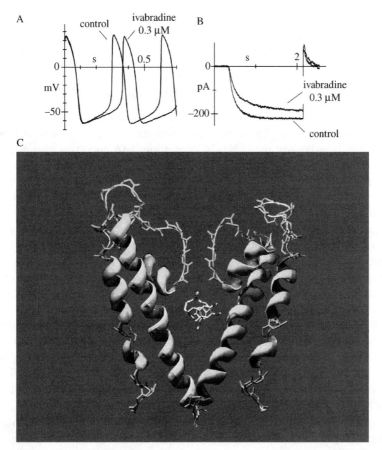

Figure 3.3. (**A**) Ivabradine (0.3 µM) slows spontaneous activity of SAN myocytes by reducing specifically the rate of diastolic depolarization. (**B**) Steady-state inhibition of I_f by ivabradine 0.3 µM during repetitive voltage-clamp steps to $-100/+5$ mV (1/6 Hz). (**C**) Hypothetical position of ivabradine in the hydrophilic cavity of HCN4 channels. The 3D reconstruction of the HCN4 pore region (S5, S6, and S5-S6 linker) was modeled on by homology with the KscA K^+ channel X-ray structure [95]. For clarity, only two of the four HCN4 subunits are shown.

respiratory problems, and rebound phenomena [185]. A limited reduction of blood pressure and visual symptoms, generally mild and well tolerated, are the only adverse events from ivabradine treatment. The visual effects are likely to be related to the presence of HCN channels in the retina. Results from a large clinical trial investigating the efficacy of ivabradine in patients with coronary artery disease (CAD) and left ventricular dysfunction (BEAUTIFUL) have been recently announced [188, 189]. These data show that whereas ivabradine does not improve cardiovascular death or heart failure, which are endpoints for the generic CAD patient, it improves coronary endpoints (i.e., hospitalization for myocardial infarction or revascularization) for the subpopulation of CAD patients with a rate >70 bpm [188, 189]. This means that

CAD patients with relatively high heart rate have a significantly higher risk of cardiovascular events and that ivabradine-induced I_f inhibition, and the associated rate slowing, can substantially reduce myocardial infarction.

3.4.5 Effects of the Heart Rate Reducing Agents on HCN Isoforms

More detailed molecular insight into the mechanisms of f-channel inhibition by heart-rate-reducing agents has been achieved by the investigation of their action in heterologously expressed individual HCN isoforms. An important goal of this approach is to provide information useful to help design more potent and more HCN4-specific molecules, because HCN4 is by large the main expressed isoform in the SAN.

Although it is true that the brain (where HCN-channel expression is high) is protected against undesired effects of ivabradine by the blood-brain barrier, a problem common to almost all heart-rate-reducing agents includes visual effects caused by the block of HCN channels of retinal cells [190]. Despite the growing relevance of specific heart-rate-reducing agents in clinical therapy, only a few studies have evaluated differential effects of these drugs on individual HCN isoforms. Some of the knowledge gained so far is summarized as follows:

a) The effects of cilobradine, ivabradine, and zatebradine have been tested on all human HCN isoforms expressed in HEK cells, and a comparison among the dose-response relationships does not indicate any subtype specificity. All drugs have a similar IC_{50} (in the μM range) and Hill slope factors close to 1; these values are similar to those reported for the native SAN I_f current [168].

b) The mode of action of ivabradine on HCN4 and HCN1 isoforms has been characterized [191]. Even though no obvious isoform specificity is found for the steady-state block, important differences exist in the mechanism of the block. HCN4 channels, like native f-channels, are blocked by ivabradine according to an open-channel type of block, whereas the block of HCN1 can occur only when the channels are closed [191].

c) Three residues (Y355, M357, and V359) of the lower (cytoplasmic) side of the S6 TM domain of the mHCN1 isoform seem to be critical for ZD7288 binding [94].

d) The residues A425 and I432, located in the S6 domain of mHCN2, are critical for ZD7288 binding [192]; for example, replacing I432 with an alanine residue induces a 100-fold decrease of drug sensitivity. The same amino acids were also found to affect the block of cilobradine.

3.5 GENETICS OF HCN CHANNELS

3.5.1 HCN-KO Models

The understanding of the mechanisms that control the genesis and modulation of the cardiac spontaneous activity is an important issue in the biomedical field. Since the funny current was originally described in 1979 [9], a wealth of evidence has been collected to support its role in generation of spontaneous activity and control of heart rate.

Recently, the use of HCN4 knock-out mice has provided important information on the functional and pathological implications of a reduced contribution of HCN channels to the electrical activity of the SAN. In particular, data from global and cardiac-specific HCN4 knock-out mice have been reported [193]. According to these data, the heart develops normally up to the E9.5-E11.5 day; after this period, however, death ensues because of lack of development of the cardiac pacemaker. It is interesting to note that this corresponds roughly to the time when cardiogenesis is near completion. An additional piece of information comes from the finding that the cardiac pacemaker tissue develops from cardiac progenitor cells of the "second heart field" after the activation of a specific gene activation program, and that HCN4 is one of the genes that undergo early activation [194–196].

To overcome the embryonic death of HCN4 KO mice, two models of inducible HCN4 knock-out mice were developed. In these models, the functional elimination of the gene can be obtained by targeted excision of the gene of interest at any time during life, and therefore, the relevance of HCN4 to cardiac chronotropism can be evaluated also in the adult mice [197, 198]. Experiments carried out both *in vivo* and in single cells isolated from the SAN showed that the adult homozygous HCN4$^{-/-}$ mice have cardiac arrhythmia characterized by recurrent sinus pauses and that the SAN I_f is almost fully abolished (about 80% reduction). However, no impairment of sympathetic-induced rate acceleration was observed in mutant mice.

Constitutive HCN2 KO mice have also been developed. This model shows that a lack of HCN2 does not impair embryonic development, but in the adult animals, the cardiac phenotypic alterations were sinus arrhythmia and a reduction of about 30% of the sinoatrial node pacemaker current [199].

KO studies therefore suggest the following: 1) The I_f current in murine SAN cells is predominantly generated by HCN4 channels (contributing to about 80% of total current), and the remaining fraction is mediated by other subunits, presumably mainly by HCN2; 2) HCN4 is necessary to maintain a stable cardiac rhythm; and 3) sympathetic acceleration of heart rate cannot be explained as a mechanism solely controlled by either HCN4 or HCN2 channels.

3.5.2 Pathologies Associated with HCN Dysfunctions

Cardiovascular diseases represent a major cause of worldwide mortality, and the relevance of the genetic component of such diseases has recently become more apparent. Considerable efforts have therefore recently been devoted to the identification and investigation of cardiac pathologies caused by defective ion channels (channelopathies, [200]), that is, ion channels whose contribution to electrical activity and/or excitation-contraction (EC) coupling is altered because of mutations leading to functional modifications (typically either loss or gain of function). The relevance of f-channels to cardiac pacemaking naturally points to HCN4, the molecular correlate of f-channels, as an obvious candidate for mutations associated with rhythm disturbances. To date, several genetic alterations of the open reading frame of HCN4 channels variously coupled to rhythm disturbances have been reported in humans. Early reports describe a single patient with bradycardia, atrial fibrillation (AF) and chronotropic incompetence [201], and a small family with several symptoms including syncope, severe bradycardia, long QT interval, and torsades de pointes. The genetic anomalies of HCN4 gene associated with these diseases were a heterozygous single base-pair deletion (1631delC) in exon 5, leading to a truncated protein that completely lacks the CNBD [201] and the missense mutation D533N [202], respectively. The problems in these reports are that the first case regarded a single patient, and the second case involved a complex array of disturbances not clearly attributable to the HCN4 mutation.

More recently, we reported that in a large Italian family, the point mutation S672R of the HCN4 channel was tightly linked to an asymptomatic bradycardic phenotype (load score of 5.47), according to an autosomal dominant pattern (Figure 3.4) [203]. Members of the family carrying the mutation had an average heart rate of 52.2 beats/min, whereas members with wild-type HCN4 had a rate of 73.2 beats/min. *In vitro* studies showed that the S672R mutation causes a hyperpolarizing shift of the HCN4 channel open probability curve of about 5 mV in heterozygosis; this effect is similar to the hyperpolarizing shift caused by parasympathetic stimulation and can fully explain a reduction of inward current during diastole and the resulting slower spontaneous rate [203].

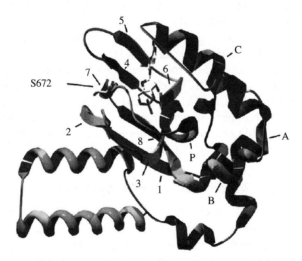

Figure 3.4. hHCN4 single-point mutation (S672R) associated with sinus bradycardia. 3-D ribbon model of the hHCN4 CNBD based on the mHCN2 CNBD crystal structure [76]. The bound cAMP molecule is shown as a stick model and is located close to the S672 residue. α-helices and β-sheets of the CNBD are indicated by letters and numbers, respectively, in accordance with previously published sequence data (see ref. 203).

A form of asymptomatic bradycardia associated with the point mutation (G480R) of the HCN4 channel was also found by Nof et al. [204]. Members carrying the mutation displayed slower heart rates (<55 beats/min) when compared with unaffected members (>63 beats/min).

The above findings confirm the role of f-channels in pacemaker activity, and at the same time, they suggest the possible involvement of f-channel dysfunction in other types of rhythm disorders such as symptomatic bradycardia, tachycardia, and atrial fibrillation. f-channel dysfunctions could also partly contribute to more complex arrhythmic syndromes such as the sick-sinus syndrome (SSS). SSS comprises a group of symptoms such as sinus tachy- and/or bradyarrhythmias including sinus pauses, reduced or absent response to autonomic modulation (chronotropic incompetence), and sinus node exit block [205]. Although SSS is known to be associated with the aging process, it may also affect young people. In this last case, the etiology of SSS cannot be simply attributed to an age-dependent degenerative process linked to an increase of fibrotic tissue, and it requires a different explanation [205].

3.6   HCN-BASED BIOLOGICAL PACEMAKERS

Several acquired or genetic cardiac diseases are characterized by life-threatening rhythm disturbances. These include severe bradycardia, SSS, atrioventricular (AV) nodal block, and heart block. Pharmacological treatment of these disorders is not always applicable, and antiarrhythmic drugs often turn out to be proarrhythmic. When a pharmacological therapy is not applicable, implantation of electronic pacemakers is often required.

Electronic devices are normally effective, but represent nonetheless a palliative cure; also, their use has limitations among which the lack of interaction with the autonomic nervous system for modulation of heart rate, the need to have an external power source, and the sensitivity to strong electrical and magnetic fields.

Gene- or cell-based biological pacemakers represent a potential means to overcome these limitations. In the last decade or so, several approaches have been pursued to induce spontaneous rhythmic activity in quiescent substrates both *in vitro* and *in vivo*. These include overexpression of β_2-adrenergic receptors [206, 207], downregulation of the inward rectifying I_{K1} current [208], virus-mediated overexpression of HCN channels [116, 209–213], and development of spontaneously contracting cells derived from human embryonic stem (hES) cells [214, 215].

Although all of these approaches proved to be feasible at least in principle, biological pacemakers based on transfer of HCN channels have been and remain today the most promising. The use of HCN channels take advantage of the fact that these channels are functional only at negative voltages, and thus even if largely overexpressed, their contribution during AP phases other than the DD is negligible.

A first "proof of principle" on the feasibility of pacemaker induction by HCN transfer was provided with the demonstration that adenovirus-mediated overexpression of HCN2 in primary cultures of neonatal ventricular myocytes causes an 83%

acceleration of spontaneous rate by increasing the steepness of the slow DD [116]. Other protocols have then been tested to generate HCN-based biological pacemakers, including. 1) adenoviral-mediated HCN channels infection [209, 210, 212, 216], 2) implant of mesenchymal stem cell overexpressing HCN2 channels [211], 3) PEG-induced fusion of HCN1-expressing fibroblasts [217], and 4) implant of spontaneously beating hES cell-derived cardiomyocytes [214, 215].

Adenoviral-Mediated HCN Channels Infection. As well as in *in vitro* experiments, adenovirus-mediated overexpression of HCN2 can be performed *in vivo* by injecting the virus directly in the left atrium or in the left bundle branch; these experiments showed that, following sinus rhythm suppression by vagal stimulation, a stable sustained spontaneous activity originating from the site of injection could pace the heart [209, 210]. In similar experiments, other groups have demonstrated that injection in the atrium of adenovirus carrying a mutated HCN1 or injection of the HCN4 gene in the ventricle of swine could also sustain a stable ectopic rhythm that was observed to originate from the site of virus injection [218, 219].

Although these data demonstrate that overexpression of pacemaker channels is by itself sufficient to drive the heart, they still showed two drawbacks: first, the relatively low basal heart rate reached after virus injection (88 beats/min in dogs [210] and 64 [218] or 69 beats/min [219] in pigs) and second, the limitations of the gene delivery system. Use of either a mutated HCN2 channel with a more depolarized activation curve or a chimeric channel (HCN212) activating with much faster kinetics could not accelerate basal heart rate, although it improved the catecholamine sensitivity [212]; however, overexpression of the chimeric HCN212 channel caused a burst of rapid action potentials followed by pauses of activity [213]. Clearly, more data will be necessary to achieve fine regulation of the effects of HCN transfer techniques on heart rate in animal models.

A different approach involved the transformation of a human voltage sensitive potassium channels (hKv1.4) into a nonselective hyperpolarization-activated channel by mutating three amino acids in the voltage-sensitive S4 transmembrane domain and one in the pore. Virus-mediated gene transfer of this synthetic pacemaker channel (SPC) was able to induce pacemaker activity in guinea pig adult ventricular myocardium and produced idioventricular rhythms on electrocardiogram (ECG) [216].

Implant of Mesenchymal Stem Cell Overexpressing HCN2 Channels. Because adenovirus-driven gene transfer presents limitations in the duration of protein expression and safety of adenoviral construct, researchers have explored the possibility to generate a biological pacemaker using a cell-based approach. To do this, undifferentiated mesenchymal stem cells were engineered to express high levels of HCN2 channels [211]. This cellular substrate was able to couple electrically to the surrounding cardiac tissue, through endogenous gap junctions, and to modify its beating rate. This system is based on mesenchymal stem cells behaving as a source of depolarizing current (as electronic pacemakers do), and it can work as long as

HCN2-expressing cells remain undifferentiated and coupled to the substrate. A possible limitation could be because of the plasticity of mesenchymal stem cells, which *in vivo* differentiate toward different phenotypes, potentially leading to a rearrangement of endogenous and exogenous gene expression.

Chemically-Induced Fusion of HCN1-Expressing Fibroblasts. Polyethylene glycol (PEG)-induced fusion of engineered HCN1-expressing guinea pig lung fibroblasts with cardiac myocytes was shown to provide enough depolarizing current during diastole to induce spontaneous activity in the heterokaryon, both *in vitro* and *in vivo* [217]. Although this strategy apparently presents several advantages over the approaches described above, such as independence from virus and stem cells and the possibility to use patient-derived fibroblasts, major concerns are the long-term ability to pace the heart and the ultimate fate of fused cells.

Implant of Spontaneously Beating hES cell-Derived Cardiomyocytes. An alternative method would be to use terminally differentiated, stem-cell-derived myocytes with electrophysiological and molecular characteristics of native pacemaker myocytes. So far, of the different types of stem cells investigated, only embryonic stem cells (ESCs) have been convincingly and reproducibly shown to differentiate into myocytes with a pacemaker phenotype. Early studies showed that murine ESCs can differentiate into cardiac myocytes when let to differentiate spontaneously through the formation of three-dimensional cell aggregates called embryoid bodies (EBs). During differentiation of EBs, some foci of autorhythmic cells appear, which include spontaneously beating cells characterized by action potentials typical of pacemaker cells and expressing the pacemaker I_f current [50, 220, 221].

Similar results were obtained also from human ESCs [48, 222, 223]. A cellular approach to biological pacemaking has been successfully attempted using human embryonic stem cells differentiated into spontaneously contracting EBs [214, 215]. The contractile portions of EBs, once isolated, were shown to integrate and pace either cultures of neonatal rat cardiac myocytes *in vitro* or whole hearts of swine [214] and guinea pigs [215] *in vivo*. Although in the above studies the molecular mechanism underlying pacemaking was not directly investigated, it is likely that an important role in the generation of rhythmic activity could be played by the I_f current. In these models, β-adrenergic receptor stimulation was effective in increasing the rate, and additionally, the f-channel blocker ZD7288 was able to slow the rate [214, 215].

Although the unrestricted use of hESC might raise concern, these data are extremely important in light of the recent finding that adult somatic cells can be reprogrammed to become induced pluripotent stem (iPS) cells with properties similar to those of hESCs [224, 225].

Although the various strategies developed so far still have several drawbacks and imperfections, yet they clearly demonstrate the feasibility of pacemaker control by

HCN channel transfer *in vivo*, and thus represent important "proofs of principle" in view of a possible therapeutic application of biological pacemakers.

REFERENCES

1. Weidmann, S. (1951). Effect of current flow on the membrane potential of cardiac muscle. Journal of Physiology, 115, 227–236.

2. Vassalle, M. (1966). Analysis of cardiac pacemaker potential using a "voltage clamp" technique. American Journal of Physiology, 210, 1335–1341.

3. Deck, K.A., Trautwein, W. (1964). Ionic currents in cardiac excitation. Pflugers Archiv— European Journal of Physiology, 280, 63–80.

4. Noble, D., Tsien, R.W. (1968). The kinetics and rectifier properties of the slow potassium current in cardiac Purkinje fibres. Journal of Physiology, 195, 185–214.

5. Peper, K., Trautwein, W. (1969). A note on the pacemaker current in Purkinje fibers. Pflugers Archiv—European Journal of Physiology, 309, 356–361.

6. Hauswirth, O., Noble, D., Tsien, R.W. (1968). Adrenaline: mechanism of action on the pacemaker potential in cardiac Purkinje fibers. Science, 162, 916–917.

7. DiFrancesco, D., McNaughton, P.A. (1979). The effects of calcium on outward membrane currents in the cardiac Purkinje fibre. Journal of Physiology, 289, 347–373.

8. Cohen, I., Daut, J., Noble, D. (1976). The effects of potassium and temperature on the pace-maker current, iK2, in Purkinje fibres. Journal of Physiology, 260, 55–74.

9. Brown, H.F., DiFrancesco, D., Noble, S.J. (1979). How does adrenaline accelerate the heart? Nature, 280, 235–236.

10. Yanagihara, K., Irisawa, H. (1980). Inward current activated during hyperpolarization in the rabbit sinoatrial node cell. Pflugers Archiv—European Journal of Physiology, 385, 11–19.

11. DiFrancesco, D., Ohba, M., Ojeda, C. (1979). Measurement and significance of the reversal potential for the pace-maker current (iK2) in sheep Purkinje fibres. Journal of Physiology, 297, 135–162.

12. DiFrancesco, D., Ojeda, C. (1980). Properties of the current if in the sino-atrial node of the rabbit compared with those of the current iK, in Purkinje fibres. Journal of Physiology, 308, 353–367.

13. DiFrancesco, D. (1981). A study of the ionic nature of the pace-maker current in calf Purkinje fibres. Journal of Physiology, 314, 377–393.

14. DiFrancesco, D. (1981). A new interpretation of the pace-maker current in calf Purkinje fibres. Journal of Physiology, 314, 359–376.

15. DiFrancesco, D. (1985). The cardiac hyperpolarizing-activated current, if. Origins and developments. Progress in Biophysics and Molecular Biology, 46, 163–183.

16. DiFrancesco, D. (1993). Pacemaker mechanisms in cardiac tissue. Annual Review of Physiology, 55, 455–472.

17. Baruscotti, M., Bucchi, A., DiFrancesco, D. (2005). Physiology and pharmacology of the cardiac pacemaker ("funny") current. Pharmacology & Therapeutics, 107, 59–79.

18. Chang, F., Cohen, I.S., DiFrancesco, D., Rosen, M.R., Tromba, C. (1991). Effects of protein kinase inhibitors on canine Purkinje fibre pacemaker depolarization and the pacemaker current i(f). Journal of Physiology, 440, 367–384.

19. Accili, E.A., Redaelli, G., DiFrancesco, D. (1997). Differential control of the hyperpo-larization-activated current (i(f)) by cAMP gating and phosphatase inhibition in rabbit sino-atrial node myocytes. Journal of Physiology, 500, 643–651.

20. Qu, J., Kryukova, Y., Potapova, I.A., Doronin, S.V., Larsen, M., Krishnamurthy, G., Cohen, I.S., Robinson, R.B. (2004). MiRP1 modulates HCN2 channel expression and gating in cardiac myocytes. Journal of Biological Chemistry, 279, 43497–43502.

21. Barbuti, A., Gravante, B., Riolfo, M., Milanesi, R., Terragni, B., DiFrancesco, D. (2004). Localization of pacemaker channels in lipid rafts regulates channel kinetics. Circulation Research, 94, 1325–1331.

22. Pian, P., Bucchi, A., Robinson, R.B., Siegelbaum, S.A. (2006). Regulation of gating and rundown of HCN hyperpolarization-activated channels by exogenous and endogenous PIP2. Journal of General Physiology, 128, 593–604.

23. Pian, P., Bucchi, A., Decostanzo, A., Robinson, R.B., Siegelbaum, S.A. (2007). Modulation of cyclic nucleotide-regulated HCN channels by PIP(2) and receptors coupled to phospholipase C. Pflugers Archiv—European Journal of Physiology, 455, 125–145.

24. DiFrancesco, D., Ferroni, A., Mazzanti, M., Tromba, C. (1986). Properties of the hyperpolarizing-activated current (if) in cells isolated from the rabbit sino-atrial node. Journal of Physiology, 377, 61–88.

25. DiFrancesco, D. (1991). The contribution of the 'pacemaker' current (if) to generation of spontaneous activity in rabbit sino-atrial node myocytes. Journal of Physiology, 434, 23–40.

26. Yu, H., Chang, F., Cohen, I.S. (1993). Phosphatase inhibition by calyculin A increases i(f) in canine Purkinje fibers and myocytes. Pflugers Archiv—European Journal of Physiology, 422, 614–616.

27. Wu, J.Y., Cohen, I.S. (1997). Tyrosine kinase inhibition reduces i(f) in rabbit sinoatrial node myocytes. Pflugers Archiv—European Journal of Physiology, 434, 509–514.

28. DiFrancesco, D. (1995). Cardiac pacemaker: 15 years of "new" interpretation. Acta Cardiologica, 50, 413–427.

29. Yu, H., Chang, F., Cohen, I.S. (1993). Pacemaker current exists in ventricular myocytes. Circulation Research, 72, 232–236.

30. DiFrancesco, D., Ferroni, A. (1983). Delayed activation of the cardiac pacemaker current and its dependence on conditioning pre-hyperpolarizations. Pflugers Archiv—European Journal of Physiology, 396, 265–267.

31. DiFrancesco, D., Noble, D. (1985). A model of cardiac electrical activity incorporating ionic pumps and concentration changes. Philosophical Transactions of The Royal Society B, 307, 353–398.

32. McCormick, D.A., Pape, H.C. (1990). Properties of a hyperpolarization-activated cation current and its role in rhythmic oscillation in thalamic relay neurones. Journal of Physiology, 431, 291–318.

33. Noble, D., DiFrancesco, D., Denyer, J. (1989). Ionic Mechanisms in Normal and Abnormal Cardiac Pacemaker Activity in Neuronal and Cellular Oscillators. Jacket JW, New York, pp. 59–85.

34. van Ginneken, A.C., Giles, W. (1991). Voltage clamp measurements of the hyperpolari-zation-activated inward current I(f) in single cells from rabbit sino-atrial node. Journal of Physiology, 434, 57–83.

35. Demir, S.S., Clark, J.W., Murphey, C.R., Giles, W.R. (1994). A mathematical model of a rabbit sinoatrial node cell. American Journal of Physiology, 266, C832–C852.

36. DiFrancesco, D. (1984). Characterization of the pace-maker current kinetics in calf Purkinje fibres. Journal of Physiology, 348, 341–367.

37. Altomare, C., Bucchi, A., Camatini, E., Baruscotti, M., Viscomi, C., Moroni, A., DiFrancesco, D. (2001). Integrated allosteric model of voltage gating of HCN channels. Journal of General Physiology, 117, 519–532.

38. Frace, A.M., Maruoka, F., Noma, A. (1992). External $K+$ increases $Na+$ conductance of the hyperpolarization-activated current in rabbit cardiac pacemaker cells. Pflugers Archiv—European Journal of Physiology, 421, 97–99.

39. Wollmuth, L.P., Hille, B. (1992). Ionic selectivity of Ih channels of rod photoreceptors in tiger salamanders. Journal of General Physiology, 100, 749–765.

40. Hille, B. (2001). Ionic Channels of Excitable Membranes. Sinauer Associates Inc, Sunderland, MA, pp. 337–361.

41. Bucchi, A., Baruscotti, M., DiFrancesco, D. (2002). Current-dependent block of rabbit sino-atrial node I(f) channels by ivabradine. Journal of General Physiology, 120, 1–13.

42. DiFrancesco, D., Tortora, P. (1991). Direct activation of cardiac pacemaker channels by intracellular cyclic AMP. Nature, 351, 145–147.

43. Bucchi, A., Baruscotti, M., Robinson, R.B., DiFrancesco, D. (2007). Modulation of rate by autonomic agonists in SAN cells involves changes in diastolic depolarization and the pacemaker current. Journal of Molecular and Cellular Cardiology, 43, 39–48.

44. Barbuti, A., Baruscotti, M., DiFrancesco, D. (2007). The pacemaker current: from basics to the clinics. Journal of Cardiovascular Electrophysiology, 18, 342–347.

45. Barbuti, A., Terragni, B., Brioschi, C., DiFrancesco, D. (2007). Localization of f-channels to caveolae mediates specific beta2-adrenergic receptor modulation of rate in sinoatrial myocytes. Journal of Molecular and Cellular Cardiology, 42, 71–78.

46. Robinson, R.B., Yu, H., Chang, F., Cohen, I.S. (1997). Developmental change in the voltage-dependence of the pacemaker current, if, in rat ventricle cells. Pflugers Archiv—European Journal of Physiology, 433, 533–535.

47. Cerbai, E., Pino, R., Sartiani, L., Mugelli, A. (1999). Influence of postnatal-development on I(f) occurrence and properties in neonatal rat ventricular myocytes. Cardiovascular Research, 42, 416–423.

48. Sartiani, L., Bettiol, E., Stillitano, F., Mugelli, A., Cerbai, E., Jaconi, M.E. (2007). Developmental changes in cardiomyocytes differentiated from human embryonic stem cells: a molecular and electrophysiological approach. Stem Cells, 25, 1136–1144.

49. Cerbai, E., Mugelli, A. (2006). I(f) in non-pacemaker cells: Role and pharmacological implications. Pharmacological Research, 53, 416–423.

50. Abi-Gerges, N., Ji, G.J., Lu, Z.J., Fischmeister, R., Hescheler, J., Fleischmann, B.K. (2000). Functional expression and regulation of the hyperpolarization activated non-selective cation current in embryonic stem cell-derived cardiomyocytes. Journal of Physiology, 523, 377–389.

51. Yasui, K., Liu, W., Opthof, T., Kada, K., Lee, J.K., Kamiya, K., Kodama, I. (2001). I(f) current and spontaneous activity in mouse embryonic ventricular myocytes. Circulation Research, 88, 536–542.

52. White, S.M., Claycomb, W.C. (2005). Embryonic stem cells form an organized, functional cardiac conduction system in vitro. American Journal of Physiology Heart and Circulatory Physiology, 288, H670–H679.

53. Qu, Y., Whitaker, G.M., Hove-Madsen, L., Tibbits, G.F., Accili, E.A. (2007). Hyperpolarization-activated cyclic nucleotide-modulated 'HCN' channels confer regular and faster rhythmicity to beating mouse embryonic stem cells. Journal of Physiology, 586, 701–716.

54. van Kempen, M., van Ginneken, A., de, G., I, Mutsaers, N., Opthof, T., Jongsma, H., van der, H.M. (2003). Expression of the electrophysiological system during murine embryonic stem cell cardiac differentiation. Cellular Physiology and Biochemistry, 13, 263–270.

55. Wang, K., Xue, T., Tsang, S.Y., Van Huizen, R., Wong, C.W., Lai, K.W., Ye, Z., Cheng, L., Au, K.W., Zhang, J., Li, G.R., Lau, C.P., Tse, H.F., Li, R.A. (2005). Electrophysiological properties of pluripotent human and mouse embryonic stem cells. Stem Cells, 23, 1526–1534.

56. Fernandez-Velasco, M., Goren, N., Benito, G., Blanco-Rivero, J., Bosca, L., Delgado, C. (2003). Regional distribution of hyperpolarization-activated current (If) and hyperpolarization-activated cyclic nucleotide-gated channel mRNA expression in ventricular cells from control and hypertrophied rat hearts. Journal of Physiology, 553, 395–405.

57. Zicha, S., Fernandez-Velasco, M., Lonardo, G., L'Heureux, N., Nattel, S. (2005). Sinus node dysfunction and hyperpolarization-activated (HCN) channel subunit remodeling in a canine heart failure model. Cardiovascular Research, 66, 472–481.

58. Wit, A.L., Fenoglio, J.J., Jr., Wagner, B.M., Bassett, A.L. (1973). Electrophysiological properties of cardiac muscle in the anterior mitral valve leaflet and the adjacent atrium in the dog. Possible implications for the genesis of atrial dysrhythmias. Circulation Research, 32, 731–745.

59. Wit, A.L., Fenoglio, J.J., Jr., Hordof, A.J., Reemtsma, K. (1979). Ultrastructure and transmembrane potentials of cardiac muscle in the human anterior mitral valve leaflet. Circulation, 59, 1284–1292.

60. Chen, Y.J., Chen, S.A., Chang, M.S., Lin, C.I. (2000). Arrhythmogenic activity of cardiac muscle in pulmonary veins of the dog: Implication for the genesis of atrial fibrillation. Cardiovascular Research, 48, 265–273.

61. Chen, Y.J., Chen, S.A., Chen, Y.C., Yeh, H.I., Chan, P., Chang, M.S., Lin, C.I. (2001). Effects of rapid atrial pacing on the arrhythmogenic activity of single cardiomyocytes from pulmonary veins: Implication in initiation of atrial fibrillation. Circulation, 104, 2849–2854.

62. Liu, J., Huang, C.X., Jiang, H., Bao, M.W., Cao, F., Wang, T. (2005). Characteristics of hyperpolarization-activated inward current in rabbit pulmonary vein muscle sleeve cells. Chinese Medical Journal (English Edition), 118, 2014–2019.

63. Perez-Lugones, A., McMahon, J.T., Ratliff, N.B., Saliba, W.I., Schweikert, R.A., Marrouche, N.F., Saad, E.B., Navia, J.L., McCarthy, P.M., Tchou, P., Gillinov, A.M., Natale, A. (2003). Evidence of specialized conduction cells in human pulmonary veins of patients with atrial fibrillation. Journal of Cardiovascular Electrophysiology, 14, 803–809.

64. Anumonwo, J.M., Delmar, M., Jalife, J. (1990). Electrophysiology of single heart cells from the rabbit tricuspid valve. Journal of Physiology, 425, 145–167.

65. Hundal, S.P., DiFrancesco, D., Mangoni, M., Brammar, W.J., Conley, E.C. (1993). An isoform of the cGMP-gated retinal photoreceptor channel gene expressed in the sinoatrial node (pacemaker) region of rabbit heart. Biochemical Society Transactions, 21, 119S.

66. Santoro, B., Grant, S.G., Bartsch, D., Kandel, E.R. (1997). Interactive cloning with the SH3 domain of N-src identifies a new brain specific ion channel protein, with homology to eag and cyclic nucleotide-gated channels. Proceedings of the National Academy of Sciences USA, 94, 14815–14820.

67. Santoro, B., Liu, D.T., Yao, H., Bartsch, D., Kandel, E.R., Siegelbaum, S.A., Tibbs, G.R. (1998). Identification of a gene encoding a hyperpolarization-activated pacemaker channel of brain. Cell, 93, 717–729.

68. Ludwig, A., Zong, X., Jeglitsch, M., Hofmann, F., Biel, M. (1998). A family of hyperpolarization-activated mammalian cation channels. Nature, 393, 587–591.

69. Gauss, R., Seifert, R., Kaupp, U.B. (1998). Molecular identification of a hyperpolariza-tion-activated channel in sea urchin sperm. Nature, 393, 583–587.

70. Jackson, H.A., Marshall, C.R., Accili, E.A. (2007). Evolution and structural diversifica-tion of hyperpolarization-activated cyclic nucleotide-gated channel genes. Physiological Genomics, 29, 231–245.

71. Robinson, R.B., Siegelbaum, S.A. (2003). Hyperpolarization-activated cation currents: from molecules to physiological function. Annual Review of Physiology, 65, 453–480.

72. Vaccari, T., Moroni, A., Rocchi, M., Gorza, L., Bianchi, M.E., Beltrame, M., DiFrancesco, D. (1999). The human gene coding for HCN2, a pacemaker channel of the heart. Biochimica et Biophysica Acta, 1446, 419–425.

73. Seifert, R., Scholten, A., Gauss, R., Mincheva, A., Lichter, P., Kaupp, U.B. (1999). Molecular characterization of a slowly gating human hyperpolarization- activated channel predominantly expressed in thalamus, heart, and testis. Proceedings of the National Academy of Sciences USA, 96, 9391–9396.

74. Ulens, C., Tytgat, J. (2001). Functional Heteromerization of HCN1 and HCN2 Pacemaker Channels. Journal of Biological Chemistry, 276, 6069–6072.

75. Chen, S., Wang, J., Siegelbaum, S.A. (2001). Properties of hyperpolarization-activated pacemaker current defined by coassembly of HCN1 and HCN2 subunits and basal modulation by cyclic nucleotide. Journal of General Physiology, 117, 491–504.

76. Zagotta, W.N., Olivier, N.B., Black, K.D., Young, E.C., Olson, R., Gouaux, E. (2003). Structural basis for modulation and agonist specificity of HCN pacemaker channels. Nature, 425, 200–205.

77. Much, B., Wahl-Schott, C., Zong, X., Schneider, A., Baumann, L., Moosmang, S., Ludwig, A., Biel, M. (2003). Role of subunit heteromerization and N-linked glycosyla-tion in the formation of functional hyperpolarization-activated cyclic nucleotide-gated channels. Journal of Biological Chemistry, 278, 43781–43786.

78. Stieber, J., Stockl, G., Herrmann, S., Hassfurth, B., Hofmann, F. (2005). Functional expression of the human HCN3 channel. Journal of Biological Chemistry, 280, 34635–34643.

79. Mistrik, P., Mader, R., Michalakis, S., Weidinger, M., Pfeifer, A., Biel, M. (2005). The murine HCN3 gene encodes a hyperpolarization-activated cation channel with slow kinetics and unique response to cyclic nucleotides. Journal of Biological Chemistry, 280, 27056–27061.

80. Altomare, C., Terragni, B., Brioschi, C., Milanesi, R., Pagliuca, C., Viscomi, C., Moroni, A., Baruscotti, M., DiFrancesco, D. (2003). Heteromeric HCN1-HCN4 channels: A comparison with native pacemaker channels from the rabbit sinoatrial node. Journal of Physiology, 549, 347–359.

81. Ishii, T.M., Takano, M., Ohmori, H. (2001). Determinants of activation kinetics in mammalian hyperpolarization-activated cation channels. Journal of Physiology, 537, 93–100.

82. Xue, T., Marban, E., Li, R.A. (2002). Dominant-negative suppression of HCN1- and HCN2-encoded pacemaker currents by an engineered HCN1 construct: Insights into structure-function relationships and multimerization. Circulation Research, 90, 1267–1273.

83. Yu, H., Wu, J., Potapova, I., Wymore, R.T., Holmes, B., Zuckerman, J., Pan, Z., Wang, H., Shi, W., Robinson, R.B., El Maghrabi, M.R., Benjamin, W., Dixon, J., McKinnon, D., Cohen, I.S., Wymore, R. (2001). MinK-related peptide 1: A beta subunit for the HCN ion channel subunit family enhances expression and speeds activation. Circulation Research, 88, E84–E87.

84. Decher, N., Bundis, F., Vajna, R., Steinmeyer, K. (2003). KCNE2 modulates current amplitudes and activation kinetics of HCN4: Influence of KCNE family members on HCN4 currents. Pflugers Archiv—European Journal of Physiology, 446, 633–640.

85. Zong, X., Eckert, C., Yuan, H., Wahl-Schott, C., Abicht, H., Fang, L., Li, R., Mistrik, P., Gerstner, A., Much, B., Baumann, L., Michalakis, S., Zeng, R., Chen, Z., Biel, M. (2005). A novel mechanism of modulation of hyperpolarization-activated cyclic nucleotide-gated channels by Src kinase. Journal of Biological Chemistry, 280, 34224–34232.

86. Arinsburg, S.S., Cohen, I.S., Yu, H.G. (2006). Constitutively active Src tyrosine kinase changes gating of HCN4 channels through direct binding to the channel proteins. Journal of Cardiovascular Pharmacology, 47, 578–586.

87. Qu, J., Altomare, C., Bucchi, A., DiFrancesco, D., Robinson, R.B. (2002). Functional comparison of HCN isoforms expressed in ventricular and HEK 293 cells. Pflugers Archiv—European Journal of Physiology, 444, 597–601.

88. Shi, W., Wymore, R., Yu, H., Wu, J., Wymore, R.T., Pan, Z., Robinson, R.B., Dixon, J.E., McKinnon, D., Cohen, I.S. (1999). Distribution and prevalence of hyperpolarization-activated cation channel (HCN) mRNA expression in cardiac tissues. Circulation Research, 85, e1–e6.

89. Moroni, A., Gorza, L., Beltrame, M., Gravante, B., Vaccari, T., Bianchi, M.E., Altomare, C., Longhi, R., Heurteaux, C., Vitadello, M., Malgaroli, A., DiFrancesco, D. (2001). Hyperpolarization-activated cyclic nucleotide-gated channel 1 is a molecular determinant of the cardiac pacemaker current I(f). Journal of Biological Chemistry, 276, 29233–29241.

90. Yamamoto, M., Dobrzynski, H., Tellez, J., Niwa, R., Billeter, R., Honjo, H., Kodama, I., Boyett, M.R. (2006). Extended atrial conduction system characterised by the expression of the HCN4 channel and connexin45. Cardiovascular Research, 72, 271–281.

91. Liu, J., Noble, P.J., Xiao, G., Abdelrahman, M., Dobrzynski, H., Boyett, M.R., Lei, M., Noble, D. (2007). Role of pacemaking current in cardiac nodes: Insights from a comparative study of sinoatrial node and atrioventricular node. Progress in Biophysics and Molecular Biology, 96, 294–304.

92. Liu, J., Dobrzynski, H., Yanni, J., Boyett, M.R., Lei, M. (2007). Organisation of the mouse sinoatrial node: Structure and expression of HCN channels. Cardiovascular Research, 73, 729–738.

93. Giorgetti, A., Carloni, P., Mistrik, P., Torre, V. (2005). A homology model of the pore region of HCN channels. Biophysical Journal, 89, 932–944.

94. Shin, K.S., Rothberg, B.S., Yellen, G. (2001). Blocker state dependence and trapping in hyperpolarization-activated cation channels: Evidence for an intracellular activation gate. Journal of General Physiology, 117, 91–101.

95. Doyle, D.A., Morais, C.J., Pfuetzner, R.A., Kuo, A., Gulbis, J.M., Cohen, S.L., Chait, B.T., MacKinnon, R. (1998). The structure of the potassium channel: Molecular basis of K+ conduction and selectivity. Science, 280, 69–77.

96. Sigworth, F.J. (1994). Voltage gating of ion channels. Quarterly Reviews of Biophysics, 27, 1–40.

97. Bezanilla, F. (2000). The voltage sensor in voltage-dependent ion channels. Physiological Reviews, 80, 555–592.

98. Chen, J., Mitcheson, J.S., Tristani-Firouzi, M., Lin, M., Sanguinetti, M.C. (2001). The S4-S5 linker couples voltage sensing and activation of pacemaker channels. Proceedings of the National Academy of Sciences USA, 98, 11277–11282.

99. Decher, N., Chen, J., Sanguinetti, M.C. (2004). Voltage-dependent gating of hyperpolarization-activated, cyclic nucleotide-gated pacemaker channels: Molecular coupling between the S4-S5 and C-linkers. Journal of Biological Chemistry, 279, 13859–13865.

100. Vaca, L., Stieber, J., Zong, X., Ludwig, A., Hofmann, F., Biel, M. (2000). Mutations in the S4 domain of a pacemaker channel alter its voltage dependence. FEBS Letters, 479, 35–40.

101. Long, S.B., Campbell, E.B., MacKinnon, R. (2005). Voltage sensor of Kv1.2: Structural basis of electromechanical coupling. Science, 309, 903–908.

102. Mannikko, R., Elinder, F., Larsson, H.P. (2002). Voltage-sensing mechanism is conserved among ion channels gated by opposite voltages. Nature, 419, 837–841.

103. Prole, D.L., Yellen, G. (2006). Reversal of HCN channel voltage dependence via bridging of the S4-S5 linker and post-S6. Journal of General Physiology, 128, 273–282.

104. Ferrer, T., Rupp, J., Piper, D.R., Tristani-Firouzi, M. (2006). The S4-S5 linker directly couples voltage sensor movement to the activation gate in the human ether-a'-go-go-related gene (hERG) K+ channel. Journal of Biological Chemistry, 281, 12858–12864.

105. Lu, Z., Klem, A.M., Ramu, Y. (2002). Coupling between voltage sensors and activation gate in voltage-gated K+ channels. Journal of General Physiology, 120, 663–676.

106. Xue, T., Li, R.A. (2002). An external determinant in the S5-P linker of the pacemaker (HCN) channel identified by sulfhydryl modification. Journal of Biological Chemistry, 277, 46233–46242.

107. Au, K.W., Siu, C.W., Lau, C.P., Tse, H.F., Li, R.A. (2008). Structural and functional determinants in the S5-P region of HCN-encoded pacemaker channels revealed by cysteine-scanning substitutions. American Journal of Physiology Cellular Physiology, 294, C136–C144.

108. DiFrancesco, D., Mangoni, M. (1994). Modulation of single hyperpolarization-activated channels (i(f)) by cAMP in the rabbit sino-atrial node. Journal of Physiology, 474, 473–482.

109. DiFrancesco, D. (1999). Dual allosteric modulation of pacemaker (f) channels by cAMP and voltage in rabbit SA node. Journal of Physiology, 515, 367–376.

110. Barbuti, A., Baruscotti, M., Altomare, C., Moroni, A., DiFrancesco, D. (1999). Action of internal pronase on the f-channel kinetics in the rabbit SA node. Journal of Physiology, 520, 737–744.

111. Wainger, B.J., DeGennaro, M., Santoro, B., Siegelbaum, S.A., Tibbs, G.R. (2001). Molecular mechanism of cAMP modulation of HCN pacemaker channels. Nature, 411, 805–810.

112. Craven, K.B., Zagotta, W.N. (2004). Salt bridges and gating in the COOH-terminal region of HCN2 and CNGA1 channels. Journal of General Physiology, 124, 663–677.

113. Zhou, L., Olivier, N.B., Yao, H., Young, E.C., Siegelbaum, S.A. (2004). A conserved tripeptide in CNG and HCN channels regulates ligand gating by controlling C-terminal oligomerization. Neuron, 44, 823–834.

114. Zhou, L., Siegelbaum, S.A. (2007). Gating of HCN channels by cyclic nucleotides: Residue contacts that underlie ligand binding, selectivity, and efficacy. Structure, 15, 655–670.

115. Tellez, J.O., Dobrzynski, H., Greener, I.D., Graham, G.M., Laing, E., Honjo, H., Hubbard, S.J., Boyett, M.R., Billeter, R. (2006). Differential expression of ion channel transcripts in atrial muscle and sinoatrial node in rabbit. Circulation Research, 99, 1384–1393.

116. Qu, J., Barbuti, A., Protas, L., Santoro, B., Cohen, I.S., Robinson, R.B. (2001). HCN2 overexpression in newborn and adult ventricular myocytes: Distinct effects on gating and excitability. Circulation Research, 89, E8–14.

117. Zolles, G., Klocker, N., Wenzel, D., Weisser-Thomas, J., Fleischmann, B.K., Roeper, J., Fakler, B. (2006). Pacemaking by HCN channels requires interaction with phosphoinositides. Neuron, 52, 1027–1036.

118. Li, C.H., Zhang, Q., Teng, B., Mustafa, S.J., Huang, J.Y., Yu, H.G. (2008). Src tyrosine kinase alters gating of hyperpolarization-activated HCN4 pacemaker channel through Tyr531. American Journal of Physiology Cellular Physiology, 294, C355–C362.

119. Kryukova, Y., Rybin, V.O., Qu, J., Steinberg, S.F., Robinson, R.B. (2008). Age-dependent differences in the inhibition of HCN2 current in rat ventricular myocytes by the tyrosine kinase inhibitor erbstatin. Pflugers Archiv—European Journal of Physiology, 457, 821–830.

120. Yu, H.G., Lu, Z., Pan, Z., Cohen, I.S. (2004). Tyrosine kinase inhibition differentially regulates heterologously expressed HCN channels. Pflugers Archiv—European Journal of Physiology, 447, 392–400.

121. Huang, J., Huang, A., Zhang, Q., Lin, Y.C., Yu, H.G. (2008). A novel mechanism for suppression of HCN pacemaker channels by receptor-like tyrosine phosphatase alpha. Journal of Biological Chemistry, 283, 29912–29919.

122. Haas, M., Askari, A., Xie, Z. (2000). Involvement of Src and epidermal growth factor receptor in the signal-transducing function of Na + /K + -ATPase. Journal of Biological Chemistry, 275, 27832–27837.

123. Huang, X., Yang, P., Du, Y., Zhang, J., Ma, A. (2007). Age-related down-regulation of HCN channels in rat sinoatrial node. Basic Research in Cardiology, 102, 429–435.

124. Stillitano, F., Lonardo, G., Zicha, S., Varro, A., Cerbai, E., Mugelli, A., Nattel, S. (2008). Molecular basis of funny current (If) in normal and failing human heart. Journal of Molecular and Cellular Cardiology, 45, 289–299.

125. Pitt, B., Zannad, F., Remme, W.J., Cody, R., Castaigne, A., Perez, A., Palensky, J., Wittes, J. (1999). The effect of spironolactone on morbidity and mortality in patients with severe heart failure. Randomized Aldactone Evaluation Study Investigators. New England Journal of Medicine, 341, 709–717.

126. Pitt, B., Williams, G., Remme, W., Martinez, F., Lopez-Sendon, J., Zannad, F., Neaton, J., Roniker, B., Hurley, S., Burns, D., Bittman, R., Kleiman, J. (2001). The EPHESUS trial: Eplerenone in patients with heart failure due to systolic dysfunction complicating acute myocardial infarction. Eplerenone Post-AMI Heart Failure Efficacy and Survival Study. Cardiovascular Drugs and Therapy, 15, 79–87.

127. Muto, T., Ueda, N., Opthof, T., Ohkusa, T., Nagata, K., Suzuki, S., Tsuji, Y., Horiba, M., Lee, J.K., Honjo, H., Kamiya, K., Kodama, I., Yasui, K. (2007). Aldosterone modulates I(f) current through gene expression in cultured neonatal rat ventricular myocytes. American Journal of Physiology, 293, H2710–H2718.

128. Kuwahara, K., Saito, Y., Takano, M., Arai, Y., Yasuno, S., Nakagawa, Y., Takahashi, N., Adachi, Y., Takemura, G., Horie, M., Miyamoto, Y., Morisaki, T., Kuratomi, S., Noma, A., Fujiwara, H., Yoshimasa, Y., Kinoshita, H., Kawakami, R., Kishimoto, I., Nakanishi, M., Usami, S., Saito, Y., Harada, M., Nakao, K. (2003). NRSF regulates the fetal cardiac gene program and maintains normal cardiac structure and function. EMBO Journal, 22, 6310–6321.

129. Kuratomi, S., Kuratomi, A., Kuwahara, K., Ishii, T.M., Nakao, K., Saito, Y., Takano, M. (2007). NRSF regulates the developmental and hypertrophic changes of HCN4 transcription in rat cardiac myocytes. Biochemical and Biophysical Research Communications, 353, 67–73.

130. Van Bogaert, P.P., Goethals, M. (1987). Pharmacological influence of specific bradycardic agents on the pacemaker current of sheep cardiac Purkinje fibres. A comparison between three different molecules. European Heart Journal, 8, 35–42.

131. BoSmith, R.E., Briggs, I., Sturgess, N.C. (1993). Inhibitory actions of ZENECA ZD7288 on whole-cell hyperpolarization activated inward current (If) in guinea-pig dissociated sinoatrial node cells. British Journal of Pharmacology, 110, 343–349.

132. Van Bogaert, P.P., Pittoors, F. (2003). Use-dependent blockade of cardiac pacemaker current (If) by cilobradine and zatebradine. European Journal of Pharmacology, 478, 161–171.

133. Yusuf, S., Camm, A.J. (2003). Sinus tachyarrhythmias and the specific bradycardic agents: a marriage made in heaven? Journal of Cardiovascular Pharmacology & Therapeutics, 8, 89–105.

134. Stockhaus, K. (1977). Problems of Drug Dependence. National Academy of Sciences, Cambridge, MA, pp. 355–366.

135. Millar, J.S., Williams, E.M. (1981). Pacemaker selectivity: Influence on rabbit atria of ionic environment and of alinidine, a possible anion antagonist. Cardiovascular Research, 15, 335–350.

136. Kobinger, W., Lillie, C., Pichler, L. (1979). N-Allyl-derivative of clonidine, a substance with specific bradycardic action at a cardiac site. Naunyn-Schmiedeberg's Archives of Pharmacology, 306, 255–262.

137. Lillie, C., Kobinger, W. (1983). Comparison of the bradycardic effects of alinidine (St 567), AQ-A 39 and verapamil on guinea-pig sinoatrial node superfused with different Ca2 + and NaCl solutions. European Journal of Pharmacology, 87, 25–33.

138. Traunecker, W., Walland, A. (1980). Haemodynamic and electrophysiologic actions of alinidine in the dog. Archives internationales de pharmacodynamie et de thérapie, 244, 58–72.

139. Satoh, H., Hashimoto, K. (1986). Electrophysiological study of alinidine in voltage clamped rabbit sino-atrial node cells. European Journal of Pharmacology, 121, 211–219.

140. Snyders, D.J., Van Bogaert, P.P. (1987). Alinidine modifies the pacemaker current in sheep Purkinje fibers. Pflugers Archiv—European Journal of Physiology, 410, 83–91.

141. van Ginneken, A.C., Bouman, L.N., Jongsma, H.J., Duivenvoorden, J.J., Opthof, T., Giles, W.R. (1987). Alinidine as a model of the mode of action of specific bradycardic agents on SA node activity. European Heart Journal, 8, 25–33.

142. Shanks, R.G. (1987). The clinical pharmacology of alinidine and its side-effects. European Heart Journal, 8, 83–90.

143. Harron, D.W., Jady, K., Riddell, J.G., Shanks, R.G. (1982). Effects of alinidine, a novel bradycardic agent, on heart rate and blood pressure in man. Journal of Cardiovascular Pharmacology, 4, 213–220.

144. Jaski, B.E., Serruys, P.W. (1985). Anion-channel blockade with alinidine: A specific bradycardic drug for coronary heart disease without negative inotropic activity? American Journal of Cardiology, 56, 270–275.

145. Hohnloser, S., Weirich, J., Homburger, H., Antoni, H. (1982). Electrophysiological studies on effects of AQ-A 39 in the isolated guinea pig heart and myocardial preparations. Arzneimittelforschung, 32, 730–734.

146. Verdouw, P.D., Bom, H.P., Bijleveld, R.E. (1983). Cardiovascular responses to increasing plasma concentrations of AQ-A 39 Cl, a new compound with negative chronotropic effects. Arzneimittelforschung, 33, 702–706.

147. Kobinger, W., Lillie, C. (1984). Cardiovascular characterization of UL-FS 49, 1,3,4,5-tetrahydro-7,8-dimethoxy-3-[3-][2-(3,4-dimethoxyphenyl)ethyl] methylimino]propyl]-2H-3-benzazepin-2-on hydrochloride, a new "specific bradycardic agent". European Journal of Pharmacology 104, 9–18.

148. Franke, H., Su, C.A., Schumacher, K., Seiberling, M. (1987). Clinical pharmacology of two specific bradycardiac agents. European Heart Journal, 8, 91–98.

149. Riley, D.C., Gross, G.J., Kampine, J.P., Warltier, D.C. (1987). Specific bradycardic agents, a new therapeutic modality for anesthesiology: Hemodynamic effects of UL-FS 49 and propranolol in conscious and isoflurane-anesthetized dogs. Anesthesiology, 67, 707–716.

150. Thollon, C., Cambarrat, C., Vian, J., Prost, J.F., Peglion, J.L., Vilaine, J.P. (1994). Electrophysiological effects of S 16257, a novel sino-atrial node modulator, on rabbit and guinea-pig cardiac preparations: Comparison with UL-FS 49. British Journal of Pharmacology, 112, 37–42.

151. Granetzny, A., Schwanke, U., Schmitz, C., Arnold, G., Schafer, D., Schulte, H.D., Gams, E., Schipke, J.D. (1998). Pharmacologic heart rate reduction: Effect of a novel, specific bradycardic agent on the heart. Thoracic and Cardiovascular Surgeon, 46, 63–69.

152. Cheng, Y., George, I., Yi, G.H., Reiken, S., Gu, A., Tao, Y.K., Muraskin, J., Qin, S., He, K.L., Hay, I., Yu, K., Oz, M.C., Burkhoff, D., Holmes, J., Wang, J. (2007). Bradycardic therapy improves left ventricular function and remodeling in dogs with coronary embolization-induced chronic heart failure. Journal of Pharmacology and Experimental Therapeutics, 321, 469–476.

153. DiFrancesco, D. (1994). Some properties of the UL-FS 49 block of the hyperpolarization-activated current (i(f)) in sino-atrial node myocytes. Pflugers Archiv—European Journal of Physiology, 427, 64–70.

154. Kobinger, W., Lillie, C. (1981). AQ-A 39 (5,6-dimethoxy-2-[3[[alpha-(3,4-dimethoxy)-phenylethyl]methylamino]propyl] phtalimidine), a specific bradycardic agent with direct action on the heart. European Journal of Pharmacology, 72, 153–164.

155. Osterrieder, W., Pelzer, D., Yang, Q.F., Trautwein, W. (1981). The electrophysiological basis of the bradycardic action of AQA 39 on the sinoatrial node. Naunyn-Schmiedeberg's Archives of Pharmacology, 317, 233–237.

156. Pelzer, D., Trautwein, W., McDonald, T.F. (1982). Calcium channel block and recovery from block in mammalian ventricular muscle treated with organic channel inhibitors. Pflugers Archiv—European Journal of Physiology 394, 97–105.

157. Goethals, M., Raes, A., Van Bogaert, P.P. (1993). Use-dependent block of the pacemaker current I(f) in rabbit sinoatrial node cells by zatebradine (UL-FS 49). On the mode of action of sinus node inhibitors. Circulation, 88, 2389–2401.

158. Doerr, T., Trautwein, W. (1990). On the mechanism of the "specific bradycardic action" of the verapamil derivative UL-FS 49. Naunyn-Schmiedeberg's Archives of Pharmacology, 341, 331–340.

159. Bois, P., Bescond, J., Renaudon, B., Lenfant, J. (1996). Mode of action of bradycardic agent, S 16257, on ionic currents of rabbit sinoatrial node cells. British Journal of Pharmacology 118, 1051–1057.

160. Valenzuela, C., Delpon, E., Franqueza, L., Gay, P., Perez, O., Tamargo, J., Snyders, D.J. (1996). Class III antiarrhythmic effects of zatebradine. Time-, state-, use-, and voltage-dependent block of hKv1.5 channels. Circulation, 94, 562–570.

161. Guth, B.D., Heusch, G., Seitelberger, R., Ross, J., Jr. (1987). Elimination of exercise-induced regional myocardial dysfunction by a bradycardiac agent in dogs with chronic coronary stenosis. Circulation, 75, 661–669.

162. Krumpl, G., Winkler, M., Schneider, W., Raberger, G. (1988). Comparison of the haemodynamic effects of the selective bradycardic agent UL-FS 49, with those of propranolol during treadmill exercise in dogs. British Journal of Pharmacology 94, 55–64.

163. Indolfi, C., Guth, B.D., Miura, T., Miyazaki, S., Schulz, R., Ross, J., Jr. (1989). Mechanisms of improved ischemic regional dysfunction by bradycardia. Studies on UL-FS 49 in swine. Circulation, 80, 983–993.

164. Frishman, W.H., Pepine, C.J., Weiss, R.J., Baiker, W.M. (1995). Addition of zatebradine, a direct sinus node inhibitor, provides no greater exercise tolerance benefit in patients with angina taking extended-release nifedipine: Results of a multicenter, randomized, double-blind, placebo-controlled, parallel-group study. The Zatebradine Study Group. Journal of the American College of Cardiology, 26, 305–312.

165. Glasser, S.P., Michie, D.D., Thadani, U., Baiker, W.M. (1997). Effects of zatebradine (ULFS 49 CL), a sinus node inhibitor, on heart rate and exercise duration in chronic stable angina pectoris. Zatebradine Investigators. American Journal of Cardiology, 79, 1401–1405.

166. Satoh, T.O., Yamada, M. (2000). A bradycardiac agent ZD7288 blocks the hyperpolarization-activated current (I(h)) in retinal rod photoreceptors. Neuropharmacology, 39, 1284–1291.

167. Gargini, C., Demontis, G.C., Bisti, S., Cervetto, L. (1999). Effects of blocking the hyperpolarization-activated current (Ih) on the cat electroretinogram. Vision Research, 39, 1767–1774.

168. Stieber, J., Wieland, K., Stockl, G., Ludwig, A., Hofmann, F. (2006). Bradycardic and proarrhythmic properties of sinus node inhibitors. Molecular Pharmacology, 69, 1328–1337.

169. Schmitz-Spanke, S., Granetzny, A., Stoffels, B., Pomblum, V.J., Gams, E., Schipke, J.D. (2004). Effects of a bradycardic agent on postischemic cardiac recovery in rabbits. Journal of Physiology and Pharmacology, 55, 705–712.

170. Maccarone, R., Izzizzari, G., Gargini, C., Cervetto, L., Bisti, S. (2004). The impact of organic inhibitors of the hyperpolarization activated current (Ih) on the electroretinogram (ERG) of rodents. Archives italiennes de biologie, 142, 95–103.

171. Marshall, P.W., Rouse, W., Briggs, I., Hargreaves, R.B., Mills, S.D., McLoughlin, B.J. (1993). ICI D7288, a novel sinoatrial node modulator. Journal of Cardiovascular Pharmacology, 21, 902–906.

172. Briggs, I., BoSmith, R.E., Heapy, C.G. (1994). Effects of Zeneca ZD7288 in comparison with alinidine and UL-FS 49 on guinea pig sinoatrial node and ventricular action potentials. Journal of Cardiovascular Pharmacology, 24, 380–387.

173. Rouse, W., Johnson, I.R. (1994). Haemodynamic actions of a novel sino-atrial node function modulator, ZENECA ZD7288, in the anaesthetized dog: a comparison with zatebradine, atenolol and nitrendipine. British Journal of Pharmacology, 113, 1064–1070.

174. Harris, N.C., Constanti, A. (1995). Mechanism of block by ZD 7288 of the hyperpolarization-activated inward rectifying current in guinea pig substantia nigra neurons in vitro. Journal of Neurophysiology, 74, 2366–2378.

175. Gasparini, S., DiFrancesco, D. (1997). Action of the hyperpolarization-activated current (Ih) blocker ZD 7288 in hippocampal CA1 neurons. Pflugers Archiv—European Journal of Physiology, 435, 99–106.

176. Williams, S.R., Turner, J.P., Hughes, S.W., Crunelli, V. (1997). On the nature of anomalous rectification in thalamocortical neurones of the cat ventrobasal thalamus in vitro. Journal of Physiology, 505, 727–747.

177. Simon, L., Ghaleh, B., Puybasset, L., Giudicelli, J.F., Berdeaux, A. (1995). Coronary and hemodynamic effects of S 16257, a new bradycardic agent, in resting and exercising conscious dogs. Journal of Pharmacology and Experimental Therapeutics 275, 659–666.

178. Thollon, C., Bidouard, J.P., Cambarrat, C., Lesage, L., Reure, H., Delescluse, I., Vian, J., Peglion, J.L., Vilaine, J.P. (1997). Stereospecific in vitro and in vivo effects of the new sinus node inhibitor (+)-S 16257. European Journal of Pharmacology, 339, 43–51.

179. Monnet, X., Ghaleh, B., Colin, P., de Curzon, O.P., Giudicelli, J.F., Berdeaux, A. (2001). Effects of heart rate reduction with ivabradine on exercise-induced myocardial ischemia and stunning. Journal of Pharmacology and Experimental Therapeutics, 299, 1133–1139.

180. Colin, P., Ghaleh, B., Hittinger, L., Monnet, X., Slama, M., Giudicelli, J.F., Berdeaux, A. (2002). Differential effects of heart rate reduction and beta-blockade on left ventricular relaxation during exercise. American Journal of Physiology Heart and Circulatory physiology, 282, H672–H679.

181. Borer, J.S., Fox, K., Jaillon, P., Lerebours, G. (2003). Antianginal and antiischemic effects of ivabradine, an I(f) inhibitor, in stable angina: A randomized, double-blind, multicentered, placebo-controlled trial. Circulation, 107, 817–823.

182. Camm, A.J., Lau, C.P. (2003). Electrophysiological effects of a single intravenous administration of ivabradine (S 16257) in adult patients with normal baseline electrophysiology. Drugs in R&D, 4, 83–89.

183. Vilaine, J.P., Bidouard, J.P., Lesage, L., Reure, H., Peglion, J.L. (2003). Anti-ischemic effects of ivabradine, a selective heart rate-reducing agent, in exercise-induced myocardial ischemia in pigs. Journal of Cardiovascular Pharmacology, 42, 688–696.

184. Colin, P., Ghaleh, B., Monnet, X., Hittinger, L., Berdeaux, A. (2004). Effect of graded heart rate reduction with ivabradine on myocardial oxygen consumption and diastolic time in exercising dogs. Journal of Pharmacology and Experimental Therapeutics, 308, 236–240.

185. Tardif, J.C., Ford, I., Tendera, M., Bourassa, M.G., Fox, K. (2005). Efficacy of ivabradine, a new selective I(f) inhibitor, compared with atenolol in patients with chronic stable angina. European Heart Journal, 26, 2529–2536.

186. Ruzyllo, W., Tendera, M., Ford, I., Fox, K.M. (2007). Antianginal efficacy and safety of ivabradine compared with amlodipine in patients with stable effort angina pectoris: a 3-month randomised, double-blind, multicentre, noninferiority trial. Drugs, 67, 393–405.

187. Lopez-Bescos, L., Filipova, S., Martos, R. (2007). Long-term safety and efficacy of ivabradine in patients with chronic stable angina. Cardiology, 108, 387–396.

188. Fox, K., Ford, I., Steg, P.G., Tendera, M., Robertson, M., Ferrari, R. (2008). Heart rate as a prognostic risk factor in patients with coronary artery disease and left-ventricular systolic dysfunction (BEAUTIFUL): A subgroup analysis of a randomised controlled trial. Lancet, 372, 817–821.

189. Fox, K., Ford, I., Steg, P.G., Tendera, M., Ferrari, R. (2008). Ivabradine for patients with stable coronary artery disease and left-ventricular systolic dysfunction (BEAUTIFUL): A randomised, double-blind, placebo-controlled trial. Lancet, 372, 807–816.

190. Cervetto, L., Demontis, G.C., Gargini, C. (2007). Cellular mechanisms underlying the pharmacological induction of phosphenes. British Journal of Pharmacology, 150, 383–390.

191. Bucchi, A., Tognati, A., Milanesi, R., Baruscotti, M., DiFrancesco, D. (2006). Properties of ivabradine-induced block of HCN1 and HCN4 pacemaker channels. Journal of Physiology, 572, 335–346.

192. Cheng, L., Kinard, K., Rajamani, R., Sanguinetti, M.C. (2007). Molecular mapping of the binding site for a blocker of hyperpolarization-activated, cyclic nucleotide-modulated pacemaker channels. Journal of Pharmacology and Experimental Therapeutics, 322, 931–939.

193. Stieber, J., Herrmann, S., Feil, S., Loster, J., Feil, R., Biel, M., Hofmann, F., Ludwig, A. (2003). The hyperpolarization-activated channel HCN4 is required for the generation of pacemaker action potentials in the embryonic heart. Proceedings of the National Academy of Sciences USA, 100, 15235–15240.

194. Christoffels, V.M., Mommersteeg, M.T., Trowe, M.O., Prall, O.W., Gier-de Vries, C., Soufan, A.T., Bussen, M., Schuster-Gossler, K., Harvey, R.P., Moorman, A.F., Kispert, A. (2006). Formation of the venous pole of the heart from an Nkx2-5-negative precursor population requires Tbx18. Circulation Research, 98, 1555–1563.

195. Moretti, A., Caron, L., Nakano, A., Lam, J.T., Bernshausen, A., Chen, Y., Qyang, Y., Bu, L., Sasaki, M., Martin-Puig, S., Sun, Y., Evans, S.M., Laugwitz, K.L., Chien, K.R. (2006). Multipotent embryonic isl1 + progenitor cells lead to cardiac, smooth muscle, and endothelial cell diversification. Cell, 127, 1151–1165.

196. Mommersteeg, M.T., Hoogaars, W.M., Prall, O.W., Gier-de Vries, C., Wiese, C., Clout, D.E., Papaioannou, V.E., Brown, N.A., Harvey, R.P., Moorman, A.F., Christoffels, V.M. (2007). Molecular pathway for the localized formation of the sinoatrial node. Circulation Research, 100, 354–362.

197. Herrmann, S., Stieber, J., Stockl, G., Hofmann, F., Ludwig, A. (2007). HCN4 provides a 'depolarization reserve' and is not required for heart rate acceleration in mice. EMBO Journal, 26, 4423–4432.

198. Hoesl, E., Stieber, J., Herrmann, S., Feil, S., Tybl, E., Hofmann, F., Feil, R., Ludwig, A. (2008). Tamoxifen-inducible gene deletion in the cardiac conduction system. Journal of Molecular and Cellular Cardiology, 45, 62–69.

199. Ludwig, A., Budde, T., Stieber, J., Moosmang, S., Wahl, C., Holthoff, K., Langebartels, A., Wotjak, C., Munsch, T., Zong, X., Feil, S., Feil, R., Lancel, M., Chien, K.R., Konnerth, A., Pape, H.C., Biel, M., Hofmann, F. (2003). Absence epilepsy and sinus dysrhythmia in mice lacking the pacemaker channel HCN2. EMBO Journal, 22, 216–224.

200. Ashcroft, F.M. (2006). From molecule to malady. Nature, 440, 440–447.

201. Schulze-Bahr, E., Neu, A., Friederich, P., Kaupp, U.B., Breithardt, G., Pongs, O., Isbrandt, D. (2003). Pacemaker channel dysfunction in a patient with sinus node disease. Journal of Clinical Investigation, 111, 1537–1545.

202. Ueda, K., Nakamura, K., Hayashi, T., Inagaki, N., Takahashi, M., Arimura, T., Morita, H., Higashiuesato, Y., Hirano, Y., Yasunami, M., Takishita, S., Yamashina, A., Ohe, T., Sunamori, M., Hiraoka, M., Kimura, A. (2004). Functional characterization of a trafficking-defective HCN4 mutation, D553N, associated with cardiac arrhythmia. Journal of Biological Chemistry, 279, 27194–27198.

203. Milanesi, R., Baruscotti, M., Gnecchi-Ruscone, T., DiFrancesco, D. (2006). Familial sinus bradycardia associated with a mutation in the cardiac pacemaker channel. New England Journal of Medicine, 354, 151–157.

204. Nof, E., Luria, D., Brass, D., Marek, D., Lahat, H., Reznik-Wolf, H., Pras, E., Dascal, N., Eldar, M., Glikson, M. (2007). Point mutation in the HCN4 cardiac ion channel pore affecting synthesis, trafficking, and functional expression is associated with familial asymptomatic sinus bradycardia. Circulation, 116, 463–470.

205. Benditt, D.G., Sakaguchi, S., Goldstein, M.A., et al. Sinus node dysfunction: Pathophysiology, clinical features, evaluation, and treatment, In Zipes, D.P., Jalife, J., eds. Cardiac Electrophysiology. From Cell to Bedside, WB Saunders. Philadelphia, PA, 1995, pp. 1215–1237.

206. Edelberg, J.M., Aird, W.C., Rosenberg, R.D. (1998). Enhancement of murine cardiac chronotropy by the molecular transfer of the human beta2 adrenergic receptor cDNA. Journal of Clinical Investigation, 101, 337–343.

207. Edelberg, J.M., Huang, D.T., Josephson, M.E., Rosenberg, R.D. (2001). Molecular enhancement of porcine cardiac chronotropy. Heart, 86, 559–562.

208. Miake, J., Marban, E., Nuss, H.B. (2002). Biological pacemaker created by gene transfer. Nature, 419, 132–133.

209. Qu, J., Plotnikov, A.N., Danilo, P., Jr., Shlapakova, I., Cohen, I.S., Robinson, R.B., Rosen, M.R. (2003). Expression and function of a biological pacemaker in canine heart. Circulation, 107, 1106–1109.

210. Plotnikov, A.N., Sosunov, E.A., Qu, J., Shlapakova, I.N., Anyukhovsky, E.P., Liu, L., Janse, M.J., Brink, P.R., Cohen, I.S., Robinson, R.B., Danilo, P., Jr., Rosen, M.R. (2004). Biological pacemaker implanted in canine left bundle branch provides ventricular escape rhythms that have physiologically acceptable rates. Circulation, 109, 506–512.

211. Potapova, I., Plotnikov, A., Lu, Z., Danilo, P., Jr., Valiunas, V., Qu, J., Doronin, S., Zuckerman, J., Shlapakova, I.N., Gao, J., Pan, Z., Herron, A.J., Robinson, R.B., Brink, P.R., Rosen, M.R., Cohen, I.S. (2004). Human mesenchymal stem cells as a gene delivery system to create cardiac pacemakers. Circulation Research, 94, 952–959.

212. Bucchi, A., Plotnikov, A.N., Shlapakova, I., Danilo, P., Jr., Kryukova, Y., Qu, J., Lu, Z., Liu, H., Pan, Z., Potapova, I., KenKnight, B., Girouard, S., Cohen, I.S., Brink, P.R., Robinson, R.B., Rosen, M.R. (2006). Wild-type and mutant HCN channels in a tandem biological-electronic cardiac pacemaker. Circulation, 114, 992–999.

213. Plotnikov, A.N., Bucchi, A., Shlapakova, I., Danilo, P., Jr., Brink, P.R., Robinson, R.B., Cohen, I.S., Rosen, M.R. (2008). HCN212-channel biological pacemakers manifesting ventricular tachyarrhythmias are responsive to treatment with I(f) blockade. Heart Rhythm, 5, 282–288.

214. Kehat, I., Khimovich, L., Caspi, O., Gepstein, A., Shofti, R., Arbel, G., Huber, I., Satin, J., Itskovitz-Eldor, J., Gepstein, L. (2004). Electromechanical integration of cardiomyocytes derived from human embryonic stem cells. Nature Biotechnology, 22, 1282–1289.

215. Xue, T., Cho, H.C., Akar, F.G., Tsang, S.Y., Jones, S.P., Marban, E., Tomaselli, G.F., Li, R.A. (2005). Functional integration of electrically active cardiac derivatives from genetically engineered human embryonic stem cells with quiescent recipient ventricular cardiomyocytes: insights into the development of cell-based pacemakers. Circulation, 111, 11–20.

216. Kashiwakura, Y., Cho, H.C., Barth, A.S., Azene, E., Marban, E. (2006). Gene transfer of a synthetic pacemaker channel into the heart: A novel strategy for biological pacing. Circulation, 114, 1682–1686.

217. Cho, H.C., Kashiwakura, Y., Marban, E. (2007). Creation of a biological pacemaker by cell fusion. Circulation Research, 100, 1112–1115.

218. Tse, H.F., Xue, T., Lau, C.P., Siu, C.W., Wang, K., Zhang, Q.Y., Tomaselli, G.F., Akar, F.G., Li, R.A. (2006). Bioartificial sinus node constructed via in vivo gene transfer of an engineered pacemaker HCN Channel reduces the dependence on electronic pacemaker in a sick-sinus syndrome model. Circulation, 114, 1000–1011.

219. Cai, J., Yi, F.F., Li, Y.H., Yang, X.C., Song, J., Jiang, X.J., Jiang, H., Lin, G.S., Wang, W. (2007). Adenoviral gene transfer of HCN4 creates a genetic pacemaker in pigs with complete atrioventricular block. Life Sciences, 80, 1746–1753.

220. Maltsev, V.A., Wobus, A.M., Rohwedel, J., Bader, M., Hescheler, J. (1994). Cardiomyocytes differentiated in vitro from embryonic stem cells developmentally express cardiac-specific genes and ionic currents. Circulation Research, 75, 233–244.

221. Hescheler, J., Fleischmann, B.K., Lentini, S., Maltsev, V.A., Rohwedel, J., Wobus, A.M., Addicks, K. (1997). Embryonic stem cells: a model to study structural and functional properties in cardiomyogenesis. Cardiovascular Research, 36, 149–162.

222. Kehat, I., Kenyagin-Karsenti, D., Snir, M., Segev, H., Amit, M., Gepstein, A., Livne, E., Binah, O., Itskovitz-Eldor, J., Gepstein, L. (2001). Human embryonic stem cells can differentiate into myocytes with structural and functional properties of cardiomyocytes. Journal of Clinical Investigation, 108, 407–414.

223. He, J.Q., Ma, Y., Lee, Y., Thomson, J.A., Kamp, T.J. (2003). Human embryonic stem cells develop into multiple types of cardiac myocytes: action potential characterization. Circulation Research, 93, 32–39.

224. Takahashi, K., Yamanaka, S. (2006). Induction of pluripotent stem cells from mouse embryonic and adult fibroblast cultures by defined factors. Cell, 126, 663–676.

225. Yu, J., Vodyanik, M.A., Smuga-Otto, K., Antosiewicz-Bourget, J., Frane, J.L., Tian, S., Nie, J., Jonsdottir, G.A., Ruotti, V., Stewart, R., Slukvin, I.I., Thomson, J.A. (2007). Induced pluripotent stem cell lines derived from human somatic cells. Science, 318, 1917–1920.

CHAPTER 4

Arrhythmia Mechanisms in Ischemia and Infarction

RUBEN CORONEL, WEN DUN, PENELOPE A. BOYDEN, and
JACQUES M.T. DE BAKKER

4.1 INTRODUCTION

Sudden cardiac death presents a large burden to Western societies [1]. In most cases, death is unexpected and occurs in the absence of preexisting precipitating factors and therefore is probably related to ventricular tachyarrhythmias [1]. Townsend Porter in 1894 already identified coronary occlusion as a main factor for ventricular arrhythmias: He observed cardiac standstill accompanied by fibrillar contraction within minutes after ligation [2]. Although knowledge about the mechanisms of these life-threatening arrhythmias has increased considerably during the last decades, it is still unclear why some patients under otherwise similar conditions die from arrhythmias and others do not [3]. Hereditary factors seem to play a role [3], and environmental conditions also contribute (for example, the composition of the diet and the presence of other diseases). Antiarrhythmic drugs, with the exception of β-adrenergic receptor blocking drugs, are largely ineffective or even harmful [4]. Therefore, knowledge of the mechanisms of life-threatening arrhythmias resulting from ischemia and infarction is important for risk stratification of patients and for the development of interventions to decrease mortality caused by coronary artery disease.

This chapter covers some topics so excellently described previously by Janse and Wit [5]. To make the content of this chapter as current as possible, we have endeavored to incorporate the recent scientific advances that may be of relevance for the development of new therapeutic approaches of arrhythmias related to acute myocardial ischemia and infarction. This chapter is subdivided into three sections, each representing the episodes of specific arrhythmias occurring during the progression of ischemia into infarction as described by Harris [6].

Novel Therapeutic Targets for Antiarrhythmic Drugs, Edited by George Edward Billman
Copyright © 2010 John Wiley & Sons, Inc.

4.1.1 Modes of Ischemia, Phases of Arrhythmogenesis

Myocardial ischemia, which is the disequilibrium of oxygen supply and oxygen demand of cardiac myocardium, comes in many shapes and shades. In clinical cardiology, a complete obstruction of coronary blood flow is often preceded by months or even years of partial occlusion. The latter may remain unnoticed until the full-blown occlusion (total ischemia) occurs. The partial ischemia may lead to intermittent insufficiency of the coronary blood flow or stuttering ischemia, and it may be characterized by diminished coronary blood flow (low-flow ischemia) rather than a complete cessation of blood flow (no-flow ischemia). Although the myocardium has a low oxygen pressure in both cases, metabolites from the ischemic myocardium accumulate in the latter case, whereas washout of these products is still present in the former. Moreover, preceding episodes of transient ischemia may yield the myocardium less vulnerable to subsequent episodes of ischemia. This phenomenon, preconditioning [7], therefore is usually present in patients with angina pectoris, and it may impact on the lethality of the subsequent episode of irreversible ischemia.

Typically, ischemia takes place in only part of the heart, usually the part that depends on blood flow through the stenotic artery. The resulting regional ischemia is in contrast to global ischemia, which affects the entire heart. Global ischemia may result from a pulmonary embolus, asphyxia, or loss of circulation by bleeding or rapid tachyarrhythmias. We will show that, although global ischemia is often used as an experimental model for myocardial ischemia, it strikingly differs from regional ischemia in time course, severity, and mechanism of arrhythmogenesis.

Also, the presence of collateral arteries is a major determinant of the dimensions of the ischemic area and therefore of its propensity to generate arrhythmias [8]. In young patients with a myocardial infarction, lethal arrhythmias occur more often than in older patients with more collateral vessels [9].

Therefore, ventricular arrhythmias occurring during myocardial ischemia depend on many factors, among which are the cause of ischemia and the status of collateral circulation. For the study of arrhythmogenesis, the choice of the mode of ischemia and of the model in which ischemia is studied is important. Extrapolation of experimentally obtained data to the clinical setting strongly depends on the choice of these factors.

Ischemic myocardium does not die immediately, but it can be salvaged by reperfusion. In the absence of relevant reperfusion, necrosis occurs, followed eventually by replacement of viable myocardium by connective tissue: An infarct has developed.

Notwithstanding these admonitions, a generalization can be made with respect to the phases of arrhythmogenesis during myocardial ischemia and infarction.

Harris wrote in his 1943 paper: "Almost all fibrillations occurred within the first 10 min, or not at all during the period of occlusion [10]." If the first phase of arrhythmogenesis was circumvented by application of the "Harris two-stage ligation," whereby a total occlusion was preceded by 30 min of partial occlusion of the coronary artery, a delayed phase of arrhythmogenesis became evident. [6] Thus, the following three periods were described by Harris: 1) an immediate phase of the first 10 minutes after occlusion, 2) an intermediate period of little ectopic activity of 4.5 to 8 h duration, and 3) the delayed ("persistent") period of arrhythmias [6].

The first phase of arrhythmogenesis has been subdivided after the observations by Kaplinsky et al. [11] in dogs. Within the Harris phase 1, Kaplinsky described the immediate-type ventricular arrhythmias (IVA) and the delayed-type ventricular arrhythmias (DVA). The IVAs occurred within 8 min after coronary occlusion, whereas the DVAs occurred between 12 and 15 min of ischemia. Today, these early phases are termed 1a and 1b type arrhythmias [5, 12, 13]. Because the type 1a arrhythmias are often severe, it is difficult to arrive at phase 1b of arrhythmogenesis without using preconditioning protocols [6, 14, 15] or, for example, maintaining a slow cardiac rhythm during phase 1a [16]. This is probably the reason why phase 1b arrhythmias have not been extensively studied. However, the initial description by Kaplinsky et al. [11] makes clear that, despite the substantial risks during phase 1a, relatively more animals die during the 1b phase.

Whether the distinctive phases described in dog and pigs are also found in humans has never been definitely resolved. Rodents usually lack the distinction between phases 1a and 1b [17].

This chapter comprises three parts, each dedicated to a specific period of arrhythmogenesis. The first section deals with the combined phases 1a and 1b of arrhythmias (during the first hour of ischemia), and the second deals with the arrhythmias several days post-occlusion. The last part of this chapter deals with the arrhythmias occurring during chronic infarction, months of years after the acute ischemic event.

4.1.2 Trigger-Substrate-Modulating Factors

According to Coumel [18], arrhythmias occur when a trigger and a substrate coincide. The arrhythmogenic trigger is defined as a single incident that may set off an arrhythmia. An arrhythmogenic substrate is a preexisting condition that facilitates arrhythmogenesis given the presence of a trigger. Both the trigger and substrate are influenced by modulating factors. When discussing arrhythmogenic mechanisms, we have to distinguish between mechanisms underlying the trigger, the substrate, and those of the modulating factors, although the difference between the three sometimes is not clear. The trigger can take the form of a premature beat, which in the setting of regional heterogeneities (the "substrate") may set the stage for reentrant activation and ventricular fibrillation. Alternatively, triggers may consist of acceleration of the heart rate, slowing of heart rate, myocardial stretch, release of sympathetic neurohormones, and so on. A substrate may be formed by the structural changes caused by interstitital fibrosis, the remodeling by hypertrophy and heart failure, changes in calcium handling, dispersion of repolarization caused by regional ischemia, and so forth. Each of these factors may be modulated among others by the autonomic nervous system, the presence of drugs, fever, or dietary components.

4.2 ARRHYTHMOGENESIS IN ACUTE MYOCARDIAL ISCHEMIA

4.2.1 Phase 1A

Acute myocardial ischemia is associated with a plethora of changes in metabolism [19], the composition of the intracellular and extracellular spaces [20–29], and mechanical function [30, 31]. These changes develop within the first seconds or minutes of the onset of ischemia. Each of these changes in isolation may affect the occurrence of arrhythmias. To define the critical ischemia-induced electrophysiological changes that underlie arrhythmogenesis, attempts have been made to isolate individual factors related to ischemia that alone or in combination reproduce the changes observed *in vivo* [32, 33]. The combination of hypoxia, hyperkalemia (11.5 mM), and acidosis was able to more or less reproduce the action potential configuration observed after 5 min of regional ischemia in pig hearts [33]. The definition of the "ischemic" perfusate allowed the study of simulated ischemia in isolated myocardial tissue and myocytes, although it is often difficult to obtain a low enough pO_2. Other methods to study "simulated ischemia" have been used as well by metabolic inhibition (e.g., by the use of cyanide and metabolic uncouplers). In whatever manner ischemia is simulated, the interventions cannot faithfully imitate the absence of perfusion and the inherent accumulation of metabolites in the extracellular space in combination with all the other consequences of ischemia, including the heterogeneities thereof.

Janse et al.[40] have demonstrated the heterogeneities within the myocardium deprived of coronary blood flow. Figure 4.1 is a demonstration of the electrophysiologic and metabolic gradients that occur across the ischemic border of a pig heart [34]. Gradients also exist in the extracellular potassium concentration inside the ischemic myocardium of isolated pig hearts [20, 35]. When the remainder of the heart was perfused with perfusate containing a higher potassium concentration than existed in the ischemic myocardium, the gradient could be reversed, indicating that exchange between the extracellular space of the nonischemic and the ischemic tissue was possible even in the absence of collateral flow (nonexistent in pig) [36]. This exchange is responsible for the gradients in extracellular potassium. In the border zone (inside the ischemic area), the extracellular potassium normalizes after an initial increase [35]. For all other constituents of the extracellular space during ischemia, probably the same holds true. Indeed, gradients in pH have been demonstrated [37, 38].

Heterogeneities caused by ischemia play a decisive role in arrhythmogenesis. This has been shown in experiments in which part of the heart was perfused with a hyperkalemic, hypoxic acidotic perfusate [39]. Although regional simulated ischemia did not always result in ventricular fibrillation (VF) true ischemia superimposed on regional simulated ischemia invariably caused VF and heterogeneities in $[K^+]_o$ within seconds [39].

4.2.1.1   *Mechanisms of Arrhythmias in Phase 1a: Trigger and Substrate.*
The classic epicardial mapping experiments by Janse et al. [40] have contributed significantly to the understanding of the mechanisms of ischemia-induced arrhythmias. These experiments have shown that the electrophysiological mechanism for the maintenance of ischemia-induced ventricular tachycardia and fibrillation is reentry within the ischemic myocardial tissue and that the initiating beat (the "trigger") of the arrhythmia almost always originated from the nonischemic tissue [40]. The multiple reentrant waves circle around temporarily functionally inexcitable tissue. Once the

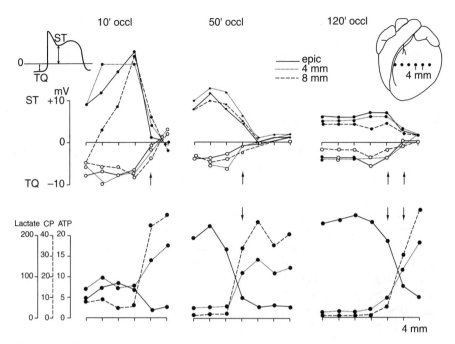

Figure 4.1. Epicardial and intramural T-Q (open circles) and S-T segment (closed circles) potentials after occlusions lasting 10, 50, and 120 min. Electrodes were placed in a row (see inset) and were separated by 4 mm. The moments of the cardiac cycle at which measurements were made are indicated in the upper left inset. Lower panel: tissue content of lactate, CP, and ATP at the electrode sites are indicated in μ moles per gram dry weight. Upward-pointing arrows indicate electrical border sites; downward-pointing arrows indicate metabolic border sites. Note that metabolic measurements at the electrical border site were normal. Reproduced with permission from ref. 34.

reentrant arrhythmia is set up, the normal tissue maintains the reentrant activation even when the ischemic tissue has become fully inexcitable. Reentrant but also non-reentrant beats have been documented by Pogwizd and Corr [41] during early ischemia. Rotating spiral waves are most likely the underlying mechanism of VF, and the changes in the frequency content of local electrograms during VF can be explained by the dynamic changes of these spirals [42].

Slow conduction and a short refractory period facilitate the occurrence of a reentrant arrhythmia [43]. For the initiation of the arrhythmia, unidirectional block is a prerequisite [43]. In the following section, we will show that ischemic myocardial tissue is characterized by large heterogeneities in excitability and refractoriness and by slow conduction. Overall, most studies report an increase in refractory period [44], although hypoxic tissue is characterized by a decrease in refractoriness [32]. The latter can occur at the margin of the ischemic zone. The coincidence between the end of repolarization and the refractory period that exists in normal, nonischemic tissue is lost during ischemia, where refractoriness extends beyond the moment of repolarization (post-repolarization refractoriness). Thus, in ischemia, measures of action potential duration (activation recovery intervals, monophasic action potentials) cannot be used as an estimate of the refractory period. It may occur that the action potential duration decreases, whereas the refractory period prolongs substantially.

The experiments by Janse et al. also have shed light on the mechanism of the initiating premature beat, the trigger. Figure 4.2 shows superimposed action potentials from the normal and ischemic zones after about 5 min of regional ischemia in a pig heart. The ischemic zone is activated with a long delay, and consequently, the action potential plateau of the ischemic zone coincides with the diastole of the normal tissue. This will give rise to a current of injury flowing intracellularly from the ischemic to the normal zone. This "injury" current will be reflected in the extracellular electrograms as a deeply negative T-wave recorded from the ischemic tissue [45]. Then, the same current of injury will tend to depolarize the normal zone and will facilitate the occurrence of premature beats from that site [5]. Janse and van Capelle [46] have demonstrated in computer model studies that, if a degree of uncoupling is present between the two zones, premature beats originate from the nondepolarized tissue [46]. We have shown that the diastolic stimulation threshold at the nonischemic side of the border is decreased by about 20% as a result of the current of injury [47]. It can be argued that during a negative T-wave, the amplitude of the current of injury is several fold higher, leading to a premature beat in the normal tissue [40, 47].

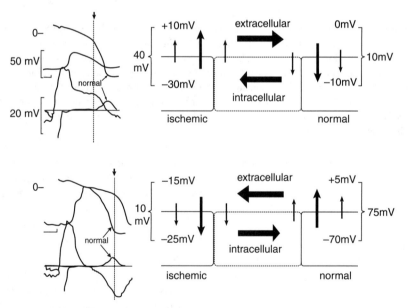

Figure 4.2. Relationship between transmembrane potential and DC extracellular electrogram during regional ischemia. The signals from ischemic and nonischemic potentials are superimposed. In the diagram, the relationship is given among transmembrane potential, extracellular potential, and current flow at a time indicated by the arrows in the superimposed potentials. In the upper panel, electrotonic current has a depolarizing effect on the ischemic cells; in the lower panel, the electrotonic current exerts a depolarizing effect on the normal cells. Reproduced with permission from ref. 45.

A focal origin of a premature beat was demonstrated at the normal side of the border between the normal and the ischemic zone [39], preceded by a large positive T-wave, indicative of the flow of "injury" current. This is in line with the simulation studies by Janse and van Capelle [46]. The high-density mapping experiments by Pogwizd et al. and those of Janse et al. have unequivocally demonstrated that even reentry itself can be the mechanism of the initiating premature beat [46]. In the experiments of Pogwizd and Corr [41] and Janse et al. [48], they even constituted most cases (in about 75%).

4.2.1.2 Role of Extracellular Potassium, Anoxia, $I_{K, ATP}$

4.2.1.2.1 Extracellular Potassium. Changes in the extracellular potassium concentration cause changes in the resting membrane potential of the cardiac myocyte after the Nernst equation [49]. The resting membrane potential in turn determines sodium channel function in a sigmoid manner [21, 49], with a depolarization of the resting membrane leading to less available sodium current, decrease of excitability, slowing of the upstroke of the action potential, and decrease of conduction velocity [50]. A small depolarization of the resting membrane, however, leads to increased excitability and to paradoxical increase of conduction velocity, because the resting membrane potential is brought closer to the threshold potential for excitation [51]. The increased $[K^+]_{out}$ also accounts for action potential shortening [52].

Because the extracellular potassium concentration is a major determinant of the electrocardiographic and arrhythmogenic changes during acute myocardial ischemia, much attention has been given to the time course of change of extracellular potassium and its modifying factors. The mechanism of the potassium loss has been subject to intense discussions about the nature of the accompanying "other" ion to compensate for the charge associated with the K^+ transport, but it is outside the scope of this chapter. Most likely the cellular K^+-loss is compensated by a gain in intracellular Na^+ [53]. A rise in extracellular potassium concentration is one of the first signs of ischemia: It starts within seconds after the onset of ischemia together with the loss of contractility [54, 55]. It is directly related to the decrease in free energy of adenosine triphosphate (ATP) hydrolysis [56]. Because the ATP levels decrease in a biphasic fashion, extracellular potassium rise also occurs in a biphasic fashion [20]. After a steady rise in the first 5 min of ischemia up to a concentration of about 12 mM, the extracellular potassium concentration reaches a plateau that lasts until about 15 min of ischemia. Next, a secondary rise takes place, which leads the myocardium into the phase of irreversible changes. During the plateau phase, a small decrease in $[K^+]_{out}$ can sometimes be observed [57]. Reperfusion during the first 15 min usually restores cardiac function completely, whereas it does not after that period. The secondary rise in extracellular potassium concentration is associated with the increase in resting tension of the muscle. Arrhythmogenesis during phase 1a therefore is linked to the first phase of rise in $[K^+]_{out}$ [20, 58]. The above description of the rise in ischemia-induced $[K^+]_{out}$ is observed in globally ischemic myocardium or in the core of regionally ischemic myocardium [20, 35, 59, 60]. In the lateral border zone, the time course is altogether different, with an initial rise to much lower values and a normalization during the plateau phase [14, 35]. The changes in $[K^+]_{out}$ (and intracellular $[Na^+]$) are modulated by the alterations in osmolality caused by the creation of intracellular osmotically active particles that cause a "contraction" of the extracellular space and an increase of the intracellular space [22, 23].

The lateral gradients of K-rise during ischemia are caused by the exchange between the interstitial space of the ischemic and nonischemic areas [35]. Indeed, an elevation of potassium concentration can be detected in coronary sinus blood during regional myocardial ischemia in pigs [61]. However, diffusion constants are extremely low in ischemic myocardial tissue and cannot account for these changes [62]. The gradients of potassium during ischemia are much steeper at the endocardial and epicardial border zone [59, 63], probably because of a lack of contiguous myocardial tissue, and are approximately 600 μm wide. These gradients can be modulated by the oxygen content of the surroundings [59].

As expected [34], there is a high correlation between the changes in the TQ-segment of local electrograms and extracellular potassium concentration [35]. The gradients across the border zone in $[K^+]_{out}$ are directly reflected in the amount of TQ depression in the ischemic zone. The occurrence of activation block is associated with extracellular concentrations of potassium of 8 mM and higher [58]. Ventricular fibrillation, however, does not occur when a large enough part of the ischemic myocardium has reached a $[K^+]_{out}$ of above 13 mM [38]. At this concentration, the resting membrane potential of the ischemic zone is about -60 mV, which completely inactivates the fast sodium channels. A critical range of $[K^+]_{out}$ between 8 and 12 mM therefore is present in the ischemic region during phase 1a of arrhythmogenesis. The tissue, in which these K^+-concentrations occur, constitutes the substrate for arrhythmogenesis. When the conditions are present in insufficient tissue, phase 1a ends [64].

Across the lateral border zone, changes in excitability take place: Within the ischemic tissue, a smaller rise in $[K^+]_{out}$ occurs than in the central ischemic tissue [47], and at the margins of the ischemic tissue, the resting membrane potential is closer to the threshold potential for activation. Immediately outside the ischemic tissue, where no rise in $[K^+]_{out}$ has occurred, diastolic stimulation threshold is also decreased (by about 20%). This is probably caused by the flow of injury current [47].

Thus, after about 5 min of myocardial ischemia, closely juxtaposed regions of inexcitable myocardium, and myocardium with reduced excitability and increased excitability, set the stage for the occurrence of focal and reentrant arrhythmias.

4.2.1.2.2 Anoxia. Immediately after coronary occlusion, the residual oxygen available in the ischemic zone is used. Any oxygen entering the ischemic zone will be bound immediately, and therefore, the gradient of pO_2 across the ischemic borders is acute [65], contrary to the gradient of potassium and pH. Thus, the ischemic tissue is homogeneously anoxic [65]. This is also reflected by the sharp transition between glycogen-rich tissue and tissue devoid of glycogen across the ischemic border [34].

Myocardial tissue subjected to anoxia demonstrates a dramatic shortening of the action potential, maybe by opening of K_{ATP} channels [32, 66]. Under these circumstances, the relation between recovery of excitability (end of refractoriness) and the end of repolarization is maintained [32]. Because the gradients of oxygen and potassium across the ischemic border are disparate, the changes in action potential configuration, excitability, and refractoriness vary substantially between adjacent sites. Figure 4.3 schematically illustrates that close to the ischemic border hypoxic changes prevail, whereas deeper into the ischemic tissue truly ischemic electrophysiological changes occur [67]. Thus, within the ischemic tissue, all the conditions necessary for the initiation of reentry coexist: short refractory period, decreased excitability, slow conduction, and large heterogeneities.

4.2.1.2.3 *Sarcolemmal* $I_{K, ATP}$.
The ATP-sensitive potassium channel is closed under normal conditions in ventricular myocardium, but it may give rise to substantial outward current when intracellular ATP falls below 1 mM. [68]. The current causes extreme shortening of the cardiac action potential [69]. During early ischemia, the ATP levels during ischemia do not pass below this threshold level during the first several minutes of ischemia [56], but intracellular compartmentalization of ATP may lead to lower subsarcolemmal ATP levels [50, 70] and may explain the early action potential

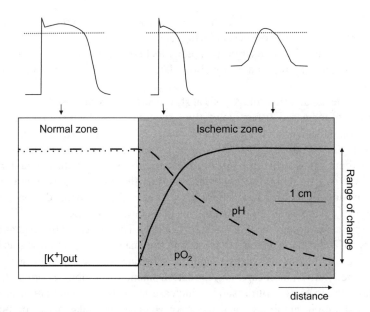

Figure 4.3. Schematic representation of the gradients of extracellular potassium concentration ($[K^+]_{out}$), pH and pO_2 across the lateral border zone during regional ischemia (phase 1a). The associated action potential configurations are schematically shown above. After Coronel (thesis, 1988) [67].

shortening observed during ischemia. Also, after anoxic superfusion of myocytes, action potential shortening took place only after 8–15 min as well [71].

The contribution of $I_{K, ATP}$ to arrhythmias occurring during phase 1a are unresolved, although in mice homogeneously deficient of the Kir6.2 gene (which encodes the pore-forming subunit of sarcolemmal K_{ATP} channels), ischemia-induced ST-segment elevation was completely abolished [72].

4.2.1.2.4 Other Ischemia Related Factors. Many other contributors to the ischemia-induced arrhythmias have been studied. For example, pH falls during ischemia during the first 15 min and reaches a plateau [38]. The acidosis leads to a small depolarization of the resting membrane and a prolongation of the action potential [52, 73].

Other factors include accumulation of lysophosphoglycerides, fatty acids, and arachidonic acid [52, 74], as well as the formation of reactive oxygen species [52, 75].

4.2.1.3 Modulating Factors. Cardiac electrophysiology can be modulated by a plethora of drugs and compounds, the occurrence of a preceding episode of ischemia in the same myocardial tissue (preconditioning) [76, 77] or elsewhere in the body (remote preconditioning), or stretch of the myocardium by reactive oxygen species and many other factors. We limit ourselves to a few of those modulating factors.

4.2.1.3.1 Heart Rate. A fast heart rate, as well as a slow heart rate, is associated with increased arrhythmogenesis during acute myocardial ischemia [78]. The beneficial effects of β-adrenergic receptor blockers on mortality in patients with acute myocardial infarction are probably related to the prevention of high in heart rates [79].

On the one hand, arrhythmogenesis at slow heart rates is supposedly related to the occurrence of increased dispersion of repolarization [80], which is a mechanism for unidirectional block or on the occurrence of early after depolarizations. On the other hand, a slow heart rate is associated with longer refractory periods, which is *in itself* antiarrhythmic. It is difficult to determine what the result of these counteracting factors will be. An alternative explanation is that the process of ischemia-induced electrophysiological changes depends on heart rate and the associated expenditure of energy. For example, during ischemia in quiescent hearts, the rise in $[K^+]_{out}$ is considerably slower than at a higher heart rate [81]. Therefore, the time spent during the phase of ischemia in which dangerous intermediate $[K^+]_{out}$ are present is longer in bradycardia than in tachycardia, and the substrate for reentry is present over a longer period [58]. At fast heart rates, the action potential duration is shortened, which is proarrhythmic. Also, with a sudden increase in heart rate, alternation of action potential duration, amplitude, and upstroke velocity will take place, particularly during ischemia [44, 82], leading to ventricular fibrillation.

The heart is only functionally perfused during diastole. When coronary stenosis is the reason for ischemia, lowering heart rate provides a longer diastolic perfusion time of the myocardium at risk.

Heart rate is directly under the influence of the autonomic nervous system, and the proarrhythmic effects of a fast heart rate may be the indirect effect of a high sympathetic tone. heart rate turbulence is a noninvasive measure of the autonomic balance that can be used to estimate risk of sudden cardiac death [83]. However, the observation of increased arrhythmogenesis in isolated regionally ischemic hearts indicates that heart rate is also an independent factor, although the effect of higher energy consumption remains pertinent.

4.2.1.3.2 Thrombus. The presence of an intracoronary thrombus profoundly modulates the ischemia-induced electrophysiological changes [84], leading to more arrhythmias than in ischemia without a thrombus. An intracoronary thrombus is found in a large percentage of patients with sudden death [85]. Thrombin, which is one of the initiators of the coagulation cascade, has a direct effect on cardiac electrophysiology: It increases the sodium current, depolarizes the resting membrane, and leads to more increase of intracellular sodium during ischemia in atrial myocytes [86]. We introduced a thrombus into the left anterior descending artery of anaesthetized pigs before creating a total occlusion [87]. More phase 1a arrhythmias occurred in the presence of a thrombus (with no effect on phase 1b arrhythmias). The proarrhythmia was associated with more conduction slowing in the ischemic tissue than when no thrombus was present.

After preconditioning with one or more ischemic episodes, the proarrhythmic effect of a thrombus was not detectable [87].

Of course, many more components of a thrombus may be involved in its arrhythmogenic actions, which include platelet factors, coagulation factors, inflammatory factors. The individual contribution of these factors on cellular electrophysiology is unknown.

4.2.1.3.3 Autonomic Nervous System. The autonomic nervous system has an important influence on arrhythmogenesis during ischemia. This is evident from the effect of β-adrenergic receptor blocking agents on mortality [88]. The experiments of Schwartz et al. [89] provide a clear indication of the influence of the autonomic nervous system: dogs could be either susceptible or not susceptible to VF during ischemia (in the setting of a previous myocardial infarction). Baroreceptor reflex sensitivity was among the parameters that could distinguish between the two groups [89]. A similar distinction can be made in patients [89–91].

Immediately following the onset of ischemia, plasma catecholamines rise and catecholamines are released from nerve endings inside the ischemic myocardium in the course of ischemia (although not during phase 1a of arrhythmogenesis) [92, 93]. Catecholamines have a direct effect on action potential duration and upstroke velocity of ventricular myocardium [52]. Increased contractility produces an altered effect of mechanoelectrical feedback. Sympathetic stimulation or systemic catecholamines increase dispersion in refractoriness [94]. Under ischemic conditions, the response of normal and affected tissue is qualitatively different, which increases dispersion in refractory periods even more [95]. That the brain-heart axis plays an important role in cardiovascular death is clear from observations on Voodoo death and on the relation between cardiovascular mortality and depression [96, 97]. Skinner and Reed [98] have demonstrated in pigs that there are cortical brain areas that, if cooled, protect against ischemia-induced arrhythmias, whereas electrical stimulation of those brain areas produce ventricular fibrillation in the absence of ischemia [98]. The 9-11 terrorist attacks in the United States had remarkable influence on heart rate variability in highway patrol trooper [99]. The mechanisms of these influences are still unclear.

4.2.1.3.4 Diet. A Mediterranean diet is associated with a decreased incidence of death from coronary artery disease [100]. Many dietary components of the Mediterranean diet have been investigated, such as olive oil [101], wine, and free radical scavengers. Especially the use of various forms of oil has regained an interest since the 1970s of the previous century with a new surge in interest in more recent years [102]. Experimental data have indicated that the severity of arrhythmias occurring following myocardial ischemia depend on the type of dietary oil intake [103]. The observation that Greenland Inuit relatively rarely suffer from sudden cardiac death have boosted interest in the antiarrhythmic potential of fish oil fatty acids [104]. The Gruppo Italiano per lo Studio della Sopravvivenza nell'Infarto Miocardico (GISSI) and the Diet and Reinfarction Study (DART) trials have confirmed that the ingestion of omega-3 fatty acids reduces sudden cardiac death in a population of patients with prior myocardial infarction [105, 106]. A trial in patients with angina pectoris, however, did not demonstrate an antiarrhythmic effect [107], and randomized controlled trials in patients with an implanted cardioverter defibrillator even pointed to a proarrhythmic effect [108] or were inconclusive [109].

We studied the influence of a diet rich in omega-3 fatty acids to pigs on subsequent myocardial ischemia. Following acute myocardial ischemia, more arrhythmias occurred in the animals that were fed fish oil than in a control group of pigs [16], probably caused by a larger decrease in excitability. These changes were evident in both phase 1a and 1b of arrhythmias and remarkably did not differ between the fish oil group and the sunflower oil group. Earlier work on the dietary influences of fish oil on ischemia-induced arrhythmias pointed to an antiarrhythmic effect [110] in marmosets and dogs [111]. Some studies were executed by applying fish oil fatty acids acutely to myocytes [111, 112]. There is a difference in electrophysiologic effects between acutely administered fish oil fatty acids and those administered by feeding [102]. Shortening of the cardiac action potential by a diet rich in fish oil fatty acids probably contributes to proarrhythmia during ischemia [113].

4.2.1.3.5 Genetic Factors. Genetic determinants of all modifying factors mentioned above and of all causes and risk factors of coronary artery disease can modulate the arrhythmogenic effects of acute myocardial ischemia. Little is known of the influence of genetic factors, although it is clear that there is a familial occurrence of sudden cardiac death [114]. Whether a patient with acute myocardial infarction develops ventricular fibrillation is also highly determined by the family history of similar events [3]. Of course, environmental factors like diet, behavior, and risk factors may correlate with this familial association. Because coronary artery disease is a multifactorial disease, and because arrhythmogenesis is modulated by many different factors, it is not likely that a single gene underlies the familial occurrence of ischemia-induced arrhythmogenesis, although genes involved in conduction and repolarization may play a more prominent role [115].

4.2.2 Phase 1B

4.2.2.1 *Arrhythmogenic Mechanisms: Substrate.* The work of Kaplinsky et al. [11] has suggested that the mechanism of arrhythmias in phase 1b of ischemia is different from that in phase 1a. Figure 4.4, derived from their seminal paper shows that the electrograms recorded in the two periods of arrhythmogenesis differ in the presence of diastolic potentials. The authors, therefore, concluded that reentry was not the probable mechanism of the delayed ventricular arrhythmias (of phase 1b arrhythmias).

Insight into the arrhythmogenic mechanism of phase 1b arrhythmias was boosted by the observation that intercellular uncoupling occurred in this phase of ischemia [116]. Uncoupling does not occur in phase 1a. The correspondence between phase 1b arrhythmias and the increase in myocardial tissue impedance was demonstrated by Smith et al. [117]. This relation in time also existed after preconditioning of the heart [118]. The closure of gap junctions is associated with an increase in intracellular $[Ca^{2+}]$ [119, 120] and/or a decrease in intracellular pH [121], and it leads to slowing of conduction and conduction block [122, 123]. de Groot et al. [124]

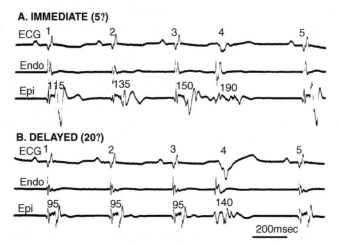

Figure 4.4. Local electrograms recorded during the early (phase 1a) and delayed (phase 1b) phase of arrhythmogenesis after acute myocardial ischemia. Note the difference in diastolic potentials preceding premature complexes between the two phases. Reproduced with permission from ref. 11.

next demonstrated that arrhythmogenesis in phase 1b occurred merely when un-coupling was moderate (up to about 40% of maximal) and terminated when uncoupling was complete [12, 124]. Moreover, they showed that epicardial reentry was the probably mechanism of the arrhythmia.

Because a considerable degree of uncoupling is needed to result in conduction slowing [123], alternative mechanisms for arrhythmogenesis have to be considered. One possibility is that uncoupling may unmask preexisting differences in action potential duration. In normal myocardium, heterogeneity in action potential duration is minimized though the high degree of electrotonic coupling between cells. When the coupling is diminished, action potential heterogeneity may become apparent [125]. This was demonstrated indirectly in isolated myocytes subjected to simulated ischemia [126], although cell pairs did not show heterogeneities before excitability was lost. Therefore, unmasking of heterogeneities does not seem to be a dominant mechanism of phase 1b arrhythmias.

During acute myocardial ischemia, parts of the heart survive. In humans, a subendocardial layer, and in pigs a subepicardial layer, of myocardium remains excitable, whereas intramural tissue becomes inexcitable. A new hypothesis was proposed for the phase 1b arrhythmias, which is related to this surviving layers of myocardium. With a moderate degree of uncoupling, the inexcitable part of the myocardium may act as a passive load for surviving and relatively normal tissue. This results in conduction slowing and unmasking of action potential heterogeneities in the surviving and intrinsically normal layers that are nevertheless depolarized by being coupled to the severely depolarized midmyocardial tissue [124]. A similar mecha-nism has been demonstrated in cell pairs [127] and in a simulation study [128]. When the uncoupling process is complete and the electrotonic interaction between the two layers ceases, the arrhythmogenic substrate disappears and phase 1b terminates. In a review on this subject, de Groot et al. [124] mention observations that are in support of this idea [124]. Nevertheless, definitive proof is still wanting. The main problem for a demonstration of a causal relation between cellular uncoupling and the interaction between the two myocardial layers on one hand and arrhythmogenesis on the other hand is that the role of uncoupling can not be studied in isolation. For that purpose, Xiao et al. [129] have executed a computer modeling study in which a surviving and a depolarized sheet of myocardium were coupled. The normal "epicardial" sheet contained heterogeneities. Indeed, epicardial reentry could be induced in the presence of moderate uncoupling, without the involvement of other ischemia-related factors [129].

4.2.3 Arrhythmogenic Mechanism: Trigger

Ischemia-induced VF in both phases 1a and 1b phase is induced by a critically timed premature beat [11]. The mechanism of this beat is not clear. Triggered activity emanating from Purkinje fibers during cellular uncoupling has been suggested [130]. Alternatively, the mechanical stretch acting exerted by the normally contracting myocardium on the rigid ischemic tissue may also play a role. We have shown that phase 1b arrhythmias were less numerous in isolated nonworking hearts than in *in situ* hearts, and arrhythmias became more prominent when a left intraventricular balloon was inflated [13]. Moreover, the site of origin of the ventricular extrasystoles was directly outside the ischemic region and postextrasystolic potentiation led to an increase in extrasystolic activity, directly related to the peak of the intraventricular pressure wave [13]. Although this indicates a role of mechanoelectrical interaction in phase 1b arrhythmias, gadolinium, which is a blocker of stretch-activated channels, did not reduce the arrhythmias [131].

4.2.4 Catecholamines

Because catecholamines are released from the terminal nerve endings at about the same time as the start of phase 1b of arrhythmias [92, 93] the autonomic nervous system has be implicated in arrhythmogenesis in this phase. Verkerk et al. [130] have found support for this idea. Application of cromakalim, which is a specific K_{ATP}-channel opener, reduced the release of catecholamines and tended to reduce ischemia-induced arrhythmias [132].

4.3 ARRHYTHMOGENESIS DURING THE FIRST WEEK POST MI

4.3.1 Mechanisms

After 24–48 h (subacute phase of infarction) post-occlusion, delayed spontaneous arrhythmias of ventricular origin (subendocardial Purkinje) occur in experimental models and may have counterparts in humans [133]. During the healing (5–7 days) infarct phase, sustained ventricular tachycardias are inducible in both animal and human hearts, suggesting that the reentrant substrate is present. The site of origin of the ventricular arrhythmias in these hearts depends on the location of the surviving cells overlying the infarcted region. In one canine myocardial infarction (MI) model, these arrhythmias have been mapped to an area described as the epicardial border zone (EBZ) [134].

The specific changes in the cell action potential (AP) configuration that occur in the canine subendocardial Purkinje fiber and the subepicardial ventricular fiber post-coronary artery occlusion are discussed in ref. [134]. Generally, by 24 to 48 h after total coronary artery occlusion, the APs of the subendocardial Purkinje fibers show reduced resting potentials, as well as an increase in total time of repolarization. However, the cells of the EBZ of the canine model show a reduction in V_{max} and a shortening and triangularization of the AP by 5 days after total artery occlusion. By 14 days post-occlusion, additional shortening of the AP occurs. Then by the time of the healed infarct (2 months), AP voltage profiles have returned to nearly normal [135], suggesting the presence of a process that might be termed "reverse remodeling." In addition, changes in conduction of the impulse at various times after coronary artery occlusion as well as the altered refractoriness of the tissue in the infarcted myocardium have been documented [134].

4.3.2 The Subendocardial Purkinje Cell as a Trigger 24–48 H Post Occlusion

4.3.2.1 Resting Potential. The origin of the delayed phase of spontaneous arrhythmias secondary to coronary artery occlusion in canine and porcine hearts is most likely in the abnormally automatic subendocardial Purkinje fibers that survive. The loss of resting potential is significant and dramatic in the multicellular preparations of these fibers. Concomitant with this dramatic loss is a reduction in intracellular ion concentrations, but this alone cannot account fully for the loss in resting potential (average change 35 mV) [134].

Importantly, the abnormalities in the resting potentials of subendocardial Purkinje fibers surviving in the 24–48 h infarcted heart persist even after they are enzymatically disaggregated and studied as single myocytes [136]. In the isolated Purkinje myocyte, a reduction in intracellular $[K^+]$ could not account for the reduced resting potential. Rather, Purkinje myocytes isolated from the infarcted zone of the myocardium (IZPCs) show an increase in the ratio of the membrane permeability of Na^+ to K^+ ions (P_{Na}/P_K) as compared with Purkinje cells from the normal zone (NZPCs) [136]. Finally, there is a persistent decrease in the density of both the outward and inward rectifying K current, I_{K1}, described for the voltage clamped IZPCs [137]. Thus, remodeling of I_{K1} underlies Purkinje cell depolarization in the post-MI heart.

4.3.2.2 Phase 0 of the Action Potential V_{max} and Na^+ Current. By virtue of the loss of resting potential, there would be a predictable change in V_{max} of the subendocardial Purkinje myocytes that survive in IZPCs. In fact, IZPCs have markedly reduced AP amplitudes and V_{max} [134]. As yet, there have been no voltage clamp studies that have identified whether the fast Na^+ current density is altered in Purkinje myocytes dispersed at this time period after coronary artery occlusion.

4.3.2.2.1 Ca^{2+} Currents. Peak L type Ca^{2+} current (I_{CaL}) density is significantly reduced in IZPCs as compared with control and with those from the 24 h infarcted heart [138]. Current density reduction is not accompanied by a shift in the current voltage relationship or a change in the time course of I_{CaL} decay but by a hyperpolarizing shift in steady state availability of the channel. Peak T type Ca^{2+} current density is also decreased in subendocardial Purkinje myocytes that survive in the 24 h infarcted heart, and more reduction occurs by 48 h. This loss in Ca^{2+} channel function could contribute to the depressed and triangular plateau phase of the APs of these arrhythmogenic Purkinje myocytes.

4.3.2.2.2 Intracellular Ca^{2+} Cycling. Reduced Ca^{2+} influx via the I_{CaL} may be partially responsible for the abnormal AP evoked global Ca^{2+} transients observed in IZPCs [139]. Many have suggested that alterations in Ca^{2+} handling could feed back to modify electrophysiology and give rise to abnormal electrical activity [140]. One cellular mechanism of triggered activity is the delayed afterdepolarization (DAD). We have shown that nonuniform Ca^{2+} transients in subendocardial Purkinje cells that have survived the infarct underlie spontaneous membrane depolarizations. Both the *amplitude* of the intracellular Ca^{2+} waves and their number and spatial extent that predict the membrane depolarization of the Purkinje cell [139]. Furthermore, electrically evoked Ca^{2+} transients in IZPCs originate faster than those in normal Purkinje cell aggregates but show substantial spatiotemporal nonuniformity within an IZPC aggregate as well as between IZPC aggregates. Most importantly, IZPCs show low amplitude, spontaneously occurring micro Ca^{2+} (μCa^2) wavelets (extent $\leq 8\,\mu m$) at *a 5-fold higher incidence* than in normal Purkinje aggregates. These μCa^{2+} wavelets seem to meander over distances $\leq 100\,\mu m$ and reduce the local Ca^{2+} transient of the next paced beat (Figure 4.5). Finally, these μCa^{2+} wavelets precede cell-wide Ca^{2+} waves. Cell-wide Ca^{2+} waves, in turn, clearly cause membrane depolarization and elicit spontaneous APs [141]. Thus, the high incidence of μCa^{2+} wavelets in IZPCs is fundamental to the abnormal Ca^{2+} handling of diseased Purkinje cells, underlying the arrhythmias originating in the subendocardial Purkinje network after a myocardial infarct.

Recently, we evaluated the reasons for the increased incidence of μCa^{2+} wavelets in IZPCs. IZPC μCa^{2+} wavelets are not affected by verapamil [142] and are insensitive to the T type Ca^{2+} channel blocker, mibefradil [143]. Because Ca^{2+} waves and resultant membrane depolarization in Purkinjes are ryanodine sensitive [142], we sought to determine whether Ca^{2+} waves in IZPCs were caused by *enhanced* spontaneous Ca^{2+} release secondary to altered activity of the sarcoplasmic reticulum (SR) Ca^{2+} release channels. Recent data have shown that in intact IZPCs, the intracellular Ca^{2+} event (Ca^{2+} sparks) rate of IZPCs is increased compared with NZPCs, but it occurs without a change in SR-Ca^{2+} content, which is consistent with an enhanced open probability of SR Ca^{2+} release channels in IZPCs. Interestingly, the enhanced Ca^{2+} release event rate in IZPCs is normalized by the experimental drug, JTV-519 (K201), without a change in cell SR content [144]. JTV-519 (K201) also reduces the incidence of cell-wide Ca^{2+} waves [142] in IZPCs and thus would be highly antiarrhythmic in this setting.

These functional data are consistent with the multiple Ca^{2+} release compartments in Purkinje cells, which we hypothesize to exist based on our immuncytochemistry data [141]. Figure 4.6 shows a set of serial frames obtained by optical sectioning of an aggregate of normal canine Purkinje cells. The reconstructed fluorescence from the respective antibodies against the Ryanodine release (RyR) channel and the channels associated with type 1 IP3 receptors (red, anti-RYR$_2$ receptor; green, anti-IP$_3$R1) is shown. Panel Aa of this figure shows the section sampled across the aggregate near the bottom edge. IP$_3$R1 positive areas are organized in bands and are readily visible, whereas RyR$_2$ red pixels are at a lower frequency. Sectioning deeper into the core of the aggregate (Panel Ab) there is less IP$_3$R1-specific staining and more RyR$_2$ (red) staining. However, green pixels still surround the cells. Pixel density analysis of RyR$_2$ and IP$_3$R1 positive regions revealed that only 5% of pixels overlapped in subcellular regions. Panel B shows a high-power section showing the regionality of the two types of Ca^{2+} release channels in the normal Purkinje cell. Note the area below the sarcolemma with no staining. These NZPC data that describe the novel microarchitecture of the Ca^{2+} release channels in Purkinje cells are consistent with our functional data above showing frequent μCa waves and sparks in areas just below

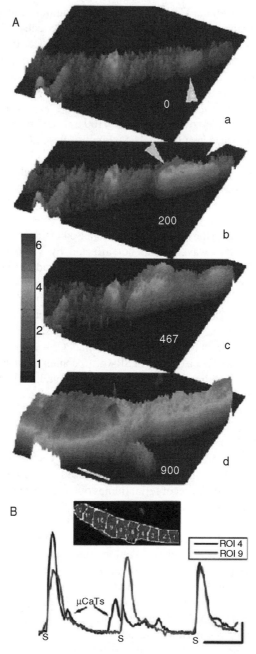

Figure 4.5. Nonuniformly occurring micro Ca^{2+} transients cause nonuniformity of the Ca^{2+} response of a paced canine IZPC aggregate. **Panel A**: Three-dimensional surface plots of IZPC just preceding and during an electrically evoked Ca^{2+} transient. [Ca^{2+}] is denoted by both the color and height of the surface. White numbers indicate time of frame relative to $t = 0$ (Aa).

the sarcolemma and mostly sparks alone in the core. Ca^{2+} waves are viewed in both functional regions [141]. However, their relationships in Purkinje cells from infarcted heart are not known at this time except that immunostaining for RyR_2 in IZPCs reveals three patterns (Figure 4.7). Type 1 Purkinje cells showed regular periodicity of staining [left, NZPCs 89% of total cells (n = 55); IZPCs 38% of total (n = 24)]; Type 2 cells (middle) lacked some periodicity [NZPCs (11%), IZPCs (42%)], whereas some IZPCs (right, 21%) showed regions of disorder throughout most of the cell. Thus, it seems that for most IZPCs showing enhanced Ca^{2+} release, structural remodeling of RyR_2 proteins is not pivotal.

4.3.2.3 *Repolarization and Refractoriness.* AP recordings of the subendocardial Purkinje fibers that survive 24 to 48 h after occlusion have a small degree of rapid phase 1 of repolarization when fibers are driven at slow rates. Pacing at fast rates causes little or no change in phase 1 of repolarization in normal Purkinje fibers; yet it has a dramatic effect on the time course of repolarization of subendocardial Purkinje myocytes surviving in the infarcted heart. In some cases, with an increase in drive rate, the rapid phase 1 of repolarization of APs in these fibers completely disappears (see Fig. 3.30 of ref. 134). Whole cell voltage clamp experiments have confirmed that the density and kinetics of I_{to}, the transient outward current, in single IZPCs is reduced by 51%, and that these changes are not caused by alterations in steady-state availability of the channel. However, I_{to} currents in IZPCs show specific kinetic changes, in that the time course of current decay is accelerated while the time course of reactivation of I_{to} is significantly delayed. This slowing of I_{to} recovery implies that less outward repolarizing current is available for APs occurring at high pacing rates or during closely spaced voltage clamp steps [145]. IZPCs have a significantly increased density of E4031 sensitive currents (a gain in function) compared with those of normal Purkinje myocytes [137]. E4031 sensitive Purkinje myocyte currents differ from those of the normal or infarcted ventricular myocytes (I_{Kr}), and its molecular identity is unknown at this time. However these data do suggest that Purkinje myocytes surviving in the infarcted heart would show an increased responsiveness to this class of antiarrhythmic drugs (methanesulfonanilides).

The aggregate was stimulated just before $t = 900$ ms (Ad). Note the presence of micro Ca^{2+} waves (arrowheads), which propagate over short distances ($t = 0$ to 467 ms) meandering from the right section of the aggregate toward the core. Subsequent stimulation causes nonuniform electrically evoked local Ca^{2+} transients ($t = 900$ ms), particularly in regions where micro Ca^{2+} waves had been. The horizontal bar indicates 50 μm. The color bar indicates ratio range. **Panel B**: Changes in intensity of fluorescence (F/F_0) at two selected specific regions of interest (ROIs) in IZPC aggregate of panel A. Stimuli are indicated (S). Each ROI is represented by a different color, and location is noted in upper image. Note that when the micro Ca^{2+} transients (μCa$_i$T) observed in ROI4 (see arrowheads of panel A) precede S, the subsequent Ca^{2+} transient of S is diminished compared with that of the previous S. Note that in ROIs where micro Ca^{2+} transients were absent (e.g., ROI 9), response to stimulation was constant. Vertical and horizontal lines are 1 F/F_0 units and 1.58 s, respectively. Reproduced with permission from ref. 139. See color insert.

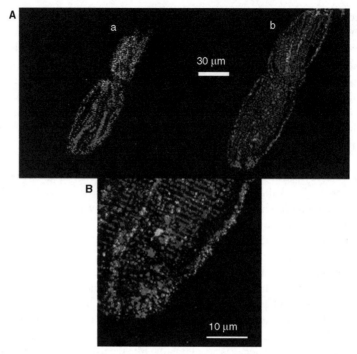

Figure 4.6. Localization of SR Ca^{2+} channels (RyR_2 and IP_3R_1) in a canine NZPC. **Panel Aa**: The superficial edge of the NZPC. Note that IP_3R_1 (green) are organized in bands and readily visible, whereas RYR_2 (red) are at a lower frequency. **Panel Ab**: The core section of the NZPC. Note that there is less IP_3R_1 (green) specific staining and more RYR_2 (red) staining; however, green pixels still surround the cells. **Panel B**: A high-power section showing the regionality of RyR_2 and IP_3R_1 in the NZPC. Scale bars were labeled in white lines. See color insert.

4.3.3 Five Days Post-Occlusion: Epicardial Border Zone

In the multicellular preparations of the myocardium isolated from the EBZ of the 5-day infarcted heart, the following abnormalities have been described: a decrease in resting potential, total AP amplitude and V_{max}, a reduction in AP duration at both 50 and 90% repolarization, and a loss in the plateau potentials [135]. However, when the EBZ cells (IZs) are dispersed and studied as isolated myocytes *in vitro* [146], the resting potential is no different than control epicardial cells (NZs), suggesting that other factors control resting membrane potential in the multicellular preparation. One likely factor may be extracellular ion accumulation, because in single cells, electrical activity is studied after it is removed from the syncytium and superfused in an environment where immediate extracellular ion accumulation and depletion are not significant.

Although resting potentials of the 5-day IZs are similar to NZ values, APs of these myocytes show changes in the repolarization particularly during the terminal portion

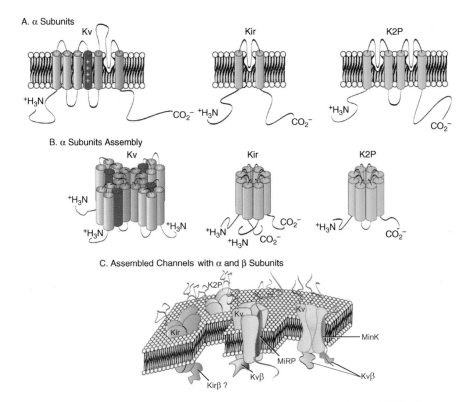

Figure 2.2. Pore-forming subunits and assembly of cardiac Kv, Kir, and K2P channels. Membrane topologies of individual Kv, Kir, and K2P pore-forming (α) subunits (**A**) and the tetrameric assembly of Kv and Kir subunits and the dimeric assembly of K2P subunits (**B**) are illustrated. (**C**) Schematic of assembled Kv, Kir, and K2P α subunits with associated transmembrane and cytoplasmic accessory subunits.

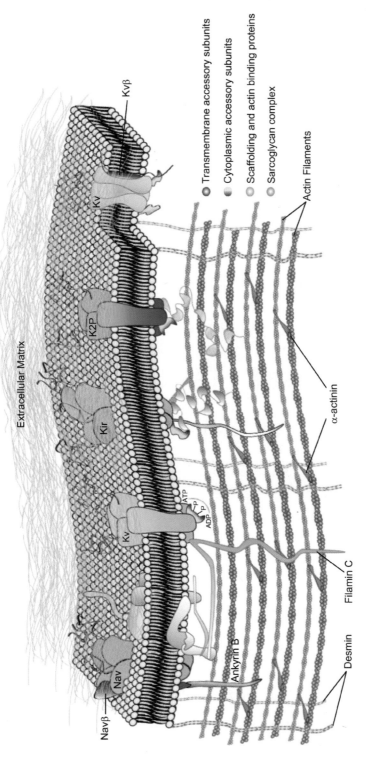

Figure 2.3. Cardiac Kv, Kir, and K2P channels function as components of macromolecular protein complexes. Schematic illustrating functional cardiac K^+ channels, composed of pore-forming α subunits and both transmembrane and cytosolic K^+ channel accessory subunits. Interactions between cardiac K^+ channels and the actin cytoskeleton are mediated through actin-binding proteins, such as filamin and α-actinin, and PDZ domain-containing scaffolding proteins.

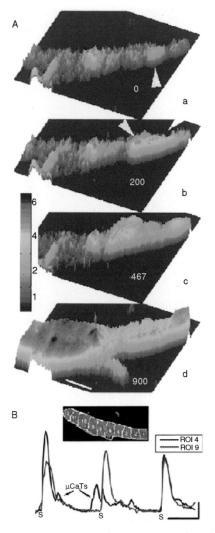

Figure 4.5. Nonuniformly occurring micro Ca^{2+} transients cause nonuniformity of the Ca^{2+} response of a paced canine IZPC aggregate. **Panel A**: Three-dimensional surface plots of IZPC just preceding and during an electrically evoked Ca^{2+} transient. $[Ca^{2+}]$ is denoted by both the color and height of the surface. White numbers indicate time of frame relative to $t = 0$ (Aa). The aggregate was stimulated just before $t = 900$ ms (Ad). Note the presence of micro Ca^{2+} waves (arrowheads), which propagate over short distances ($t = 0$ to 467 ms) meandering from the right section of the aggregate toward the core. Subsequent stimulation causes nonuniform electrically evoked local Ca^{2+} transients ($t = 900$ ms), particularly in regions where micro Ca^{2+} waves had been. The horizontal bar indicates $50 \, \mu m$. The color bar indicates ratio range. **Panel B**: Changes in intensity of fluorescence (F/F_0) at two selected specific regions of interest (ROIs) in IZPC aggregate of panel A. Stimuli are indicated (S). Each ROI is represented by a different color, and location is noted in upper image. Note that when the micro Ca^{2+} transients (μCa_iT) observed in ROI4 (see arrowheads of panel A) precede S, the subsequent Ca^{2+} transient of S is diminished compared with that of the previous S. Note that in ROIs where micro Ca^{2+} transients were absent (e.g., ROI 9), response to stimulation was constant. Vertical and horizontal lines are $1 \, F/F_0$ units and 1.58 s, respectively. Reproduced with permission from ref. 139.

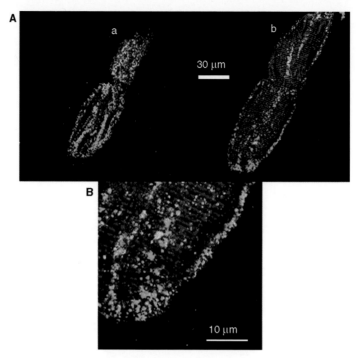

Figure 4.6. Localization of SR Ca^{2+} channels (RyR$_2$ and IP$_3$R$_1$) in a canine NZPC. **Panel Aa**: The superficial edge of the NZPC. Note that IP$_3$R$_1$ (green) are organized in bands and readily visible, whereas RYR$_2$ (red) are at a lower frequency. **Panel Ab**: The core section of the NZPC. Note that there is less IP$_3$R$_1$ (green) specific staining and more RYR$_2$ (red) staining; however, green pixels still surround the cells. **Panel B**: A high-power section showing the regionality of RyR$_2$ and IP$_3$R$_1$ in the NZPC. Scale bars were labeled in white lines.

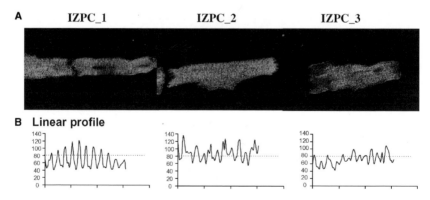

Figure 4.7. Three patterns of RYR$_2$ localization in IZPCs. **Panel A**: Three different types of RYR2 staining in IZPCs. **Panel B**: Linear profile for those cells of panel A after fluorescence intensity was averaged along longitudinal profiles through the binary images (not shown) of the cells. Note that type 1 cell shows regular periodicity of staining, type 2 cell lacks some periodicity, and type 3 cell shows the disorder. The vertical axis is fluorescence intensity; the horizontal axis is distance of pixels.

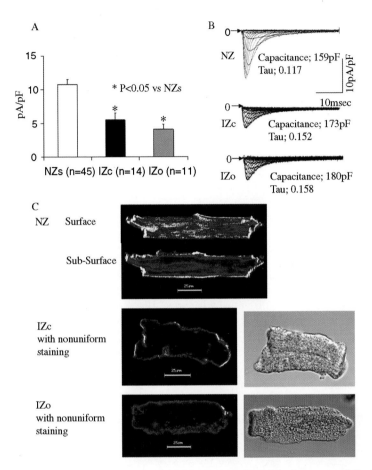

Figure 4.8. I_{Na} current recordings from NZs, IZc, and IZo. **Panel A**: Average peak I_{Na} in each of the three groups. Note that average peak I_{Na} of IZc and IZo were significantly smaller than that of NZs. **Panel B**: Family of Na^+ current tracing from a cell of each group. **Panel C**: Cell staining for the α-subunit of the cardiac sodium channel, $Na_v1.5$. Note that in the NZ, the optical plane through the surface shows cell membrane staining (pseudocolor is reddish orange) that is robust, uniform, and has a particular pattern, but no staining in the cell core. In the IZc and IZo, the cell surface staining is present but nonuniform in these core plane. The corresponding IZc and IZo micrographs (right) illustrate the morphological changes in the IZs. Note the altered shape. NZs = normal zone, epicardial cells from noninfarcted heart; IZc = Isshemic border zone epicardial cells dispersed from the center pathway of reentrant circuit; IZo = Ischemic border zone epicardial cells dispersed from adjacent outer pathway of reentrant circuit.

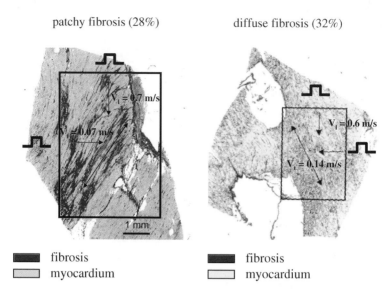

patchy fibrosis (28%)   diffuse fibrosis (32%)

fibrosis
myocardium

fibrosis
myocardium

Figure 4.11. Effect of the type of fibrosis on conduction velocity. The amount of fibrosis is similar for the tissue with patchy (left panel) and diffuse (right panel) fibrosis. Conduction parallel to the fiber direction is virtually the same. However, for activation running almost perpendicular to the fiber direction, conduction velocity in patchy fibrosis is only half of that in diffuse fibrosis. Adapted from ref. 238.

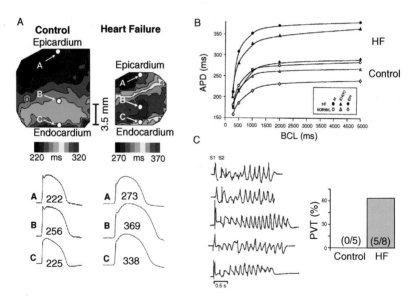

Figure 9.2. Heart Failure prolongs the AP and increases arrhythmia susceptibility **A. (Upper panel)** Representative APD contour maps recorded from the transmural surfaces of a control (left) and canine tachypacing HF wedge (right). APD was heterogeneously prolonged across all layers in HF. **(Lower panel)** Representative action potentials from subepicardial, midmyocardial, and subendocardial layers of the control and HF wedges. B. HF wedges exhibited a significant prolongation of APD in all layers of the myocardium, which was associated with a marked increase in arrhythmia inducibility (PVT%). **C.** with a single premature stimulus (modified from ref. 9).

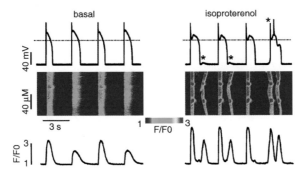

Figure 10.2. Two proarrhythmic phenotypes in HF: Calcium and action potential alternans (left) and DADs caused by spontaneous Ca^{2+} releases (right). Representative recordings of membrane potential with corresponding line-scan images and temporal profiles of Fluo-3 fluorescence in HF myocyte recorded in the absence (left panel) and in the presence (right panel) of 100 nM isoproterenol, a β-adrenergic receptor agonist. *Delayed afterdepolarizations. Dashed line marks 0 mV.

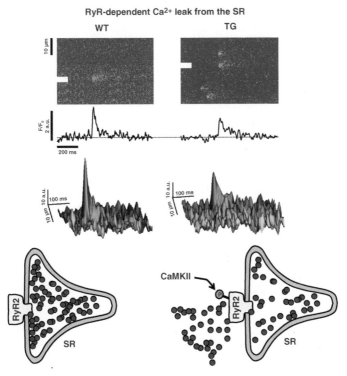

Figure 12.4. Increased SR Ca^{2+} leak caused by increased elementary SR Ca^{2+} release events (Ca^{2+} sparks). Original confocal images showing significantly increased Ca^{2+} spark frequency in CaMKIIδ_C transgenic mouse myocytes leading to a CaMKII-dependent diastolic SR Ca^{2+} leak. This leak is significantly (about four times) higher in TG than in WT. In contrast, CaMKII inhibition using KN-93 decreases Ca spark frequency back to control levels. An explanation for this increased Ca spark frequency most likely is the CaMKII-dependent hyperphosphorylation of SR Ca^{2+} release channels (RyR2; adapted from ref. 44).

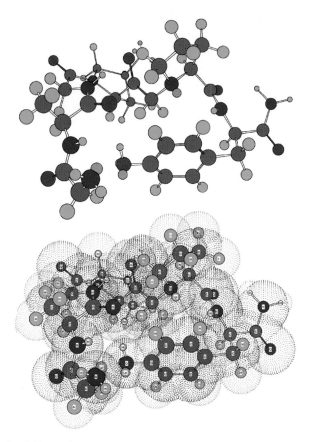

Figure 16.4. Spatial horseshoe-like semicyclic structure of AAP10 as revealed by ROESY, COSY, and computer simulation using MM2- and molecular dynamics simulation.

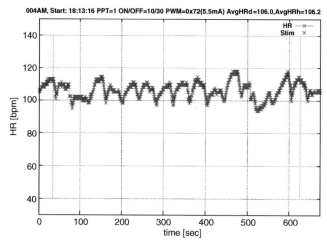

Figure 19.4. Heart rate observed during vagal stimulation (5.5 mAmp, 10 s ON time: red crosses, 30 s OFF time: blue crosses) in patient 4. A reduction of almost 10 b/min, starting from a baseline heart rate of 110 b/min occurs during the 10 s train of pulses (from ref. 55).

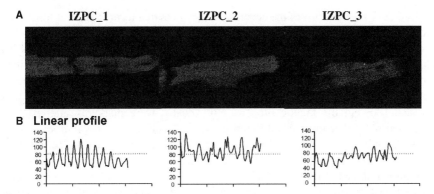

Figure 4.7. Three patterns of RYR_2 localization in IZPCs. **Panel A**: Three different types of RYR2 staining in IZPCs. **Panel B**: Linear profile for those cells of panel A after fluorescence intensity was averaged along longitudinal profiles through the binary images (not shown) of the cells. Note that type 1 cell shows regular periodicity of staining, type 2 cell lacks some periodicity, and type 3 cell shows the disorder. The vertical axis is fluorescence intensity; the horizontal axis is distance of pixels. See color insert.

of phase 3. Net membrane currents are significantly different between NZ and IZ groups, but I_{K1} appears to differ only at hyperpolarized potentials [147].

4.3.3.1 Sodium Current. Arrhythmias arise in the EBZ of the 5-day infarcted heart most likely caused by abnormalities in impulse conduction [134]. Although microelectrode recordings of IZs have shown resting potentials similar to those of NZs, the mean V_{max} of IZs remains significantly reduced when compared with NZs [146]. Steady-state availability relationships of V_{max} in IZs are shifted along the voltage axis in the hyperpolarizing direction by 10 mV [146, 148]. Lazzara and Scherlag [149] have suggested that in surviving cells in the 5-day infarcted heart, cellular inexcitability can outlast the repolarization phase of the AP or post repolarization refractoriness occurs. Clearly in NZ myocytes, the time constant of recovery of V_{max} is rapid and voltage dependent, whereas in IZ myocytes, the time course of recovery of V_{max} is significantly prolonged but remains voltage dependent [146, 148]. Whole cell voltage clamp data have confirmed that the reduced V_{max} of IZs is secondary to a decrease in I_{Na} density and altered Na^+ current kinetics [150]. In particular, a marked lag in recovery of I_{Na} seems to account in part for the cellular phenomenon of post repolarization refractoriness in these myocytes [150]. More recent studies have suggested that the altered inactivation gating kinetics of IZ I_{Na} affect the cellular action of the local anesthetic lidocaine [151]. In particular, the degree of tonic block of I_{Na} is significantly increased in IZs. Interestingly, whereas in drug-free conditions, there is a significant enhancement of use-dependent reduction of I_{Na} in IZs, the differences in rates of loss and recovery of availability of I_{Na} between NZs and IZs are minimized with lidocaine [151].

Studies of mechanisms of the decrease in I_{Na} in IZs that form the line of functional block during EBZ reentry have recently been completed. When IZ myocytes are dispersed from the central common pathway (IZc) and from the outer pathway (IZo) of mapped figure-of-eight reentrant circuits of the EBZ, we found that regional differences in several ionic currents of IZc and IZo cells help to form the line of functional block in this EBZ substrate [152]. In fact, I_{Na} density was reduced in both IZc and IZo, but the kinetic properties of IZc I_{Na} were markedly altered. This suggested to us that there are differences in the level of phosphorylation of Na^+ channels and/or regulation of β subunits on Na^+ channels between IZc and IZo. Furthermore, immunocytochemistry experiments indicate that the α-subunit, $Na_v1.5$ protein, is reduced at the IZ surface in both IZo and IZc, which is consistent with reduced peak I_{Na} in these areas (Figure 4.8). Another study using pharmacological techniques [153] also suggests that in the basal state, Na^+ channel proteins are already phosphorylated in IZs. This would interrupt trafficking of Na^+ channel proteins to the cell surface partially leading to the observed decrease in I_{Na} of IZs. Ankyrins are a family of intracellular adaptor proteins involved in targeting diverse proteins to specialized membrane domains. Ankyrin-G protein showed a time-dependent (24 h, 48 h, 5 day) significant increase in EBZ versus Remote tissues, whereas $Na_v1.5$ protein expression decreased in the EBZ. Ankyrin-G cell immunostaining was increased just below the sarcolemma in 5-day IZ cells [154]. Thus, we hypothesize that the increase in ankyrin-G protein expression may be an attempt of the cell to compensate for reduced $Na_v1.5$ protein levels in the IZ cells, because it is known that $Na_v1.5$ channel targeting in the heart requires the ankyrin-G dependent cellular pathway [155]. Finally, a more recent study shows that Ca^{2+}/calmodulin-dependent protein kinase II (CaMKII) is hyperactivated in the EBZ tissues [156]. Furthermore, in simulations, this CaMKII hyperactivity decreases peak I_{Na} during pacing (increased use dependence similar to experiments [151]) because of a depolarizing shift in sodium channel availability and a slowing of recovery from inactivation, leading to a reduction in the maximal upstroke velocity observed in simulated cell APs of the EBZ. Therefore, diverse intracellular components participate in Na^+ channel remodeling of the cells of the EBZ.

4.3.3.2 Ca^{2+} *Currents.*

The peak I_{CaL} density of IZ cells from the 5-day infarcted heart is reduced by 36% compared with control [157]. This density reduction is not caused by a decrease in steady-state availability or a prolonged time course of recovery of I_{CaL}. However, the time course of decay of these currents is significantly faster than control. These findings may be related to a decrease in the number of functioning channels as well as an acceleration of inactivation of the remaining channels. Unlike findings in the subendocardial Purkinje myocytes studies (see above), no significant differences were found between peak density and frequency of T type Ca^{2+} currents in IZs surviving in the 5-day infarcted heart versus NZs. Our knowledge of altered sensitivity to transmitters of the autonomic system in diseased myocytes is derived from comparisons of the effects of adrenergic agonists on specific ionic currents. Commonly, adrenergic sensitivity is assessed by the effects of the adrenergic agonist, isoproterenol, on I_{CaL}. In normal ventricular myocytes,

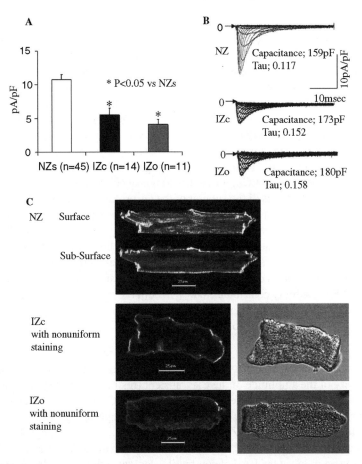

Figure 4.8. I_{Na} current recordings from NZs, IZc, and IZo. **Panel A**: Average peak I_{Na} in each of the three groups. Note that average peak I_{Na} of IZc and IZo were significantly smaller than that of NZs. **Panel B**: Family of Na^+ current tracing from a cell of each group. **Panel C**: Cell staining for the α-subunit of the cardiac sodium channel, $Na_v1.5$. Note that in the NZ, the optical plane through the surface shows cell membrane staining (pseudocolor is reddish orange) that is robust, uniform, and has a particular pattern, but no staining in the cell core. In the IZc and IZo, the cell surface staining is present but nonuniform in these core plane. The corresponding IZc and IZo micrographs (right) illustrate the morphological changes in the IZs. Note the altered shape. NZs = normal zone, epicardial cells from noninfarcted heart; IZc = Isshemic border zone epicardial cells dispersed from the center pathway of reentrant circuit; IZc = Ischemic border zone epicardial cells dispersed from adjacent outer pathway of reentrant circuit. See color insert.

isoproterenol depolarizes the resting membrane potential by inhibiting I_{K1} [158] and prolongs the action potential by increasing the I_{CaL} [159, 160]. Mimicry of isoproterenol effects using forskolin and cyclic adenosine $3',5'$-monophosphate (cAMP) has provided information regarding additional defects in the adrenergic complex.

Sympathetic stimulation produces minimal AP shortening in areas overlying the infarct and the border zone, whereas in areas remote from the arrhythmia substrate pronounced AP shortening occurs [161]. Furthermore, catecholamine-induced increases of the plateau phase of action potentials is absent in the fibers of the EBZ of the 5-day and 14-day infarcted heart [162]. Similar abbreviated responses to catecholamines have been documented in the ischemic human ventricle [163]. From voltage clamp data and when compared with normal cells, isoproterenol produces a smaller increase in I_{CaL} in IZs from the 5-day and 2-month-old infarct, independent of calcium dependent inactivation [164, 165]. This is consistent with multiple defects in components of the adrenergic receptor complex in IZs of the 5-day old infarct, including decreases in adrenergic receptor density; diminished basal, guanine nucleotide, isoproterenol, forskolin, and manganese-dependent adenylyl cyclase activities; increases in the EC_{50} for isoproterenol-dependent activation of adenylate cyclase; diminished levels of the subunit of the Gs protein; and elevated levels of the subunit of the Gi protein [166]. Therefore, an interesting question put forward is whether other signaling pathways are involved in the remodelled basal Ca^{2+} currents and isoproterenol-stimulated Ca^{2+} current function of the 5-day IZs. Protein tyrosine kinases (PTKs) have been shown to modulate basal as well as β-adrenergic-stimulated Ca^{2+} current function in cardiac cells from normal hearts [167]. A recent study has shown that PKA activity contributes to I_{CaL} in both NZs and IZs, but dysregulation of PTK activity cannot account for the reduced basal Ca^{2+} currents or hyporesponsiveness of I_{CaL} to isoproterenol in the IZs [168].

4.3.3.3 Intracellular Ca^{2+} in IZs.
In the NZ, an increase in rate is associated with an increase in Ca_i transient amplitude whereas in IZs it is not [169]. In addition, the recovery of the amplitude of the Ca_i transient (restitution) is markedly slowed in the IZs, although there is marked rest potentiation of Ca_i transients in IZ myocytes versus rest depression of the Ca_i transients in the NZ. Importantly, despite the smaller amplitude Ca_i transients in the IZ, little or no cell shortening exists, suggesting that the lack of cell shortening in the IZ may be related to dramatic alterations in excitation-contraction coupling at the level of contractile element activation and/or to an altered production of microtubules. Furthermore, when clamping the transmembrane voltage with the AP profile, we found that abnormal Ca_i transients in voltage clamped IZs persist [170]. In these experiments, in the NZ, Ca_i transients showed the expected voltage dependence while the IZ did not. Thus, the abnormalities in Ca_i handling in the IZ appear not to arise secondary to changes in AP configuration nor do they appear to be due to disease-induced alterations in NaCa exchanger function. Interestingly, the abnormal Ca_i transients of IZs are "rescued" when cells are superfused with the L-type calcium channel agonist, Bay5959 [171]. This effect on the remodeled cells may underlie Bay5959 antiarrhythmic effect in this model of VT in the post infarcted heart [172].

4.3.3.4 Repolarization.
Even though post repolarization refractoriness exists in both the single-cell and multiple-cell preparations of the 5-day EBZ, these cells repolarize abnormally, suggesting defects in K^+ currents.

Transient outward current (I_{to}). APs recorded from IZs usually show no phase 1or reduced phase 1 of repolarization, suggesting a loss in the voltage-dependent Ito [146]. This is in contrast to APs recorded from epicardial NZs, which show a large and prominent spike and dome morphology. Voltage clamp studies confirm that the density and kinetics of the voltage-dependent and non-$Ca^{2+}{}_i$ dependent I_{to} in the IZ myocytes demonstrating the loss in the notch are reduced [146]. Transcriptional regulation of the KChIP2 gene is a primary determinant of I_{to} expression in canine ventricle and KChIP2 coexpressed with Kv4.3 channel increases the density of expressed I_{to} [173]. We have found that I_{to} densities were significantly increased by injection of adenoviral constructs of KChIP2 (AdKChIP2) to the EBZ and thus "rescued" by AdKChIP2 (Figure 4.9D), suggesting a new therapy for rescue of remodeled potassium channels; one that is based on increasing the availability of an important accessory subunit of a remodeled ion channel. This so-called rescue therapy may also apply to other channels remodeled post infarction (i.e., the beta subunits of sodium channel proteins).

Delayed rectifier K current (I_K). Similarly, densities of I_{Ks} and I_{Kr} (the two components of I_K) are reduced significantly in IZ myocytes dispersed from the 5-day infarcted heart [174]. Our kinetic analysis suggested that I_{Kr} activation and I_{Ks} deactivation were accelerated in IZ myocytes. Messenger RNA (mRNA) levels of I_{Kr} and I_{Ks} channel subunits (ERG, KCNE1, and KCNQ1) are all reduced 2 days after total coronary artery occlusion. By day 5, the KCNQ1 mRNA level returns to normal, whereas the ERG and KCNE1 levels remain reduced [174]. Interestingly, a "lone" KCNQ1 type current, which is an isoproterenol- stimulated azimilide-sensitive current, voltage-dependent and fast activated, is upregulated in some of IZs [175], which is consistent with the transcript findings above (a completely recovered KCNQ1 and still decreased KCNE1 mRNA levels by day 5 after total coronary artery occlusion). These changes, if occurring alone, would retard action potential repolarization.

Ca^{2+}-dependent outward currents. Studies using normal myocytes of some species have shown the presence of two types of transient outward currents. One is transient, voltage dependent, and 4-AP sensitive (I_{to}, see above). The other is Ca^{2+} dependent (I_{to2}) [176–179]. It is thought that for normal myocytes, the source of intracellular Ca^{2+} activating $I_{to,2}$ results from Ca^{2+} released from the sarcoplasmic reticulum. In IZs, pronounced changes in $Ca^{2+}{}_i$ cycling persist (see above) [169]. Furthermore, these Ca_i cycling changes are reflected in the characteristics of the Ca_i dependent outward currents(I_{to2}) of these cells [180]. Namely, the difference between the magnitude of I_{to2} in IZ versus NZ myocytes is exaggerated with constant pacing. Generally, for NZs, beat to beat change in I_{to2} tracked frequency dependent changes in $I_{Ca,L}$ [180] and the globally assessed $Ca^{2+}{}_i$ transient amplitude [169]. For IZs, $Ca^{2+}{}_i$ transients varied in amplitude, as I_{to2} amplitude and I_{CaL} decreased with the fast pacing rate. Thus, differences in $I_{to,2}$ observed in response to pacing in the two cell types led to heterogeneity of AP repolarization within the infarcted heart.

Na^+/Ca^2-currents. In normal myocytes with normal $Ca^{2+}{}_i$ cycling, it is well established that currents generated by the Na^+/Ca^{2+} exchanger can play an important role in the electrical activity of a myocyte [181]. The Na^+/Ca^{2+} current is either outward (normal mode) as the transporter protein exchanges $Ca^{2+}{}_i$ for external Na^+ ions, or inward (reverse mode) as the transporter causes Ca^{2+} influx by exchanging external Ca^{2+} ions for $Na^+{}_i$. Therefore, the time course of the exchanger current is related to the time course of $Ca^{2+}{}_i$ cycling. There have been several reports of

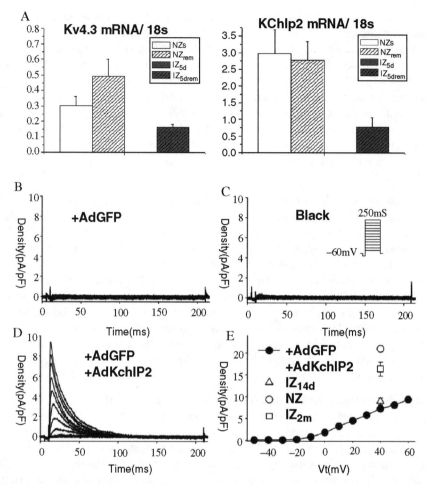

Figure 4.9. Effect of "rescue" of KChIP2 on the α-subunit of the cardiac I_{to}, K_v4. 3, in the IZs. **Panel A**: average Kv4.3 mRNA/18S mRNA (left) and KChIP2 mRNA/18S mRNA (right) in the EBZ and remote slices from control noninfarcted canine hearts (CON) and the same from the 5-day infarcted hearts. Note that there is a significant decrease in both Kv4.3 and KChIP2 mRNA in the EBZ and remote regions of the 5-day hearts **Panel B**: Current tracings of 4AP sensitive currents (Ito) from + AdGFP(adeno virus with GFP) (Panel B), black (Panel C) and + AdGFP + AdKChIP2(virus with KChIP2) (Panel D) IZ5d. Currents were elicited by membrane depolarization from a holding voltage (Vh) of −60 mV to various test voltages (Vt: from −50 to +60 mV in 10 mV increments) for 210 ms once every 10 s (see inset). Panel E shows the current-voltage relations of 4AP sensitive Ito density from + AdGFP + AdKChIP2 IZ5d and average densities for NZs, IZ14d and IZ2m [233]. Note that in + AdGFP + AdKChIP2 IZ5d), there is a marked increase in amplitude of Ito current (Panel D). In fact, the "rescued" current in this IZ5d approached the Ito value of IZ14d (triangle) but still was reduced compared with NZ and IZ2m average values (circle and square). Consistent with our published data [146] about this substrate, black IZ5d (n = 3) and + AdGFP IZ5d (n = 1) show no 4AP sensitive currents.

abnormal Ca^{2+}_i cycling in cells that have survived in the infarcted heart [182–186]. In IZs, both current clamp [169] and voltage clamp studies [170] show that the diminished globally (whole cell) assessed Ca^{2+}_i transient of the IZ has a slow relaxation (decay) phase. Furthermore, these cells have an altered phase 3 of their APs. These changes are consistent with changes in the Na^+/Ca^{2+} exchanger current. However, when studied under strict conditions that isolate only Ca^{2+}_i and ionic current changes secondary to the Na^+/Ca^{2+} exchanger, both Ca^{2+} entry (via the reverse exchanger) and Ni^{2+} sensitive IZ currents as well as Ca^{2+} extrusion (via normal mode exchanger) in IZ myocyte are similar to those of the NZ, no matter what the Na^+_i load [170]. Thus, in these cells where L type Ca^{2+} channels are down-regulated (see above), the Na^+/Ca^{2+} exchanger has a reserve efficiency and continues to contribute current to the transmembrane AP.

Connexins. In addition to the numerous ion channels that contribute to transmembrane voltage profile, ion channels that form at gap junctions between two cells play a role in impulse propagation and perhaps repolarization. In the EBZ of the 5-day infarcted heart, reentrant arrhythmias occur in fibers where impulse propagation shows accentuated anisotropic properties [187]. Subcellular redistribution of the gap junction protein connexin 43 (Cx43) has been observed and correlated with the likelihood of sustained ventricular tachycardias in both the healing (5 day) and chronically infarcted myocardium [188, 189]. Recently the *functional* consequences of these changes in Cx43 proteins have been determined using cell IZ and NZ cell pairs [190]. Gap junctional conductance (Gj) between IZ pairs connected side to side was reduced to 10% of its control value, whereas Gj between IZ cell pairs connected end to end was reduced to 30% of its control value [190]. Gj of end-to-end-coupled IZs is not different from end-to-end-coupled NZs. Furthermore, the heterogeneous structural remodeling of Cx43 has been studied in cells dispersed from either side of the line of functional block localized by mapping the reentrant circuits [191] in an attempt to understand how the line of functional block is formed during this reentry. The transverse (side-to-side) coupling (gap junction conductance) is markedly decreased in outer path cell (IZo) pairs compared with that of center path (IZc) pair Gj that is similar to NZ pairs [191]. Longitudinal (end-to-end) coupling in both IZc and IZo does not differ from NZs. Interestingly, the marked functional changes in gap junctional conductance in IZo pairs are NOT accompanied by Cx43 protein lateralization along the cell membrane (structural remodeling). Rather, and in contrast to IZc cells and tissues where prominent Cx43 lateralization has occurred, functional changes in gap conductance have not occurred. We suggest then that lateralization of Cx43 protein may be a compensatory cellular response to *restore* the reduced coupling conductance. However, we think it is more likely that lateralized Cx43 protein found at the IZc lateral membranes does not form functional gap junctions between IZs. In this case, the Cx43 lateralization that occurs in IZc cells would not be expected to have an effect in transverse conductance [191].

4.3.3.4.1 Structural Anatomy EBZ. Both histologic images and magnetic resonance imaging (MRI) indicate that the region of central common pathway of the reentry circuit of the 5 day EBZ is much thinner than that of the outer [135, 192]. The functional block lines of the reentry circuit are formed along the central pathway lateral edges where a transition from thin to thick structures happens, leading to a large impedance mismatch. Thus, the unique three-dimensional anatomical structure of the EBZ may also contribute to forming the reentry circuits in 5-day infarcted hearts.

4.4 ARRHYTHMIA MECHANISMS IN CHRONIC INFARCTION

4.4.1 Reentry and Focal Mechanisms

Studies carried out in animal models of chronic infarction and in humans suggest that reentry is the major mechanism of ventricular tachycardia in the healed phase of myocardial infarction. The anatomical structure of the chronically infarcted heart provides an ideal substrate for reentrant circuits. Various studies present evidence for the existence of surviving myocardial strands that traverse (part of) the infarcted zone [193, 194]. These reentrant pathways may be located subepicardially, subendocardially or even intramurally. In the human heart, surviving areas are frequently found at the subendocardium, whereas in experimental models they are often present in the subepicardial border zone. The reentrant pathways involve channels with various diameter, which are ideally suited to set-up unidirectional conduction block at sites where a discontinuity arises because of sudden change in channel diameter [195]. Although conduction slowing in hearts as large as the human heart is not a prerequisite for reentry, conduction slowing often arises in the infarcted zone, [193, 196, 197]. In sporadic cases, activation revolving around the infarct scar has been observed at close to normal conduction velocity [193], but in most instances, surviving tracts in the infarct area are involved. In the healed phase of myocardial infarction, the surviving myocardial tracts within the infarcted zone reveal close to normal electrophysiological characteristics [195, 198]. Conduction slowing arises because of the increased route activation has to travel through the labyrinth of merging and diverging myocardial bundles. The resulting zig-zag route of activation causes apparent conduction slowing [195, 199]. Additional conduction slowing may arise at sites with tissue discontinuities [200]. Fiber direction is another factor that profoundly affects conduction velocity. In myocardium remote from the infarcted site, anisotropy may increase because interstitial fibrosis is enhanced. In the infarcted area and the border zone, sudden changes in fiber direction may arise and affect conduction. Spach et al. [201] have shown that sudden changes in fiber orientation are preferential sites for conduction slowing and block. In hypertrophic myocardium (remote from the infarct), conduction velocity may even be faster than normal as a result of the larger dimensions of the myocyte and the resulting fewer cell-cell transitions encountered per unit of distance [202].

Although reentry seems to be the key player for ventricular arrhythmias in the chronic phase of myocardial infarction, Pogwizd et al. [203] demonstrated by applying three dimensional intraoperative mapping in patients with healed myocardial infarction, that 50% of the sustained ventricular tachycardias were initiated in the subendocardium by a focal mechanism. There were no significant conduction delays at adjacent sites 1–2 cm away from sites revealing focal activity. In another study of isolated superfused preparations, the investigators showed that microreentry could occur within areas as small as 0.05 cm^2 [204]. In the human study, activation delays in the order of 100 ms over a span of 1–2 cm had been observed. Therefore, the authors felt it unlikely that the focal mechanism was based on microreentry. Histological analysis of the site of focal origin showed extensively thickened and fibrotic subendocardial tissue with residual small subendocardial bundles and Purkinje fibers in a number of cases. However, similar histological characteristics were found in hearts from patients revealing reentry as mechanism for ventricular tachycardia (VT) [203].

An extensive overview of the mechanism of ventricular tachycardias in the healing and healed phase of myocardial infarction has been provided by Janse and Wit in ref. [5].

Although the infarct structure consisting of an intermingling of fibrotic and surviving myocardial bundles probably represents the basis for infarct-related ventricular tachycardias, various other factors will add to arrhythmogenesis. These factors not only include the anisotropic characteristics and structural complexity of the heart but also involve heterogeneities that already exist in the healthy, non-compromised, heart like heterogeneity in ion and gap junction channel expression in the ventricles. In addition, these parameters are often modified after cardiac disease in such a way that conduction and/or repolarization are impaired and arrhythmia vulnerability is increased.

4.4.2 Heterogeneity of Ion Channel Expression in the Healthy Heart

Local cardiac repolarization is determined by the combination of local activation time and local action potential duration. The healthy, noncompromised heart is character-ized by regional heterogeneity of the action potential configuration and duration. These differences are caused by variations in the density of the underlying trans-membrane ion currents between different areas of the heart. Action potentials recorded at the epicardium have a prominent spike and dome configuration that is absent in the subendocardially recorded action potentials [205, 206]. The notch of the action potential is caused by the relatively large transient outward current I_{to} in the subepicardial layers. A transmural gradient in action potential duration has been reported with longer durations in midmyocardial cells. Although the transmural gradient in action potential duration has been documented in isolated cells and isolated canine left ventricular wedge preparations, it does not occur in intact tissue [64, 207–210]. The gradient in the intrinsic action potential duration has been explained by differences in the slowly activating component of the delayed rectifier potassium current I_{Kr} between the sub-epicardial and mid-myocardial cells Liu et al. [205]. The rapidly activating component I_{Ks} of the delayed rectifier and the inward rectifier current I_{K1} seem to be similar in the different layers. However, Volders et al. [211] have shown that I_{Ks} is larger in the right than the left ventricular midmyocardium of the canine heart.

A gradient in action potential duration that is also reflected in heterogeneity in repolarization times may be of more importance for arrhythmia vulnerability because of its propensity to lead to unidirectional block. Szentadrassy et al. [212] demonstrated the existence of a marked apicobasal gradient in ionic currents and ion channel proteins in both canine and human ventricular myocardium. Especially the densities of I_{to} and I_{Ks} currents proved to be 2 times as large in apical compared with basal cardiomyocytes, which could explain the shorter action potential duration at the apex of the heart compared with the base (Figure 4.10).

Electrophysiological heterogeneity in the heart is not limited to transmural and apicobasal gradients of potassium channels. The interventricular septum is molecularly and electrically heterogeneous. Messenger RNA levels of the β-subunit of I_{to} and the α-subunit of I_{Ks} are higher in cells of the right ventricular septum as compared to the left ventricular septum [213]. These differences in mRNA expression were associated with small differences in action potential duration and configuration. Action potential duration in cells of the left ventricular septum is longer than in the right side of the interventricular septum.

Another ion channel gradient that is present in the normal human heart is sodium channel density. Ashamalla et al. [214] showed in the rat heart that sodium current density is significantly lower in epicardial cells of the left ventricle compared with those present in endocardial cells of the same ventricle. The biophysical characteristics of these channels were, however, similar for both cell populations, suggesting that the gradient is not attributed to differential distribution of sodium channel isoforms. The sodium calcium exchanger too is differentially expressed in the heart and proved to be greatest at the epicardium and least in subendocardial myocytes [215].

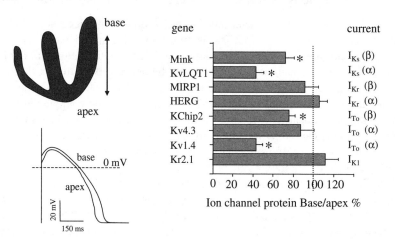

Figure 4.10. Left panel: apex-basal gradient in action potential duration. The action potential duration of ventricular cells is shorter at the apex compared with the base. Right panel: Ratio of potassium channel proteins of base and apex. Note that the lower expression of the α and β subunits of most of the potassium channels at the base of the heart results in a longer action potential at the base. Adapted from ref. 212.

The gap junction protein Cx43 does not escape heterogeneity. Several studies have shown that cell-to-cell coupling, which is mediated by Cx43 in ventricular working myocardium, shortens action potential duration and reduces its intrinsic differences [125, 216]. Tight cell-to-cell coupling that is present in the healthy, noncompromised, heart, attenuates these heterogeneities. Because several studies reveal a transmural gradient in action potential duration, Poelzing et al. [217] hypothesized that heterogeneous Cx43 expression could be the cause of this. Using wedge preparations of the dog heart, the investigators demonstrated that Cx43 expression was indeed lower in the subepicardial layers of the left ventricular wall as compared with the subendocardium and intramural layers. Yamada et al. [218] did find a similar transmural gradient in which the subepicardial Cx43 expression was about 50% of that in the midendocardial and subendocardial layers of the mouse heart. Interestingly, such a transmural gradient of Cx43 was not seen in rat hearts [218]. Wiegerinck et al. [219] documented intramural loss of Cx43 in association with increased dispersion of refractoriness in a rabbit model of heart failure. In another study in rabbit hearts, the lowest Cx43 expression was also found in the midmyocardial layers [220]. These observations indicate that there is a high variability among species. The differences in gap junction channel expression may increase heterogeneity in action potential duration and enhance arrhythmogenesis. Data about the human heart are currently lacking.

Action potential characteristics are modulated by the amplitude and duration of the intracellular Ca-transient. Transmural heterogeneity exists in the shape of the Ca-transient and in the underlying Ca-handling proteins [221]. Evidence exists that these transmural heterogeneities play a role in action potential alternation, especially at rapid heart rates. Alternation in action potential duration is important for the initiation of reentry [222].

4.4.3   Remodeling in Chronic Myocardial Infarction

Cardiac disease is associated with structural, electrical, and (para)sympathetic remodeling, which may initially be adaptive in nature but finally may have maladaptive consequences leading to cardiac arrhythmias. Electrical remodeling involves changes in ion channel expression and/or function as well as alterations in gap junction expression and/or distribution.

4.4.3.1   *Ion Channel Remodeling.*   Valdivia et al. [223] showed that in hearts from patients with heart failure undergoing heart transplantation, the peak I_{Na} density was decreased by 57%, although the kinetics were not different from control hearts (hearts from donors of whom the hearts were not used for technical reasons). A 50% reduction of the sodium current has been shown to reduce conduction velocity by approximately 20%, which indicates that this "loss of function" could facilitate reentrant arrhythmia [224]. In addition, the study by Valdivia et al. showed that the late or persistent I_{Na} current was significantly increased. This current may contribute to action potential prolongation and in that way may promote the occurrence of triggered

arrhythmias. Similar observations in human failing myocytes have been made by Undrovinas et al. [225].

In heart failure, which is often the result of myocardial infarction, the action potential duration of the surviving myocardium is usually increased, and next to decreased cell-to-cell coupling, alterations in potassium current may underlie these changes. In a rat study of chronic myocardial infarction caused by ligation of the left anterior descending coronary artery, it was shown that in isolated left ventricular myocytes (from noninfarcted myocardium) the transient outward currents I_{to-f} and I_{to-s} were significantly reduced, but kinetics of both currents were similar to controls [226]. Also in the failing human heart, I_{to} has been shown to be downregulated [227].

Studies of the calcium current in post myocardial infarction have yielded variable results, some showing a decrease, whereas others did not find any difference [228, 229]. This may be because of differences in infarct size or heterogeneity of regional responses, where the remote and adjacent regions may differ. Kim et al. [230] showed that in sheep with anteroseptal myocardial infarction the contractile function, calcium transients and the L-type calcium current were reduced 8 weeks after onset. Changes occurred both in the border zone and at remote sites but were largest in regions adjacent to the infarction. The authors suggest that the impaired excitation-contraction coupling underlies the dysfunction of noninfarcted, remodeled myocardium. The decrease in L-type calcium current may result in action potential prolongation as shown in the study of Santos et al. [229]. Next to reduction of the calcium current, slowing of inactivation of the current has been observed in rat hearts with chronic infarcts [231]. These changes in the biophysical characteristics of the calcium current may contribute to the disturbance in cellular electrical behavior and increase arrhythmia vulnerability in the chronically infarcted heart.

Decreases in I_{K1} and the delayed-rectifier currents I_{Ks} and I_{Kr} have also been observed in the rabbit hearts with healed myocardial infarction [232]. These changes resulted in action potential prolongation and the occurrence of early after depolarizations in cells isolated from the rabbit hearts.

Dun et al. [233] have studied potassium and calcium currents in surviving epicardial myocytes at various times following myocardial infarction. Changes in these currents occur at least up to 14 days after occlusion. By 2 months post occlusion, there is somewhat of a normalization of the action potential duration, but action potential duration (APD) is now governed by a slightly different balance of current densities.

4.4.3.2 Gap Junction Remodeling.

Marked changes in connexin43 expression and distribution occur in healed myocardial infarction in both patients and animal models [234]. Kostin et al. [235] showed that in myocytes bordering regions of healed myocardial infarction, connexin43 labeling was highly disrupted instead of being confined to the intercalated discs. In myocardium distant from the infarct region, Cx43 distribution was normal at the intercalated discs, but the Cx43 area per myocyte surface was significantly decreased by 30% as compared with normal human myocardium.

Although the heart has a great redundancy with regard to connexin43 expression, the focal disorganization of gap junction distribution in concert with the down-regulation of Cx43 could play a role in the development of an arrhythmogenic substrate in the healed phase of myocardial infarction. The redundancy of Cx43 has been emphasized by a study on mice heterozygous for connexin43 [236]. *In vivo* and *in vitro* studies on wild-type and Cx43-deficient mice 10 weeks after induced myocardial infarction revealed no statistical difference in spontaneous and induced ventricular arrhythmias. There was only a trend toward increased arrhythmia vulnerability with regard to the incidence of nonsustained ventricular tachycardias in the isolated heart.

4.4.4 Structural Remodeling

Myocardial infarction is accompanied by loss of necrotic cardiomyocytes, which presents a reparative process to maintain structural integrity of the heart. In the initial process, inflammatory cells invade the site of injury, regulatory peptides are activated, angiogenesis is initiated, and fibroblast-like cells (myofibroblasts) appear and replicate. The early inflammatory phase results in granulation tissue and is followed by a fibrogenic phase, which leads to scar tissue. In case of large transmural infarction, the entire heart is involved in the repair process, and unwanted collagen deposition occurs at sites remote from the infarcted zone. Although the healing process is considered to be completed 6 to 8 weeks after the onset of myocardial infarction in humans, the remodeling process does not stop at this time [72]. The myofibroblasts are persistent at the infarct site and continue to produce fibrillar type 1 collagen. This ongoing process is reflected by the increase of fractionated electrograms, which has been shown to occur after onset of infarction [237].

Tissue fibrosis is the result of an altered balance between collagen synthesis and degradation, the latter being mediated by metalloproteinases. Thus, collagen is continuously synthesized and deposited in the infarct scar and is not a transient but an ongoing, slow process. Although the infarcted tissue may consist entirely of collagen, this is often not the case. Collateral vessels that are present may cause parts of the compromised myocardial area to survive, giving rise to patchy or diffuse fibrosis consisting of an intermingling of myocardial and fibrotic fibers. This structure of a mixture of excitable and nonexcitable fibers is highly arrhythmogenic, mainly because activation has to follow a tortuous route through the resulting labyrinth. This results in apparent conduction slowing; conduction within the surviving fibers is usually close to normal [195, 198].

Although the amount of fibrosis is to some extent related to the amount of conduction slowing, it is not the complete story. The type of fibrosis also has an impact on conduction slowing, the effect of patchy fibrosis being greater than that of diffuse fibrosis [238] (Figure 4.11). As mentioned, the arrhythmogenic substrate for reentry usually involves the infarct region or at least part of it, but reentry encircling the infarct scar has been observed occasionally.

patchy fibrosis (28%)   diffuse fibrosis (32%)

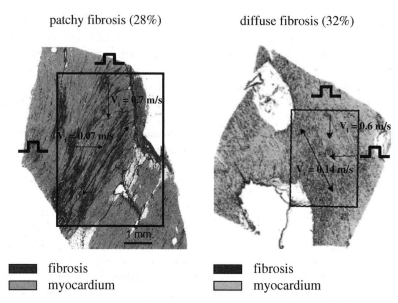

Figure 4.11. Effect of the type of fibrosis on conduction velocity. The amount of fibrosis is similar for the tissue with patchy (left panel) and diffuse (right panel) fibrosis. Conduction parallel to the fiber direction is virtually the same. However, for activation running almost perpendicular to the fiber direction, conduction velocity in patchy fibrosis is only half of that in diffuse fibrosis. Adapted from ref. 238. See color insert.

4.4.4.1 *Role of the Autonomic Nervous System.*

Next to electrical and structural remodeling, neural remodeling plays an important role in arrhythmogenicity in the chronic phase of myocardial infarction. Various clinical and experimental studies have shown that after myocardial infarction, diminished vagal activity, sympathetic hyperinnervation, heterogeneous cardiac nerve sprouting, and sympathetic imbalance are important players in arrhythmia vulnerability [239–242]. In the noncompromised heart, significant functional asymmetry exists between left and right sympathetic innervation [242]. The left and right sympathetic imbalance has been linked to the sudden infant death syndrome by Schwarz [243], who suggested that prolongation of the QT interval in these patients depends on alterations in sympathetic innervation. The mammalian peripheral nervous system can regenerate after injury. Nori et al. [244] showed that denervation occurred directly after injury of the myocardium, but that proliferative regeneration of nerve fibers followed. Similar observations of denervation followed by reinnervation have been made in humans and dog models of myocardial infarction [245]. Nerve sprouting after myocardial infarction may help increase hemodynamic performance of remaining myocardium, but excessive sprouting may give rise to abnormal patterns of myocardial innervation and increase arrhythmia vulnerability.

Indeed, several studies showed that an abnormal increase in sympathetic nerve sprouting was responsible for ventricular arrhythmogenesis after myocardial infarction [240, 245]. This was supported by infusion of nerve growth factor to the left stellate ganglion in infarcted dog hearts, which profoundly increased nerve generation and the incidence of sudden cardiac death. Jiang et al. [246], in a study carried out in rabbit hearts at 8 weeks after myocardial infarction, describe that the magnitude of sympathetic nerve sprouting was associated with local transmural dispersion of repolarization, which might provide an arrhythmogenic component.

4.4.5 Role of the Purkinje System

Several tachycardias arise at the subendocardium because this area often survives because of the presence of a subendocardial plexus [247]. Studies by Fenoglio et al. [194] and Friedman et al. [248] showed that subendocardial Purkinje fibers at the infarcted region remain virtually intact [194]. Animal studies, however, revealed that the surviving Purkinje fibers exhibited increased action potential duration and spontaneous depolarization or reentry [248]. In a clinical study, Bogun et al. [249] selected 9 patients from a group of 81 post-infarct patients with monomorphic ventricular tachycardias. The ventricular arrhythmias had a relatively narrow QRS complex, mimicking fascicular tachycardias. Catheter mapping of the tachycardias demonstrated reentry in the inferior left ventricular wall. At the exit site of the tachycardia, Purkinje activity was recorded that preceded the QRS complex during sinus rhythm. The exit site was located within the scar region, and conduction was slow at sites with contiguous Purkinje signals. Classic bundle branch reentry was excluded. Ablation at the exit site abolished the tachycardias.

Szumowski et al. [250] showed that the Purkinje system may also play a role in triggering and maintenance of polymorphic ventricular tachycardias. In three of five patients with recurrent episodes of ventricular tachycardia following anterior MI, the polymorphic tachycardias occurred in the early phase after myocardial infarction (4 to 8 days after onset), whereas in two other patients the arrhythmias arose in the chronic phase (150 and 170 days after MI). In all cases, ventricular premature beats, which initiated the polymorphic tachycardia, were preceded by Purkinje potentials along the border zone of scar tissue. Purkinje activity preceded the QRS complex by 20 to 60 ms. Ablation of the associated Purkinje network resulted in suppression of the tachyarrhythmias.

More support for a role of the Purkinje system in initiating and maintaining polymorphic ventricular tachycardias was provided by Berenfeld and Jalife [251]. These investigators used a three-dimensional model of the mammalian ventricles, in which an extensive Purkinje network was incorporated. In their model, propagation of the electrical activity from Purkinje to muscle was slower than in the opposite direction, which could lead to undirectional conduction block and reentrant activity. In the initial stage, maintenance of reentry depended on the coexistence of myocardium and Purkinje, but at a later stage reentry persisted even without the Purkinje system. These studies indicate that the Purkinje system plays a role in several tachycardias related to remote myocardial infarction.

4.4.5.1 Molecular Markers of Arrhythmogenicity. Recently it has been found that microRNAs (miRNAs) play a crucial role in regulating cardiac arrhythmogenicity [252]. miRNAs are about 22 nucleotides in length and mediate posttranscriptional gene silencing. They regulate a variety of physiological functions, which include development, proliferation, and apoptosis. Up to now, more than 300 miRNA genes have been identified of which miR-1 and miR-133 are considered to be muscle specific. Most commonly, the miRNAs pair with the 3' untranslated region of the microRNA to repress or completely silence protein formation. Yang et al. [253] recently showed that microRNA miR-1 expression is upregulated in structurally diseased human hearts and in the infarct border zone of a rat model of myocardial infarction. The investigators provided evidence that this upregulation is associated with electrical remodeling and arrhythmias.

Increased miR-1 proved to be related with reduced expression of connexin43 and decreased Kir2.1, which is the α-subunit of the inward rectifier current I_{K1}. The reduction in cell-to-cell coupling may promote reentry arrhythmias, whereas the reduced potassium current will lengthen action potential duration and may cause afterdepolarizations. On the one hand, the role of miR-1 was elucidated even more by transfecting the microRNA into healthy hearts, which resulted in widening of the QRS complex and prolonged QT interval, indicating conduction slowing and increased action potential duration. On the other hand, blocking miR-1 in the infarcted heart with antisense oligonucleotides normalized connexin43 and Kir2.1 expression. These studies underscore the important role of miR-1 in arrhythmogenesis in the infarcted heart. The role of miR-1 in hypertrophy, however, is still unclear [254].

REFERENCES

1. Podrid, P.J., Myerburg, R.J. (2005). Epidemiology and stratification of risk for sudden cardiac death. Clinical Cardiology, 28, I3–I11.
2. Porter, W.T. (1894). On the results of ligation of the coronary arteries. Jouranl of Physiology, 15, 121–138.
3. Dekker, L.R.C., Bezzina, C.R., Henriques, J.P.S., Tanck, M.W., Koch, K.T., Alings, M. W., Arnold, A.E.R., de Boer, M.J., Gorgels, A.P.M., Michels, H.R., Verkerk, A., Verheugt, F.W.A., Zijlstra, F., Wilde, A.A.M. (2006). Familial sudden death is an important risk factor for primary ventricular fibrillation: A case-control study in acute myocardial infarction patients. Circulation, 114, 1140–1145.
4. Akhtar, M., Breithardt, G., Camm, A.J., Coumel, P., Janse, M.J., Lazarra, R., Myerburg, R.J., Schwartz, P.J., Waldo, A.L., Wellens, H.J.J., Zipes, D.P. (1990). CAST and beyond: Implications of the cardiac arrhythmia suppression trial. Circulation, 81, 1123–1127.
5. Janse, M.J., Wit, A.L. (1989). Electrophysiological mechanisms of ventricular arrhythmias resulting from myocardial ischemia and infarction. Physiological Reviews, 69, 1049–1169.
6. Harris, A.S. (1950). Delayed development of ventricular ectopic rhythms following experimental coronary occlusion. Circulation, 1, 1318–1328.

7. Garcia-Dorado, D., Ruiz-Meana, M., Padilla, F., Rodriguez-Sinovas, A., Mirabet, M. (2002). Gap junction-mediated intercellular communication in ischemic preconditioning. Cardiovascular Research, 55, 456–465.

8. Skelton, R.B., Gergely, N., Manning, G.W., Coles, J.C. (1962). Mortality studies in experimental coronary occlusion. Journal of Thoracic Cardiovascular Surgery, 44, 90–96.

9. David, G.K. (1979). Myocardial Infarction in Young Adults. A Clinical and Angiographic Study. Tulp, Zwolle, The Netherlands.

10. Harris, A.S., Rojas, A.G. (1943). The initiation of ventricular fibrillation due to coronary occlusion. Experimental Medicine and Surgery, 1, 105–111.

11. Kaplinsky, E., Ogawa, S., Blake, C.W., Dreifus, L.S. (1979). Two periods of early ventricular arrhythmias in the canine acute myocardial infarction model. Circulation, 60, 397–403.

12. de Groot, J.R., Wilms-Schopman, F.J.G., Opthof, T., Remme, C.A., Coronel, R. (2001). Late ventricular arrhythmias during acute regional ischemia in the isolated blood perfused pig heart. Role of electrical cellular coupling. Cardiovascular Research, 50, 362–372.

13. Coronel, R., Wilms-Schopman, F.J.G., de Groot, J.R. (2002). Origin of ischemia-induced phase 1b ventricular arrhythmias in pig hearts. Journal of the American College of Cardiology, 39, 166–167.

14. Coronel, R., Fiolet, J.W.T., Wilms-Schopman, F.J.G., Opthof, T., Schaapherder, A.F.M., Janse, M.J. (1989). Distribution of extracellular potassium and electrophysiologic changes during two-stage coronary ligation in the isolated, perfused canine heart. Circulation, 80, 165–177.

15. Kabell, G., Scherlag, B.J., Hope, R.R., Lazzara, R. (1982). Regional myocardial blood flow and ventricular arrhythmias following one-stage and two-stage coronary artery occlusion in anesthetized dogs. American Heart Journal, 104, 537–544.

16. Coronel, R., Wilms-Schopman, F.J.G., den Ruijter, H.M., Belterman, C.N., Schumacher, C.A., Opthof, T., Hovenier, R., Lemmens, A.G., Terpstra, A.H.M., Katan, M. B., Zock, P. (2007). Dietary n-3 fatty acids promote arrhythmias during acute regional myocardial ischemia in isolated pig hearts. Cardiovascular Research, 73, 386–394.

17. Curtis, M.J. (1998). Characterisation, utilisation and clinical relevance of isolated perfused heart models of ischaemia-induced ventricular fibrillation. Cardiovascular Research, 39, 194–215.

18. Coumel, P. (1987). The management of clinical arrhythmias. An overview on invasive versus non-invasive electrophysiology. European Heart Journal, 8, 92–99.

19. Corr, P.B., Snyder, D.W., Cain, M.E., Crafford, W.A. Jr., Gross, R.W., Sobel, B.E. (1981). Electrophysiological effects of amphiphiles on canine purkinje fibers. Implications for dysrhythmia secondary to ischemia. Circulation Research, 49, 354–363.

20. Hill, J.L., Gettes, L.S. (1980). Effect of acute coronary artery occlusion on local myocardial extracellular K^+ activity in swine. Circulation, 61, 768–777.

21. Gettes, L.S., Reuter, H. (1974). Slow recovery from inactivation of inward currents in mammalian myocardial fibres. Journal of Physiology, 240, 703–723.

22. Krieger, W.J.G., Ter Welle, H.F., Fiolet, J.W.T., Janse, M.J. (1984). Tissue osmolality, metabolic response, and reperfusion in myocardial ischemia. Basic Research in Cardiology, 79, 562–571.

23. Tranum-Jensen, J., Janse, M.J., Fiolet, J.W.T., Krieger, W.J.G., Naumann d'Alnoncourt, C., Durrer, D. (1981). Tissue osmolality, cell swelling, and reperfusion in acute

regional myocardial ischemia in the isolated porcine heart. Circulation Research, 49, 364–381.

24. Hearse, D.J., Crome, R., Yellon, D.M., Wyse, R. (1983). Metabolic and flow correlates of myocardial ischaemia. Cardiovascular Research, 17, 452–458.

25. Shattock, M.J., Matsuura, H., Hearse, D.J. (1991). Functional and electrophysiological effects of oxidant stress on isolated ventricular muscle: A role for oscillatory calcium release from sarcoplasmic reticulum in arrhythmogenesis? Cardiovascular Research, 25, 645–651.

26. Downar, E., Janse, M.J., Durrer, D. (1977). The effect of acute coronary artery occlusion on subepicardial transmembrane potentials in the intact porcine heart. Circulation, 56/2, 217–224.

27. Wiggers, C.J., Wegria, R., Pineda, B. (1940). The effects of myocardial ischemia on the fibrillation threshold—The mechanism of spontaneous ventricular fibrillation following coronary occlusion. American Journal of Physiology, 131, 309–316.

28. Gettes, L.S., Hill, J.L., Saito, T., Kagiyama, Y. (1982). Factors related to vulnerability to arrhythmias in acute myocardial infarction. American Heart Journal, 103, 667–672.

29. Cinca, J., Janse, M.J., Morena, H., Candell, J., Valle, V., Durrer, D. (1980). Mechanism and time course of the early electrical changes during acute coronary artery occlusion. An attempt to correlate the early ECG changes in man to the cellular electrophysiology in the pig. Chest, 77, 499–505.

30. Franz, M.R., Cima, R., Wang, D., Profitt, D., Kurz, R. (1992). Electrophysiological effects of myocardial stretch and mechanical determinants of stretch-activated arrhythmias. Circulation, 86, 968–978.

31. Burton, F.L., Cobbe, S.M. (1998). Effect of sustained stretch on dispersion of ventricular fibrillation intervals in normal rabbit hearts. Cardiovascular Research, 39, 351–359.

32. Kodama, I., Wilde, A., Janse, M.J., Durrer, D., Yamada, K. (1984). Combined effects of hypoxia, hyperkalemia and acidosis on membrane action potential and excitability of guinea-pig ventricular muscle. Journal of Molecular and Cellular Cardiology, 16, 247–259.

33. Morena, H., Janse, M.J., Fiolet, J.W.T., Krieger, W.J.G., Crijns, H., Durrer, D. (1980). Comparison of the effects of regional ischemia, hypoxia, hyperkalemia, and acidosis on intracellular and extracellular potentials and metabolism in the isolated porcine heart. Circulation Research, 46, 634–646.

34. Janse, M.J., Cinca, J., Morena, H., Fiolet, J.W.T., Kléber, A.G., Vries, G.P., Becker, A. E., Durrer, D. (1979). The "border zone" in myocardial ischemia. An electrophysiological, metabolical, and histochemical correlation in the pig heart. Circulation Research, 44, 576–588.

35. Coronel, R., Fiolet, J.W.T., Wilms-Schopman, F.J.G., Schaapherder, A.F.M., Johnson, T.A., Gettes, L.S., Janse, M.J. (1988). Distribution of extracellular potassium and its relation to electrophysiologic changes during acute myocardial ischemia in the isolated perfused porcine heart. Circulation, 77, 1125–1138.

36. Patterson, R.E., Kirk, E.S. (1983). Analysis of coronary collateral structure, function and ischemic border zones in pigs. American Journal of Physiology, 244, H23–H31.

37. Johnson, T.A., Engle, C.L., Kusy, R.P., Knisley, S.B., Graebner, C.A., Gettes, L.S. (1990). Fabrication, evaluation, and use of extracellular K^+ and H^+ ion-selective electrodes. American Journal of Physiology, 258, H1224–H1231.

38. Coronel, R., Wilms-Schopman, F.J.G., Fiolet, J.W.T., Opthof, T., Janse, M.J. (1995). The relation between extracellular potassium concentration and pH in the border zone during regional ischemia in isolated porcine hearts. Journal of Molecular and Cellular Cardiology, 27, 2069–2073.

39. Coronel, R., Wilms-Schopman, F.J.G., Dekker, L.R.C., Janse, M.J. (1995). Heterogeneities in [K +](0) and TQ potential and the inducibility of ventricular fibrillation during acute regional ischemia in the isolated perfused porcine heart. Circulation, 92, 120–129.

40. Janse, M.J., Van Capelle, F.J.L., Morsink, H., Kléber, A.G., Wilms-Schopman, F., Cardinal, R., Naumann d'Alnoncourt, C., Durrer, D. (1980). Flow of "injury" current and patterns of excitation during early ventricular arrhythmias in acute regional myocardial ischemia in isolated porcine and canine hearts. Evidence for two different arrhythmogenic mechanisms. Circulation Research, 47, 151–165.

41. Pogwizd, S.M., Corr, P.B. (1987). Reentrant and nonreentrant mechanisms contribute to arrhythmogenesis during early myocardial ischemia: Results using three dimensional mapping. Circulation Research, 61, 352–371.

42. Mandapati, R., Asano, Y., Baxter, W.T., Gray, R., Davidenko, J., Jalife, J. (1998). Quantification of effects of global ischemia on dynamics of ventricular fibrillation in isolated rabbit heart. Circulation, 98, 1688–1696.

43. Mines, G.R. (1914). On circulating excitation in heart muscles and their possible relation to tachycardia and fibrillation. Transactions of the Royal Society of Canada, IV 43–52.

44. Janse, M.J., Capucci, A., Coronel, R., Fabius, M.A.W. (1985). Variability of recovery of excitability in the normal canine and the ischemic porcine heart. European Heart Journal, 6, 41–52.

45. Kléber, A.G., Janse, M.J., van Capelle, F.J.L., Durrer, D. (1978). Mechanism and time course of S-T and T-Q segment changes during acute regional myocardial ischemia in the pig heart determined by extracellular and intracellular recordings. Circulation Research, 42, 603–613.

46. Janse, M.J., Van Capelle, F.J.L. (1982). Electrotonic interactions across an inexcitable region as a cause of ectopic activity in acute regional myocardial ischemia. A study in intact porcine and canine hearts and computer models. Circulation Research, 50, 527–537.

47. Coronel, R., Wilms-Schopman, F.J.G., Opthof, T., Van Capelle, F.J.L., Janse, M.J. (1991). Injury current and gradients of diastolic stimulation threshold, TQ potential, and extracellular potassium concentration during acute regional ischemia in the isolated perfused pig heart. Circulation Research, 68, 1241–1249.

48. Janse, M.J., Kléber, A.G., Capucci, A., Coronel, R., Wilms-Schopman, F.J.G. (1986). Electrophysiological basis for arrhythmias caused by acute ischemia. Role of the subendocardium. Journal of Molecular and Cellular Cardiology, 18, 339–355.

49. Weidmann, S. (1955). The effect of the cardiac membrane potential on the rapid availability of the sodiumcarrying system. Journal of Physiology, 127, 213–224.

50. Kléber, A.G., Rudy, Y. (2004). Basic mechanisms of cardiac impulse propagation and associated arrhythmias. Physiological Reviews, 84, 431–488.

51. Dominguez, G., Fozzard, H.A. (1970). Influence of extracellular K^+ concentration on cable properties and excitability of sheep cardiac Purkinje fibers. Circulation Research, 26, 565–574.

52. Carmeliet, E. (1999). Cardiac ionic currents and acute ischemia: From channels to arrhythmias. Physiological Reviews, 79, 917–1017.

53. Ramasamy, R., Liu, H., Oates, P.J., Schaefer, S. (1999). Attenuation of ischemia induced increases in sodium and calcium by the aldose reductase inhibitor Zopolrestat. Cardiovascular Research, 42, 130–139.

54. Cascio, W.E., Yan, G.X., Kléber, A.G. (1990). Passive electrical properties, mechanical activity, and extracellular potassium in arterially perfused and ischemic rabbit ventricular muscle. Effects of calcium entry blockade or hypocalcemia. Circulation Research, 66, 1461–1473.

55. Cascio, W.E., Yan, G., Kléber, A.G. (1992). Early changes in extracellular potassium in ischemic rabbit myocardium: The role of extracellular carbon dioxide accumulation and diffusion. Circulation Research, 70, 409–422.

56. Fiolet, J.W.T., Baartscheer, A., Schumacher, C.A., Coronel, R., Welle, H.F. (1985). The change of free energy of ATP hydrolysis during global ischemia and anoxia in the rat heart: Its possible relation in the regulation of transsarcolemmal sodium and potassium gradients. Journal of Molecular and Cellular Cardiology, 17, 1023–1036.

57. Wilde, A.A.M., Peters, R.J.G., Janse, M.J. (1988). Catecholamine release and potassium accumulation in the isolated globally ischemic rabbit heart. Journal of Molecular and Cellular Cardiology, 20, 887–896.

58. Coronel, R. (1994). Heterogeneity in extracellular potassium concentration during early myocardial ischaemia and reperfusion. Implications for arrhythmogenesis. Cardiovascular Research, 28, 770–777.

59. Schaapherder, A.F.M., Schumacher, C.A., Coronel, R., Fiolet, J.W.T. (1990). Transmural inhomogeneity of extracellular [K(+)] and pH and myocardial energy metabolism in the isolated rat heart during acute global ischemia;dependence on gaseous environment. Basic Research Cardiology, 85, 33–44.

60. Weiss, J., Shine, K.I. (1982). [K +]o accumulation and electrophysiologic alterations during early myocardial ischemia. American Journal of Physiology, 243, H318–H327.

61. Aksnes, G., Kirkeboen, K.A., Lanse, K., Ilebek, A. (1992). Myocardial potassium balance associated with regional ischaemia in the pig: Effects of B-adrenoceptor blockade, duration of ischaemia and preceding ischaemic period. Acta Physiological Scandinavian, 145, 39–48.

62. Haunso, S., Sejrsen, P., Svendsen, J.H. (1991). Transport of Beta-blockers and calcium antagonists by diffusion in cat myocardium. Journal of Cardiovascular Pharmacology, 17, 357–364.

63. Wilensky, R.L., Tranum-Jensen, J., Coronel, R., Wilde, A.A.M., Fiolet, J.W.T., Janse, M.J. (1986). The subendocardial border zone during acute ischemia of the rabbit heart: an electrophysiologic, metabolic, and morphologic correlative study. Circulation, 74, 1137–1146.

64. Coronel, R., Opthof, T., Taggart, P., Tytgat, J., Veldkamp, M. (1997). Differential electrophysiology of repolarisation from clone to clinic. Review. Cardiovascular Research, 33, 503–517.

65. Walfridsson, H., Odman, S., Lund, N. (1985). Myocardial oxygen pressure across the lateral border zone after acute coronary occlusion in the pig heart. Advanas in Experimental Medicine and Biology, 191, 203–210.

66. Wilde, A.A.M., Janse, M.J. (1994). Electrophysiological effects of ATP sensitive potassium channel modulation—implications for arrhythmogenesis. Cardiovascular Research, 28, 16–24.

67. Coronel, R. (1988). Distribution of extracellular potassium during acute myocardial ischemia. Thesis. ICG Printing, Dordrecht, The Netherlands.

68. Noma, A. (1983). ATP-regulated K^+ channels in cardiac muscle. Nature, 305, 147–148.

69. Flagg, T.P., Nichols, C.G. (2005). Sarcolemmal KATP channels: What do we really know? Journal of Molecular and Cellular Cardiology, 39, 61–70.

70. Tsuchiya, K., Horie, M., Watanuki, M., Albrecht, C.A., Obayashi, K., Fujiwara, H., Sasayama, S. (1997). Functional compartmentalization of ATP is involved in angiotensin II mediated closure of cardiac ATP-sensitive K^+ channels. Circulation, 96, 3129–3135.

71. Verkerk, A.O., Veldkamp, M.W., van Ginneken, A.C., Bouman, L.N. (1996). Biphasic response of action potential duration to metabolic inhibition in rabbit and human ventricular myocytes: Role of transient outward current and ATP-regulated potassium current. Journal of Molecular and Cellular Cardiology, 28, 2443–2456.

72. Sun, Y., Weber, K.T. (2000). Infarct scar: A dynamic tissue. Cardiovascular Research, 46, 250–256.

73. Pierce, G.N., Meng, H. (1992). The role of sodium-proton exchange in ischemic/ reperfusion injury in the heart. Na(+)-H+ exchange and ischemic heart disease. American Journal of Cardiovascular Pathology, 4, 91–102.

74. Sobel, B.E., Corr, P.B., Robison, A.K., Goldstein, R.A., Witkowski, F.X., Klein, M.S. (1978). Accumulation of lysophosphoglycerides with arrhythmogenic properties in ischemic myocardium. Journal of Clinical Investigation, 62, 546–553.

75. Fukuda, K., Davies, S.S., Nakajima, T., Ong, B.H., Kupershmidt, S., Fessel, J., Amarnath, V., Anderson, M.E., Boyden, P.A., Viswanathan, P.C., Roberts, L.J. II, Balser, J.R. (2005). Oxidative mediated lipid peroxidation recapitulates proarrhythmic effects on cardiac sodium channels. Circulation Research, 97, 1262–1269.

76. Evrengul, H., Seleci, D., Tanriverdi, H., Kaftan, A. (2006). The antiarrhythmic effect and clinical consequences of ischemic preconditioning. Coronary Artery Disease, 17, 283–288.

77. Shiki, K., Hearse, D.J. (1987). Preconditioning of ischemic myocardium: Reperfusion-induced arrhythmias. American Journal of Physiology, 253, H1470–H1476.

78. Chadda, K.D., Banka, V.S., Helfant, R.H. (1974). Heart rate dependent ventricular ectopia following acute coronary occlusion: The concept of optimal antiarrhythmic heart rate. Circulation, 49, 654–658.

79. Fox, K., Borer, J.S., Camm, A.J., Danchin, N., Ferrari, R., Lopez Sendon, J.L., Steg, P. G., Tardif, J.C., Tavazzi, L., Tendera, M. (2007). Resting heart rate in cardiovascular disease. Journal of the American College of Cardiology, 50, 823–830.

80. Han, J., Moe, G.K. (1964). Nonuniform recovery of excitability in ventricular muscle. Circulation Research, 14, 44–61.

81. Wilde, A.A.M., Escande, D., Schumacher, C.A., Thuringer, D., Mestre, M., Fiolet, J.W.T., Janse, M.J. (1990). Potassium accumulation in the globally ischemic mammalian heart. A role for the ATP-sensitive potassium channel. Circulation Research, 67, 835–843.

82. Downar, E., Janse, M.J., Durrer, D. (1977). The effect of "ischemic" blood on transmembrane potentials of normal porcine ventricular myocardium. Circulation, 55/ 3, 455–462.

83. Cygankiewicz, I., Zareba, W., Vazquez, R., Vallverdu, M., Gonzalez-Juanatey, J. R., Valdes, M., Almendral, J.M., Cinca, J., Caminal, P., Bayes de Luna, A., on behalf of the MUSIC Investigators. (2008). Heart rate turbulence predicts all-cause mortality and sudden death in congestive heart failure patients. Heart Rhythm, 5, 1095–1102.

84. Goldstein, J.A., Butterfield, M.C., Ohnishi, Y., Shelton, T.J., Corr, P.B. (1994). Arrhythmogenic influence of intracoronary thrombosis during acute myocardial ischemia. Circulation, 90, 139–147.

85. Davies, M.J. (1981). Pathological view of sudden cardiac death. British Heart Journal, 45, 88–96.

86. Pinet, C., Le Grand, B., John, G.W., Coulombe, A. (2002). Thrombin facilitation of voltage-gated sodium channel activation in human cardiomyocytes: Implications for ischemic sodium loading. Circulation, 106, 2098–2103.

87. Coronel, R., Wilms-Schopman, F.J.G., Janse, M.J. (1997). Profibrillatory effects of intracoronary thrombus in acute regional ischemia of the in situ porcine heart. Circulation, 96, 3985–3991.

88. Dorian, P. (2005). Antiarrhythmic action of β-blockers: Potential mechanisms. Journal of Cardiovascular Pharmacology and Therapeutics, 10, S15–S22.

89. Schwartz, P.J., Vanoli, E., Stramba-Badiale, M., De Ferrari, G.M., Billman, G.E., Foreman, R.D. (1988). Autonomic mechanisms and sudden death. New insights from analysis of baroreceptor reflexes in conscious dogs with and without a myocardial infarction. Circulation, 78, 969–979.

90. La Rovere, M.T., Pinna, G.D., Maestri, R., Mortara, A., Capomolla, S., Febo, O., Ferrari, R., Franchini, M., Gnemmi, M., Opasich, C., Riccardi, P.G., Traversi, E., Cobelli, F. (2003). Short-term heart rate variability strongly predicts sudden cardiac death in chronic heart failure patients. Circulation, 565–570.

91. Passariello, G., Peluso, A., Moniello, G., Maio, A., Mazo, S., Boccia, G., Passariello, N., Lettieri, B., Chiefari, M. (2007). Effect of autonomic nervous system dysfunction on sudden death in ischemic patients with anginal syndrome died during electrocardiographic monitoring in Intensive Care Unit. Minerva Anestesiologica, 73, 207–212.

92. Schömig, A., Dart, A.M., Dietz, R., Mayer, E., Kübler, W. (1984). Release of endogenous catecholamines in the ischemic myocardium of the rat. Part A: Locally mediated release. Circulation Research, 55, 689–701.

93. Dart, A.M., Schömig, A., Dietz, R., Mayer, E., Kubler, W. (1984). Release of endogeneous catecholamines in the ischemic myocardium of the rat. Part B: Effect of sympathetic nerve stimulation. Circulation Research, 55, 702–706.

94. Opthof, T., Ramdat Misier, A.R., Coronel, R., Vermeulen, J.T., Verberne, H.J., Frank, R. G.J., Moulijn, A.C., Van Capelle, F.J.L., Janse, M.J. (1991). Dispersion of refractoriness in canine ventricular myocardium: Effects of sympathetic stimulation. Circulation Research, 68, 1204–1215.

95. Opthof, T., Dekker, L.R.C., Coronel, R., Vermeulen, J.T., Van Capelle, F.J.L., Janse, M. J. (1993). Interaction of sympathetic and parasympathetic nervous system on ventricular refractoriness assessed by local fibrillation intervals in canine heart. Cardiovascular Research, 27, 753–759.

96. Cannon, W.B. (1942). "Voodoo" death. American Anthropologist, 44/2, 169–181.

97. Bremmer, M.A., Hoogendijk, W.J.G., Deeg, D.J.H., Schoevers, R.A., Schalk, B.W.M., Beekman, A.T.F. (2006). Depression in older age is a risk factor for first ischemic cardiac events. American Journal of Geriatric Psychiatry, 14, 523–530.

98. Skinner, J.E., Reed, J.C. (1981). Blockade of frontocortical-brain stem pathway prevents ventricular fibrillation of ischemic heart. American Journal of Physiology Heart and Circulatory Physiology, 240, H156–H163.

99. Riedeker, M., Herbst, M.C., Devlin, R.B., Griggs, T.R., Bromberg, P.A., Cascio, W.E. (2005). Effect of the September 11, 2001 terrorist attack on a state highway patrol trooper's heart rate variability. Annals of Noninvasive Electrocardiology, 10, 83–85.

100. de Lorgeril, M., Salen, P., Paillard, F., Laporte, F., Boucher, F., de Leiris, J. (2002). Mediterranean diet and the French paradox: Two distinct biogeographical concepts for one consolidated scientific theory on the role of nutrition in coronary heart disease. Cardiovascular Research, 54, 503–515.

101. Lairon, D. (2007). Intervention studies on Mediterranean diet and cardiovascular risk. Molecular Nutrition & Food Research, 51, 1209–1214.

102. Den Ruijter, H.M., Berecki, G., Opthof, T., Verkerk, A.O., Zock, P.L., Coronel, R. (2007). Pro- and antiarrhythmic properties of a diet rich in fish oil. Cardiovascular Research, 73, 316–325.

103. Isensee, H., Jacob, R. (1994). Differential effects of various oil diets on the risk of cardiac arrhythmias in rats. Journal of Cardiovascular Risk, 1, 353–359.

104. Bang, H.O., Dyerberg, J., Hjoome, N. (1976). The composition of food consumed by Greenland eskimos. Acta Medica Scandinavica, 200, 69–73.

105. Marchioli, R., et al. (2002). Early protection against sudden death by n-3 polyunsaturated fatty acids after myocardial infarction. Time course analysis of the results of the Gruppo Italiano per lo Studio della Sopravvivenza nel'Infarto Miocardico (GISSI)-Prevenzione. Circulation, 105, 1897–1903.

106. Burr, M.L., Fehily, A.M., Gilbert, J.F., Rogers, S., Holliday, R.M., Sweetnam, P.M., Elwood, P.C., Deadman, N.M. (1989). Effects of changes in fat, fish, and fibre on death myocardial reinfarction: diet and reinfarction trial (DART). Lancet, 2, 757–761.

107. Burr, M.L., Ashfield-Watt, P.A., Dunstan, F.F.A.M., Breay, P., Zotos, P.C., Haboubi, N. A., Elwood, P.C. (2003). Lack of benefit of dietary advice to men with angina: results of a controlled trial. European Journal of Clinical Nutrition, 57, 193–200.

108. Raitt, M.H., Connor, W.E., Morris, C., Kron, J., Halperin, B., Chugh, S., McClelland, J., Cook, J., MacMurdy, K., Swenson, R., Connor, S.L., Gerhard, G., Kraemer, D.F., Oscran, D., Marchant, C., Calhoun, D., Shriner, R., McAnulty, J. (2005). Fish oil supplementation and risk of ventricular tachycardia and ventricular fibrillation in patients with implantable defibrillators. JAMA, 293, 2884–2891.

109. Brouwer, I.A., Zock, P., Camm, A.J., Böcker, D., Hauer, R.N.W., Wever, E.F.D., Dullemeijer, C., Ronden, J.E., Katan, M.B., Lubinski, A., Buschler, H., Schouten, E.G., for the SOFA study Group. (2006). Effect of fish oil on ventricular tachyar-rhythmia and death in patients with implantable cardioverter defibrillators. The study on omega-3 fatty acids and ventricular arrhythmia (SOFA) randomized trial. JAMA, 295, 2613–2619.

110. McLennan, P.L., Abeywardena, M.Y., Charnock, J.S. (1988). Dietary fish oil prevents ventricular fibrillation following coronary artery occlusion and reperfusion. American Heart Journal, 116, 709–717.

111. Billman, G.E., Kang, J.X., Leaf, A. (1999). Prevention of sudden death by dietary pure n-3 polyunsaturated fatty acids in dogs. Circulation, 99, 2452–2457.

112. Xiao, Y.-F., Kang, J.X., Morgan, J.P., Leaf, A. (1995). Blocking effects of polyunsaturated fatty acids on Na^+ channels of neonatal rat ventricular myocytes. Proceedings of the National Academy of Sciences USA, 92, 11000–11004.

113. Verkerk, A.O., van Ginneken, A.C.G., Berecki, G., Den Ruijter, H.M., Schumacher, C. A., Veldkamp, M.W., Baartscheer, A., Casini, S., Opthof, T., Hovenier, R., Fiolet, J.W., Zock, P., Coronel, R. (2006). Incorporated sarcolemmal fish oil fatty acids shorten pig ventricular action potentials. Cardiovascular Research, 70, 509–520.

114. Kannel, W.B., Plehn, J.F., Cupples, L.A. (1988). Cardiac failure and sudden death in the Framingham Study. American Heart Journal, 115, 869–875.

115. Wolf, C.M., Berul, C.I. (2006). Inherited conduction system abnormalities. One group of diseases, many genes. Journal of Cardiovascular Electrophysiology, 17, 446–455.

116. Kléber, A.G., Riegger, C.B., Janse, M.J. (1987). Electrical uncoupling and increase of extracellular resistance after induction of ischemia in isolated, arterially perfused rabbit papillary muscle. Circulation Research, 61, 271–279.

117. Smith IV, W.T., Fleet, W.F., Johnson, T.A., Engle, C.L., Cascio, W.E. (1995). The 1B phase of ventricular arrhythmias in ischemic in situ porcine heart is related to changes in cell-to-cell coupling. Circulation, 92, 3051–3060.

118. Cinca, J., Warren, M., Carreno, A., Tresanchez, M., Armadans, L., Gomez, P., Soler-Soler, J. (1997). Changes in myocardial electrical impedance induced by coronary artery occlusion in pigs with and without preconditioning. Correlation with local ST segment potential and ventricular arrhyhtmias. Circulation, 96, 3079–3086.

119. Dekker, L.R.C., Fiolet, J.W.T., VanBavel, E., Opthof, T., Coronel, R., Spaan, J.A.E., Janse, M.J. (1995). Intracellular calcium concentration and cellular uncoupling during ischemia in the perfused rabbit papillary muscle. Circulation, 92, I–188.

120. De Mello, W.C. (1975). Effect of intracellular injection of calcium and strontium on cell communication in heart. Journal of Physiology, 250, 231–245.

121. Yan, G.X., Kléber, A.G. (1992). Changes in extracellular and intracellular pH in ischemic rabbit papillary muscle. Circulation Research, 71, 460–470.

122. Weingart, R., Maurer, P. (1988). Action potential transfer in cell pairs isolated from adult rat and guinea pig ventricles. Circulation Research, 63, 72–80.

123. Jongsma, H.J., Wilders, R. (2000). Gap junctions in cardiovascular disease. Circulation Research, 86, 1193–1197.

124. de Groot, J.R., Coronel, R. (2004). Acute ischemia-induced gap junctional uncoupling and arrhythmogenesis. Cardiovascular Research, 62, 323–334.

125. Lesh, M.D., Pring, M., Spear, J.F. (1989). Cellular uncoupling can unmask dispersion of action potential duration in ventricular myocardium. A computer modeling study. Circulation Research, 65, 1426–1440.

126. de Groot, J.R., Schumacher, C.A., Verkerk, A.O., Baartscheer, A., Fiolet, J.W., Coronel, R. (2003). Intrinsic heterogeneity in repolarization is increased in isolated failing rabbit cardiomyocytes during simulated ischemia. Cardiovascular Research, 59, 705–714.

127. Tan, R.C., Joyner, R.W. (1990). Electrotonic influences on action potentials from isolated ventricular cells. Circulation Research, 67, 1071–1081.

128. Pollard, A.E., Cascio, W.E., Fast, V.G., Knisley, S.B. (2002). Modulation of triggered activity by uncoupling in the ischemic border: A model study with phase 1b-like conditions. Cardiovascular Research, 56, 381–392.

129. Xiao, J., Rodriguez, B., de Groot, J.R., Coronel, R., Trayanova, N. (2008). Reentry in survived subepicardium coupled to depolarized and inexcitable midmyocardium: Insights into arrhythmogenesis in ischemia phase 1B. Heart Rhythm, 7, 1036–1044.

130. Verkerk, A.O., Veldkamp, M.W., Coronel, R., Wilders, R., van Ginneken, A.C.G. (2001). Effects of cell-to-cell uncoupling and catecholamines on Purkinje and ventricular action potentials: implications for phase-1b arrhythmias. Cardiovascular Research, 51, 30–40.

131. Barrabes, J.A., Garcia-Dorado, D., Agullo, L., Rodriguez-Sinovas, A., Padilla, F., Trobo, L., Soler-Soler, J. (2006). Intracoronary infusion of Gd3 + into ischemic region does not suppress phase Ib ventricular arrhythmias after coronary occlusion in swine. American Journal of Physiology Heart and Circulatory Physiology, 290, H2344–H2350.

132. Remme, C.A., Schumacher, C.A., de Jong, J.W., Fiolet, J.W., Coronel, R., Wilde, A.A. (2001). K(ATP) channel opening during ischemia: effects on myocardial noradrenaline release and ventricular arrhythmias. Journal of Cardiovascular Pharmacology, 38, 406–416.

133. Bigger, J.T. Jr., Dresdale, R.J., Heissenbuttel, R.H., Weld, F.M., Wit, A.L. (1977). Ventricular arrhythmias in ischemic heart disease: Mechanism, prevalence, significance, and management. Progress in Cardiovascular Disease, 19, 255–300.

134. Wit, A.L., Janse, M.J. (1993). The Ventricular Arrhythmias of Ischemia and Infarction. Electrophysiological Mechanisms. Futura Publishing Co, Mount Kisco, NY.

135. Ursell, P.C., Gardner, P.I., Albala, A., Fenoglio, J.J. Jr., Wit, A.L. (1985). Structural and electrophysiological changes in the epicardial border zone of canine myocardial infarcts during infarct healing. Circulation Research, 56, 436–451.

136. Boyden, P.A., Albala, A., Dresdner, K. (1989). Electrophysiology and ultrastructure of canine subendocardial Purkinje cells isolated from control and 24 hour infarcted hearts. Circulation Research, 65, 955–970.

137. Pinto, J.M.B., Boyden, P.A. (1998). Reduced inward rectifying and increased E4031 sensitive K^+ channel function in arrhythmogenic subendocardial Purkinje myocytes from the infarcted heart. Journal of Cardiovascular Electrophysiology, 9, 299–311.

138. Boyden, P.A., Pinto, J.M.B. (1994). Reduced calcium currents in subendocardial Purkinje myocytes that survive in the 24 and 48 hour infarcted heart. Circulation, 89, 2747–2759.

139. Boyden, P.A., Barbhaiya, C., Lee, T., Ter Keurs, H.E.D.J. (2003). Nonuniform Ca^{2+} Transients in Arrhythmogenic Purkinje Cells that survive in the infarcted canine heart. Cardiovascular Research, 57, 681–693.

140. Ter Keurs, H.E.D.J., Boyden, P.A. (2007). Calcium and arrhythmogenesis. Physiological Reviews, 87, 457–506.

141. Stuyvers, B.D., Dun, W., Matkovich, S.J., Sorrentino, V., Boyden, P.A., Ter Keurs, H.E.D.J. (2005). Ca^{2+} sparks and Ca^{2+} waves in Purkinje Cells: A triple layered system of activation. Circulation Research, 97, 35–43.

142. Boyden, P.A., Dun, W., Barbhaiya, C., Ter Keurs, H.E.D.J. (2004). 2APB- and JTV519 (K201) sensitive micro Ca^{2+} waves in arrhythmogenic Purkinje cells that survive in infarcted canine heart. Heart Rhythm, 1, 218–226.

143. Pinto, J.M.B., Sosunov, E.A., Gainullin, R.Z., Rosen, M.R., Boyden, P.A. (1999). The effects of Mibefradil a T type calcium channel current antagonist on the electrophysiology of Purkinje fibers that have survived in the infarcted heart. Journal of Cardiovascular Electrophysiology, 10, 1224–1235.

144. Hirose, M., Stuyvers, B.D., Dun, W., Ter Keurs, H.E.D., Boyden, P.A. (2008). Function of Ca^{2+} release channels in Purkinje cells that survive in the infarcyed canine heart;a mechanism for triggered Purkinje ectopy. Circulation. Arrhythmia and Electrophysiology, 1, 387–395.

145. Jeck, C., Pinto, J.M.B., Boyden, P.A. (1995). Transient outward currents in subendocardial Purkinje myocytes surviving in the 24 and 48 hr infarcted heart. Circulation, 92, 465–473.

146. Lue, W.-M., Boyden, P.A. (1992). Abnormal electrical properties of myocytes from chronically infarcted canine heart. Alterations in Vmax and the transient outward current. Circulation, 85, 1175–1188.

147. Pinto, J.M.B., Boyden, P.A. (1999). Electrophysiologic remodeling in ischemia and infarction. Cardiovascular Research, 42, 284–297.

148. Patterson, E., Scherlag, B.J., Lazzara, R. (1993). Rapid inward current in ischemically-injured subepicardial myocytes bordering myocardial infarction. Journal of Cardiovascular Electrophysiology, 4, 9–22.

149. Lazzara, R., Scherlag, B.J. (1984). Electrophysiologic basis for arrhythmias in ischemic heart disease. American Journal of Cardiology, 53, 1B–7B.

150. Pu, J., Boyden, P.A. (1997). Alterations of Na^+ currents in myocytes from epicardial border zone of the infarcted heart. A possible ionic mechanism for reduced excitability and postrepolarization refractoriness. Circulation Research, 81, 110–119.

151. Pu, J., Balser, J., Boyden, P.A. (1998). Lidocaine action on sodium currents of ventricular myocytes from the epicardial border zone of the infarcted heart. Circulation Research, 83, 431–440.

152. Baba, S., Dun, W., Cabo, C., Boyden, P.A. (2005). Remodeling in cells from different regions of the reentrant circuit during ventricular tachycardia. Circulation, 112, 2386–2396.

153. Baba, S., Dun, W., Boyden, P.A. (2004). Can PKA Activators rescue Na channel function in epicardial border zone cells that survive in the infarcted canine heart? Cardiovascular Research, 64, 260–267.

154. Dun, W., Robinson, R.B., Lowe, J.S., Mohler, P.J., Boyden, P.A. (2008). Ankyrin-G participates in remodeling of I_{Na} in myocytes from the epicardial border zone of infarcted canine heart. Biophysical Journal, 94, 3105.

155. Lowe, J.S., Palygin, O., Bhasin, N., Hund, T.J., Boyden, P.A., Shibata, E.F., Anderson, M.E., Mohler, P.J. (2007). Voltage gated Na channel targeting in heart requires an ankyrin G dependent cellular pathway. Journal of Cellular Biology, 180, 173–186.

156. Hund, T.J., Decker, K.F., Kanter, E., Mohler, P.J., Boyden, P.A., Schuessler, R.B., Yamada, K.A., Rudy, Y. (2008). Role of activated CaMKII in abnormal calcium homeostasis and I_{Na} remodeling after myocardial infarction: Insights from mathematical modeling. Journal of Molecular and Cellular Cardiology, 45, 420–428.

157. Aggarwal, R., Boyden, P.A. (1995). Diminished calcium and barium currents in myocytes surviving in the epicardial border zone of the 5 day infarcted canine heart. Circulation Research, 77, 1180–1191.

158. Koumi, S.I., Backer, C.L., Arentzen, C.E., Sato, R. (1995). Beta-adrenergic modulation of the inwardly rectifying potassium channel in isolated human ventricular myocytes. Journal of Clinical Investigation, 96, 2870–2881.

159. Kameyama, M., Hofmann, F., Trautwein, W. (1985). On the mechanism of beta-adrenergic regulation of the Ca channel in the guinea-pig heart. Pfluegers Archive, 405, 285–293.

160. Tsien, R.W., Bean, B.P., Hess, P., Lansman, J.B., Nilius, B., Nowycky, M.C. (1986). Mechanisms of calcium channel modulation by beta adrenergic agents and dihydropyridine calcium agonist. Journal of Molecular Cellular Cardiology, 18, 691–710.

161. Gaide, M.S., Myerburg, R.J., Kozlovskis, P.L., Bassett, A.L. (1983). Elevated sympathetic response of epicardial proximal to healed myocardial infarction. American Journal of Physiology, 245, H646–H652.

162. Boyden, P.A., Gardner, P.I., Wit, A.L. (1988). Action potentials of cardiac muscle in healing infarcts: Response to norepinephrine and caffeine. Journal of Molecular and Cellular Cardiology, 20, 525–537.

163. Mubagwa, K., Flameng, W., Carmeliet.E. (1994). Resting and action potentials of nonischemic and chronically ischemic human ventricular muscle. Journal of Cardiovascular Electrophysiology, 5, 659–671.

164. Pinto, J.M.B., Yuan, F., Wasserlauf, B.J., Bassett, A.L., Myerburg, R.J. (1997). Regional gradation of L-type calcium currents in the feline heart with a healed myocardial infarct. Journal of Cardiovascular Electrophysiology, 8, 548–560.

165. Aggarwal, R., Boyden, P.A. (1996). Altered pharmacologic responsiveness of reduced L-type calcium currents in myocytes surviving in the infarcted heart. Journal of Cardiovascular Electrophysiology, 7, 20–35.

166. Steinberg, S.F., Zhang, H., Pak, E., Pagnotta, G., Boyden, P.A. (1995). Characteristics of the beta-adrenergic receptor complex in the epicardial border zone of the 5-day infarcted canine heart. Circulation, 91, 2824–2833.

167. Davis, M.J., Wu, X., Nurkiewicz, T.R., Kawasaki, J., Gui, P., Hill, M.A., Wilson, E. (2001). Regulation of ion channels by protein tyrosine phosphorylation. American Journal of Physiology Heart and Circulatory Physiology, 281, H1835–H1862.

168. Yagi, T., Boyden, P.A. (2002). The function of protein tyrosine kinases and L type Ca^{2+} currents in cells that have survived in the canine infarcted heart. Journal of Cardiovascular Pharmacology, 40, 669–677.

169. Licata, A., Aggarwal, R., Robinson, R.B., Boyden, P.A. (1997). Frequency dependent effects on Cai transients, cell shortening in myocytes that survive in the infarcted heart. Cardiovascular Research, 33, 341–350.

170. Pu, J., Robinson, R.B., Boyden, P.A. (2000). Abnormalities in Ca_i handling in myocytes that survive in the infarcted heart are not just due to alterations in repolarization. JMCC, 32, 1509–1523.

171. Pu, J., Ruffy, F., Boyden, P.A. (1999). Effects of bay Y5959 on Ca^{2+} currents and intracellular Ca^{2+} in cells that have survived in the epicardial border zone of the infarcted canine heart. Journal of Cardiovascular Pharmacology, 33, 929–937.

172. Cabo, C., Schmitt, H., Wit, A.L. (2000). New mechanism of antiarrhythmic drug action: Increasing inward L type calcium current prevents reentrant tachycardia in the infarcted canine heart. Circulation, 102, 2417–2425.

173. Rosati, B., Grau, F., Rodriguez, S., Li, H., Nerbonne, J.M., McKinnon, D. (2003). Concordant expression of KChIP2 mRNA, protein and transient outward current throughout the canine ventricle. Journal of Physiology, 548, 815–822.

174. Jiang, M., Cabo, C., Yao, J.-A., Boyden, P.A., Tseng, G.-N. (2000). Delayed rectifier K currents have reduced amplitudes and altered kinetics in myocytes from infarcted canine ventricle. Cardiovascular Research, 48, 34–43.

175. Dun, W., Baba, S., Boyden, P.A. (2005). Diverse phenotypes of outward currents in epicardial border zone cells of the 5 day infarcted heart. American Journal of Physiology, 289, H667–H673.

176. Hiraoka, M., Kawano, S. (1989). Calcium-sensitive and insensitive transient outward current in rabbit ventricular myocytes. Journal of Physiology, 410, 187–212.

177. Kawano, S., Hirayama, Y., Hiraoka, M. (1995). Activation mechanism of Ca sensitive transient outward current in rabbit ventricular myocytes. Journal of Physiology, 486, 593–604.

178. Siegelbaum, S., Tsien, R.W. (1980). Calcium-activated transient outward current in calf cardiac Purkinje fibres. Journal of Physiology, 299, 485–506.

179. Sipido, K.R., Callewaert, G., Carmeliet, E.E. (1993). Ca_i^{2+} transients and Ca_i^{2+} dependent chloride current in single Purkinje cells from rabbit heart. Journal of Physiology, 468., 641–667.

180. Aggarwal, R., Pu, J., Boyden, P.A. (1997). Ca^{2+} dependent outward currents in myocytes from the epicardial border zone of the 5 day infarcted heart. American Journal of Physiology, 273, H1386–H1394.

181. Janvier, N.C., Boyett, M.R. (1996). The role of NaCa exchange current in the cardiac action potential. Cardiovascular Research, 32, 69–84.

182. Zhang, X.-Q., Tillotson, D.L., Moore, R.L., Cheung, J.Y. (1996). Na/Ca exchange currents and SR Ca^{2+} contents in postinfarction myocytes. American Journal of Physiology, 271, C1800–C1807.

183. Zhang, X.-Q., Moore, R.L., Tenhave, T., Cheung, J.Y. (1995). Ca_i^{++} transients in hypertensive and postinfarction myocytes1. American Journal of Physiology, 269, C632–C640.

184. Cheung, J.Y., Musch, T.I., Misawa, H., Semanchick, A., Elensky, M., Yelamarty, R.V., Moore, R.L. (1994). Impaired cardiac function in rats with healed myocardial infarction: cellular vs. myocardial mechanisms. American Journal of Physiology, 266, C29–C36.

185. Pu, J., Robinson, R.B., Boyden, P.A. (1998). Na/Ca exchanger density/function is unchanged in myocytes from the epicardial border zone of the 5 day infarcted heart. Circulation, 98, I-680-

186. Litwin, S.E., Bridge, J.H.B., (1997). Enhanced NaCa exchange in the infarcted heart. Implications for excitation contraction coupling. Circulation Research, 81, 1083–1093.

187. Dillon, S., Allessie, M.A., Ursell, P.C., Wit, A.L. (1988). Influences of anisotropic tissue structure on reentrant circuits in the epicardial border zone of subacute canine infarcts. Circulation Research, 63, 182–206.

188. Peters, N.S., Coromilas, J., Severs, N.J., Wit, A.L. (1997). Disturbed Connexin43 Gap junction distribution correlates with the location of reentrant circuits in the epicardial border zone of healing canine infarcts that cause ventricular tachycardia. Circulation, 95, 988–996.

189. Peters, N.S., Wit, A.L. (1998). Myocardial architecture and ventricular arrhythmogenesis. Circulation, 97, 1746–1754.

190. Yao, J.-A., Hussain, W., Patel, P., Peters, N.S., Boyden, P.A., Wit, A.L. (2003). Remodeling of gap junctional channel function in epicardial border zone of healing canine infarcts. Circulation Research, 92, 437–443.

191. Cabo, C., Yao, J.A., Boyden, P.A., Chen, S., Hussain, W., Duffy, H.S., Ciaccio, E.J., Peters, N.S., Wit, A.L. (2006). Heterogeneous Gap junction structural and functional remodeling influences conduction in central common pathway of reentrant circuits of the Epicardial Border zone of the healing canine infarct. Cardiovascular Research, 72, 241–249.

192. Ciaccio, E.J., Chow, A.W., Kaba, R.A., Davies, D.W., Segal, O.R., Peters, N.S. (2008). Detection of the diastolic pathway, circuit morphology, and inducibility of human postinfarction ventricular tachycardia from mapping in sinus rhythm. Heart Rhythm, 5, 981–991.

193. de Bakker, J.M., van Capelle, F.J., Janse, M.J., Wilde, A.A., Coronel, R., Becker, A.E., Dingemans, K.P., van Hemel, N.M., Hauer, R.N. (1988). Reentry as a cause of ventricular tachycardia in patients with chronic ischemic heart disease: electrophysiologic and anatomic correlation. Circulation, 77, 589–606.

194. Fenoglio, J.J. Jr., Albala, A., Silva, F.G., Friedman, P.L., Wit, A.L. (1976). Structural basis of ventricular arrhythmias in human myocardial infarction: a hypothesis. Human Pathology, 7, 547–563.

195. de Bakker, J.M., van Capelle, F.J., Janse, M.J., Tasseron, S., Vermeulen, J.T., de Jonge, N., Lahpor, J.R. (1993). Slow conduction in the infarcted human heart. 'Zigzag' course of activation. Circulation, 88, 915–926.

196. Downar, E., Saito, J., Doig, J.C., Chen, T.C., Sevaptsidis, E., Masse, S., Kimber, S., Mickleborough, L., Harris, L. (1995). Endocardial mapping of ventricular tachycardia in the intact human ventricle. III. Evidence of multiuse reentry with spontaneous and induced block in portions of reentrant path complex. Journal of the American College of Cardiology, 25, 1591–1600.

197. Kaltenbrunner, W., Cardinal, R., Dubuc, M., Shenasa, M., Nadeau, R., Tremblay, G., Vermeulen, M., Savard, P., Page, P.L. (1991). Epicardial and endocardial mapping of ventricular tachycardia in patients with myocardial infarction. Is the origin of the tachycardia always subendocardially localized? Circulation, 84, 1058–1071.

198. Spear, J.F., Horowitz, L.N., Hodess, A.B., MacVaugh, H. III, Moore, E.N. (1979). Cellular electrophysiology of human myocardial infarction. 1. Abnormalities of cellular activation. Circulation, 59, 247–256.

199. Gardner, P.I., Ursell, P.C., Fenoglio, J.J. Jr., Wit, A.L. (1985). Electrophysiologic and anatomic basis for fractionated electrograms recorded from healed myocardial infarcts. Circulation, 72, 596–611.

200. Fast, V.G., Kléber, A.G. (1995). Cardiac tissue geometry as a determinant of unidirectional conduction block: assessment of microscopic excitation spread by optical mapping in patterned cell cultures and in a computer model. Cardiovascular Research, 29, 697–707.

201. Spach, M.S., Miller, W.T. III, Dolber, P.C., Kootsey, J.M., Sommer, J.R., Mosher, C.E. Jr. (1982). The functional role of structural complexities in the propagation of depolarization in the atrium of the dog. Cardiac conduction disturbances due to discontinuities of effective axial resistivity. Circulation Research, 50, 175–191.

202. Wiegerinck, R.F., Verkerk, A.O., Belterman, C.N., van Veen, T.A., Baartscheer, A., Opthof, T., Wilders, R., de Bakker, J.M., Coronel, R. (2006). Larger cell size in rabbits with heart failure increases myocardial conduction velocity and QRS duration. Circulation, 113, 806–813.

203. Pogwizd, S.M., Hoyt, R.H., Saffitz, J.E., Corr, P.B., Cox, J.L., Cain, M.E. (1992). Reentrant and focal mechanisms underlying ventricular tachycardia in the human heart. Circulation, 86, 1872–1887.

204. Zuanetti, G., Hoyt, R.H., Corr, P.B. (1990). Beta-adrenergic-mediated influences on microscopic conduction in epicardial regions overlying infarcted myocardium. Circulation Research, 67, 284–302.

205. Liu, D.W., Gintant, G.A., Antzelevitch, C. (1993). Ionic bases for electrophysiological distinctions among epicardial, midmyocardial, and endocardial myocytes from the free wall of the canine left ventricle. Circulation Research, 72, 671–687.

206. Drouin, E., Charpentier, F., Gauthier, C., Laurent, K., Le, M.H. (1995). Electrophysiologic characteristics of cells spanning the left ventricular wall of human heart: evidence for presence of M cells. Journal of the American College of Cardiology, 26, 185–192.

207. Conrath, C.E., Wilders, R., Coronel, R., de Bakker, J.M.T., Taggart, P., de Groot, J.R., Opthof, T. (2004). Intercellular coupling through gap junctions masks M cells in the human heart. Cardiovascular Research, 62, 407–414.

208. Opthof, T., Coronel, R., Wilms-Schopman, F.J.G., Plotnikov, A.N., Shlapakova, I.N., Danilo, P. Jr., Rosen, M.R., Janse, M.J. (2007). Dispersion of repolarization in canine ventricle and the electrocardiographic T wave: Tp-e interval does *not* reflect transmural dispersion. Heart Rhythm, 4, 341–348.

209. Coronel, R., Opthof, T., Plotnikov, A.N., Wilms-Schopman, F.J.G., Shlapakova, I.N., Danilo, P. Jr., Sosunov, E.A., Anyukhovsky, E.P., Janse, M.J., Rosen, M.R. (2007). Long-term cardiac memory in canine heart is associated with the evolution of a transmural repolarization gradient. Cardiovascular Research, 74, 416–425.

210. Anyukhovsky, E.P., Sosunov, E.A., Gainullin, R.Z., Rosen, M.R. (1999). The controversial M Cell. Journal of Cardiovascular Electrophysiology, 10, 244–260.

211. Volders, P.G., Sipido, K.R., Carmeliet, E., Spatjens, R.L., Wellens, H.J., Vos, M.A. (1999). Repolarizing K^+ currents ITO1 and IKs are larger in right than left canine ventricular midmyocardium. Circulation, 99, 206–210.

212. Szentadrassy, N., Banyasz, T., Biro, T., Szabo, G., Toth, B.I., Magyar, J., Lazar, J., Varro, A., Kovacs, L., Nanasi, P.P. (2005). Apico-basal inhomogeneity in distribution of ion channels in canine and human ventricular myocardium. Cardiovascular Research, 65, 851–860.

213. Ramakers, C., Stengl, M., Spatjens, R.L., Moorman, A.F., Vos, M.A. (2005). Molecular and electrical characterization of the canine cardiac ventricular septum. Journal of Molecular and Cellular Cardiology, 38, 153–161.

214. Ashamalla, S.M., Navarro, D., Ward, C.A. (2001). Gradient of sodium current across the left ventricular wall of adult rat hearts. Journal of Physiology, 536, 439–443.

215. Xiong, W., Tian, Y., Disilvestre, D., Tomaselli, G.F. (2005). Transmural heterogeneity of Na + -Ca2 + exchange: evidence for differential expression in normal and failing hearts. Circulation Research, 97, 207–209.

216. Joyner, R.W., Picone, J., Veenstra, R., Rawling, D. (1983). Propagation through electrically coupled cells. Effects of regional changes in membrane properties. Circulation Research, 53, 526–534.

217. Poelzing, S., Akar, F.G., Baron, E., Rosenbaum, D.S. (2004). Heterogeneous connexin43 expression produces electrophysiological heterogeneities across ventricular wall. American Journal of Physiology Heart and Circulatory Physiology, 286, H2001–H2009.

218. Yamada, K.A., Kanter, E.M., Green, K.G., Saffitz, J.E. (2004). Transmural distribution of connexins in rodent hearts. Journal of Cardiovascular Electrophysiology, 15, 710–715.

219. Wiegerinck, R.F., van Veen, A.A., Belterman, C.N., Schumacher, C.A., Noorman, M., de Bakker, J.M., Coronel, R. (2008). Transmural dispersion of refractoriness and conduction velocity is associated with heterogeneously reduced connexin43 in a rabbit model of heart failure. Heart Rhythm, 5, 1178–1185.

220. Ripplinger, C.M., Li, W., Hadley, J., Chen, J., Rothenberg, F., Lombardi, R., Wickline, S.A., Marian, A.J., Efimov, I.R. (2007). Enhanced transmural fiber rotation and connexin 43 heterogeneity are associated with an increased upper limit of vulnerability in a transgenic rabbit model of human hypertrophic cardiomyopathy. Circulation Research, 101, 1049–1057.

221. Wan, X., Laurita, K.R., Pruvot, E.J., Rosenbaum, D.S. (2005). Molecular correlates of repolarization alternans in cardiac myocytes. Journal of Molecular and Cellular Cardiology, 39, 419–428.

222. Rosenbaum, D.S., Jackson, L.E., Smith, J.M., Garan, H., Ruskin, J.N., Cohen, R.J. (1994). Electrical alternans and vulnerability to ventricular arrhythmias. New England Journal of Medicine, 330, 235–241.

223. Valdivia, C.R., Chu, W.W., Pu, J., Foell, J.D., Haworth, R.A., Wolff, M.R., Kamp, T.J., Makielski, J.C. (2005). Increased late sodium current in myocytes from a canine heart failure model and from failing human heart. Journal of Molecular and Cellular Cardiology, 38, 475–483.

224. van Veen, T.A., Stein, M., Royer, A., Le, Q.K., Charpentier, F., Colledge, W.H., Huang, C.L., Wilders, R., Grace, A.A., Escande, D., de Bakker, J.M., van Rijen, H.V. (2005). Impaired impulse propagation in Scn5a-knockout mice: combined contribution of excitability, connexin expression, and tissue architecture in relation to aging. Circulation, 112, 1927–1935.

225. Undrovinas, A.I., Maltsev, V.A., Kyle, J.W., Silverman, N., Sabbah, H.N. (2002). Gating of the late Na^+ channel in normal and failing human myocardium. Journal of Molecular and Cellular Cardiology, 34, 1477–1489.

226. Qin, D., Zhang, Z.H., Caref, E.B., Boutjdir, M., Jain, P., el-Sherif, N. (1996). Cellular and ionic basis of arrhythmias in postinfarction remodeled ventricular myocardium. Circulation Research, 79, 461–473.

227. Zicha, S., Xiao, L., Stafford, S., Cha, T.J., Han, W., Varro, A., Nattel, S. (2004). Transmural expression of transient outward potassium current subunits in normal and failing canine and human hearts. Journal Physiology, 561, 735–748.

228. Zhang, X.Q., Moore, R.L., Tillotson, D.L., Cheung, J.Y. (1995). Calcium currents in postinfarction rat cardiac myocytes. American Journal of Physiology, 269, C1464–C1473.

229. Santos, P.E., Barcellos, L.C., Mill, J.G., Masuda, M.O. (1995). Ventricular action potential and L-type calcium channel in infarct-induced hypertrophy in rats. Journal of Cardiovascular and Electrophysiology, 6, 1004–1014.

230. Kim, Y.K., Kim, S.J., Kramer, C.M., Yatani, A., Takagi, G., Mankad, S., Szigeti, G.P., Singh, D., Bishop, S.P., Shannon, R.P., Vatner, D.E., Vatner, S.F. (2002). Altered

excitation-contraction coupling in myocytes from remodeled myocardium after chronic myocardial infarction. Journal of Molecular Cellular Cardiology, 34, 63–73.

231. Aimond, F., Alvarez, J.L., Rauzier, J.M., Lorente, P., Vassort, G. (1999). Ionic basis of ventricular arrhythmias in remodeled rat heart during long-term myocardial infarction. Cardiovascular Research, 42, 402–415.

232. Liu, N., Niu, H., Li, Y., Zhang, C., Zhou, Q., Ruan, Y., Pu, J., Lu, Z. (2004). The changes of potassium currents in rabbit ventricle with healed myocardial infarction. Journal of Huazhong University of Science and Technology, 24, 128–131.

233. Dun, W., Baba, S., Yagi, T., Boyden, P.A. (2004). Dynamic remodeling of K^+ and Ca^{2+} currents in cells that survived in the epicardial border zone of canine healed infarcted heart. American Journal of Physiology Heart and Circulatory Physiology, 287, H1046–H1054.

234. Peters, N.S. (1995). Myocardial gap junction organization in ischemia and infarction. Microscopy Research and Technique, 31, 375–386.

235. Kostin, S., Rieger, M., Dammer, S., Hein, S., Richter, M., Klovekorn, W.P., Bauer, E.P., Schaper, J. (2003). Gap junction remodeling and altered connexin43 expression in the failing human heart. Molecular and Cellular Biochemistry, 242, 135–144.

236. Betsuyaku, T., Kanno, S., Lerner, D.L., Schuessler, R.B., Saffitz, J.E., Yamada, K.A. (2004). Spontaneous and inducible ventricular arrhythmias after myocardial infarction in mice. Cardiovascular Pathology, 13, 156–164.

237. Bogun, F., Krishnan, S., Siddiqui, M., Good, E., Marine, J.E., Schuger, C., Oral, H., Chugh, A., Pelosi, F., Morady, F. (2005). Electrogram characteristics in postinfarction ventricular tachycardia: effect of infarct age. Journal of the American College of Cardiology, 46, 667–674.

238. Kawara, T., Derksen, R., de, G. Jr., Coronel, R., Tasseron, S., Linnenbank, A.C., Hauer, R.N., Kirkels, H., Janse, M.J., de Bakker, J.M. (2001). Activation delay after premature stimulation in chronically diseased human myocardium relates to the architecture of interstitial fibrosis. Circulation, 104, 3069–3075.

239. La Rovere, M.T., Bigger, J.T. Jr., Marcus, F.I., Mortara, A., Schwartz, P.J. (1998). Baroreflex sensitivity and heart-rate variability in prediction of total cardiac mortality after myocardial infarction. ATRAMI (Autonomic Tone and Reflexes After Myocardial Infarction) Investigators. Lancet, 351, 478–484.

240. Cao, J.M., Chen, L.S., KenKnight, B.H., Ohara, T., Lee, M.H., Tsai, J., Lai, W.W., Karagueuzian, H.S., Wolf, P.L., Fishbein, M.C., Chen, P.S. (2000). Nerve sprouting and sudden cardiac death. Circulation Research, 86, 816–821.

241. Chang, C.M., Wu, T.J., Zhou, S., Doshi, R.N., Lee, M.H., Ohara, T., Fishbein, M.C., Karagueuzian, H.S., Chen, P.S., Chen, L.S. (2001). Nerve sprouting and sympathetic hyperinnervation in a canine model of atrial fibrillation produced by prolonged right atrial pacing. Circulation, 103, 22–25.

242. Schwartz, P.J. (2001). QT prolongation, sudden death, and sympathetic imbalance: the pendulum swings. Journal of Cardiovascular Electrophysiology, 12, 1074–1077.

243. Schwartz, P.J. (1976). Cardiac sympathetic innervation and the sudden infant death syndrome. A possible pathogenetic link. American Journal of Medicine, 60, 167–172.

244. Nori, S.L., Gaudino, M., Alessandrini, F., Bronzetti, E., Santarelli, P. (1995). Immunohistochemical evidence for sympathetic denervation and reinnervation after necrotic injury in rat myocardium. Cellular & Molecular Biology, 41, 799–807.

245. Chen, P.S., Chen, L.S., Cao, J.M., Sharifi, B., Karagueuzian, H.S., Fishbein, M.C. (2001). Sympathetic nerve sprouting, electrical remodeling and the mechanisms of sudden cardiac death. Cardiovascular Research, 50, 409–416.

246. Jiang, H., Lu, Z., Yu, Y., Zhao, D., Yang, B., Huang, C. (2007). Relationship between sympathetic nerve sprouting and repolarization dispersion at peri-infarct zone after myocardial infarction. Autonomic Neuroscience, 134, 18–25.

247. Estes, E.H. Jr., Entman, M.L., Dixon, H.B., Hackel, D.B. (1966). The vascular supply of the left ventricular wall. Anatomic observations, plus a hypothesis regarding acute events in coronary artery disease. American Heart Journal, 71, 58–67.

248. Friedman, P.L., Stewart, J.R., Wit, A.L. (1973). Spontaneous and induced cardiac arrhythmias in subendocardial Purkinje fibers surviving extensive myocardial infarction in dogs. Circulation Research, 33, 612–626.

249. Bogun, F., Good, E., Reich, S., Elmouchi, D., Igic, P., Tschopp, D., Dey, S., Wimmer, A., Jongnarangsin, K., Oral, H., Chugh, A., Pelosi, F., Morady, F. (2006). Role of Purkinje fibers in post-infarction ventricular tachycardia. Journal of the American College of Cardiology, 48, 2500–2507.

250. Szumowski, L., Sanders, P., Walczak, F., Hocini, M., Jais, P., Kepski, R., Szufladowicz, E., Urbanek, P., Derejko, P., Bodalski, R., Haissaguerre, M. (2004). Mapping and ablation of polymorphic ventricular tachycardia after myocardial infarction. Journal of the American College of Cardiology, 44, 1700–1706.

251. Berenfeld, O., Jalife, J. (1998). Purkinje-muscle reentry as a mechanism of polymorphic ventricular arrhythmias in a 3-dimensional model of the ventricles. Circulation Research, 82, 1063–1077.

252. Wang, Z., Luo, X., Lu, Y., Yang, B. (2008). miRNAs at the heart of the matter. Journal of Molecular Medicine, 86, 771–783.

253. Yang, B., Lin, H., Xiao, J., Lu, Y., Luo, X., Li, B., Zhang, Y., Xu, C., Bai, Y., Wang, H., Chen, G., Wang, Z. (2007). The muscle-specific microRNA miR-1 regulates cardiac arrhythmogenic potential by targeting GJA1 and KCNJ2. Nature Medicine, 13, 486–491.

254. van Rooij, E., Sutherland, L.B., Liu, N., Williams, A.H., McAnally, J., Gerard, R.D., Richardson, J.A., Olson, E.N. (2006). A signature pattern of stress-responsive micro-RNAs that can evoke cardiac hypertrophy and heart failure. Proceedings of the National Academy of Sciences USA, 103, 18255–18260.

CHAPTER 5

Antiarrhythmic Drug Classification

CYNTHIA A. CARNES

5.1 INTRODUCTION

The goals in treating cardiac rhythm disorders are to minimize symptoms and prolong survival. Although rhythm disorders have classically been treated with pharmacologic therapy, arrhythmias are increasingly treated through nonpharmacologic means. Nonpharmacologic treatments of arrhythmias include devices such as pacemakers and implantable cardioverter defibrillators, or procedures to reduce the initiation and/ or propagation of arrhythmias (e.g., ablation procedures).

Drugs used to treat cardiac rhythm disorders are typically blockers of sarcolemmal ion channels. This chapter will provide an introduction and overview of drugs used to treat cardiac arrhythmias. The modified Vaughan Williams classification (see Table 5.1) is traditionally used to group antiarrhythmic medications. However, this approach is limited because 1) many drugs have multiple pharmacologic effects, 2) drugs are classified based on effects on normal ventricular or Purkinje fiber preparations, 3) some antiarrhythmics do not fit into a single drug class, and 4) some antiarrhythmic actions are not included in the classification. Alternative classification systems have been proposed, e.g., The Sicilian Gambit [1], but the Vaughan Williams classification [2, 3] remains the most common. In this chapter, the Vaughan Williams class is therefore noted where applicable.

5.2 SODIUM CHANNEL BLOCKERS

Sodium channel blocking drugs may be classified by their specificity for the sodium channel or the state(s) of the channel within a cardiac cycle during which they bind or unbind, which contributes to more or less drug effect at faster (i.e., use-dependent blockers) or slower (reverse use-dependent blockers) rates of activation. The time

Novel Therapeutic Targets for Antiarrhythmic Drugs, Edited by George Edward Billman

Table 5.1. Vaughan Williams Classification of Antiarrhythmic Drugs [2, 3]

Class I (Sodium Channel Blockers)
Ia (Intermediate kinetics and action potential prolongation)
Quinidine
Procainamide
Disopyramide

Ib (Rapid kinetics)
Lidocaine
Mexiletine

Ic (Slow kinetics)
Flecainide
Propafenone

II
Beta-adrenergic receptor blockers

III (Action Potential Prolonging)
Amiodarone
Dofetilide
Ibutilide
Sotalol

Class IV (Calcium Channel Blockers)
Diltiazem
Verapamil

required for binding and/or unbinding of the drug to the channel (kinetics of action) also varies, and it may also serve as a means to group sodium channel blocking drugs. Another complexity of these drugs is related to the pharmacokinetics of these compounds. These salient features of sodium-channel-blocking antiarrhythmic drugs are reviewed below (Table 5.2).

5.2.1 Mixed Sodium Channel Blockers (Vaughan Williams Class Ia)

The mixed sodium-channel blockers are not specific for sodium channels. Notably, the kinetics of interaction (τ-on) with sodium channels, and the time for recovery of the sodium channels from drug block, are intermediate to other types of blockers, as described below [4–6].

5.2.1.1 Quinidine. An early antiarrhythmic medication was quinidine, which is a plant-derived alkaloid whose antiarrhythmic activity was initially described in 1749 [7]. Quinidine is the prototype of antiarrhythmic drugs thought to act primarily through inhibition of the rapid inward sodium current with affinity for both open and inactivated channels [8], while also prolonging repolarization of the cardiac

Table 5.2. Electrocardiographic Effects of Antiarrhythmic Drugs at Physiologic Heart Rates

Drug	Heart Rate	PR	QRS	QT
Adenosine	0	↑	0	0
Amiodarone	↓	↑	↑	↑
Beta-adrenergic receptor blockers	↓	↑	0	0
Digoxin	↓	↑	0	0
Diltiazem	↓	↑	0	0
Disopyramide	↑↓	↑↓	↑	↑
Dofetilide	0 or ↓	0	0	↑
Flecainide	0	↑	↑	0
Ibutilide	0	0	0	↑
Lidocaine	0	0	0	0
Mexiletine	0	0	0	0
Procainamide	↓	↑↓	↑	↑
Propafenone	0	↑	↑	0
Quinidine	↑↓	↑↓	↑	↑
Sotalol	↓	↑	0	↑
Verapamil	↓	↑	0	0

myocardium via inhibition of the repolarizing K^+ current, I_{Kr}. This combination of effects results in slowing of conduction in the atrial and ventricular myocardium while prolonging repolarization throughout the heart. Quinidine also has effects on the autonomic system: inhibition of α-adrenergic receptors and inhibition of muscarinic receptors [9, 10]. These effects can result in the reduction in blood pressure and consequent hypotension, as well as in the acceleration of the sinus rate and the acceleration of atrioventricular (AV) nodal conduction (an effect that can unfortunately accelerate the ventricular response rate during atrial tachyarrhythmias). The clinical use of quinidine in human medicine is therefore limited because of its known risk of proarrhythmia [11] and other (e.g., gastrointestinal) adverse effects. Notably, quinidine is a potent inhibitor of the hepatic CYP2D6 metabolic pathway [12], which may increase the concentrations of other medications, e.g., beta-adrenergic receptor blockers.

5.2.1.2 Procainamide. Procainimide is similar to quinidine in that it inhibits both the fast sodium current and I_{Kr}. Procainamide also inhibits muscarinic receptors, although less potently than quinidine; however, it also has the potential to accelerate the sinus rate and AV nodal conduction during atrial tachyarrhythmias. Procainamide is also a ganglionic bocker; this action reduces peripheral vascular resistance and blood pressure, which is an effect that occurs primarily when administered intravenously and is dependent on the rate of drug administration. The N-acetylation metabolic pathway is genetically polymorphic with the human population divided into rapid and slow acetylators [13]. Acetylation of procainamide results in the formation of N-acetylprocainamide, which is a pharmacologically active metabolite that is renally eliminated. N-acetylprocainamide is a blocker of I_{Kr} and therefore prolongs cardiac repolarization. Thus, sustained therapy with procainamide results in therapeutically relevant concentrations of both procainamide and the active metabolite, N-acetylprocainamide, although the relative concentrations of the parent drug and metabolite are regulated (in part) by acetylator status [14]. Potential adverse effects (e.g., drug-induced lupus—particularly in slow acetylators, proarrhythmia, anticholinergic effects, and blood dyscrasias) limit the clinical utility of procainamide.

5.2.1.3 Disopyramide. Disopyramide is similar to quinidine and procainamide, in that it inhibits both fast sodium current and I_{Kr}. In addition, disopyramide is a highly potent anticholinergic drug [9], and it can accelerate sinus rate and AV nodal conduction. Disopyramide is administered as a racemic mixture with stereoselective effects on repolarization, whereas the effects on depolarization and contractility are nonstereoselective [15]. The use of disopyramide is limited by its anticholinergic, negative inotropic, and potential proarrhythmic effects.

5.3 INHIBITORS OF THE FAST SODIUM CURRENT WITH RAPID KINETICS (VAUGHAN WILLIAMS CLASS IB)

These sodium-channel blockers have a rapid rate constant for block of the current and a rapid recovery from block (τ 200–500 ms). Thus, these drugs exhibit little beat-to-beat accumulation of block of the fast inward sodium current, unless the rate of activation is abnormally rapid.

5.3.1 Lidocaine

Lidocaine primarily inhibits the fast inward sodium current. Lidocaine blocks the inactivated state of the sodium channel, resulting in increased current block at faster heart rates (use-dependent block). At physiologic human heart rates, in normal hearts, there is little apparent lidocaine effect on conduction velocity. Because of the affinity of lidocaine for the inactivated state of the fast inward cardiac sodium current, there is an increased effect in ischemic tissue, which is attributable to depolarization of the resting potential (increasing sodium channel inactivation). The activity of lidocaine is also increased during ischemia because of the lower pH in ischemic tissue as this alters the ratio of neutral to charged lidocaine. Lidocaine does cause shortening of the ventricular action potential, which is attributed to blocking of the relatively small, slowly inactivating sodium current, which is activated during plateau potentials (plateau current, recently demonstrated in canine Purkinje cells) [16]. Action potential shortening by lidocaine is particularly advantageous in situations where early afterdepolarizations trigger arrhythmias [17]. Lidocaine has been thought to have minimal effects on atrial electrophysiology, which has been attributed to the relatively abbreviated atrial action potential [18], although the ventricular specificity of lidocaine's effects has recently been called into question [19].

The utility of lidocaine is limited by its narrow therapeutic window combined with complex pharmacokinetics [20]. Circulating lidocaine is bound to albumin and alpha-1-acid glycoprotein, an acute phase reactant; thus, the free or active portion of total lidocaine is difficult to predict based on dose or measured total plasma concentration. Lidocaine has multiple active (sodium-channel-blocking) metabolites. The hepatic clearance of lidocaine is dependent on hepatic blood flow and hepatic metabolic activity, and lidocaine concentrations increase after prolonged therapy in an unpredictable manner. Significant concentration-dependent central nervous system adverse effects are possible with lidocaine therapy (including seizures and coma). In summary, because of the potential toxicity of lidocaine, which may be attributed to the impact of complex pharmacokinetics on the risk:benefit ratio, lidocaine is no longer used for routine prophylaxis of ventricular tachyarrhythmias, but it is reserved for the acute treatment of life-threatening ventricular arrhythmias.

5.3.2 Mexiletine

Mexiletine is similar in cardiac electrophysiologic effects to lidocaine and inhibits both the fast sodium current and the plateau sodium current [21]. Specifically, the interaction of mexiletine with the sodium channel is minimal at physiologic heart rates, and increased at rapid rates or during depolarization of the resting potential (e.g., during ischemia) [22]. Unlike lidocaine, mexiletine may be administered orally. Potential adverse effects during mexiletine therapy include effects on the nervous system (e.g., paresthesias, tremor, and loss of coordination) and the gastrointestinal tract. Multiple pharmacokinetic interactions occur between mexiletine and other medications [23], which are notable given the narrow therapeutic index of antiarrhythmic medications.

5.4 INHIBITORS OF THE FAST SODIUM CURRENT WITH SLOW KINETICS (VAUGHAN WILLIAMS CLASS IC)

This group of antiarrhythmic drugs exhibits a slow onset of block and a prolonged recovery from block ($\tau > 12$ s) [4, 6]. Thus, drugs with these characteristics exhibit accumulating sodium current block at fast heart rates with minimal diastolic recovery.

5.4.1 Flecainide

When compared with lidocaine- or quinidine-like drugs, flecainide has a much slower rate of onset and offset of block of the cardiac sodium channels. This effect results in slowing of conduction in the atrium, His-Purkinje system, and ventricle; this effect is more prominent at rapid heart rates. Notably, the extent of block is increased during diastolic depolarization (e.g., see ref. 24) and augmented sympathetic tone [25]. This, combined with the slow offset kinetics, is thought to contribute to the well-known proarrhythmic potential of this drug in patients with underlying ischemic cardiac disease [26]. Flecainide is therefore contraindicated in patients with ischemic heart disease or structural heart disease because of the increased risk of proarrhythamia.

5.4.2 Propafenone

Propafenone is similar to flecainide in its electrophysiologic effects on the fast inward sodium current. A notable difference is the β-adrenergic-receptor-blocking activity of propafenone. Propafenone inhibits both β-1 and β-2 adrenergic receptors. Even though the potency of propafenone is ~50-fold lower than that of propranolol on a molar basis, the circulating concentrations of propafenone are many-fold higher than those of propranolol [27]. Thus, propafenone may exhibit nonselective β-adrenergic-blocking activity in addition to inhibitory effects on sodium current. As with flecainide, propafenone is contraindicated in patients with known ischemic heart disease or structural heart disease, because of the increased risk of proarrhythmia.

5.5 INHIBITORS OF REPOLARIZING K$^+$ CURRENTS (VAUGHAN WILLIAMS CLASS III)

There are multiple repolarizing currents in the myocardium as described in Chapter 2. By prolonging repolarization, and therefore refractoriness, reentrant arrhythmias can be terminated.

5.5.1 Dofetilide

Dofetilide is a selective I_{Kr} blocker with minimal extracardiac effects. Dofetilide prolongs repolarization of atrial and ventricular myocardium. Thus, dofetilide prolongs the action potential duration and the QT and QTc intervals on the electrocardiogram. The effects of dofetilide on I_{Kr} are reverse use dependent, thus exhibiting a larger effect at slower heart rates; however, this is not a consistent finding and may be dependent on [K$^+$] [28–31]. Dofetilide may also have mild negative chronotropic effects, which may result from prolonged repolarization in the sinoatrial (SA) node, thereby reducing the rate of spontaneous activity [32, 33].

Pharmacodynamic interactions with dofetilide may occur with any medication that prolongs repolarization or the QT interval. Dofetilide undergoes a relatively small amount of inactivation by CYP3A4 metabolism but is primarily renally eliminated. Significant pharmacokinetic drug interactions occur with other medications eliminated via the renal cation transporter (e.g., cimetidine, trimethoprim, or ketoconazole) and may occur with inhibitors of CYP3A4 (notably verapamil); because of the narrow therapeutic index of dofetilide, coadministration of such medications is contraindicated. The initial dosing and dosing adjustments of dofetilide are based on estimated renal function and post-dose QT intervals. In patients with left ventricular dysfunction or heart failure, the risk of torsades de pointes during dofetilide therapy is highest in the initial 3 days after initiation of treatment [34]. Thus, in-hospital monitoring is recommended for the first 3 days of therapy.

5.5.2 Sotalol

Sotalol inhibits I$_{Kr,}$ and is a nonselective antagonist of β_1- and $\beta2$-adrenergic receptors. The l-sotalol isomer is responsible for the β-adrenergic receptor antagonism of racemic sotalol. A trial of d-sotalol in post-myocardial infarction patients with reduced left ventricular systolic function found an increase in mortality, suggesting that there is some antiarrhythmic benefit from the addition of beta-adrenergic receptor activity to the APD prolonging effects of I$_{Kr}$ inhibition [35]. Notably, the inhibition of I$_{Kr}$ by sotalol exhibits reverse use dependence [36] and thus is increased at lower heart rates.

Bradycardia (which may occur with β-adrenergic receptor inhibition) increases the risk of sotalol-induced torsades de pointes, as does hypokalemia, hypomagnesemia, long baseline QT interval, severe left ventricular systolic failure, or female sex. In addition to the risk of torsades de pointes, adverse effects of sotalol include those previously described with beta-adrenergic receptor blockers (e.g., bradycardia and bronchospasm in patients with underlying asthma). Sotalol is renally eliminated, and doses must be adjusted based on renal impairment and prolongation of the QT interval on the electrocardiogram.

5.5.3 Amiodarone

Amiodarone was initially developed as an antianginal drug [37] and was later found to have antiarrhythmic efficacy. Initially described as a Vaughan Williams class III drug (an effect resulting from lengthening of the action potential duration via inhibition of I$_{Kr}$), amiodarone has a broad spectrum of antiarrhythmic activity across each of the four Vaughan Williams drug classes. With respect to its sodium-channel-blocking activity, amiodarone exhibits frequency-dependent block [38, 39] and rapid kinetics of blocking and recovery from inactivation [40]. Amiodarone is a noncompetitive and nonselective antagonist of beta-adrenergic receptors, and it has also been shown to reduce the expression of myocardial beta-adrenergic receptors [41, 42]. Amiodarone also acts as a blocker of sarcolemmal calcium channels in a frequency-dependent manner [43].

Amiodarone is unique and has a long half-life (average of more than 50 days) [44]. Amiodarone is highly lipophilic and highly protein bound with an extremely large volume of distribution [44], and it is highly concentrated in many organs (e.g., liver, lungs, and skin). Loading regimens are required to shorten the time to reach an effective drug concentration. Amiodarone is hepatically metabolized and has a pharmacologically active metabolite (desethyl-amiodarone). Amiodarone is an inhibitor of the CYP2C9 hepatic metabolic pathway giving rise to an interaction with warfarin [45]; amiodarone interacts with multiple other medications both pharmacokinetically and pharmacodynamically.

Amiodarone is more effective than other antiarrhythmic medications, but it has the potential for significant extracardiac adverse effects, some of which may result in significant morbidity (e.g., pulmonary fibrosis, hyperthyroidism, and hepatitis). Amiodarone may cause either hyperthyroidism or hypothyroidism [46]; the complex nature of effects on thyroid function are thought to occur because amiodarone is 37% iodine by molecular weight, and it inhibits the conversion of thyroxine to triiodothyronine.

The adverse effects of amiodarone therapy are dose related, and the maintenance doses used for atrial arrhythmias (i.e., 200 mg per day) are safer than the higher doses used for ventricular tachyarrhythmias. In addition to electrocardiograms, careful monitoring for ophthalmologic, pulmonary, hepatic, and thyroid toxicities are recommended for patients chronically treated with amiodarone [47]. Other extracardiac adverse effects include photosensitivity and a slate-blue skin discoloration after sun exposure.

5.5.4 Ibutilide

Ibutilide prolongs repolarization and refractoriness by inhibition of I_{Kr} current [48]. It can also augment late sodium current [49], which may contribute to prolonged repolarization. Ibutilide is used for acute conversion of atrial arrhythmias, and it is only available for intravenous use. Ibutilide reportedly results in torsades de pointes in ~4% of patients and is more common in females [50]; monitoring is therefore required for up to 6 h after dosing to monitor for the development of torsades de pointes.

5.6 I_{KUR} BLOCKERS

I_{Kur}, the ultra-rapid delayed rectifier potassium current, has been described as an "atrial-selective" current in large mammals including humans. Thus, drugs targeting this current would hypothetically avoid the risks of ventricular proarrhythmia, which occur with other drugs that block repolarizing currents. Currently, there are mixed blockers of I_{Kur}, I_{to}, and other currents in development for the treatment of atrial tachyarrhythmias [51–53]. However, as discussed in Chapter 18, additional validation is needed to ensure atrial selectivity of this therapeutic approach in patients.

5.7 INHIBITORS OF CALCIUM CHANNELS

5.7.1 Verapamil and Diltiazem

Two pharmacologically distinct types of calcium channel blockers are dihydropyridines and nondihydropyridines (exemplified by diltiazem and verapamil). Dihydropyridines are relatively selective for vascular calcium channels and have minimal effects on cardiac calcium channels at typical therapeutic concentrations. In contrast, diltiazem and verapamil affect both vascular and cardiac calcium channels; the latter effect provides use in the treatment of cardiac arrhythmias.

Verapamil and diltiazem block activated and inactivated sarcolemmal L-type calcium channels and therefore slow phase-zero depolarization of SA and AV nodal cells [54, 55]. Thus, these drugs can be used to slow the sinus node rate (useful in the treatment of sinus tachycardias) or to slow conduction through the AV node [56]. Slowing conduction through the AV node is beneficial for controlling ventricular response rates during atrial tachyarrhythmias, to treat junctional tachyarrhythmias, or for any reentrant arrhythmias where the AV node forms part of the reentrant circuit.

Potential adverse cardiac effects associated with antiarrhythmic calcium channel blockers include bradycardia, AV blocks, and impaired cardiac contractility, which is most significant in patients with impaired systolic function. Potential extracardiac adverse effects include hypotension, constipation, and peripheral edema. Verapamil undergoes extensive metabolism via CYP3A4, and it inhibits CYP3A4, providing a basis for multiple pharmacokinetic drug and food interactions [57, 58]. Similarly, diltiazem is a substrate for CYP3A4 metabolism but is a weak inhibitor of CYP3A4.

5.8 INHIBITORS OF ADRENERGICALLY-MODULATED ELECTROPHYSIOLOGY

The sympathetic nervous system is an important modulator of cardiovascular function. Antagonists of the β-adrenergic receptors modulate cardiac electrophysiology in a manner that can be antiarrhythmic. β-adrenergic receptor antagonists are antiarrhythmic by modulating the function of the pacemaker current, I_f, and by modulating calcium signaling.

5.8.1 Funny Current (I_f) Inhibitors

For detailed information on I_f and the current-encoding (HCN) channels, the reader is referred to recent reviews [59, 60]. The pacemaker current, I_f, is a nonselective cationic (K^+ and Na^+) current that is inward at hyperpolarized membrane potentials and confers automaticity (spontaneous depolarization) to specific regions of the normal mammalian heart. Recently, it has been reported that HCN channels are also permeant to Ca^{2+} ions [61].

As an aside, the "f" in I_f is from the "funny" nature of the channel, i.e., the nonselectivity of the channel, and the very hyperpolarized range of activation. In mammalian hearts, I_f is encoded by the hyperpolarization-activated cationic nucleoside-modulated (HCN) channels, and multiple isoforms, HCN1, HCN2, HCN3, and HCN4, have been described in cardiac tissue. In normal hearts, I_f is restricted to SA and AV nodal cells and to the His-Purkinje, with the greatest density in the SA nodal cells. Adrenergic stimulation accelerates current activation and thus accelerates diastolic depolarization, thus accelerating SA nodal activity and heart rate; this process is opposed by muscarinic activation. Thus, the physiologic heart rate is governed by the intrinsic sinus rate, which is dependent on the balance of adrenergic and muscarinic influences.

During the process of aging and during pathologic processes such as hypertension and heart failure, I_f expression is no longer restricted in location and has been shown to be expressed in the heart outside the conduction system. This pathologic increase in expression of the current, combined with the enhanced adrenergic tone that often accompanies these conditions, may provide a source of arrhythmogenic activity [62–65].

Multiple investigational I_f antagonists, e.g., ivabradine, may have utility in the treatment of tachyarrhythmias, ischemic heart disease, or heart failure. These are discussed more in Chapter 3.

5.8.2 Beta-Adrenergic Receptor Antagonists

Beta-adrenergic receptor antagonists are proven to reduce mortality after myocardial infarction [66] and have utility in the treatment of some congenital forms of long QT syndrome (for a recent review, see ref. 67). These drugs are antiarrhythmic by inhibition of I_f and by inhibition of sarcolemmal L-type calcium current (as described above). The effects of β-adrenergic receptor blockers on I_f are most likely to be antiarrhythmic when there is an elevated sympathetic tone. In addition to the effects on I_f-mediated arrhythmias described above, there is the potential to reduce arrhythmias caused by calcium overload (see Chapters 19 and 20).

Through effects on the L-type calcium current, β-adrenergic receptor blockers can be used to slow the sinus node rate (useful in the treatment of sinus tachycardias) or to slow conduction through the AV node. Thus, they are beneficial for controlling ventricular response rates during atrial tachyarrhythmias, treatment of junctional tachyarrhythmias, or for any reentrant arrhythmias where the AV node forms part of the reentrant circuit.

Even though β-adrenergic receptor blockers are effective for many forms of adrenergically mediated arrhythmias, their usefulness may be limited by adverse effects. In specific, patients with reversible airway disease (asthma) may be unable to tolerate $β_2$-adrenergic receptor antagonism. The use of a $β_1$-adrenergic receptor "selective" drug may limit the occurrence of bronchospasm, but selectivity is concentration dependent and may be lost at higher concentrations. Patients with SA nodal disease (sick sinus syndrome) may not tolerate β-blockers without an electronic pacemaker. The use of a β-adrenergic receptor blocker with intrinsic sympathomimetic activity (e.g., acebutelol or pindolol) may reduce bradycardia by exerting a sympathetic effect when endogenous sympathetic activity is low. Most β-adrenergic receptor blockers are metabolized by CYP2D6, which is subject to both genetic polymorphisms and modulation by other drugs. The tolerability and efficacy of β-adrenergic receptor blockers may be in part determined by pharmacogenomic differences [68–71].

5.9 ADENOSINE

Adenosine is a naturally occurring nucleoside. The circulating half-life of adenosine is less than 30 s, and therefore, pharmacologic doses are given by the intravenous route for the acute treatment of arrhythmias. Adenosine exerts its antiarrhythmic effect on the AV node and is used for the termination of narrow complex supraventricular tachyarrhythmias. Adenosine is reported to activate an inwardly rectifying time-independent potassium current in AV nodal myocytes via activation of the AV nodal A1 adenosine receptor [72]. This current hyperpolarizes the sarcolemmal membrane to inhibit AV node activation. In addition, adenosine inhibits calcium current, which also inhibits AV node conduction [73].

Potential adverse effects of adenosine include those related to vasodilation (i.e., headache and flushing), proarrhythmia, and bronchoconstriction. Other than bronchoconstriction, these effects are typically short lived because of the short half-life.

5.10 DIGOXIN

Although digoxin has long been recognized as a positive inotrope, it acts indirectly as an antiarrhythmic drug. Digoxin exerts antiarrhythmic effects by slowing the sinus node rate and by inhibiting the AV node. These effects occur via increased vagal stimulation and decreased sympathetic discharge, rather than through direct effects on the electrophysiology of the nodal tissues. Consequently, these antiarrhythmic effects of digoxin may be antagonized when there are increases in endogenous sympathetic tone.

Results from the Atrial Fibrillation Follow-up Investigation of Rhythm Management (AFFIRM) trial indicate that digoxin is reasonably effective for rate-control in patients with atrial fibrillation [74]. Digoxin is the best choice for control of ventricular response rate during atrial tachyarrhythmias in patients with impaired systolic function; however, for the general patient population, other approaches such as β-blockers or calcium channel blockers may be more effective [75].

5.11 CONCLUSIONS

Drug therapy remains an important approach to managing patients with cardiac arrhythmias. Current drug therapy of arrhythmias is limited by modest efficacy and the risk of significant drug-induced morbidity and even mortality. Nonpharmacologic approaches such as implantable devices and ablation procedures are becoming increasingly more prevalent in the treatment of rhythm disorders. Often, a combination of pharmacologic and nonpharmacologic therapies is required for adequate rhythm control in many patients. Potential future directions for antiarrhythmic drug development include chamber-selective therapies or therapies to reduce or reverse pathologic electrophysiologic remodeling.

REFERENCES

1. Task Force of the Working Group on Arrhythmias of the European Society of Cardiology. (1991). The Sicilian gambit. A new approach to the classification of antiarrhythmic drugs based on their actions on arrhythmogenic mechanisms. Circulation, 84, 1831–1851.

2. Vaughan Williams E.M. (1984). A classification of antiarrhythmic actions reassessed after a decade of new drugs. Journal of Clinical Pharmacology, 24, 129–147.

3. Harrison D.C. (1986). A rational scientific basis for subclassification of antiarrhythmic drugs. Transactions of the American Clinical and Climatological Association, 97, 43–52.

4. Hondeghem L.M. (2000). Classification of antiarrhythmic agents and the two laws of pharmacology. Cardiovascular Research, 45, 57–60.

5. Weirich J., Antoni H. (1990). Differential analysis of the frequency-dependent effects of class 1 antiarrhythmic drugs according to periodical ligand binding: implications for antiarrhythmic and proarrhythmic efficacy. Journal of Cardiovascular Pharmacology, 15, 998–1009.

6. Campbell T.J. (1983). Kinetics of onset of rate-dependent effects of Class I antiarrhythmic drugs are important in determining their effects on refractoriness in guinea-pig ventricle, and provide a theoretical basis for their subclassification. Cardiovascular Research, 17, 344–352.

7. Luderitz B. History of the Disorders of Cardiac Rhythm. 2nd ed. Armonk, NY: Futura Publishing Company, 1994.

8. Hondeghem L.M., Matsubara T. (1988). Quinidine blocks cardiac sodium channels during opening and slow inactivation in guinea-pig papillary muscle. British Journal of Pharmacology, 93, 311–318.

9. Mirro M.J., Manalan A.S., Bailey J.C., Watanabe A.M. (1980). Anticholinergic effects of disopyramide and quinidine on guinea pig myocardium. Mediation by direct muscarinic receptor blockade. Circulation Research, 47, 855–865.

10. Waelbroeck M., De Neef P., Robberecht P., Christophe J. (1984). Inhibitory effects of quinidine on rat heart muscarinic receptors. Life Science, 35, 1069–1076.

11. Morganroth J., Goin J.E. (1991). Quinidine-related mortality in the short-to-medium-term treatment of ventricular arrhythmias. A meta-analysis. Circulation, 84, 1977–1983.

12. Branch R.A., Adedoyin A., Frye R.F., Wilson J.W., Romkes M. (2000). In vivo modulation of CYP enzymes by quinidine and rifampin. Clinical Pharmacology & Therapeutics, 68, 401–411.

13. Weber W.W., Hein D.W. (1985). N-acetylation pharmacogenetics. Pharmacological Reviews, 37, 25–79.

14. Coyle J.D., Boudoulas H., Lima J.J. (1991). Acecainide pharmacokinetics in normal subjects of known acetylator phenotype. Biopharmaceutics & Drug Disposition, 12, 599–612.

15. Kidwell G.A., Lima J.J., Schaal S.F., Muir W.W. III. (1989). Hemodynamic and electrophysiologic effects of disopyramide enantiomers in a canine blood superfusion model. Journal of Cardiovascular Pharmacology, 13, 644–655.

16. Bocchi L., Vassalle M. (2008). Characterization of the slowly inactivating sodium current INa2 in canine cardiac single Purkinje cells. Experimental Physiology, 93, 347–361.

17. Roden D.M. (1993). Early after-depolarizations and torsade de pointes: Implications for the control of cardiac arrhythmias by prolonging repolarization. European Heart Journal, 14, 56–61.

18. Langenfeld H., Weirich J., Kohler C., Kochsiek K. (1990). Comparative analysis of the action of class I antiarrhythmic drugs (lidocaine, quinidine, and prajmaline) in rabbit atrial and ventricular myocardium. Journal of Cardiovascular Pharmacology, 15, 338–345.

19. Burashnikov A., Di Diego J.M., Zygmunt A.C., Belardinelli L., Antzelevitch C. (2008). Atrial-selective sodium channel block as a strategy for suppression of atrial fibrillation. Annals of NY Academy Sciences, 1123, 105–112.

20. Nattel S., Gagne G., Pineau M. (1987). The pharmacokinetics of lignocaine and beta-adrenoceptor antagonists in patients with acute myocardial infarction. Clinical Pharmacokinetics, 13, 293–316.

21. Saint D.A. (2008). The cardiac persistent sodium current: an appealing therapeutic target? British Journal of Pharmacology, 153, 1133–1142.

22. Ducceschi V., Di Micco G., Sarubbi B., Russo B., Santangelo L., Iacono A. (1996). Ionic mechanisms of ischemia-related ventricular arrhythmias. Clinical Cardiology, 19, 325–331.

23. Labbe L., Turgeon J. (1999). Clinical pharmacokinetics of mexiletine. Clinical Pharmacokinetics, 37, 361–384.

24. Cragun K.T., Johnson S.B., Packer D.L. (1997). Beta-adrenergic augmentation of flecainide-induced conduction slowing in canine Purkinje fibers. Circulation, 96, 2701–2708.

25. Packer D.L., Munger T.M., Johnson S.B., Cragun K.T. (1997). Mechanism of lethal proarrhythmia observed in the Cardiac Arrhythmia Suppression Trial: Role of adrenergic modulation of drug binding. Pacing and Clinical Electrophysiology, 20, 455–467.

26. Echt D.S., Liebson P.R., Mitchell L.B., Peters R.W., Obias-Manno D., Barker A.H., Arensberg D., Baker A., Friedman L., Greene H.L. (1991). Mortality and morbidity in patients receiving encainide, flecainide, or placebo. The Cardiac Arrhythmia Suppression Trial. New England Journal of Medicine, 324, 781–788.

27. McLeod A.A., Stiles G.L., Shand D.G. (1984). Demonstration of beta adrenoceptor blockade by propafenone hydrochloride: Clinical pharmacologic, radioligand binding and adenylate cyclase activation studies. Journal of Pharmacology and Experimental Therapeutics, 228, 461–466.

28. Yang T., Tande P.M., Lathrop D.A., Refsum H. (1992). Effects of altered extracellular potassium and pacing cycle length on the class III antiarrhythmic actions of dofetilide (UK-68,798) in guinea-pig papillary muscle. Cardiovascular Drugs and Therapy, 6, 429–436.

29. Yuan S., Wohlfart B., Rasmussen H.S., Olsson S., Blomstrom-Lundqvist C. (1994). Effect of dofetilide on cardiac repolarization in patients with ventricular tachycardia. A study using simultaneous monophasic action potential recordings from two sites in the right ventricle. European Heart Journal, 15, 514–522.

30. Tran A., Vichiendilokkul A., Racine E., Milad A. (2001). Practical approach to the use and monitoring of dofetilide therapy. American Journal of Health System Pharmacy, 58, 2050–2059.

31. Knobloch K., Brendel J., Peukert S., Rosenstein B., Busch A.E., Wirth K.J. (2002). Electrophysiological and antiarrhythmic effects of the novel I(Kur) channel blockers, S9947 and S20951, on left vs. right pig atrium in vivo in comparison with the I(Kr) blockers dofetilide, azimilide, d,l-sotalol and ibutilide. Naunyn Schmiedebergs Archives of Pharmacology, 366, 482–487.

32. Lei M., Brown H.F. (1996). Two components of the delayed rectifier potassium current, IK, in rabbit sino-atrial node cells. Experimental Physiology, 81, 725–741.

33. Yang T., Tande P.M., Refsum H. (1991). Negative chronotropic effect of a novel class III antiarrhythmic drug, UK-68,798, devoid of beta-blocking action on isolated guinea-pig atria. British Journal of Pharmacology, 103, 1417–1420.

34. Torp-Pedersen C., Moller M., Bloch-Thomsen P.E., Kober L., Sandoe E., Egstrup K., Agner E., Carlsen J., Videbaek J., Marchant B., Camm A.J. (1999). Dofetilide in patients with congestive heart failure and left ventricular dysfunction. Danish Investigations of Arrhythmia and Mortality on Dofetilide Study Group. New England Journal of Medicine, 341, 857–865.

35. Waldo A.L., Camm A.J., deRuyter H., Friedman P.L., MacNeil D.J., Pauls J.F., Pitt B., Pratt C.M., Schwartz P.J., Veltri E.P. (1996). Effect of d-sotalol on mortality in patients with left ventricular dysfunction after recent and remote myocardial infarction. The SWORD Investigators. Survival With Oral d-Sotalol. Lancet, 348, 7–12.

36. Marschang H., Beyer T., Karolyi L., Kubler W., Brachmann J. (1998). Differential rate and potassium-dependent effects of the class III agents d-sotalol and dofetilide on guinea pig papillary muscle. Cardiovascular Drugs and Therapy, 12, 573–583.

37. Singh B.N., Vaughan Williams E.M. (1970). The effect of amiodarone, a new anti-anginal drug, on cardiac muscle. British Journal of Pharmacology, 39, 657–667.

38. Mason J.W., Hondeghem L.M., Katzung B.G. (1983). Amiodarone blocks inactivated cardiac sodium channels. Pflugers Archiv—European Journal of Physiology, 396, 79–81.

39. Varro A., Nakaya Y., Elharrar V., Surawicz B. (1985). Use-dependent effects of amiodarone on Vmax in cardiac Purkinje and ventricular muscle fibers. European Journal of Pharmacology, 112, 419–422.

40. Honjo H., Kodama I., Kamiya K., Toyama J. (1991). Block of cardiac sodium channels by amiodarone studied by using Vmax of action potential in single ventricular myocytes. British Journal of Pharmacology, 102, 651–656.

41. Disatnik M.H., Shainberg A. (1991). Regulation of beta-adrenoceptors by thyroid hormone and amiodarone in rat myocardiac cells in culture. Biochemical Pharmacology, 41, 1039–1044.

42. Chatelain P., Meysmans L., Matteazzi J.R., Beaufort P., Clinet M. (1995). Interaction of the antiarrhythmic agents SR 33589 and amiodarone with the beta-adrenoceptor and adenylate cyclase in rat heart. British Journal of Pharmacology, 116, 1949–1956.

43. Nishimura M., Follmer C.H., Singer D.H. (1989). Amiodarone blocks calcium current in single guinea pig ventricular myocytes. Journal of Pharmacology and Experimental Therapeutics, 251, 650–659.

44. Gillis A.M., Kates R.E. (1984). Clinical pharmacokinetics of the newer antiarrhythmic agents. Clinical Pharmacokinetics, 9, 375–403.

45. Almog S., Shafran N., Halkin H., Weiss P., Farfel Z., Martinowitz U., Bank H. (1985). Mechanism of warfarin potentiation by amiodarone: Dose—and concentration—dependent inhibition of warfarin elimination. European Journal of Clinical Pharmacology, 28, 257–261.

46. Basaria S., Cooper D.S. (2005). Amiodarone and the thyroid. American Journal of Medicine, 118, 706–714.

47. Goldschlager N., Epstein A.E., Naccarelli G.V., Olshansky B., Singh B., Collard H.R., Murphy E. (2007). A practical guide for clinicians who treat patients with amiodarone: 2007. Heart Rhythm, 4, 1250–1259.

48. Yang T., Snyders D.J., Roden D.M. (1995). Ibutilide, a methanesulfonanilide antiarrhythmic, is a potent blocker of the rapidly activating delayed rectifier K + current (IKr) in AT-1 cells. Concentration-, time-, voltage-, and use-dependent effects. Circulation, 91, 1799–1806.

49. Lee K.S. (1992). Ibutilide, a new compound with potent class III antiarrhythmic activity, activates a slow inward Na + current in guinea pig ventricular cells. Journal of Pharmacology and Experimental Therapeutics, 262, 99–108.

50. Gowda R.M., Khan I.A., Punukollu G., Vasavada B.C., Sacchi T.J., Wilbur S.L. (2004). Female preponderance in ibutilide-induced torsade de pointes. International Journal of Cardiology, 95, 219–222.

51. Knobloch K., Brendel J., Rosenstein B., Bleich M., Busch A.E., Wirth K.J. (2004). Atrial-selective antiarrhythmic actions of novel Ikur vs. Ikr, Iks, and IKAch class Ic drugs and beta blockers in pigs. Medical Science Monitor, 10, BR221–BR228.

52. Wettwer E., Hala O., Christ T., Heubach J.F., Dobrev D., Knaut M., Varro A., Ravens U. (2004). Role of IKur in controlling action potential shape and contractility in the human atrium: influence of chronic atrial fibrillation. Circulation, 110, 2299–2306.

53. Stump G.L., Wallace A.A., Regan C.P., Lynch J. J. Jr. (2005). In vivo antiarrhythmic and cardiac electrophysiologic effects of a novel diphenylphosphine oxide IKur blocker (2-isopropyl-5-methylcyclohexyl) diphenylphosphine oxide. Journal of Pharmacology and Experimental Therapeutics, 315, 1362–1367.

54. Henry P.D. (1980). Comparative pharmacology of calcium antagonists: nifedipine, verapamil and diltiazem. American Journal of Cardiology, 46, 1047–1058.

55. Triggle D.J. (1990). Calcium, calcium channels, and calcium channel antagonists. Canadian Journal of Physiology and Pharmacology, 68, 1474–1481.

56. Nademanee K., Singh B.N. (1988). Control of cardiac arrhythmias by calcium antagonism. Annals of the NY Academy of Sciences, 522, 536–552.

57. Bailey D.G., Malcolm J., Arnold O., Spence J.D. (1998). Grapefruit juice-drug interactions. British Journal of Clinical Pharmacology, 46, 101–110.

58. Fuhr U. (1998). Drug interactions with grapefruit juice. Extent, probable mechanism and clinical relevance. Drug Safety, 18, 251–272.

59. Barbuti A., Difrancesco D. (2008). Control of cardiac rate by "funny" channels in health and disease. Annals of the NY Academy of Sciences, 1123, 213–223.

60. Wahl-Schott C., Biel M. (2009). HCN channels: Structure, cellular regulation and physiological function. Cellular and Molecular Life Sciences, 66, 470–494.

61. Michels G., Brandt M.C., Zagidullin N., Khan I.F., Larbig R., van Aaken S., Wippermann J., Hoppe U.C. (2008). Direct evidence for calcium conductance of hyperpolarization-activated cyclic nucleotide-gated channels and human native If at physiological calcium concentrations. Cardiovascular Research, 78, 466–475.

62. Sridhar A., Dech S.J., Lacombe V.A., Elton T.S., McCune S.A., Altschuld R.A., Carnes C.A. (2006). Abnormal diastolic currents in ventricular myocytes from spontaneous hypertensive and heart failure (SHHF) rats. American Journal of Physiology Heart Circulatory Physiology, 291, 42192–42198.

63. Stillitano F., Lonardo G., Zicha S., Varro A., Cerbai E., Mugelli A., Nattel S. (2008). Molecular basis of funny current (If) in normal and failing human heart. Journal of Molecular and Cellular Cardiology, 45, 289–299.

64. Cerbai E., Barbieri M., Mugelli A. (1994). Characterization of the hyperpolarization-activated current, I(f), in ventricular myocytes isolated from hypertensive rats. Journal Physiology, 481, 585–591.

65. Cerbai E., Barbieri M., Mugelli A. (1996). Occurrence and properties of the hyperpolarization-activated current If in ventricular myocytes from normotensive and hypertensive rats during aging. Circulation, 94, 1674–1681.

66. Freemantle N., Cleland J., Young P., Mason J., Harrison J. (1999). beta Blockade after myocardial infarction: systematic review and meta regression analysis. BMJ, 318, 1730–1737.

67. Goldenberg I., Zareba W., Moss A.J. (2008). Long QT syndrome. Current Problems in Cardiology, 33, 629–694.

68. Terra S.G., Hamilton K.K., Pauly D.F., Lee C.R., Patterson J.H., Adams K.F., Schofield R.S., Belgado B.S., Hill J.A., Aranda J.M., Yarandi H.N., Johnson J.A. (2005). Beta1-adrenergic receptor polymorphisms and left ventricular remodeling changes in response to beta-blocker therapy. Pharmacogenetics and Genomics, 15, 227–234.

69. Terra S.G., Pauly D.F., Lee C.R., Patterson J.H., Adams K.F., Schofield R.S., Belgado B. S., Hamilton K.K., Aranda J.M., Hill J.A., Yarandi H.N., Walker J.R., Phillips M.S., Gelfand C.A., Johnson J.A. (2005). beta-Adrenergic receptor polymorphisms and responses during titration of metoprolol controlled release/extended release in heart failure. Clinical Pharmacology & Therapeutics, 77, 127–137.

70. Beitelshees A.L., Zineh I., Yarandi H.N., Pauly D.F., Johnson J.A. (2006). Influence of phenotype and pharmacokinetics on beta-blocker drug target pharmacogenetics. Pharmacogenomics Journal, 6, 174–178.

71. Shin J., Johnson J.A. (2008). beta-Blocker pharmacogenetics in heart failure. Heart Failure Reviews.

72. Rankin A.C., Martynyuk A.E., Workman A.J., Kane K.A. (1997). Ionic mechanisms of the effect of adenosine on single rabbit atrioventricular node myocytes. Canadian Journal of Cardiology, 13, 1183–1187.

73. Martynyuk A.E., Kane K.A., Cobbe S.M., Rankin A.C. (1997). Role of nitric oxide, cyclic GMP and superoxide in inhibition by adenosine of calcium current in rabbit atrioventricular nodal cells. Cardiovascular Research, 34, 360–367.

74. Olshansky B., Rosenfeld L.E., Warner A.L., Solomon A.J., O'Neill G., Sharma A., Platia E., Feld G.K., Akiyama T., Brodsky M.A., Greene H.L. (2004). The Atrial Fibrillation Follow-up Investigation of Rhythm Management (AFFIRM) study: Approaches to control rate in atrial fibrillation. Journal of the American College Cardiology, 43, 1201–1208.

75. Boriani G., Biffi M., Diemberger I., Martignani C., Branzi A. (2003). Rate control in atrial fibrillation: Choice of treatment and assessment of efficacy. Drugs, 63, 1489–1509.

CHAPTER 6

Repolarization Reserve and Proarrhythmic Risk

ANDRÁS VARRÓ

6.1 DEFINITIONS AND BACKGROUND

The concept and terminology of repolarization reserve was put forward by Roden [1] in a preliminary form in an editorial in 1998:

> The greater problem is predicting the development of torsade de pointes in the absence of high doses or plasma concentrations. We have developed the concept of "**repolarization reserve**" to address this issue. We postulate that there exist in the normal ventricle and conducting system mechanisms to effect orderly and rapid repolarization that runs essentially no risk of setting up re-entrant circuits or of generating EADs [early after depolarizations]. Indeed, the normal function of the delayed rectifier currents I_{Kr} and I_{Ks} is a major contributor to such stable repolarization, or a large **repolarization reserve**. Identified risk factors for torsades de pointes reduce this repolarization reserve, making it more likely that the further added stress of, for e.g. an I_{Kr} blocking drug or a subtle genetic defect, is sufficient to precipitate torsades de pointes in individual patients.

At that time, this concept was not based on specific experimental evidence, but it represented a way of creative speculation using general knowledge about cardiac repolarization. Regardless of that, the immediate impact of this editorial was substantial, and it was widely appreciated. It earned 16 citations the next year and more than 250 since then. During subsequent years, it became an important principle to understand unexpected proarrhythmic complications associated with genetical disorders, diseases, and drug effects. In addition, this concept also serves as a theoretical background for safety pharmacology related to drug-induced QT prolongation. Subsequently, this concept was given a more specific definition [2], as follows:

Novel Therapeutic Targets for Antiarrhythmic Drugs, Edited by George Edward Billman
Copyright © 2010 John Wiley & Sons, Inc.

The concept of **repolarization reserve** provides a unifying framework for analysis of these risk factors and their clinical mechanisms. We propose that normal hearts include multiple, redundant mechanisms to accomplish normal repolarization. As a result, lesions in one of these mechanisms may be insufficient to elicit a full-blown LQTS phenotype, and this applies to both the drug-induced form and the congenital form.

More recently, some 10 years after the concept of repolarization reserve was first proposed, the definition was revised again [3].

The concept of "repolarization reserve," the idea is that the complexity of repolarization includes some redundancy. As a consequence, loss of 1 component (such as I_{Kr}) ordinarily will not lead to failure of repolarization (i.e., marked QT prolongation); as a corollary, individuals with subclinical lesions in other components of the system, say I_{Ks} or calcium current, may display no QT change until I_{Kr} block is superimposed.

In 1998, around the same time the term "repolarization reserve" was first proposed and after fairly acceptable specific inhibitors (chromanol 293B, L-735,821, and HMR-1556) of the slow delayed rectifier potassium current (I_{Ks}) became available, we performed experiments on dog papillary muscles and Purkinje fibers in our laboratory. The original aim of those investigations was to test the hypothesis put forward earlier by Jurkiewicz and Sanguinetti [4] regarding specific I_{Ks} block. According to the speculation of Jurkiewicz and Sanguinetti, I_{Ks} inhibition was expected to lengthen cardiac repolarization and refractoriness in a nonreverse, rate-dependent manner that would be explained by I_{Ks} accumulation at fast frequencies. In general, both academics and the pharmaceutical industry considered I_{Ks} block to have beneficial class III antiarrhythmic effects. In contrast to the rapid delayed rectifier potassium current (I_{Kr}) inhibition, inhibiton of I_{Ks} was expected to cause less or negligible proarrhythmic complications. Based on this belief, several drug companies launched projects to develop new and specific I_{Ks} inhibitors. Enthusiastically, we speculated that the I_{Ks} block would lengthen repolarization mainly in the ventricular muscle but less so in the Purkinje fibre recognizing the latter had its plateau phase in a relatively negative potential range, which is below the threshold of I_{Ks} activation. If our speculation proved to be correct, then I_{Ks} block would be even more attractive as an antiarrhythmic intervention compared with blocking I_{Kr} by causing reduced dispersion and/or heterogeneity of repolarization. Surprisingly, neither in dog papillary muscle nor in Purkinje fibres did I_{Ks} block elicit any measurable effects on repolarization [5, 6]. This observation (Figure 6.1) contradicted some already published studies [7, 8], as well as the general belief that the decrease of a major and important potassium current should substantionally delay cardiac repolarization. Therefore, to understand our findings more accurately, we examined the property of I_{Ks} in dog ventricular myocytes more quantitatively. We came to the conclusion [5, 6] that contrary to what had been observed regarding I_{Kr}, the activation of I_{Ks} in the plateau ranges was too slow and its amplitude was too small to produce a robust current during the time course of the action potential, which would have had a strong impact on the repolarization process (Figure 6.2). The question about the possible role of I_{Ks} in cardiomyocytes had not been answered until we lengthened

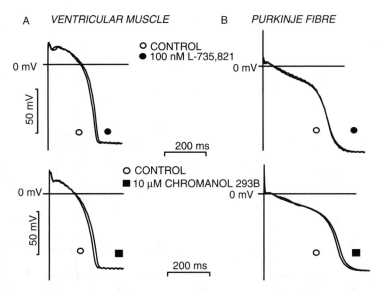

Figure 6.1. The lack of marked prolongation after I_{Ks} block by L-735,821 and chromanol 293B on the right ventricular papillary muscle of the dog and Purkinje fibers at 1 Hz stimulation frequency. (From ref. 6 with permission.)

ventricular action potential duration, thereby allowing more I_{Ks} to be activated (Figure 6.2), and we studied the effect of I_{Ks} block in these conditions. In these preparations, I_{Ks} inhibition lengthened repolarization even more (Figure 6.3). Based on these results, we speculated that the slowly activating and relatively small I_{Ks} represented a negative feedback mechanism that would limit excessive repolarization lengthening. We stated in the corresponding paper that:

> Although I_{Ks} may have little role in normal action potential repolarization, it probably plays a vital role when cardiac APD is abnormally lengthened by other means (e.g. by reductions in I_{Kr} or I_{k1} or increases in I_{Na} or I_{Ca}). As such, pharmacological block of I_{Ks} might be expected to have severe detrimental consequences when this protective mechanism is eliminated. For example, if repolarization is excessively lengthened due to drug-induced I_{Kr} block, hypokalaemia, genetic abnormality, or bradycardia, the subsequent increase in APD would favour I_{Ks} activation and provide a negative feedback mechanism to limit further APD lengthening.

The principle of repolarization reserve was thereby experimentally demonstrated directly for the first time [5, 6], and in the conclusion of this paper, the concept was defined using similar words short of mentioning the term "repolarization reserve."

> This study indicated that in normal dog ventricular muscle I_{Ks} plays a minor role in control of APD. This current, however, could provide an important means of limiting excessive APD lengthening when action potentials are increased beyond normal by other mechanisms.

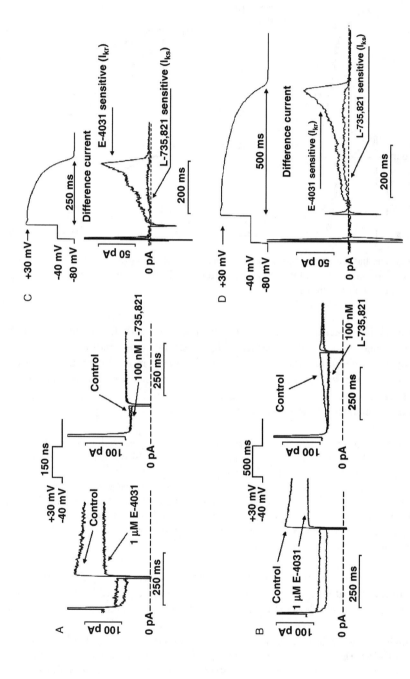

Figure 6.2. Comparison of the magnitude of I_{Kr} and I_{Ks} after short and long square and action potential-like voltage clamp pulses. As panels **A** and **C** show, short voltage clamp pulses corresponding to "normal action potential" elicit relatively large I_{Kr} (E-4031 sensitive current) but small I_{Ks} (L-735,821 sensitive current). Increasing the duration of the voltage clamp pulses beyond "normal" (**B** and **D**) did not change the density of I_{Kr} but increased that of I_{Ks}. (From ref. 6 with permission.)

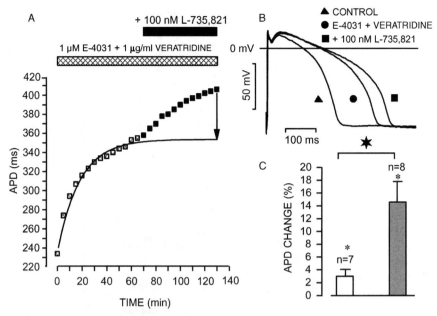

Figure 6.3. Effect of I_{Ks} block on dog ventricular action potential duration, which was lengthened previously by application of E-4031 (I_{Kr} block) and veratridine (augmented late I_{Na}). Note that in preparations where repolarization was lengthened, inhibition of I_{Ks} resulted in significant APD prolongation. (From ref. 6 with permission.)

This paper, in which repolarization reserve was demonstrated experimentally directly for the first time, represented an example of "serendipity research" not uncommon in pharmacology. Initially, it had a well-defined goal to clarify the mechanism of a drug's action but resulted in a completely different discovery in ion channel physiology that also had important safety pharmacology implications.

6.2 THE MAJOR PLAYERS CONTRIBUTING TO REPOLARIZATION RESERVE

The repolarization in cardiac muscle is caused by the simultaneous and balanced function (activation and inactivation) of several inward and outward currents flowing through distinctly different ion channels or electrogenic ion pumps (Figure 6.4). In this chapter, we focus on ventricular tissue; however, it is well known that there are differences between various parts of the heart (atria, sinoatrial [SA]-node, and atrioventricular [AV]-node), and we should also point out that the concept of repolarization reserve can be extended from the ventricle to other cardiac regions.

6.2.1 Inward Sodium Current (I_{Na})

After the large fast sodium current is inactivated within a few milliseconds, the sodium current does not vanish completely during the plateau phase. In a limited

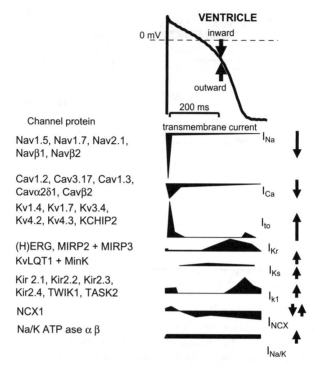

Figure 6.4. Ventricular action potential (top) and schematic representation of the most important underlying transmembrane ionic currents and electrogenic pumps (bottom). Channel proteins, which are responsible for mediating the respective current, are indicated on the left. Upward and downward deflections and arrows denote outward and inward currents, respectively.

range of potentials where activation and inactivation overlap, a relatively small steady-state sodium current can be recorded that is called "Na$^+$—window current" [9]. In addition, a small fraction of the sodium current inactivates slowly during the plateau phase [10]. This so-called persistent sodium current opposes the function of repolarizing potassium currents and delays repolarization. In certain situations, such as the long QT3 (LQT3) syndrome or heart failure, this persistent sodium current is augmented [11], further opposing the function of outward currents. If there is compensation for this current, then the net result is only a diminished repolarization reserve. However, when the magnitude of this inward current increase is substantial, prolongation of repolarization may occur.

6.2.2 Inward L-Type Calcium Current ($I_{Ca,L}$)

The function of inward calcium current on the repolarization is more complex than that of I_{Na} and still not fully understood. The calcium current, similar to I_{Na}, expresses both slowly inactivating and window components, but the inactivation of the current is dependent on the free cytosolic calcium concentration ($[Ca^{2+}]_i$) as well. Because

$[Ca^{2+}]_i$ is dynamically changing during the action potential and is regulated by many factors [12] such as SERCA, phospholamban, ryanodine receptor, calmodulin, and protein kinase A (PKA) and C (PKC), the impact of inward calcium current on the repolarization is difficult to predict accurately and represents one of the most problematic target for mathematical action potential modeling. Also, if inward currents (both I_{Na} and I_{Ca}) are augmented, then the plateau voltage is shifted toward more positive values that may result in the activation of more outward potassium currents that can shorten repolarization, depending on the actual balance of currents.

6.2.3   Rapid Delayed Rectifier Outward Potassium Current (I_{Kr})

I_{Kr} activates rapidly on depolarization [13] that is more positive than $-30\,\text{mV}$ ($\tau \sim 40\,\text{ms}$ at $+30\,\text{mV}$), but its inactivation precedes the activation upon depolarization [14]. This has the consequence that I_{Kr} channels are largely closed during the plateau phase and only are open when membrane potential returns to around $0\,\text{mV}$. After recovery from inactivation, which is also rapid, as membrane potential slowly changes toward negative values, the channels open again and then slowly deactivate (close) resulting in the transient nature of I_{Kr}. It should be noted that it is difficult to measure the fast inactivation of I_{Kr} in native myocytes because of overlap with other currents. However, the inactivation of I_{Kr} has been elegantly demonstrated in human ether a-go-go related gene (hERG) channel expressing cell lines [14]. In native cells, unlike in cell lines, there is a small but persistent I_{Kr} current on depolarisation, which suggests that some I_{Kr} operates during the plateau [6, 15], probably reflecting incomplete inactivation. This can be because the I_{Kr} alpha hERG protein is coexpressed with beta subunits such as MinK; MIRP1, 2, 3, 4, and 5; and KChIP2 [16]. These latter proteins may modify gating, and their variability can also explain known species differences in I_{Kr}. The modulation of I_{Kr} is not well explored [16]. It has been shown in guinea pig ventricular myocytes that after phosphorylation by Ca^{2+}-dependent PKC, because of reductions in the inactivation of this channel, I_{Kr} current is enhanced at positive potentials and can shorten repolarization [17]. This important pathway, however, should be confirmed in other preparations. More research is needed to characterize the exact function of I_{Kr}. It is also known that opposite to what one would expect from the Nernst equation, increased extracellular K^+ concentration enhances, whereas decreased extracellular K^+ concentration reduces I_{Kr}. Because of its peculiar gating properties, i.e., its fast inactivation and recovery from inactivation, an apparent inward rectification (see also I_{k1} later) occurs. I_{Kr} may play a role as a positive feedback mechanism and may contribute to repolarization lengthening when repolarization is already prolonged [18] by other factors, such as LQT3 or slow heart rate. In this situation, as shown on Figure 6.5. during longer action potentials, less I_{Kr} (and also less I_{k1}, see later) develops at isochronal points, further weakening the force of repolarization [18]. This makes repolarization more vulnerable when depolarizing factors (I_{Na}, I_{Ca}, and N_{CX}) are augmented or repolarizing factors (I_{k1}, I_{Ks}, and Na/K) are diminished. Therefore, even a small decrease in I_{Kr} may lead to substantial APD prolongation at slow rates or may have an additive effect to other interventions lengthening repolarization. In general, it is well appreciated that I_{Kr} is

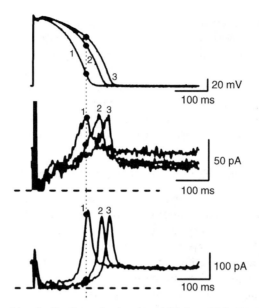

Figure 6.5. The positive feedback mechanism by which I_{Kr} and I_{k1} augment repolarization delay if action potential duration had been prolonged previously by other means.

one of the most important outward currents to control repolarization. A marked decrease or loss of this current results in substantial repolarization lengthening in many species, including humans [6, 19, 20]. When the decrease of I_{Kr} is only fractional, the action potential duration is not necessarily prolonged. This is because of the possible compensatory function by other outward currents. However, any additional impairment of the current may have detrimental consequences, such as excessive repolarization lengthening, which can lead to torsades de pointes arrhythmia. This is the most likely reason why relatively weak I_{Kr} inhibition by certain noncardiac drugs provokes arrhythmias related to repolarization abnormalities.

Therefore, it is obvious that I_{Kr} is not only a robust outward current determining the course of apparent repolarization but itself is the most important contributor to repolarization reserve.

6.2.4 Slow Delayed Rectifier Outward Potassium Current (I_{Ks})

I_{Ks}, which flows through KvLQT1 + MinK + MIRP protein constituted channels, activates slowly (500–1000 ms) during the plateau phase and deactivates rapidly (100–200 ms) at negative membrane potentials [21]. Because of its relatively small amplitude between 0 mV and 20 mV and slow activation kinetics, there is relatively little current activating during the normal course of the action potential [6, 19] and thereby has little influence on repolarization [6, 19]. However, when action potential is lengthened and plateau voltage is shifted to the more positive voltage, I_{Ks} [22] "creates an available reserve of channels that are ready to open on demand" [23].

This shift forms a transmembrane current that has the main function of participating in repolarization reserve (Figure 6.3), and it opposes excessive action potential duration lengthening [6, 19]. I_{Ks} is activated by PKC and by sympathetic stimulation because of PKA. The latter has important consequences, because the increase in the amplitude of I_{Ks} and the shift in its activation voltage toward negative potentials would enhance I_{Ks} current density during elevated sympathetic tone. Also, sympathetic stimulation enhances $I_{Ca, L}$ that in turn shifts the plateau toward more positive voltage and lengthening repolarization as well. These changes would activate I_{Ks}, which, as a negative feedback, limits the effect of the enhancement of $I_{Ca, L}$ [22, 24]. Based on this feedback cycle, it becomes evident that impairment of I_{Ks} because of the loss of function mutation (LQT1) or I_{Ks} blocking drugs in the presence of elevated sympathetic tone leaves the repolarization lengthening caused by augmented $I_{Ca,L}$ unopposed and substantial prolongation of action potential duration can develop. Therefore, I_{Ks} does not necessarily contribute to repolarization in normal settings and at low sympathetic tone. However, under certain conditons (e.g., enhanced sympathetic activation), this current provides a protective mechanism that creates a repolarization reserve, such that it counterbalances repolarization lengthening only when necessary. I_{Ks} was reported to show transmural expression differences [25] that can contribute to enhanced repolarization heterogeneity as well.

6.2.5   Inward Rectifier Potassium Current (I_{k1})

I_{k1} flows through a mixture of Kir 2.1, 2.2, 2.3, and possible TASK-1 and TWIK-1 channels showing strong inward rectification. This means that the I_{k1} current is decreasing close to zero at potentials more positive than -30 mV, and it reopens rapidly again when membrane potentials reach more negative values. The inward rectification is caused by channel block by Mg^{2+} and polyamines from the intracellular site after depolarization [26]. When the positive membrane potential is changing to the negative direction, the Mg^{2+} and polyamine-induced channel block is relieved and I_{k1} increases. This process forms a negative feedback during the repolarization making it a regenerative process. This phenomenon is similar to that mentioned in connection with I_{Kr}, but the potential range of I_{k1} is more negative than that of I_{Kr}. I_{k1} plays a similar role to I_{Kr} in the self-limiting repolarization process after APD lengthening (Figure 6.5) following, for example, slow heart rates [18]. These channels are fully open at rest, that is, during diastole. Therefore I_{k1} opposes any kind of depolarization due to enhanced pacemaker activity and Ca^{2+} overload-related delayed afterdepolarizations (DADs). This feature represents a special form of repolarization reserve. Consequently, the impairment of I_{k1} may have a proarrhythmic potential by not opposing depolarization that can thereby reach a threshold for propagating extrasystoles. In addition, smaller I_{k1} also increases duration of repolarization and its heterogeneity. The density of I_{k1} shows considerable variations among species. It is relatively weak in human ventricles [27] but is strong in the dog, rabbit, and guinea pig [28]. As a possible consequence in humans, a moderate I_{k1} defect or block does not manifest in significant repolarization lengthening. However, I_{k1} as part of the repolarization reserve together with the malfunction of other ion channels can lead to excessive action potential duration lengthening. Indeed, the loss of function mutation of Kir 2.1 channels in LQT7 (Andersen-Tawil-syndrome), although substantially decreasing I_{k1}, does not result in marked QTc lengthening [29]; yet it can greatly enhance the proarrhythmic risk of these patients (29). Based on these speculations, it is likely that I_{k1} in an important contributor to repolarization reserve both in diastole and during the final repolarization phase.

6.2.6   Transient Outward Potassium current (I_{to})

I_{to} flows through channels formed by Kv 4.3, 1.4, and KChIP2 proteins, which show large species variations. Ito has not been recorded in the guinea pig. In humans [30] and dogs [31], Kv 4.3 is considered to provide the alpha subunit, whereas in rabbits, Kv 1.4 seems to be the dominant protein [32]. In general, I_{to} is a huge and rapidly activating ($\tau \sim 1$–2 ms) and inactivating (5–10 ms) outward current at depolarization more positive than -20 Mv [33]. Therefore, I_{to} contributes to the initial, i.e., phase 1, repolarization, and its influence on the action potential duration is believed to be limited. It must be emphasized that I_{to} can alter the amplitude of the plateau and thereby indirectly change the activation, inactivation, and deactivation of other transmembrane currents. In addition, I_{to} (Kv 4.3 current) has a second, slower phase of inactivation during the plateau ($\tau \sim 15$–30 ms), which has a reasonable amplitude (Figure 6.6), and its activation and inactivation may overlap producing a similar type of window current during the final repolarization as described for I_{Ca} or I_{Na} (Figure 6.6). Thus, one can suspect that although changes in I_{to} current may not lead to marked changes in repolarization, but as part of the repolarization reserve together with other currents, I_{to} may also have an impact on repolarization. Because I_{to} has been shown to vary among subendrocardial, subepicardial, and midmyocardial layers, it may contribute to repolarization heterogeneity as well.

6.2.7   Sodium—Potassium Pump Current ($I_{Na/K}$)

The $I_{Na/K}$ is caused by the function of the sodium-potassium pump that consumes adenosine triphosphate (ATP) and is stimulated by intracellular cyclic adenosine 3',5'-monophosphate (cAMP). This electrogenic ion transport mechanism pumps out 3 Na^+ from the cell coupled to the inward movement of 2 K^+. In the range of membrane potentials corresponding to the action potential and diastole, the pump current is outward and therefore contributes to the repolarization reserve both during systole and diastole. The magnitude of this current depends primarily on intracellular Na^+, which also explains why $I_{Na/K}$ is so sensitive to frequency of stimulation. Diseases like heart failure may alter its expression, and $I_{Na/K}$ also shows characteristic transmural distribution [34].

6.2.8   Sodium–Calcium Exchanger Current (NCX)

NCX is responsible for maintaining the physiological low level of intracellular calcium. Because three Na^+ and one Ca^{2+} are transported per cycle, the transport

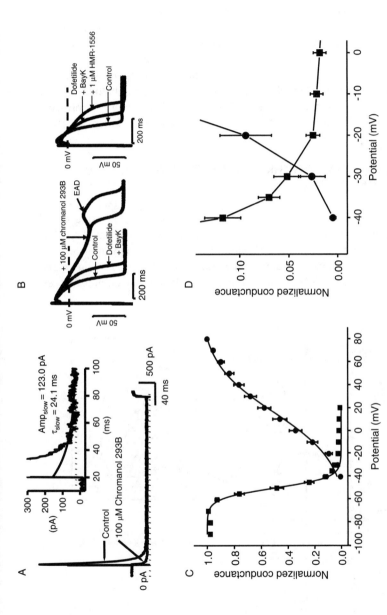

Figure 6.6. Illustration that I_{to} is not only important in determining phase 1 repolarization but may also contribute to late repolarization and that of during the plateau phase. In **A**, near full block of I_{to} by 100 μM chromanol 293B depresses a second slow component of I_{to}, which has an amplitude of more than 100 pA. The corresponding time constant of inactivation is more than 20 ms at +50 mV. This current can be expected to influence repolarization directly during the plateau. In **C** and **D**, the activation and inactivation of I_{to} suggest a small but persistent window current between −40 and −10 mV which may contribute to late repolarization. Panel **B** shows dog preparation where action potential duration was increased by I_{Kr} block (dofetilide); I_{Ca} stimulation (BayK8644) and I_{Ks} block (HMR-1556) action potential duration was lengthened substantially, but EAD did not occur. However, additional I_{to} inhibition (by 100 μM chromanol 293B) decreased the repolarization reserve, and additional excessive APD prolongation developed resulting in EAD formation.

181

is electrogenic and critically depends on the membrane potential and intracellular calcium, both of which change dynamically during the action potential. Therefore, it is difficult to estimate the actual and accurate current magnitude produced by NCX, and these efforts are also hampered by the fact that we still lack sufficiently specific inhibitors. On the one hand, at the beginning of the action potential when intracellular calcium is low and voltage is positive, NCX current is outward. On the other hand, later during the plateau phase, in early and late repolarization and also during diastole, it is inward. If calcium overload develops, then NCX can carry a depolarizing current that in the presence of decreased repolarization reserve may provoke both DADs and EADs contributing to arrhythmogenesis. NCX also has transmural expression differences [35], and it is known that NCX is upregulated in heart failure [36].

6.3 MECHANISM OF ARRHYTHMIA CAUSED BY DECREASED REPOLARIZATION RESERVE

As previously mentioned, transmembrane potassium channels show transmural and regional differences in their expression. This would create a relatively small repolarization heterogeneity that can be greatly enhanced by impaired repolarization reserve.

The hypothetical mechanism of arrhythmia development caused by increased repolarization heterogeneity is shown on Figure 6.7. In normal circumstansces,

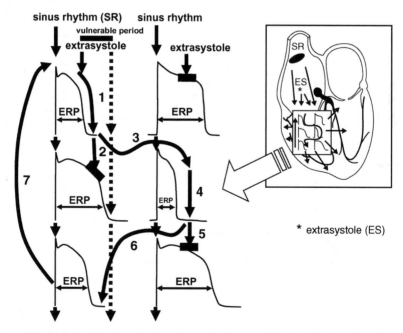

Figure 6.7. The simplified mechanism of arrhythmia caused by lengthening of repolarization and decrease of repolarization reserve. Detailed explanation can be found in the text.

conduction in the heart is fast (1–2 m/s), and the duration of myocardial cell action potential is long (200–300 ms). Thus, these cells cannot become stimulated early, because they are in a refractory state. The length of refractoriness can be characterized by the effective refractory period (ERP). Importantly, in the normal setting the difference between the action potential duration and consequently the ERPs of adjacent cells is small, and as a consequence, repolarization heterogeneity is small. Fast conduction and relatively homogenous repolarization prevents the circular reentry of excitation, and arrhythmia will not develop. However, when the duration of repolarization, and consequently the refractory period of the myocardium, are prolonged, or the repolarization reserve is decreased, the differences in the repolarization of adjacent cells also become larger, which leads to increased spatial repolarization heterogeneity. As a consequence, an extrasystole generated after a normal sinus stimulus can propagate in the direction of cell with shorter action potential duration, but its propagation will be blocked in the direction of cells with longer action potential durations (Figure 6.7). Thus, this extra stimulus can travel, usually with reduced conduction velocity, back in a complicated path toward the site of its origin and everywhere else where excitability is regained, leading to the generatation of chaotic tachycardia or even ventricular fibrillation. Ventricular fibrillation does not revert back to sinus rhythm spontaneously in humans and leads to sudden cardiac death without intervention in a few minutes. It is very important to note that two independent factors are needed for the arrhythmia described above and illustrated on Figure 6.7 to develop. Heterogeneity of repolarization following prolongation of repolarization is itself not sufficient for arrhythmia development, establishing only the possibility of an arrhythmia ("substrate"). To induce arrhythmia, an extrasystole in the vulnerable period is needed ("trigger") that can travel the reentry paths created by the heterogeneous repolarization. The timing of this trigger extrasystole is critical, because before the vulnerable period its conduction is blocked and after the vulnerable period it does not lead to tachycardia or fibrillation, only to a harmless single extrasystole. The larger the repolarization heterogeneity, the longer the vulnerability period and the more frequent the extrasystoles, the bigger the chance becomes for serious arrhythmia development. Thus, decreased repolarization reserve facilitate arrhythmias by both in the substrate and trigger levels by increasing repolarization heterogeneity and by decreasing the repolarization force during diastole, which consequently would help subthreshold depolarizations to reach threshold and to produce propagating extrasystoles.

6.4 CLINICAL SIGNIFICANCE OF THE REDUCED REPOLARIZATION RESERVE

It is known that certain factors and diseases may decrease repolarization reserve. In these cases, therefore, it is possible to recognize the consequence of the diminished repolarization reserve. However, such situations are usually more complex, and attenuated repolarization reserve can be recognized only retrospectively, sometimes only after the fatal outcome. Some patients with a QTc interval within the normal

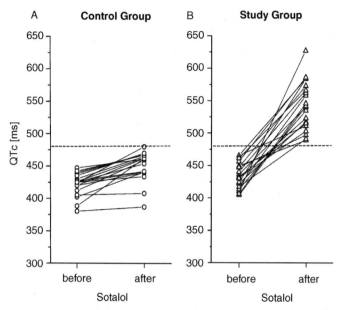

Figure 6.8. Individual QTc intervals in control and study groups before and after administration of sotalol. The dotted line indicates a cut-off value of 480 ms that distinguished best between the study population and the control group. More explanation in the text. (From ref. 37 with permission.)

range may respond to drug treatment with excessive lengthening of repolarization and arrhythmias, occasionally leading to sudden cardiac death. In other patients, these drugs do not even prolong cardiac action potential duration or only lengthen it moderately. In accordance with these observations, Kääb et al. [37] reported that patients who experienced torsades de pointes arrhythmia with QT prolonging drugs developed more QTc lengthening after intravenous sotalol, which is an I_{Kr} blocking drug, than those of the control group consisting of patients without history of torsades de pointes. An interesting observation of this study showed that in both groups the baseline QTc was normal and did not differ from each other (Figure 6.8). Therefore, it can be assumed that the striking differences in the responses to the administered drug were caused by the differences in the repolarization reserve between the two groups.

6.4.1   Genetic Defects

A recent study from Boulet et al. [38] described a loss of function mutation in the KCNQ1 gene underlying the pore-forming subunit of I_{Ks} channel in a 40-year-old woman. This woman had experienced torsades de pointes arrhythmia with a QTc interval of 430 ms (well within the normal range), which may indicate that a genetic loss of I_{Ks} functions does not necessarily prolong repolarization, as shown by the normal QTc of the patient. However, under some unfavorable conditions (e.g., hypokalemia, drug effects, and possible downregulation of potassium channels), the impairment of repolarization reserve diminished the necessary protection, making this patient more susceptible to arrhythmia than those who lack defective I_{Ks} channels.

This case highlights the importance of "silent," "subclinical," or "concealed" long QT syndrome [39], where the repolarization process is not apparently affected as measured by conventional diagnostic tools but the repolarization reserve is impaired.

6.4.2 Heart Failure

Heart failure is still one of the most devastating diseases with a worse 5-year life expectancy than cancer. Approximately, half of heart failure patients die from sudden cardiac death caused by lethal arrhythmias and not from end-stage pump failure. It has been shown that both electrophysiological and structural remodeling occurs during the progression of heart failure. This includes the substantial degree of reduction of the repolarization reserve, because of downregulation of different types of potassium channels. The results obtained so far regarding the nature of potassium channel downregulation are conflicting, depending on the form of the disease (hypertrophic vs dilated), experimental model (pacing vs valve destruction) and the species studied (rat, rabbit, and dog). In general, it has been reported that I_{k1}, I_{Ks}, I_{to}, and I_{Kr} channels were downregulated [40–42]. The persistent or slowly inactivating sodium current is also increased in heart failure [43]. This latter change in the presence of reduced repolarization reserve results in action potential duration lengthening and increased repolarization heterogeneity, which is a substrate for arrhythmias. The upregulation of NCX, pacemaker current (I_f), and malfunction of the ryanodine receptor proteins [44, 45] enhance ectopic activity, because transient depolarizations are not opposed properly during diastole caused by impaired repolarization reserve. This latter effect would increase the arrhythmia by trigger mechanisms as well.

6.4.3 Diabetes Mellitus

Repolarization abnormalities, including mild prolongation of the QT interval, have been observed in patients with diabetes mellitus [46]. Both type 1 and type 2 diabetes mellitus are associated with increased risk for sudden cardiac death [47], which cannot be attributed to general pathophysiological changes, such as atherosclerosis, hyperlipidemia, or hypertension, which are commonly observed in diabetes. The mechanisms responsible for repolarization abnormalities in long-term chronic diabetes are not well explored. The reduction of I_{to}, I_{Ks}, and I_{Kr} in different diabetic animal models [48, 49] of short term type 1 diabetes suggests that decreased density of these currents may contribute to reduced repolarization reserve in diabetes mellitus. In accordance with these experimental data, increased beat-to-beat QT variability was also recently reported [50] in patients with type 1 diabetes mellitus (Figure 6.9).

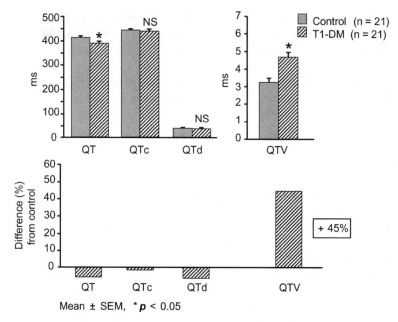

Figure 6.9. Repolarization lengthening was not detectable in 21 patients with type 1 diabetes mellitus (T1-DM) by measuring QT, QTc, and QT dispersion (QTd). The short term variability of QT (QTV), however, was markedly enhanced in diabetic patients compared to those of age and sex matched controls.

6.4.4 Gender

It is well known that women are at a significantly greater risk than men for developing torsades de pointes arrhythmia in response to drugs that prolong cardiac repolarization. This is likely related to the fact that women have longer QTc and reduced repolarization reserve than men.

The basis for the gender differences in risk of torsades de pointes and QTc is unclear. This topic is currently under intensive investigation [51–54], and it can be assumed that these differences are related to the influence of sex hormones on cardiac repolarization and the underlying transmembrane currents.

Evidence suggests that estrogene reduces I_{Kr} and prolongs repolarization [54], whereas testosterone increases I_{Kr}. [53] Sex hormones can also alter the interactions of drugs with these potassium channels [52, 54].

Interestingly, when studying I_{Kr} block-induced QTc prolongation in women at different stages of the menstrual cycle, drug-induced QTc prolongation was greatest during menses and at the ovulatory stage of the cycle, compared with the luteal phase (Figure 6.10); in despite the pre-drug condition, the QTc did not differ in the cycle [51]. This observation suggests that progesterone may be protective by opposing repolarization lengthening caused by I_{Kr} inhibition. In a recent study, it was shown that testosterone activated hERG channels via androgen receptors [53]. This finding

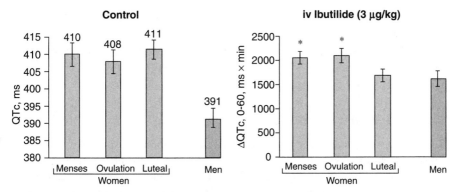

Figure 6.10. The possible influence of hormonal changes during the menstrual cycle on the repolarization reserve. On the left, mean change in QTc interval area under the curve is shown during the first hour after ibutilide (I_{Kr} block) infusion. On the right, baseline QTc intervals in women during the different phases of the menstrual cycle and there in men are shown. These suggest that progesterone may oppose I_{Kr} block induced repolarization lengthening in women. (From ref. 51 with permission.)

emphasizes the possibility of gender-based adverse consequences of drug-receptor interactions.

6.4.5 Renal Failure

It is known that patients with chronic renal failure are at increased risk for ventricular arrhythmia and sudden death [55]. It was also shown that in chronic renal failure, QT dispersion [56] and the QT variability index were increased compared with normal subjects. These results suggest the presence of impairment of repolarization reserve. However, it must be noted that chronic renal failure patients are usually comorbid patients, i.e., they have additional diseases such as diabetes, coronary artery sclerosis, hypertension, and cardiac hypertrophy, and are on variable medications. All these factors may affect repolarization, making it difficult to determine the contribution of renal dysfunction to alterations in repolarization reserve in these patients.

6.4.6 Hypokalemia

Hypokalemia is a common factor that can decrease repolarization reserve. Low extracellular potassium increases I_{Ks} and I_{k1} according to the Nernst equation but paradoxically reduces I_{Kr} and prolongs QT interval. Furthermore, lowering of extracellular potassium increased drug-induced I_{Kr} block [57], although this latter observation was questioned recently [58].

6.4.7 Hypothyroidism

Hypothyroidism decreases (i.e., downregulates) many different potassium currents [59, 60] and pacemaker channels [59], resulting in lengthened cardiac repolarization [61] and bradycardia [61]. Even in its subclinical form, it decreases repolarization reserve as reflected by an increased QTc dispersion and prolonged QTc [61]. The reduction of repolarization reserve induced by hypothyroidism is also associated with an increased number of reported torsades de pointes arrhythmias [62].

6.4.8 Competitive Athletes

Top athletes may represent a special example. Competitive sport activities elicit reversible cardiac hyperthrophy (athletes' heart) where downregulation of certain potassium channels can be expected [63]. In these athletes, mild changes in repolarization reserve probably do not represent a significant risk, but together with otherwise mild factors, such as different drugs, bradycardia, and food ingredients, early and undiagnosed cardiomyopathy and doping agents (steroids or amphetamines) can be additive and cause repolarization abnormality that occasionally lead to sudden death [64]. Indeed, despite that regular exercise has been shown to protect against ischemic arrhythmias [65] and tissue damage [66], top athletes have two to four times the mortality of sudden cardiac death than age and sex-matched controls not involved in sports activities [67].

6.5 REPOLARIZATION RESERVE AS A DYNAMICALLY CHANGING FACTOR

Recent research indicates that repolarization reserve is not a static behavior of cardiac tissue but a dynamically changing factor. After 24 h incubation with dofetilide, a potent I_{Kr} blocker, continuously paced dog ventricular myocytes elicited shorter action potential duration and blunted dofetilide response [68]. Patch clamp measurements revealed enhancement of I_{Ks} in cultured myocytes incubated with dofetilide compared with I_{Ks} in control cells. Accordingly, the KvLQT1 and MinK protein levels were increased. Interestingly, the messengerRNA (mRNA) for both KvLQT1 and MinK did not change, suggesting regulatory events at the posttranslational level. In the same experiments, the expression of microRNA 133a and 133b (miR-1330 and miR-133b) were diminished in cells previously incubated with dofetilide. In another earlier study, it was shown that muscle specific miR-133 depressed KvLQT1 protein expression without changing KvLQT1 mRNA [69]. Based on these results, it was proposed that sustained reduction of I_{Kr} leads to compensatory upregulation of I_{Ks}, data that are consistent with a feedback control of ion channel expression. This newly recognized modulation of the repolarization reserve might happen via changes of microRNA at the translational level. In fact, an enhanced miR-133 expression was associated with a decreased density of ERG protein and I_{Kr} in diabetic rabbit hearts [70]. Although these novel results are not without controversies and more studies are needed to confirm them, they suggest that repolarization reserve might be regulated by disease and drug treatment, a factor that should be taken into account for the development of future therapies.

6.6   HOW TO MEASURE THE REPOLARIZATION RESERVE

Despite its potential importance, the estimation of cardiac repolarization reserve of individual patients is not a common procedure in clinical practice. One may argue that it would be more appropriate to test individuals for their status of repolarization reserve and apply drugs accordingly, rather than restrict drug development if the compound is suspected to cause hERG inhibition or QTc lengthening. It is likely that patients with normal repolarization reserve would not respond to drugs that produce mild-to-moderate K^+ channel inhibition with arrhythmias and fatalities. Patients, however, with diminished repolarization reserve may do so. Therefore, good predictive noninvasive tests in clinical settings and easy to use animal models are badly needed.

Because of the complex nature of repolarization reserve, its accurate measurement in a quantitative manner is difficult. In the experimental preclinical level, the repolarization reserve based on theoretical considerations should be estimated by drugs that increase depolarization force, as would be produced by veratridine or toxin, ATXII. In this case, the degree of repolarization prolongation caused by these agents would be expected to be opposed by the sum of repolarizing potassium currents. If limited action potential duration prolongation is observed, then a strong repolarization reserve would be predicted. Conversely, substantial action potential duration lengthening argues for weak repolarization reserve. For a pragmatic reason it would be more appropriate to test hERG/I_{Kr} channel inhibition and analyze the evoked repolarization lengthening. This is based on the common experience that most drugs reported to cause torsades de pointes arrhythmias inhibit I_{Kr}, and the repolarization reserve in this case would include repolarizing currents largely other than I_{Kr}. Figure 6.11 illustrates that I_{Kr} block caused by full I_{Kr} block after dofetilide caused a different degree of action potential duration prolongation in various species. The large action potential duration prolongation induced by I_{Kr} inhibition in human and rabbit ventricular muscle suggests weak repolarization reserve, whereas the moderate action potential duration lengthening in dog and guinea pig ventricle suggests relatively strong repolarization reserve. These data imply that rabbit papillary muscle should be the preferred preparation for drug testing for safety pharmacology purposes. Also, preparations in which repolarization reserve had been previously attenuated by ion channel remodeling [71] or by pharmacological means [72] would also have particular value. Special techniques based on action potential configurations were also described to assess proarrhythmic drug effects based on repolarization instability [73] at the preclinical level.

At the clinical level, as Figure 6.8 suggests, simple QTc measurements from electrocardiographic (ECG) recordings are not sufficient to measure repolarization reserve. Applying other ECG parameters such as QTc dispersion, T_{peak} to T_{end}, and T vave morphology analysis also give uncertain results. Provocative pharmacological tests have been suggested [74], but this may raise ethical concerns. As Figure 6.12 shows, intravenous application of a short acting I_{Kr} blocking class III antiarrhythmic drug, ibutilide-lengthened QTc, and the magnitude of this effect had a good gaussian distribution. Furthermore, the long QTc edge of the curve (indicated by squares) and

190

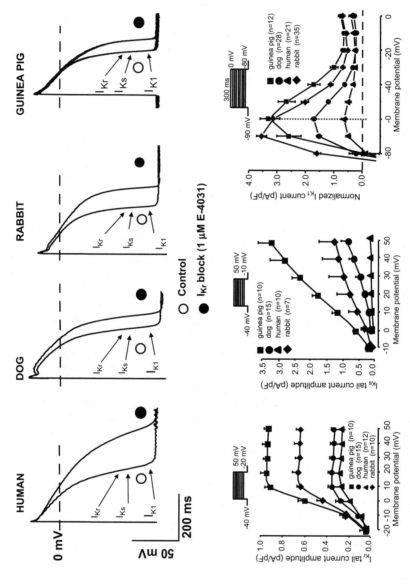

Figure 6.11. The possible influence of the repolarization reserve on the repolarization lengthening seen after full inhibition of I_{Kr}, in ventricular tissue of different species. Explanation in the text.

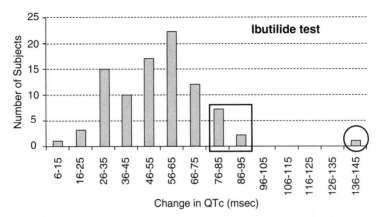

Figure 6.12. Clinical manifestation of the possibility of the reduced repolarization reserve. An extensive explanation is available in the text. (From ref. 74 with permission.)

the subjects far out of the range (indicated by circles) may identify patients with decreased repolarization reserve and increased risk for proarrhythmia after possible drug treatment [74].

Differences in the QT intervals of consecutive heart beats, measured as the variability index [75] or short-term beat-to-beat QT variability [76], was also suggested as a measure of proarrhythmic risk related to changes in repolarization reserve the collected results are encouraging. These studies [72, 75] suggest that the development of torsades de pointes arrhythmia in dogs correlated more with the short-term QT variability than with the QTc changes in general (Figure 6.13).

6.7 PHARMACOLOGICAL MODULATION OF THE REPOLARIZATION RESERVE

As mentioned previously in this chapter, decreasing repolarization reserve by drugs would have detrimential consequences by increasing the risk of proarrhythmia. As such, decreasing repolarization reserve represents an important adverse side effect of drug treatment. In addition, it must also be emphasized that drugs which block multiple potassium channels—without decreasing inward currents such as I_{Na} or I_{Ca}—are expected to have higher proarrhythmic risk than selective potassium channel inhibitors because they would depress repolarization reserve more [77, 78].

Therapeutically, it would be useful to enhance repolarization reserve and thereby attenuate the proarrhythmic risk caused by repolarization abnormalities.

Inhibition of inward sodium and calcium currents indirectly represent an example of pharmacological interventions that may have positive effects on repolarization reserve. Amiodarone, which is a drug that inhibits both I_{Na} and I_{Ca}, is one of the best examples that illustrate this beneficial action on repolarization. Amiodarone lengthens repolarization substantially, but its proarrhythmic effect is much less than those of class III antiarrrhythmics that exert their action potential duration lengthening

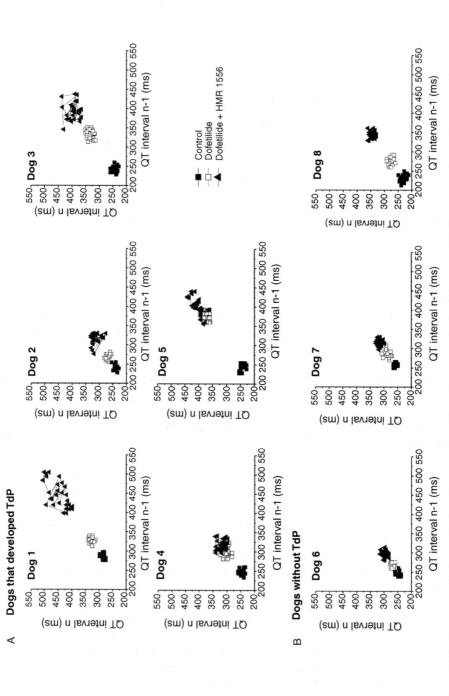

Figure 6.13. Better correlation of the development of torsades de Pointes arrhythmia in dogs with short term QT variability than with QTc changes in general. Individual Poincare plots showing increased short term variability of QT following combined I_{Ks} (HMR-1556) + I_{Kr} (dofetilide) block in dogs that later developed torsades de pointes arrhythmia (TdP) compared with those where TdP did not occur. (From ref. 72 with permission.)

by inhibiting only outward potassium currents. One may speculate that for this purpose relatively weak I_{Na} and I_{Ca} block would be sufficient, because persistent or window inward currents seem more sensitive to drug-induced inhibition than the corresponding peak currents [78]. In addition, if peak inward currents are substantially affected, then impairment of impulse conduction both at the ventricular and atrioventricular levels would be expected with a concomitant decrease of force of contraction. These effects may have detrimental consequences, especially in diseased hearts.

Another option is to enhance repolarization reserve by increasing outward potassium currents. The best candidate should be I_{Ks}, because stimulating this current would not be expected to abbreviate repolarization markedly when action potential duration is in the normal range, but as a negative feedback mechanism, it would limit excessive proarrhythmic repolarization lengthening (i.e., the desirable effect). There are reports that a benzodiazepine derivative L-364,373 enhanced I_{Ks} in guinea pig and rabbit myocytes [79, 80], but this effect was not confirmed in the dog [81]. More studies are needed to have proper conclusion regarding the effect and potency of L-364,373.

Data are available that I_{Kr} is augmented by certain drugs (NS-3623 and NS-1643) developed deliberately for an antiarrhythmic purpose. These drugs enhance I_{Kr} and shorten ventricular action potentials in different preparations [82–85]. NS-3623 was also shown to elicit postrepolarization refractoriness as an additional antiarrhythmic mechanism [84].

Repolarization reserve can be enhanced by opening the ATP sensitive potassium channels as well. Several compounds are described that act via this mechanism [86, 87], but these compounds are not selective for heart muscle. Therefore, side effects (like hypotension and diabetes mellitus) resulting from actions on other organs that also express ATP-sensitive potassium channels can be expected.

The therapeutically available option at present with actions on potassium channels is to increase serum potassium by adding potassium supplements. This intervention increases I_{Kr}; however, there is only a narrow therapeutic margin for this treatment, and it most likely would be applied only if serum potassium is below normal.

6.8 CONCLUSION

Repolarization reserve is a new concept that helps understand drug-induced proarrhythmia. According to this concept, inhibition or impairment of one transmembrane ion channel would not result in excessive repolarization changes because other currents may compensate. Reduced repolarization reserve, which is common during certain diseases, is not readily detected by conventional *in vivo* or *in vitro* electrophysiological measurements. However, reduction in repolarization reserve can lead to marked repolarization lengthening and proarrhythmia after drug treatment. Therefore, better predictive methods and new compounds are needed to quantify this phenomenon as well as to prevent arrhythmias caused by impaired repolarization reserve.

REFERENCES

1. Roden, D.M. (1998). Taking the idio out of idiosyncratic-predicting torsades de pointes. Pacing Clinical Electrophysiology, 21, 1029–1034.

2. Roden, D.M. (2006). Long QT syndrome: Reduced repolarization reserve and the genetic link. Journal of Internal Medicine, 259, 59–69.

3. Roden, D.M. (2008). Repolarization reserve. A moving target. Circulation, 118, 981–982.

4. Jurkiewicz, N.K., Sanguinetti, M.C. (1993). Rate-dependent prolongation of cardiac action potentials by a methanesulfonanilide class III antiarrhythmic agent. Specific block of rapidly activating delayed rectifier K^+ current by dofetilide. Circulation Research, 72, 75–83.

5. Iost, N., Virág, L., Opincariu, M., Szécsi, J., Varró, A., Papp, J.Gy. (1999). Does I_{Ks} play an important role in the repolarization in normal human ventricular muscle? Circulation, 100, I-495.

6. Varró, A., Baláti, B., Iost, N., Takács, J., Virág, L., Lathrop, D.A., Lengyel, C., Tálosi, L., Papp, J.Gy. (2000). The role of I_{Ks} in dog ventricular muscle and Purkinje fibre repolarisation. Journal of Physiology, 523, 67–81.

7. Bosch, R.F., Gaspo, R., Busch, A.E., Lang, H.J., Li, G.R., Nattel, S. (1998). Effects of the chromanol 293B, a selective blocker of the slow component of the delayed rectifier K^+ current, on repolarisation in human and guinea pig ventricular myocytes. Cardiovascular Research, 38, 441–450.

8. Cordeiro, J.M., Spitzer, K.W., Giles, W.R. (1998). Repolarizing K^+ currents in rabbit heart Purkinje cells. Journal of Physiology, 508, 811–823.

9. Attwell, D., Cohen, I., Eisner, D., Ohba, M., Ojeda, C. (1979). The steady state TTX-sensitive ("window") sodium current in cardiac Purkinje fibres. Pfügers Archiv: European Journal of Physiology, 379, 137–142.

10. Carmeliet, E. (1987). Slow inactivation of the sodium current in rabbit cardiac Purkinje fibres. Pfügers Archiv: European Journal of Physiology, 408, 18–26.

11. Schwartz, P.J., Priori, S.G., Locati, E.H., Napolitano, C., Cantu, F., Towbin, J.A., Keating, M.T., Hammoude, H., Brown, A.M., Chen, L.S. (1995). Long QT syndrome patients with mutations of the SCN5A and HERG genes have differential responses to Na^+ channel blockade and to increases in heart rate. Implications for gene-specific therapy. Circulation, 92, 3381–3386.

12. Bers, D.M. (2001). Excitation-contraction coupling and cardiac contractile force. 2nd Ed. Kluwer Academic Publishers, Dordrecht, The Netherlands

13. Gintant, G.A. (1996). Two components of delayed rectifier current in canine atrium and ventricle: Does I_{Ks} play a role in the reverse rate dependence of class III agents?. Circulation Research, 78, 26–37.

14. Spector, P.S., Curran, M.E., Zou, A., Keating, M.T., Sanguinetti, M.C. (1996). Fast inactivation causes rectification of the I_{Kr} channel. Journal of General Physiology, 107, 611–619.

15. Hancox, J.C., Levi, A.J., Witchel, H.J. (1998). Time course and voltage dependence of expressed HERG current compared with native "rapid" delayed rectifier K^+ current during the cardiac ventricular action potential. Pflügers Archiv: European Journal of Physiology, 436, 843–853.

16. Pourrier, M., Schram, G., Nattel, S. (2003). Properties, expression and potential roles of cardiac K^+ channel accessory subunits: MinK, MiRPs, KChlP, and KChAP. Journal of Membrane Biology, 194, 141–152.

17. Heath, B.M., Terrar, D.A. (2000). Protein kinase C enhances the rapidly activating delayed rectifier potassium current, I_{Kr}, through a reduction in C-type inactivation in guinea-pig ventricular myocytes. Journal of Physiology, 522, 391–402.

18. Virág, L., Acsai, K., Hála, O., Bitay, M., Bogáts, G., Papp, J.G., Varró, A. (2009). Self augmentation of the repolarization lengthening is related to the shape of the action potential: The role of the intrinsic properties of I_{Kr} and I_{k1} and its implication to reverse rate dependency. British Journal of Pharmacology,

19. Jost, N., Virág, L., Bitay, M., Takács, J., Lengyel, C., Biliczki, P., Nagy, Z., Bogáts, G., Lathrop, D.A., Papp, J.G., Varró, A. (2005). Restricting excessive cardiac action potential and QT prolongation: A vital role for I_{Ks} in human ventricular muscle. Circulation, 112, 1392–1399.

20. Lengyel, C., Iost, N., Virág, L., Varró, A., Lathrop, D.A., Papp, J.G. (2001). Pharmacological block of the slow component of the outward delayed rectifier current (I_{Ks}) fails to lengthen rabbit ventricular muscle QTc and action potential duration. British Journal of Pharmacology, 132, 101–110.

21. Jost, N., Papp, J.G., Varró, A. (2007). Slow delayed rectifier potassium current (I_{Ks}) and the repolarization reserve. Annals of Noninvasive Electrocardiology, 12, 64–78.

22. Han, W., Wang, Z., Nattel, S. (2001). Slow delayed rectifier current and repolarization in canine cardiac Purkinje cells. American Journal of Physiology, 280, H1075–1080.

23. Carmeliet, E. (2006). Repolarization reserve in cardial cells. Journal of Medical and Biological Engineering, 26, 97–105.

24. Volders, P.G.A., Stengl, M., van Opstal, J.M., Gerlach, U., Spätjens, R.L., Beekman, J.D.M., Sipido, K., Vos, M.A. (2003). Probiting the contribution of I_{Ks} to canine ventricular repolarization. Key role for β-adrenergic receptor stimulation. Circulation, 107, 2753–2760.

25. Gintant, G.A. (1995). Regional differences in I_K densitiy in canine left ventricle: role of I_{Ks} in electrical heterogeneity. American Journal of Physiology, 268, H604–H613.

26. Matsuda, H., Saigusa, A., Irisawa, H. (1987). Ohmic conductance through the inwardly rectifying K^+ channel and blocking by internal Mg^{2+}. Nature, 325, 156–158.

27. Jost, N., Varró, A., Szűts, V., Kovacs, P.P., Seprenyi, G., Biliczki, P., Lengyel, C., Prorok, J., Bitay, M., Ördög, B., Szabad, J., Varga-Orvos, Z., Puskas, L., Cotella, D., Papp, J.G., Virag, L., Nattel, S. (2008). Molecular basis of repolarization reserve differences between dogs and man. Circulation, 118, 18

28. Varró, A., Lathrop, D.A., Hester, S.B., Nánási, P.P., Papp, J.G. (1993). Ionic currents and action potentials in rabbit, rat, and guinea pig ventricular myocytes. Basic Research in Cardiology, 88, 93–102.

29. Zhang, L., Benson, D.W., Tristani-Firouzi, M., Ptacek, L.J., Tawil, R., Schwartz, P.J., George, A.L., Horie, M., Andelfinger, G., Snow, G.L., Fu, Y.H., Ackerman, M.J., Vincent, G.M. (2005). Electrocardiographic features in Andersen-Tawil syndrome patients with KCNJ2 mutations: Characteristic T-U-wave patterns predict the KCNJ2 genotype. Circulation, 111, 2720–2726.

30. Gaborit, N., Le Bouter, S., Szűts, V., Varró, A., Escande, D., Nattel, S., Demolombe, S. (2007). Regional and tissue specific transcript signatures of ion channel genes in the non-diseased human heart. Journal of Physiology, 582, 675–693.

31. Fülöp, L., Bányász, T., Szabó, G., Tóth, G., Biró, T., Lőrincz, I., Balogh, A., Pető, K., Mikó, I., Nánási, P.P. (2006). Effects of sex hormones on ECG parameters and expression of cardiac ion channels in dogs. Acta Physiologica, 188, 163–171.

32. Wang, Z., Feng, J., Shi, H., Pond, A., Nerbonne, J.M., Nattel, S. (1999). Potential molecular basis of different physiological properties of the transient outward K$^+$ current in rabbit and human atrial myocytes. Circulation Research, 84, 551–561.

33. Patel, S.P., Cambell, D.L. (2005). Transient outward potassium current, "I_{to}", phenotypes in the mammalian left ventricle: underlying molecular, cellular and biophysical mechanisms. Journal of Physiology, 569, 7–39.

34. Gao, J., Wang, W., Cohen, I.S., Mathias, R.T. (2005). Transmural gradients in Na/K pump activity and [Na$^+$]i in canine. Biophysical Journal, 89, 1700–1709.

35. Xiong, W., Tian, Y., DiSilvestre, D., Tomaselli, G.F. (2005). Transmural heterogeneity of Na$^+$-Ca^{2+} exchange: Evidence for differential expression in normal and failing hearts. Circulation Research, 97, 207–209.

36. Schillinger, W., Janssen, P.M., Emami, S., Henderson, S.A., Ross, R.S., Teucher, N., Zeitz, O., Philipson, K.D., Prestie, J., Hasenfuss, G. (2000). Impaired contractile performance of cultured rabbit ventricular myocytes after adenoviral gene transfer of Na$^+$-Ca^{2+} exchanger. Cirulation Research, 87, 581–587.

37. Kääb, S., Hinterseer, M., Näbauer, M., Steinbeck, G. (2003). Sotalol testing unmasks altered repolarization in patients with suspected acquired long-QT-syndrome-a case-control pilot study using i.v. sotalol. European Heart Journal, 24, 649–657.

38. Boulet, I.R., Raes, A.L., Ottschytsch, N., Snyders, D.J. (2006). Functional effects of a KCNQ1 mutation associated with the long QT. Cardiovascular Research, 70, 466–474.

39. Varro, A., Papp, J.G., Low penetrance, subclinical congenital LQTS: Concealed LQTS or silent LQTS?. Cardiovascular Research, 70, 404–406.

40. Kääb, S., Dixon, J., Duc, J., Ashen, D., Näbauer, M., Beuckelmann, D.J., Steinbeck, G., McKinnon, D., Tomaselli, G.F. (1998). Molecular basis of transient outward potassium current downregulation in human heart failure: A decrease in Kv4.3 mRNA correlates with a reduction in current density. Circulation, 98, 1383–1393.

41. Näbauer, M., Kääb, S. (1998). Potassium channel down-regulation in heart failure. Cardiovascular Research, 37, 324–334.

42. Li, G.R., Lau, C.P., Ducharme, A., Tardif, J.C., Nattel, S. (2002). Transmural action potential and ionic current remodeling in ventricles of failing canine hearts. American Journal of Physiology Heart Circulation Physiology, 283, 1031–1041.

43. Valdivia, C.R., Chu, W.W., Pu, J., Foell, J.D., Haworth, R.A., Wolff, M.R., Kamp, T.J., Makielski, J.C. (2005). Increased late sodium current in myocytes from a canine heart failure model and from failing human heart. Journal of Molecular and Cellular Cardiology, 38, 475–483.

44. Stillitano, F., Lonardo, G., Zicha, S., Varró, A., Cerbai, E., Mugelli, A. (2008). Molecular basis of funny current (I$_f$) in normal and failing human heart. Journal of Molecular and Cellular Cardiology, 45, 289–299.

45. Tateishi, H., Yano, M., Mochizuki, M., Suetomi, T., Ono, M., Xu, X., Uchinoumi, H., Okuda, S., Oda, T., Kobayashi, S., Yamamoto, T., Ikeda, Y., Ohkusa, T., Ikemoto, N., Matsuzaki, M. (2009). Defective domain-domain interactions within the ryanodine receptor as a critical cause of diastolic Ca^{2+} leak in failing hearts. Cardiovascular Research, 81, 536–545.

46. Giunti, S., Bruno, G., Lillaz, E., Gruden, G., Lolli, V., Chaturvedi, N., Fuller, J.H., Vaglio, M., Cavallo-Perin, P., EURODIAB IDDM Complications Study Group (2007). Incidence and risk factors of prolonged QTc interval in type 1 diabetes: The EURODIAB Prospective Complications Study. Diabetes Care, 30, 2057–2063.

47. Gill, G.V., Woodward, A., Casson, I.F., Weston, P.J. (2008). Cardiac arrhythmia and noctural hypoglycaemia in type 1 diabetes—the "dead in bed" syndrome revisited. Diabetologia, 52, 42–45.

48. Shimoni, Y., Ewart, H.S., Severson, D. (1998). Type I and II models of diabetes produce different modifications of K^+ currents in rat heart: role of insulin. Journal of Physiology, 507, 485–496.

49. Lengyel, C., Virág, L., Bíró, T., Jost, N., Magyar, J., Biliczki, P., Kocsis, E., Skoumal, R., Nánási, P.P., Tóth, M., Kecskeméti, V., Papp, J.Gy., Varró, A. (2007). Diabetes mellitus attenuates the repolarization reserve in mammalian heart. Cardiovascular Research, 73, 512–520.

50. Lengyel, C., Orosz, A., Takács, R., Várkonyi, T.T., Baczkó, I., Wittmann, T., Papp, J.Gy., Varró, A. (2008). Short-term QT variability in patients with long-standing type 1 diabetes mellitus. Diabetologia, 51, S556

51. Rodriguez, I., Kilborn, M.J., Liu, X.-K., Pezzullo, J.C., Woosley, R.L. (2001). Drug-induced QT prolongation in woman during the menstrual cycle. Journal of American Medical Association, 285, 1322–1326.

52. James, A.F., Hancox, J.C. (2003). Sex, drugs and arrhythmia: Are gender differences in risk of torsades de pointes simply a matter of testosterone?. Cardiovascular Research, 57 1–4.

53. Ridley, J.M., Shuba, Y.M., James, A.F., Hancox, J.C. (2008). Modulation by testosterone of an endogenous hERG potassium channel current. Journal of Physiology and Pharmacology, 59, 395–407.

54. Kurokawa, J., Tamagawa, M., Harada, N., Honda, S., Bai, C.X., Bai, C.X., Nakaya, H., Furukawa, T. (2008). Acute effects of oestrogen on the guinea pig and human I_{Kr} channels and drug-induced prolongation of cardiac repolarization. Journal of Physiology, 586, 2961–2973.

55. Johansson, M., Gao, S.A., Friberg, P., Annerstedt, M., Bergström, G., Carlström, J., Ivarsson, T., Jensen, G., Ljungman, S., Mathillas, Ö., Nielsen, F.-D. (2004). Elevated temporal QT variability index in patients with chronic renal failure. Clinical Science, 107, 583–588.

56. Lőrincz, I., Mátyus, J., Zilahi, Z., Kun, C., Karányi, Z., Kakuk, G. (1999). QT dispersion in patients with end-stage renal failure and during hemodialysis. Journal of the American Society Nephrology, 10, 1297–1302.

57. Yang, T., Roden, D.M. (1996). Extracellular potassium modulation of drug block of I_{Kr}. Implications for torsade de pointes and reverse use-dependence. Circulation, 93, 207–411.

58. Limberis, J.T., Su, Z., Cox, B.F., Gintant, G.A., Martin, R.L. (2006). Altering extracellular potassium concentration does not modulate drug block of human ether-a-go-go-related gene (hERG) channels. Clinical Experimental Pharmacology and Physiology, 33, 1059–1065.

59. Le Bouter, S., Demolombe, S., Chambellan, A., Bellocq, C., Aimond, F., Toumaniantz, G., Lande, G., Siavoshian, S., Baró, I., Pond, A.L., Nerbonne, J.M., Léger, J.J., Escande, D.,

Charpentier, F. (2003). Microarray analysis reveals complex remodelling of cardiac ion channel expression with altered thyroid status: relation to cellular and integrated electrophysiology. Circulation Research, 92, 234–242.

60. Bosch, R.F., Wang, Z., Li, G.R., Nattel, S. (1999). Electrophysiological mechanisms by which hypothyroidism delays repolarization in guinea pig hearts. American Journal of Physiology, 277, H211–220.

61. Galetta, F., Franzoni, F., Fallahi, P., Tocchini, L., Braccini, L., Santoro, G., Antonelli, A. (2008). Changes in heart rate variability and QT dispersion in patients with overt hypothyroidism. European Journal of Endocrinology, 158, 85–90.

62. Fredlund, B.O., Olsson, S.B. (1983). Long QT interval and ventricular tachycardia of "torsade de pointe" type in hypothyroidism. Acta Medica Scandinavica, 213, 231–235.

63. Hart, G. (2003). Exercise-induced cardiac hypertrophy: A substrate for sudden death in athletes?. Experimental Physiology, 88, 639–644.

64. Maron, B.J. (2007). Hypertropic cardiomyopathy and other causes of sudden cardiac death in young competitive athletes, with considerations for preparticipation screening and criteria for disqualification. Cardiology Clinics, 25, 399–414.

65. Szekeres, L., Papp, J.G., Szilvássy, Z., Udvary, E., Végh, A. (1993). Moderate stress by cardiac pacing may induce both short term and long term cardioprotection. Cardiovascular Research, 27, 593–596.

66. Das, M., Das, D.K. (2008). Molecular mechanism of preconditioning. IUBMB Life, 60, 199–203.

67. Corrado, D., Michieli, P., Basso, C., Schiavon, M., Thiene, G. (2007). How to screen athletes for cardiovascular diseases. Cardiology Clinics, 25, 391–397.

68. Xiao, L., Xiao, J., Luo, X., Lin, H., Wang, Z., Nattel, S. (2008). Feedback remodelling of cardiac potassium current expression. A novel potential mechanism for control of repolarization reserve. Circulation, 118, 983–992.

69. Luo, X., Xiao, J., Lin, H., Li, B., Lu, Y., Yang, B., Wang, Z. (2007). Transcriptional activation by stimulating protein 1 and post-transcriptional repression by muscle-specific microRNAs of I_{Ks}-encoding genes and potential implications in regional heterogeneity of their expressions. Journal of Cell Physiology, 212, 358–367.

70. Xiao, J., Luo, X., Lin, H., Zhang, Y., Lu, Y., Wang, N., Zhang, Y., Yang, B., Wang, Z. (2009). MicroRNA miR-133 represses HERG K^+ channel expression contributing to QT prolongation in diabetic hearts. Journal of Biological Chemistry, 282, 12363–12367.

71. Volders, P.G., Sipido, K.R., Vos, M.A., Spätjens, R.L., Leunissen, J.D., Carmeliet, E., Wellens, H.J. (1999). Downregulation of delayed rectifier K^+ currents in dogs with chronic complete atrioventricular block and acquired torsades de pointes. Circulation, 100, 2455–2461.

72. Lengyel, Cs., Varró, A., Tábori, K., Papp, J.G., Baczkó, I. (2007). Combined pharmacological block of I_{Kr} and I_{Ks} increases short-term QT interval variability and provokes torsades de pointes. British Journal of Pharmacology, 151, 941–951.

73. Hondeghem, L.M., Carlsson, L. (2001). Instability and triangulation of the action potential predict serious proarrhythmia, but action potential duration prolongation is antiarrhythmic. Circulation, 103, 2004–2013.

74. Kilborn, M.J., et al. (2000). Determination of QT response phenotype with low-dose ibutilide. Circulation, 102, II-673.

75. Thomsen, M.B., Verduyn, S.C., Stengl, M., Beekman, J.D., de Pater, G., van Opstal, J., Volders, P.G., Vos, M.A. (2004). Increased short-term variability of repolarization predicts d-sotalol-induced torsades de pointes in dogs. Circulation, 110, 2453–2459.

76. Berger, R.D. (2003). QT variability. Journal of Electrocardiology, 36, 83–87.

77. Biliczki, P., Virág, L., Iost, N., Papp, J.G., Varró, A. (2002). Interaction of different potassium channels in cardiac repolarization in dog ventricular preparations: role of repolarization reserve. British Journal of Pharmacology, 137, 361–368.

78. Kodama, I., Kamiya, K., Toyama, J. (1999). Amiodarone: Ionic and cellular mechanisms of action of the most promising class III agent. American Journal of Cardiology, 84, 20R–28R.

79. Salata, J.J., Jurkiewicz, N.K., Wang, J., Evans, B.E., Orme, H.T., Sanguinetti, M.C. (1998). A novel benzodiazepine that activates cardiac slow delayed rectifier K^+ currents. Molecular Pharmacology, 54, 220–230.

80. Xu, X., Salata, J.J., Wang, J., Wu, Y., Yan, G.X., Liu, T., Marinchak, R.A., Kowey, P.R. (2002). Increasing I_{Ks} corrects abnormal repolarization in rabbit models of acquired LQT2 and ventricular hypertrophy. American Journal of Physiology, 283, H664–670.

81. Magyar, J., Horváth, B., Bányász, T., Szentandrássy, N., Birinyi, P., Varró, A., Szakonyi, Z., Fülöp, F., Nánási, P.P. (2006). L-364,373 fails to activate the slow delayed rectifier K^+ current in canine ventricular cardiomyocytes. Naunyn-Schmiedeberg's Archives of Pharmacology, 373, 85–90.

82. Hansen, R.S., Diness, T.G., Christ, T., Demnitz, J., Ravens, U., Olesen, S.P., Grunnet, M. (2006). Activation of human ether-a-go-go-related gene potassium channels by the diphenylurea 1,3-bis-(2-hydroxy-5-trifluoromethyl-phenyl)-urea (NS1643). Molecular Pharmacology, 69, 266–277.

83. Hansen, R.S., Diness, T.G., Christ, T., Wettwer, E., Ravens, U., Olesen, S.P., Grunnet, M. (2006). Biophysical characterization of the new human ether-a-go-go-related gene channel opener NS3623 [N-(4-bromo-2-(1H-tetrazol-5-yl)-phenyl)-N′-(3′-trifluoromethylphenyl) urea]. Molecular Pharmacology, 70, 1319–1329.

84. Hansen, R.S., Olesen, S.P., Grunnet, M. (2007). Pharmacological activation of rapid delayed rectifier potassium current suppresses bradycardia-induced triggered activity in the isolated guinea pig heart. Journal of Pharmacology and Experimental Therapy, 321, 996–1002.

85. Diness, T.G., Yeh, Y.H., Qi, X.Y., Chartier, D., Tsuji, Y., Hansen, R.S., Olesen, S.P., Grunnet, M., Nattel, S. (2008). Antiarrhythmic properties of a rapid delayed-rectifier current activator in rabbit models of acquired long QT syndrome. Cardiovascular Research, 79, 61–69.

86. Lathrop, D.A., Nánási, P., Varró, A. (1990). In vitro cardiac models of dog Purkinje fibre triggered and spontaneous electrical activity: effects of nicorandil. British Journal of Pharmacology, 99, 119–123.

87. Carlsson, L., Abrahamsson, C., Drews, L., Duker, G. (1992). Antiarrhythmic effects of potassium channel openers in rhythm abnormalities related to delayed repolarization. Circulation, 85, 1627–1629.

CHAPTER 7

Safety Challenges in the Development of Novel Antiarrhythmic Drugs

GARY GINTANT and ZHI SU

7.1 INTRODUCTION

There remains an urgent need for effective antiarrhythmic drugs. This unmet medical need applies to drugs to treat atrial arrhythmias (including atrial fibrillation, the most common arrhythmia in clinical practice affecting over 2.5 million people in the United States) as well as ventricular arrhythmias (such as ventricular tachycardia and ventricular fibrillation responsible for sudden cardiac death). In light of disappointing results from earlier large-scale clinical trials evaluating various pharmacologic approaches, an emphasis on cardiac (as well as noncardiac) safety concerns must be maintained when developing novel antiarrhythmic drugs. Complicating the search even more for the ideal antiarrhythmic agent is the recognition that the drug target may be a complex proarrhythmic substrate reflecting dynamic electrophysiologic changes associated with advancing cardiac disease that may be modulated by neurohumoral influences. This complex milieu enables proarrhythmia after an immediate precipitating (triggering) event and may promote its perpetuation. This chapter will briefly review selected key clinical study results over the last 20 years that have directed the field of antiarrhythmic drug development, along with basic nonclinical electrophysiologic studies that provide insights into the likely mechanisms responsible for the clinical trial results. We will be considering so-called "downstream" interventions aimed at minimizing existing (or evolving) electrophysiological instability. Last, we will discuss some present-day approaches being employed to discover more effective (and safe) atrial antiarrhythmic drugs. We start our journey with a primer on basic functional cardiac electrophysiology.

Novel Therapeutic Targets for Antiarrhythmic Drugs, Edited by George Edward Billman
Copyright © 2010 John Wiley & Sons, Inc.

7.2   REVIEW OF BASIC FUNCTIONAL CARDIAC ELECTROPHYSIOLOGY

To consider the challenges of antiarrhythmic drug discovery efforts, it is instructive first to understand some key aspects of cardiac cellular electrophysiology that determine and control normal cardiac function. The efficient mechanical function of the heart depends on intrinsic electrical properties that set the appropriate heart rate and the orderly timing of excitation and contraction of the atria and ventricles. The normal heart beat originates silently as an electrical impulse arising in the sinoatrial node (SAN), which is also known as the pacemaker of the heart. This impulse propagates from the SAN (located in the right atrial roof) to excite the atria while traversing functionally distinct specialized conduction pathways leading to the atrioventricular node (AVN), the only electrical connection between atrial and ventricular chambers. The impulse slowly propagates through the AVN, invading the rapidly conducting bundles of the His and the Purkinje system that lead to the ventricular myocardium. The AVN and the His-Purkinje systems are latent pacemakers that may exhibit automaticity and override the SA node if it is suppressed. The intrinsic pacemaking rate is fastest in the SA node and slowest in the His-Purkinje system: SA node > AV node > His-Purkinje. Action potential conduction velocity also varies among different cardiac tissues, with the Purkinje system being the fastest and the AVN the slowest: His-Purkinje (2.2 m/s) > atrial muscle (1.1 m/s) > ventricular muscle (0.3 m/s) > AV node (0.05 m/s).

The integrated electrical activity of the heart is manifested on electrocardiograms (ECGs) recorded from the body surface. Electrical activation (depolarization) of the atria is registered as the P wave. The P-R interval encompasses the time required for impulse propagation from the initial activation of working atrial myocardium to electrical activation of ventricular endocardium, and it includes conduction through the atria, the AVN, and specialized conduction tissues (Purkinje fibers) in the ventricles. Slow conduction through the AVN represents most of the P-R interval. Excitation of the ventricular myocardium is reflected in the QRS complex, whereas ventricular repolarization is reflected in the ST segment and T wave. Differences in the timing of repolarization across the ventricular wall and the left versus right ventricles are responsible for rendering the ST and T wave morphologies. Although the ECG is the gold standard biomarker for the noninvasive monitoring of cardiac electrical activity, it must be recognized that it represents the sum of all cardiac electrical activity as filtered through the chest wall and recorded on the body surface. As a consequence, many details of the electrophysiologic events (including details of impulse initiation and propagation from the SAN as well as conduction through the AVN and specialized ventricular conduction system) remain largely hidden from view and must be inferred from the surface ECG. In ventricular myocardium, the influx of calcium ions during the action potential is responsible for initiating cardiac contraction by triggering release of intracellular calcium stores from the sarcoplasmic reticulum (SR); this calcium is largely returned to the SR by pumps within the SR membranes, leading to relaxation and the termination of each heart beat. Intracellular calcium concentrations have been shown to affect multiple additional cellular processes complexly (including ion channels and intracellular second messenger signaling cascades), which may contribute to arrhythmogenesis.

7.2.1 Normal Pacemaker Activity

The electrophysiological basis for the specialized pacemaker activity of SAN is its faster intrinsic rate of depolarization (termed phase 4 depolarization) along with its less negative maximal diastolic potential (MDP). A key inward current contributing to phase 4 spontaneous depolarization is a nonselective cation current termed the pacemaker current (I_f) [1]. Inward (depolarizing) Ca^{2+} current activation (including L-type and T-type) and outward K^+ current deactivation also contribute to phase-4 depolarization [2].

Autonomic regulation of I_f and the L-type Ca^{2+} current (I_{CaL}) controls the pacemaking activity of SAN and thus the heart rate (normal heart rate = 60 to 100 beats/min in humans and similar large mammals). β-adrenergic stimulation increases SAN pacemaker activity by enhancing I_f and I_{CaL}. Muscarinic acetylcholine receptor stimulation (mainly M_2) slows SAN pacemaker activity by reducing I_f, activating the acetylcholine-sensitive K^+ current (I_{KACh}), and reducing I_{CaL} [2, 3]). Accordingly, β-adrenergic receptor antagonists such as metoprolol are highly effective in the management of sinus tachycardia, and it is also the case for cholinergic receptor antagonists such as atropine in the treatment of sinus bradycardia. However, excessive blockade of β-adrenergic receptors and M-receptors can cause bradycardia and tachycardia, respectively. L-type calcium channel blockers are also effective in the treatment of sinus tachycardia. These are often combined with β-adrenergic receptor blockers in the management of angina pectoris and hypertension. However, severe bradycardia may occur in patients on the combination of β-adrenergic receptor blockers and calcium channel antagonists because of their additive negative chronotropic effects. Given the wide distribution of β-adrenergic receptors and L-type calcium channels, it is obvious that neither β-adrenergic receptor blockers nor calcium channel antagonists are "selective" heart-rate-lowering drugs.

Based on its physiological role in pacemaking, the I_f current is a natural target in the search for drugs aimed specifically at controlling heart rate. Recently, a novel heart-rate-lowering agent ivabradine has been developed. This drug selectively inhibits spontaneous pacemaker activity of the sinus node by specifically inhibiting I_f current, thus slowing the heart rate without affecting myocardial contractility and peripheral vascular resistance [4]. Recognized adverse cardiovascular effects for ivabradine are sinus bradycardia (directly caused by its mechanism of action) and QT interval prolongation (secondary to the decreased heart rate). However, the incidence of severe sinus bradycardia is low, likely because of a "ceiling" effect with ivabradine. It is intriguing to note that a reduction in heart rate (elicited with β-adrenergic receptor blockade) after myocardial infarction has been associated with the ability of these drugs to prevent sudden cardiac death [5, 6]. However, it remains to be determined whether chronic ivabradine reduces mortality in this setting. In this regard, it is important to note that chronic amiodarone, which is a potent bradycardic agent with chronic oral administration, does not seem to reduce mortality [7] in the absence of coadministration of β-adrenergic receptor blocking agents.

7.2.2 Atrioventricular Conduction

Similar to SAV cells, the upstrokes of the AVN action potentials are mediated by I_{CaL}. There is minimal functional inward rectifier current (I_{K1}) in AVN cells, which is consistent with its less negative MDP [8]. Contrary to the SAV, where both I_{Kr} and I_{Ks} are important, I_{Kr} predominates in the AVN. Action potentials from AVN cells have small amplitudes and slow upstrokes (i.e., slow phase 0 depolarization) that are largely responsible for slow impulse conduction through the AVN. Cells within the central region of the AVN (so-called N cells) also demonstrate low excitability and postrepolarization refractoriness, which limit the maximum number of impulses that can traverse to the ventricles and prevents dangerously rapid ventricular rates in response to supraventricular tachyarrhythmias [2, 9]. The cardiac action potential conduction velocity is fastest in the Purkinje system (2.2 m/s) and slowest in the AVN: His-Purkinje (2.2 m/s) > atrial muscle (1.1 m/s) > ventricular muscle (0.3 m/s) > AV node (0.05 m/s). Delayed AV conduction inscribes the P-R interval (normal human P-R interval = 120–200 ms) and allows the time of ventricular filling before ventricular contraction. AV conduction is modulated by the autonomic nervous system, with adrenergic stimulation increasing AV conduction by enhancing I_{CaL} and cholinergic stimulation decreasing conduction by reducing the I_{CaL}.

The specialized electrophysiologic properties and the anatomic location of the AVN provide a convenient target for certain antiarrhythmic drugs (adenosine, calcium channel blockers, β-adrenergic receptor blockers) in the treatment of supraventricular tachyarrhythmias (including rapid atrial and AVN arrhythmias [10, 11]). These drugs may be useful in controlling ventricular rate in the presence of atrial tachycardia and in converting AVN tachycardia to normal sinus rhythm by either directly or indirectly reducing I_{CaL}. Adenosine, which is a drug administered intravenously to facilitate the rapid conversion of paroxysmal supraventricular tachycardia (PSVT) to normal sinus rhythm, acts to slow AVN conduction by binding to adenosine A1 receptors directly coupled to ligand-gated GIRK channels to increase repolarizing K^+ current and refractoriness (a negative dromotropic effect). The drug is considered particularly safe (in part) because of its rapid clearance from the blood (half-life in whole blood less than 10 s) and the absence of any long-lived active metabolites [12].

7.2.3 Ventricular Repolarization: Effects on the QT Interval

Electrical activity (depolarization and repolarization) of the ventricular myocardium (VM) is reflected as the QT interval on the ECG. In humans at rest, the QT interval normally ranges from approximately 250 to 550 ms [13] and is strongly dependent on heart rate (faster rates associated with shorter QT intervals). This necessitates the use of correction formulas to normalize for different heart rates. For any given heart rate, QT prolongation is generally considered as contributing proarrhythmic risk, and is associated with the potential of a rare but potentially lethal arrhythmia torsades de pointes. Changes in the QT interval reflect, in a general manner, changes in the ventricular action potential configuration, which is a waveform that involves multiple ion currents through cardiac channels, exchangers, and transporters. Depolarization (phase 0) of the human ventricular myocardium is mediated by inward I_{Na} and repolarization by the activities of multiple channels (I_{Na}, I_{to}, I_{Ca}, I_{Kr}, I_{Ks}, and I_{K1}). Phase 1 repolarization mainly results from the inactivation of I_{Na} and activation of I_{to}; the plateau phase is mainly produced by the balance between the inward I_{Ca} and the outward I_K (mainly I_{Kr}); I_{Kr} is the major repolarization current of phases 2 and 3; I_{Ks} and I_{K1} also contribute to the ventricular repolarization, with I_{Ks} being active during phases 2 and 3 (during rapid rhythms and adrenergic stimulation) and I_{K1} being mainly active during (and beyond) the late stage of phase 3. (Readers should refer to Chapter 2 in this volume for more details.)

7.2.4 Electrophysiologic Lessons Learned from Long QT Syndromes

Genetic defects of cardiac ion channels (including I_{Na}, I_{Ca}, I_{Kr}, I_{Ks}, and I_{K1}) may cause either congenital long QT syndrome (LQTS) or short QT syndrome (SQTS) depending on the type of defects (loss- or gain-of-function mutation) and channel type (depolarizing or repolarizing current [14, 15]). Extensive progress has been made in studying congenital LQT syndromes, characterized by long QT interval (>450 ms), Torsade de Pointes, syncope, and sudden death from ventricular fibrillation [14, 16]. In contrast, much less is known about congenital genetic SQTS, characterized by abnormally short QT intervals (<300 ms), atrial fibrillation, palpitations, syncope, and sudden death from ventricular fibrillation [15, 17]. Studies of congenital QT syndromes have guided many aspects of antiarrhythmic drug development.

More commonly, delayed ventricular repolarization is caused by various medications, including cardiovascular (such as class IA and III antiarrhythmic drugs) and a wide range of noncardiovascular drugs [18–20]; drug-induced QT prolongation is often referred to as acquired (or drug-induced) LQTS [18, 21]. Theoretically, block of any type of potassium channel current (I_{Kr}, I_{Ks}, I_{K1}, and I_{to}/I_{sus}) might delay cardiac repolarization and lead to QT interval prolongation. However, the most likely mechanism for drug-induced LQTS is inhibition of I_{Kr} (hERG) current (somewhat analogous to LQT2 [21]). This is because the I_{Kr} channel has unique structural and biophysical properties that render it vulnerable to block by a variety of structurally different drugs [20, 22, 23].

In contrast to acquired LTQS, knowledge concerning drug-induced SQTS is sparse, with only one publication suggesting that digitalis intoxication in some patients can shorten the QT interval, and acquired short QT interval has been associated with major ventricular arrhythmias such as polymorphic ventricular tachycardia [24]. Theoretically, enhancement of any type of outward potassium currents (such as hERG channel activators) during action potential might accelerate cardiac repolarization (i.e., shortening of QT interval). However, no drug-induced SQTS has yet been documented since the first congenital SQTS case was published in 2000 [17], and no hERG enhancers or activators have been reported among marketed drugs. Interestingly, several small molecule activators of hERG channel have been recently identified among discovery compounds. It has been proposed that selective enhancement of hERG current could prove to be antiarrhythmic for inherited LQTS [25–27]; this attractive concept has yet to be proven clinically. In contrast to the potentially useful application of hERG activators in LQTS, hERG activation could be an unwanted off-target effect of noncardiovascular drugs and pose a risk of acquired SQTS; more investigations are required to clarify this potential risk.

7.3 SAFETY PHARMACOLOGY PERSPECTIVES ON DEVELOPING ANTIARRHYTHMIC DRUGS

7.3.1 Part A. On-Target (Primary Pharmacodynamic) versus Off-Target (Secondary Pharmacodynamic) Considerations

It is convenient to consider drug safety in terms of on-target and off-target effects. The term "on-target" may be more precisely termed the "primary pharmacodynamic effect" and defined as "studies on the mode of action and/or effects of a substance in relation to its desired therapeutic target" [28]. On-target effects must be considered in regard to drug exposure and the electrophysiologic substrate. For example, in the case of atrial fibrillation, progressive block of L-type calcium current with excessive verapamil concentrations can lead from proper control of ventricular rate to third-degree heart block. In addition, verapamil may be used with caution in some patients with left ventricular dysfunction because of its negative inotropic effect.

The term "off-target," which is more precisely referred to as a "secondary pharmacodynamic effect," has been defined as the effects of a substance not related to the desired therapeutic target. Off-target effects invariably increase with increasing drug concentrations, as higher concentrations promote interactions with additional cellular processes, and few drugs are so selective as to affect a single molecular target. Although off-target effects are typically linked to adverse effects, such is not always the case. Indeed, it has been argued that block of multiple cardiac ion channels may explain the efficacy (and safety) of some class IV antiarrhythmic drugs (for example, block of calcium current providing antiarrhythmic benefit while simultaneously offsetting the potentially dangerous class III effects of block of I_{Kr} (hERG, Kv11.1) with verapamil (see [29]; also [19] and [30] for reviews)).

Sometimes, serendipity and off-target effects join forces to direct antiarrhythmic drug development. Amiodarone, which is an antiarrhythmic drug widely used today to treat atrial and ventricular arrhythmias, was originally developed as an antianginal drug based on its properties as a potent vasodilator and bradycardic agent. Later, it was determined that the drug displayed class III effects (delayed cardiac repolarization) that likely contribute to its antiarrhythmic efficacy, and only later were additional electrophysiologic activities (block of sodium and calcium currents, as well as beta-adrenergic receptor blocking effects) recognized as contributing to its efficacy (and safety, [31, 32]). Indeed, a similar story seems to be unfolding with the antianginal drug ranolazine some 40 years later (see below). The nonlinear (and sometimes cyclic) nature of scientific research is recognized by some scientific historians, but oftentimes it is neither understood nor appreciated by most others.

7.3.2 Part B. General Considerations

The development of any successful drug requires consideration of potential benefits versus potential risks. For antiarrhythmic drugs, the stakes are high, as benefits may be life saving while risks from potential off-target cardiac effects may be life threatening. One goal of preclinical studies is to characterize the pharmacodynamic/pharmacokinetic relationship of a drug in relation to its efficacy as well as its adverse effects. This information provides initial estimates of a clinical therapeutic index or safety margin. In practice, this goal is rendered difficult by the fact that 1) preclinical models may not adequately reflect the complexity of dynamic cardiac disease processes in patients and 2) biomarkers used to evaluate early efficacy or adverse effects are often imperfect and may be misleading. In the case of antiarrhythmic drugs, on-target and off-target effects may be manifest in the heart because of interactions of compounds with multiple (on- and off-target) cardiac ion channels. In some instances, the on-target response itself may be proarrhythmic (as a result of erroneous target assumptions, changing electrophysiologic substrate) or possibly caused by improper or inadequate dose selection. Obviously, an understanding of 1) the physiology of the therapeutic target (both distribution and function) and 2) how pathophysiology may change the characteristics and function of that target would prove ideal in predicting efficacy and safety. The importance of considering the dynamic nature of the electrophysiologic substrate (in terms of on-target and off-target drug effects) cannot be overemphasized (for example, see Chapter 4 in this volume for a discussion of the mechanisms responsible for ventricular arrhythmia in the setting of ischemia).

Drugs may have different on-target or off-target effects in normal versus pathologic settings (see below). This argues strongly for the use of *in vivo* models and their inherent (and daunting) level of complexity, in addition to more "standard" physiologic assays, to predict both the efficacy and safety of novel antiarrhythmic drugs. Capitalizing on differences in the distribution of ionic currents in atrial versus ventricular tissues is one approach to avoid proarrhythmia specifically in chambers not targeted for drug effects (for example, selectively targeting atrial tissues to avoid potential ventricular proarrhythmia). Such an approach is exemplified in the search for drugs that block I_{Kur}, which is an atrial-specific repolarizing current, as a strategy to treating atrial fibrillation. Another strategy for pharmacologic therapy targets ionic channels that are specifically modulated or altered (electrical remodeling) by pathology or disease. Such may be the case with ranolazine, which is a drug initially developed as an antianginal agent that was subsequently demonstrated to block late sodium current, a depolarizing current that may be involved (enhanced?) in ventricular arrhythmias, thus representing a pharmacologic target for antiarrhythmic drug development. At the other end of the spectrum are strategies employed to develop drugs affecting multiple cardiac channels. Dronedarone is an analog of the antiarrhythmic drug amiodarone, which was an agent in clinical use for over 20 years against multiple arrhythmias that blocks multiple cardiac ion channels [33]. Drone-darone was developed to have similar cardiac effects to amiodarone but with fewer secondary pharmacodynamic effects [34]. Despite earlier concerns regarding inade-quate safety data, results from the ATHENA trial demonstrated a highly significant 24% relative risk reduction in time to first cardiovascular hospitalization or death with dronedarone [35, 36]. In addition, no significant difference in treatment-emergent adverse events was noted between dronedarone and placebo. Dronedarone is pres-ently under priority review by the U.S. Food and Drug Administration (FDA) for the prevention and treatment of atrial fibrillation or atrial flutter.

The following sections provide historical perspectives on several pharmacologic approaches that have shaped our understanding of present-day antiarrhythmic drug therapies and their limitations, emphasizing key, large-scale clinical trials that have shaped the antiarrhythmic drug development landscape. Regarding ventricular proarrhythmia, we start by reviewing the Cardiac Arrythmia Suppression Trial (CAST) study (ostensibly testing the utility of sodium channel blockade) and the Survival with Oral D-sotalol (SWORD) study (ostensibly tested the utility of delaying repolarization). The story of ranolazine is also discussed, an evolving antianginal drug that was tested for efficacy (and proarrhythmic safety) in the Metabolic Efficiency with Ranolazine for Less Ischemia in Non-ST Elevation Acute Coronary Syndrome-Thrombolysis in Myocardial Infarction (MERLIN-TIMI) 36 study, demonstrating potential antiarrhythmic properties. Finally, we discuss some examples of approaches used in evaluating the safety and efficacy of novel atrial antiarrhythmic drugs in clinical development.

7.4 PROARRHYTHMIC EFFECTS OF VENTRICULAR ANTIARRHYTHMIC DRUGS

7.4.1 Sodium Channel Block Reduces the Incidence of Ventricular Premature Depolarizations But Increases Mortality

The CAST [37] was designed to test the hypothesis that suppression of ventricular premature depolarizations improves survival free of arrhythmic death in patients with prior myocardial infarction. Before CAST, pharmacologic treatment of ventricular arrhythmias was largely empiric; premature ventricular beats were considered markers (harbingers) of proarrhythmia, and sodium channel blockers (such as lidocaine and quinidine) were largely used as antiarrhythmic agents. This pivotal trial challenged the assumption that pharmacological suppression of ventricular ectopy (proarrhythmic triggers) after myocardial infarction was beneficial and led to improved survival [38]. From a mechanistic perspective, the drugs tested in CAST (primarily class I sodium channel blockers, see Chapter 5) were expected to decrease myocardial excitability and hence slow (or block) conduction of premature beats, thereby preventing reentry (see below). Preceding (and in support of) CAST was the Cardiac Arrhythmia Pilot Study CAPS [39], which was a smaller study designed to evaluate the feasibility of pharmacologically suppressing ventricular premature complexes, a surrogate risk marker for proarrhythmia in patients after acute myocardial infarction with compromised left ventricular function. Drugs selected for the CAPS study were recognized prominent blockers of fast inward sodium current (class I according to the Vaughan-Williams classification) including encainide, ethmozine, flecainide, and imipramine.

The purpose of CAST was to test whether suppression of ventricular arrhythmias with long-term antiarrhythmic drug therapy would reduce arrhythmic death after myocardial infarction. Only patients whose arrhythmias were suppressed by antiarrhythmic drug therapy [80% suppression of ventricular premature depolarization (VPDs)] were entered in the trial. Study drugs included flecainide, encainide (class IC by the Vaughan-Williams classification), and moricizine (sharing characteristics with classes IA, IB, and IC). During the study, the Safety Monitoring Board recommended the encainide and flecainide study arms be removed from CAST (subsequently termed CAST-I) based on strong evidence of increased deaths compared with placebo (increase risk of 2.5 for arrhythmic death or nonfatal cardiac arrest [37]). The initiation of pharmacologic therapy did not cause sustained but nonfatal ventricular tachycardia [40]. However, a 3-fold increase in arrhythmic death (1.6% vs. 0.5%, active drug vs. placebo) was subsequently shown to occur during the first few weeks of therapy. The CAST investigators concluded that neither encainide nor flecainide should be used in the treatment of patients with asymptomatic or minimally symptomatic ventricular arrhythmia after myocardial infarction, despite marked suppression in the frequency of ventricular premature complexes and episodes of unsustained ventricular tachycardia (the targeted biomarkers). Subsequently, the moricizine arm of the CAST trial (CAST-II) demonstrated that this drug was not only ineffective but harmful [41].

The CAST trials demonstrated that pharmacologic suppression of asymptomatic or mildly symptomatic ventricular arrhythmias after myocardial infarction with three drugs was associated with increased mortality compared with placebo, and it suggested that such patients should not be treated with class I (sodium-channel-blocking) drugs unless benefit was subsequently demonstrated in a prospective, randomized, controlled clinical trial [42]. The CAST study (when compared with the CAPS study results) also emphasized the need for large-scale controlled clinical trials to assess the long-term efficacy and safety of antiarrhythmic drugs; such an evaluation is not possible with smaller sized studies, as these are not powered to detect an effect of mortality and may be too restrictive in regard to patient enrollment compared with eventual clinical drug use.

Mechanistic hypotheses to explain the increased mortality with CAST I included 1) an adverse interaction between the drugs and ischemic tissue promoted ventricular fibrillation and 2) ventricular tachycardia promoted by drug-induced conduction slowing [43]. A subsequent statistical study concluded that although both drugs shared the common ability to suppress ventricular ectopy after myocardial infarction, the increased mortality was likely mediated by different mechanisms in different populations and emphasized the complex and poorly understood hazards associated with antiarrhythmic drug therapy [44].

Experimental studies suggest that the increased mortality observed with CAST was consistent with intended on-target pharmacologic activity (sodium-channel block affecting conduction and the incidence of VPDs) along with a dynamic, evolving electrophysiologic substrate (ischemia or infarction). For example, *in vitro* studies demonstrated that β-adrenergic receptor stimulation in the setting of membrane depolarization potentiated flecainide-induced conduction slowing in canine Purkinje fibers [45]. In a conscious dog model, flecainide administration prior to the induction of acute myocardial ischemia increased the incidence of ischemic ventricular fibrillation [46]. In an anesthetized dog study with left anterior descending coronary artery occlusion followed by perfusion, flecainide (administered prior to and during the occlusion period) elicited fibrillation in 13 of 25 dogs during occlusion (compared with 1 of 25 placebo-treated dogs); the proarrhythmic effects of flecainide during occlusion confounded interpretation of its effects during reperfusion [47]. Flecainide was also shown to promote monomorphic ventricular tachycardia following occlusion in a 3-day-old healed myocardial infarction canine model [48]. A later experimental study with an anesthetized canine model with remote myocardial infarction demonstrated that conduction slowing with flecainide increased the duration of ventricular tachycardia and the ease of inducibility of ventricular tachycardia, which is analogous to the clinical situation [49]. Based on a review of clinical trials data, Nattel [50] has argued that class IC drugs cause lethal proarrhythmia by promoting fibrillation during acute ischemia, which change typically nonlethal ischemic events in cases of sudden death by exacerbating ischemia-induced conduction delay. Weiss et al. [51, 52] have also suggested that an off-target effect may be involved in enhancing subsequent profibrillatory effects of these drugs despite their ability to prevent the initiation of ventricular tachycardia associated with the induction of fibrillation.

The dynamic nature of the changing electrophysiologic substrate for ventricular arrhythmias is well appreciated. For example, a meta-analysis of placebo-control groups from five recent clinical trials emphasized the dynamic electrophysiologic changes that occur post-myocardial infarction, concluding that the risk of arrhythmic death was highest in the first 6 months and leveled off thereafter [53]. More recently, a population-based surveillance study reported that the risk of sudden cardiac death (defined as out-of-hospital deaths whose primary cause of death was coronary heart disease) following myocardial infarction in community practice is greatest during the first month. In contrast, the risk of sudden death beyond the first 30 days is low (becoming less than expected in the general population), but is markedly increased with the occurrence of heart failure (but not recurrent ischemia [54]). Such additional complicating long-term effects are challenging to study preclinically and highlight the potential "moving target" in regards to both efficacy and safety of antiarrhythmic drugs.

7.4.2 Delayed Ventricular Repolarization with d-Sotalol Increases Mortality in Patients with Left Ventricular Dysfunction and Remote Myocardial Infarction: The SWORD and DIAMOND Trials

The SWORD trial provided the first opportunity to investigate the potential benefits of pharmacologically delaying ventricular repolarization by blocking the cardiac delayed rectifier channel (hERG). SWORD was a multinational, multicenter ($>$400), randomized, double-blind, and placebo-controlled study with the treatment group considered a relatively low-risk population of post myocardial infarction patients. The primary objective of SWORD was to determine whether d-sotalol would reduce all-cause mortality compared with placebo in patients with left ventricular dysfunction and coronary artery disease (see Pratt et al. [55]). The d-isomer was selected because of concerns about the use of β-adrenergic receptor blockade to affect left ventricular dysfunction adversely in patients with prior myocardial infarction and left ventricular dysfunction (LVEF $<$ 40%). Prior to SWORD, the antiarrhythmic activity (but not proarrhythmic potential) of d-sotalol had been assessed in various accepted models (see ref. 56 for references); earlier and smaller clinical studies had suggested that d-sotalol was effective in reducing complex symptomatic ventricular ectopy in various small sets of patients.

The SWORD trial was prematurely stopped because of excessive deaths (5% in the treatment group vs. 3.1% in the placebo group) and arrhythmic death (3.6% vs. 2.0%). It is generally assumed that the increased risk of death with d-sotalol in the SWORD trial was proarrhythmia. However, despite the known electrophysiologic effects of d-sotalol, the mechanisms responsible for the unexpected results are uncertain. Pratt et al. [55] have argued that the arrhythmic deaths associated with d-sotalol were not caused by torsades de pointes for reasons that include the following: 1) no apparent relation between low heart rate and d-sotalol–associated mortality was discovered (lower heart rate would be expected to result in greater repolarization delays because of reverse rate-dependent drug effects and is a recognized risk factor for torsades de pointes), 2) no apparent relationship was observed between d-sotalol–associated mortality to baseline QTc levels or QTc levels 2 weeks post drug therapy, and 3) no apparent relationship between mortality and d-sotalol dose or serum potassium concentration. In addition, the temporal pattern of the d-sotalol–associated mortality did not resemble the temporal profile of torsades de pointes associated mortality reported for quinidine or racemic sotalol, which occurs soon after drug exposure (SWORD demonstrated an increased mortality risk in the active treatment groups after a mean of 148 days). The only major factor supporting torsades de pointes was that women tended to have a greater risk than men.

The above arguments would suggest that additional (off-target) drug effects were responsible for the increased mortality. However, it has been suggested that electrophysiologic heterogeneity of drug effects across the ventricular wall may have contributed to the untoward effects. Sicouri et al. [57] reported that supratherapeutic sotalol concentrations elicited greater prolongation of the action potential duration of midmyocardial canine ventricular preparations *in vitro* compared with either epicardial or endocardial layers. However, it remains to be determined whether drug-induced increased dispersion of repolarization occurs in the post-infarcted tissues. D-sotalol also increases the short-term variability of repolarization that predicts d-sotalol–induced torsades de pointes in AV-blocked dogs, a proarrhythmia model of torsades de pointes [58]. Of course, these later observations do not directly assess the effects of d-sotalol on models resembling the clinical experience (namely, healed infarcts). Thus, it remains unclear as to what mechanism(s) were responsible for the failure of SWORD.

Soon after the SWORD trial, two trials evaluated the effects of dofetilide in post-myocardial infarction patients. Dofetilide is a class III antiarrhythmic drug that is a potent (low nanomolar) and selective blocker of hERG (I_{Kr}) current [59]; it elicits no negative inotropic effects and does not affect cardiac conduction at therapeutic concentrations. The DIAMOND–CHF Study (Danish Investigations of Arrhythmia and Mortality on Dofetilide with Congestive Heart Failure) evaluated whether dofetilide affected survival or morbidity among patients with reduced left ventricular function and congestive heart failure [60]. Despite expectations that the drug would be effective in treating both atrial and ventricular arrhythmias, this study showed that dofetilide was primarily effective only in patients with atrial fibrillation (converting atrial fibrillation and preventing its recurrence). Dofetilide reduced the risk of hospitalization for worsening heart failure, but it had no effect on total mortality. A second trial, the Danish Investigators of Arrhythmia and Mortality on Dofetilide in Myocardial Infarction (DIAMOND-MI) trial [61], was designed to evaluate whether long-term treatment with dofetilide affected morbidity and mortality in recent survivors of myocardial infarction with severe left ventricular dysfunction. The dose was adjusted based on either creatinine clearance or if the QTc interval increased more than 20% from baseline or exceeded 550 ms. Long term-treatment with dofetilide did not affect all-cause mortality, cardiac mortality, or total arrhythmic deaths in this patient population, but it was effective in treating atrial fibrillation or flutter.

A subsequent analysis of DIAMOND-CHF patients revealed that for baseline QTc values <429 ms, dofetilide treatment was associated with a significant reduction of mortality, but a gradually increasing mortality risk with increasing baseline QTc intervals [62]. In the DIAMOND-MI study, dofetilide also resulted in a reduction in mortality with pretreatment QTc values <429 ms. However, when QTc interval was >429 ms, dofetilide did not influence mortality significantly [63]. In DIAMOND study patients treated only with dofetilide, risk factors for torsades de pointes [female gender, baseline QTc duration, and heart disease (specifically, NY Heart Association class III or IV)] were comparable with those typically cited for acquired long QT syndrome with non-cardiovascular drugs [64]; no significant differences in potassium blood levels were found. In addition, no torsades de pointes episodes were observed in DIAMOND patients with QTc duration 400 ms.

Differences in study populations may have contributed to the disparate results between the SWORD (increased mortality) and DIAMOND studies (neutral effect on mortality). Most patients in SWORD had older myocardial infarctions (>40 days), whereas DIAMOND-MI patients had more recent infarcts (<7 days). Also, patients in DIAMOND-MI had more advance heart failure. In SWORD, treatment was initiated out of the hospital, whereas in DIAMOND-MI patients were monitored by telemetry for 3 days in hospital. To our knowledge, no class III antiarrhythmic agent has been shown to reduce mortality in any patient group [65], and concerns have been expressed regarding adverse effects of excessive QT prolongation [66]. These concerns are consistent with the proarrhythmic liabilities (torsades de pointes) associated with QT prolongation by noncardiovascular drugs (see [67, 68] for reviews). It should also be noted that drugs that demonstrate comparable delayed cardiac repolarization may not share the same proarrhythmic liability (based on either QT prolongation or apparent torsadogenic propensity). Amiodarone is a drug that prolongs the QT interval clinically and demonstrates with complex electrophysiologic effects, bridging all four Vaughan-Williams antiarrhythmic drug actions (see Chapter 5). It is likely that reduction of L-type calcium current and beta-adrenergic receptor blockade by amiodarone may have protective effects in the setting of delayed repolarization. A report by Hii et al. [69] studied 38 consecutive patients treated with either class IA agents or amiodarone for ventricular tachyarrhythmias in the setting of chronic atherosclerotic heart disease (most with depressed left ventricular function); treatment of 9/38 patients was complicated by torsades de pointes [most of cases (7/9) associated with quinidine use]. Despite comparable QT prolongation, no patient demonstrated torsades de pointes with chronic amiodarone therapy. These authors postulated that class Ia drugs cause nonhomogeneous prolongation of cardiac repolarization, in contrast to the homogeneous prolongation of cardiac repolarization with amiodarone. Multiple clinical trials have failed to demonstrate enhanced proarrhythmic risk with amiodarone in various high-risk populations; indeed, reduced arrhythmia has been demonstrated in some instances [70, 71]). Amiodarone is presently used in post-myocardial infarction patients in whom antiarrhythmic therapy is indicated (for example, atrial fibrillation, see Kamath and Mittal [72] for references).

7.4.3   Ranolazine: An Antianginal Agent with a Novel Electrophysiologic Action and Potential Antiarrhythmic Properties

Ranolazine was developed as an antianginal agent [73, 74], and its therapeutic effect was initially attributed to inhibition of fatty acid oxidative metabolism (leading to a shift in adenosine triphosphate production away from fatty acid oxidation and toward more oxygen-efficient carbohydrate oxidation). However, this effect seems to occur at concentrations much greater than therapeutic levels. Subsequent studies have instead emphasized ranolazine's effect to block late sodium current [I_{NaL}, sometimes referred to as the persistent sodium current (I_{NaP})]. I_{NaL} is a small amplitude depolarizing current that may flow during the action potential after the upstroke of fast-type action responses [75–79]. Much work follows insights gained from studies of the rare congenital long QT-3 syndrome, in which mutations of the cardiac sodium channel (hH1 or Nav1.5) disrupts current inactivation, resulting in a greater and sustained depolarizing influx of sodium ions and delayed repolarization ([80]; see ref. 81 for a recent review). The following sections describe select proarrhythmic and antiarrhythmic "signals" discerned during preclinical studies with ranolazine, along with newer clinical data supporting its safety and potential utility as an antiarrhythmic.

7.4.3.1 *Preclinical Signals of Potential Proarrhythmic Risk.* Ranolazine, like many other antiarrhythmic drugs, affects multiple cardiac ion channels. Among

its more emphasized effects is block of I_{NaL}; block of I_{NaL} in canine ventricular myocytes is characterized with an IC50 value of 5.9 uM [82]. Ranolazine also blocks native I_{Kr} in canine ventricular myocytes (IC_{50} value of 11.5 uM [82]) and 12 uM in HEK293 cells stably expressing hERG channels [83]). Ranolazine also blocks I_{Ks} in native myocytes, although at higher concentrations (17% block at 30 uM). Thus, the potency of block of native late I_{NaL} is only 2-fold greater than that for block of native I_{Kr} (5.9 uM vs. 11.5 uM) as measured in the same *in vitro* preparations. The small difference in potency of I_{NaL} and I_{Kr} block is minimized by the less steep Hill coefficient for I_{Kr} (compared with I_{NaL}) block. Thus, in the clinically encountered concentration range of 2–6 uM [84], comparable potency of I_{Kr} and I_{NaL} block is anticipated. Modest delayed ventricular repolarization is observed preclinically and clinically with ranolazine (see below), which is consistent with the potency of I_{Kr} inhibition relative to therapeutic plasma concentrations. It is interesting to note that preferential block of I_{NaL} versus peak (or fast) I_{Na} has also been shown with flecainide, although with less apparent selectivity for late versus peak sodium current compared with ranolazine [85].

It is conceivable that the reduced outward (repolarizing) potassium current(s) affected by ranolazine are off-set by block of inward (depolarizing) late sodium current, thereby reducing the extent of QT prolongation (and presumably) proarrhythmic risk. Similar arguments (with calcium current block mitigating hERG block) have been advanced for noncardiovascular drugs [30, 86, 87]. More recent studies have demonstrated rapid kinetics of development and recovery from hERG block with ranolazine [83]; it is interesting to speculate that drugs demonstrating rapid interaction kinetics with the hERG channel may pose less proarrhythmic risk (and less use-dependent block) than those demonstrating slower recovery kinetics from block (see ref. 88 for example).

Preclinical repolarization assays provide conflicting signals in regard to delayed repolarization with ranolazine. Ranolazine prolongs the action potential duration of epicardial preparations (likely because predominant I_{Kr} block) and shortens the duration of midmyocardial cells (likely because of block of the more dominant late sodium current), leading to either a reduction or no change in transmural dispersion of repolarization measured *in vitro* [82]. Ranolazine also prolongs the pseudo-QT interval recorded from such ventricular wedge preparations in a concentration-dependent manner. In an *in vivo* study using acutely-AV blocked anesthetized dogs (a model predisposed toward torsades de pointes proarrhythmia), escalating doses of ranolazine (administered intravenously) produced a 10% increase in the QT interval; this effect was minimal (10%), not statistically significant, and biphasic (occurring at the intermediate infusion rate of 3 mg/kg/h but not at 10 mg/kg/h). Ranolazine also elicited a 10% increase in the QRS interval at the highest infusion rate tested (15 mg/kg/h), which is consistent with block of fast sodium current at supratherapeutic concentrations.

7.4.3.2 Preclinical Signals Consistent with Antiarrhythmic Effects.
Ranolazine demonstrates preclinical effects consistent with antiarrhythmic efficacy and improved cardiac function. In an isolated perfused rabbit heart model of

ischemia and reperfusion, ranolazine demonstrates cardioprotective effects [89]; specifically, supratherapeutic ranolazine concentrations improved left ventricular function, reduced the release of creatine kinase, reduced tissue calcium concentrations, and minimized the decrease in tissue ATP in response to ischemia. These results suggest that any antiarrhythmic effect may be related to the drug's cardioprotective effect and improved ventricular function. Later investigations have focused on studying the electrophysiologic effects of ranolazine on cardiac sodium current, often employing sea anemone toxins (such as ATX-II) in a convenient pharmacologic model that increases I_{NaL} by promoting persistent sodium current activation [90]. *In vivo*, sea anemone toxins prolong ventricular repolarization without affecting the PQ interval, QRS duration, or heart rate of anesthetized dogs, and these toxins increase proarrhythmia induced by adrenaline in the presence of ATX-II [91], which is consistent with a proarrhythmic effect induced by enhanced slow sodium current coupled with QT prolongation in a complex experimental setting. In an *in vitro* guinea pig model, ranolazine reduced action potential prolongation and mitigated early afterdepolarizations induced with ATX-II [92]; a high ranolazine concentration (10 uM) also reduced repolarization delays elicited by ATX-II in the presence of concomitant I_{Kr} or I_{Ks} block. These (and similar) electrophysiologic studies support the hypothesis that ranolazine may directly exert antiarrhythmic effects by reducing (enhanced) late sodium current. Ischemia models suggest that I_{NaL} amplitude increases *in vitro* with hypoxia and ischemic metabolites [93, 94]; late sodium current is also increased in myocytes isolated from a canine heart failure model and from failing human heart [95]. These later studies support the hypothesis that I_{NaL} may provide part of the arrhythmogenic substrate under pathologic conditions. However, it should be noted that alfuzosin, a drug that may delay repolarization by increasing sodium current flowing after the action potential upstroke [96], is not associated with proarrhythmia or torsades de pointes. Readers are referred to Saint [97] and Maltsev and Undrovinas [98] for recent critical reviews of the late sodium current as an antiarrhythmic target.

Bellardinelli [99] has suggested that ranolazine, by reducing I_{NaL}, reduces ischemia-induced accumulation of intracellular sodium, thereby preventing sodium-induced calcium overload in ventricular myocardium in pathologic settings. The increased calcium observed following acute ischemia may lead to increased diastolic wall tension and end-diastolic pressure, leading to decreased diastolic flow (and hence decreased oxygen supply) while increasing oxygen demand. As intracellular sodium levels are complexly related to intracellular calcium concentration, it is conceivable that reducing I_{NaL} could therefore reduce intracellular calcium levels in ischemic myocardium, linking an antiarrhythmic effect with antianginal efficacy.

7.4.3.3 *Clinical Support of Ranolazine as an Antiarrhythmic Agent in Angina.*
The MERLIN-TIMI 36 trial investigated the incidence of arrhythmias with ranolazine or placebo as part of a large, randomized, double-blind trial with non-ST elevation acute coronary syndrome patients within 48 h of ischemic symptoms [84]. The primary objective of this trial was to assess the effects of ranolazine on

cardiovascular death and recurrent ischemic events. Patients were monitored for 7 days with continuous Holter recordings following drug administration to evaluate potential proarrhythmic risk. Despite a significant reduction in recurrent ischemia in the ranolazine group, there were no differences in the primary efficacy endpoint (a composite of cardiovascular death, myocardial infarction, or recurrent ischemia) during the 1-year trial. During the 7-day initiation period with continuous ECG monitoring, ranolazine elicited a significant reduction in arrhythmic events (including ventricular tachycardia, supraventricular tachycardia, and bradycardia; complete heart block; or ventricular pause). The antiarrhythmic effects are considered exploratory by some, as ranolazine reduced the incidence of nonsustained ventricular arrhythmias but did not reduce the incidence of sustained arrhythmias (such as new onset atrial fibrillation and ventricular tachycardia). These results argue against a proarrhythmic liability with ranolazine caused by QT prolongation in a high-risk set of patients.

7.4.3.4 *Clinical Support of Ranolazine as an Antiarrhythmic Agent in LQT-3 Patients.*

One form of the hereditary long QT syndrome (LQT-3) is associated with a gain of function mutation of cardiac sodium channels (SCN5A-delta KPQ) that results in sustained inward sodium current after depolarization. As ranolazine has been shown to reduce late sodium current, a pilot clinical study was conducted to determine whether ranolazine would elicit QT shortening in LQT-3 patients, thereby mitigating delayed repolarization in this syndrome. Such results would be in contrast to QT prolongation observed in anginal patients administered ranolazine [84]. In an elegant study by Moss and colleagues [100], ranolazine (administered intravenously over 8 h to achieve therapeutic concentrations) shortened the QTc interval in each of five LQT-3 patients (mean change $26 +/- 3$ ms, average slope -24 ms per 1000 ng/mL, n = 5 patients) without affecting the QRS interval. In a prior study by these investigators, oral flecainide (a drug that also blocks the late sodium current) was also shown to normalize repolarization in LQT-3 patients with the SCN5A-KPQ mutation [101]. Together, these studies provide evidence of late sodium current inhibition as a pharmacologic antiarrhythmic target in a specific subset of LQT-3 patients.

7.4.3.4.1 *Concluding Remark.*

In summary, preclinical studies are generally consistent with the notion that a block of late sodium current may contribute to ranolazine's safety by offsetting the drug's ability to block hERG current. The ability to block late sodium current may also contribute to the drug's potential antiarrhythmic effects, depending (in part) on the role of late sodium current in the setting of ischemia and evolving or healing infarcts. Whether modulation of late sodium current is the primary mechanism responsible for ranolazine's antiarrhythmic effects in anginal patients awaits additional validation. Although encouraging, future clinical studies are necessary to confirm the antiarrhythmic efficacy of ranolazine in additional patient populations and to characterize the extent of efficacy relative to any potential emerging adverse effects in these populations.

7.5 AVOIDING PROARRHYTHMIA WITH ATRIAL ANTIARRHYTHMIC DRUGS

7.5.1 Introduction

With the aging population, atrial fibrillation is fast becoming the most prominent cardiac arrhythmia. Even though primary rate control and anticoagulation therapy remain the cornerstone for treatment of elderly asymptomatic patients, this approach is suboptimal for many patients. Antiarrhythmic therapy for rhythm control represents an additional pharmacologic approach requiring careful patient selection, consideration for adverse effects, and close monitoring to provide changes in drug or dose to optimize benefits [102]. The goals of atrial antiarrhythmic therapy may include 1) cardioversion of sudden onset, sustained, symptomatic arrhythmia; 2) prevention of recurrent atrial fibrillation; and 3) ventricular rate control in the presence of long-standing atrial fibrillation [103]. Additionally, pharmacologic target(s) may be dynamically changing with the evolution of atrial fibrillation due to electrophysiologic and structural atrial remodeling (see ref. 104, also recent reviews [105, 106]). It will be challenging for any one agent to fulfill these unmet medical needs, specifically targeting atrial fibrillation without affecting either ventricular electrophysiology or inotropy. Ideally, animal models need to reflect as closely as possible the clinical scenarios to select optimized novel compounds in support of early clinical studies. As congestive heart failure promotes atrial fibrosis and is a prominent risk factor for atrial fibrillation, the ideal animal model would also include such involvement to evaluate potential ventricular proarrhythmic risk (see ref. 107 for example).

Several pharmacologic approaches for treating atrial proarrhythmia based on electrophysiologic interventions have emerged. At one end of the spectrum is dronedarone, an analogue of amiodarone that blocks multiple cardiac channels developed with a reduced toxicity (noncardiac effects) profile (see ref. 108 for a recent review). Indeed, at least four agents that block multiple atrial and ventricular cardaic channels are currently under review for treatment of atrial proarrhythmia; these are azimilide, tedisamil, dronedarone, and vernakalant (RSD-1235). At the other end of the spectrum are drugs aimed at ion channel targets specific to either the "normal complement" of atrial channels or atrial channels "modified" by atrial fibrillation. Modulation of these targets would be expected to elicit minimal ventricular proarrhythmia. The ultrarapid delayed rectifier current potassium current I_{Kur}, which is a channel present predominantly in supraventricular tissues, represents one such atrial-specific target [109]. An example of a disease-modified target is the inwardly rectifying I_{Kach} channel. This channel normally mediates vagal influences on heart rate and atrial repolarization and is constitutively upregulated in atrial fibrillation [110, 111]. Savelieva and Camm [102] have used the acronym ARDA (atrial repolarization delay agents) to describe drugs that may more precisely target atrial-specific channels (or at least affect one atrial specific channel as part of its activity against multiple ion channel targets). Table 7.1 (from ref. 112) presents an overview of the ion-channel-blocking effects of various investigational

Table 7.1. Investigational antiarrhythmic drugs (mechanisms of action)

Multichannel blockers and modification of existing compounds	Atrial-selective antiarrhythmic agents
Dronedarone (I_{Kr}, I_{Ks}, β_1, I_{Ca}, 1_{to}, I_{Na})	**Vernakalant (IK_{ur}, I_{to}, I_{Na}, I_{GIRK})**
Celivarone (I_{Kr}, I_{Ks}, β_1, I_{Ca}, 1_{to}, I_{Na})	AZD7009 (I_{Na}, I_{Kr}, I_{to}, IK_{ur})
ATI-2042 (I_{Kr}, I_{Ks}, β_1, I_{Ca}, 1_{to}, I_{Na})	AVE-0118 (IK_{ur}, I_{to}, I_{GIRK})
Tedisamil (I_{Kr}, I_{to}, I_{KATP}, I_{Na}, IK_{ur})	Xen-D0101 (IK_{ur})

Table 7.1. From ref. 112. Copyright 2008 Prous Science, S.A.U. All rights reserved.

antiarrhythmic drugs (below). Such a strategy may be particularly important in the current regulatory environment, where great emphasis is placed on reducing the potential of drugs to delay ventricular repolarization to maximize safety in the setting of uncertain therapeutic efficacy.

The following sections discuss a few select compounds in later stages of development that reflect this wide spectrum of approaches, namely azimilide (a drug that blocks both I_{Kr} and I_{Ks}) and vernakalant (RSD1235), which is a drug that blocks I_{Kur} and other potassium currents. Finally, we briefly discuss some drugs in early stages of development that more specifically target atrial channels. Discussions regarding novel (noncardiac ion channel) approaches are found in Chapters 10–12 and 15–16 of this volume.

7.5.2 Lessons Learned with Azimilide, a Class III Drug that Reduces the Delayed Rectifier Currents I_{Kr} and I_{Ks}

Azimilide has been tested in clinical trials for efficacy against a variety of arrhythmias, including atrial fibrillation, paroxysmal supraventricular tachycardia, ventricular tachycardia, and recent myocardial infarction (see ref. 113). Our discussion will focus on select studies of the efficacy and safety of azimilide for atrial fibrillation. Azimilide is a class III agent that acts to block both the rapid and slow components of the delayed rectifier potassium current [114–117]. *In vitro* studies have demonstrated functional I_{Kr} and I_{Ks} current in atrial tissues from experimental animals and humans (see for example refs. 109 and 118). However, it should also be noted that the relative contribution of I_{Ks} to cardiac repolarization in different regions of the heart, at different heart rates, and with pathologic conditions is still debated. The height and duration of the action potential plateau are important determinants in defining the contribution of I_{Ks} to (ventricular) repolarization; I_{Ks} amplitude is prominently affected by adrenergic stimulation, and repolarization in diseased hearts (with possibly altered sympathetic influences) may be quite different from normal tissues [119]. Indeed, for ventricular tissues, it has been argued that combined block of I_{Kr} and I_{Ks} current is more proarrhythmic (for commentary, see ref. 120 and Chapter 6 in this volume).

Preclinical studies demonstrate antiarrhythmic effects of azimilide against programmed electrical stimulation-induced ventricular tachycardia and sudden cardiac death [121]. Studies with an *in vivo* model of vagally stimulated atrial fibrillation demonstrate that the effects of azimilide on atrial effective refractory period were rate independent [122]. As dofetilide is a selective I_{Kr} = blocker, these results suggest a potential advantage to combined I_{Kr}/I_{Ks} blockade by azimilide caused by block of I_{Ks} (the later current thought to play a prominent role in abbreviating repolarization during rapid rhythms). The efficacy of intravenous azimilide for atrial arrhythmias was demonstrated in three dog models of atrial fibrillation and flutter: a sterile pericarditis model, a canine right atrial enlargement model resulting from tricuspid valve damage and pulmonary artery banding, and the Frame model with a surgically created atrial lesion used to enhance susceptibility to electrically induced reentrant atrial flutter (see Table 7.1 of Karam et al. [123] for references).

Clinically, the Azimilide-CardiOversion MaintenancE Trial-1 (A-COMET-1 [113]) study was a multicenter randomized placebo-controlled clinical trial designed to explore the value of azimilide in maintaining sinus rhythm after restoration in patients with atrial fibrillation. The primary efficacy analysis was performed on a subgroup of patients with structural heart disease (314/446 patients). The study demonstrated a lack of an important benefit of azimilide on reducing the risk for arrhythmia recurrence. There were 6 (2.6%) occurrences of torsades de pointes in the study, which occurred during the drug loading period. QT interval prolongation (2.5% vs. 0.5%) and syncope (1.3% vs. 0.5%) was greater in the drug-treated compared with placebo group. A subsequent study (A-COMET-II) prospectively compared the efficacy of azimilide with placebo and sotalol in maintaining sinus rhythm after electrical cardioversion in patients with persistent atrial fibrillation [124]. A-COMET-II demonstrated that the antiarrhythmic efficacy of azimilide was slightly superior to placebo but significantly inferior to sotalol in patients with persistent atrial fibrillation (AF). In regard to cardiac safety, marked QTc prolongation or torsade de pointes occurred in approximately 10% of patients on azimilide; eight patients in the sotalol group (3.5%) and 16 patients in the azimilide group (7.6%) interrupted the study because of QT prolongation, and torsades de pointes was reported in five patients of the azimilide group. In all but one case, the arrhythmia occurred in the first 72 h after drug loading; older, female patients were prevalent; and hypokalemia was documented in two cases. No episodes of torsades de pointes were observed in the placebo or sotalol groups. The investigators concluded that the modest atrial antiarrhythmic effect along with the incidence of torsades de pointes and marked QT prolongation limited the usage of azimilide in these patients.

The accentuated risk of QT prolongation and torsades de pointes with azimilide reported in A-COMET-II could be attributed to a reduction of ventricular repolarization reserve brought about by block of both I_{Kr} and I_{Ks} (see Chapter 6). In support of this notion, Pratt et al. [125] reviewed 19 clinical studies (reflecting the experience of nearly 4,000 patients administered oral azimilide for numerous indications) and concluded that azimilide-associated torsades de pointes had characteristics and risk factors similar to other I_{Kr} blockers (more frequently occurring in women and elderly patients, in the presence of digitalis or diuretic agents). However, azimilide demonstrated a distinctive temporal profile, with torsades de pointes events not concentrated in the first week of administration [only 7 of 56 (13%) of torsades de pointes events occurred in the first 3 days of azimilide exposure (4 in women, 3 in men)]. In all, 43%

of torsades de pointes patients had at least one ECG with a corrected QTc (Bazett's formula) greater than 500 ms before torsades de pointes, compared with 22% of nontorsades de pointes patients ($P = 0.0014$). A clear relationship was found between maximum QTc values >500 ms and the risk of torsades de pointes (a 5-fold increase in the risk of torsades de pointes with a maximum QTc in the range of 580 msec or higher); threshold QTc values of 500 and 550 ms were significant predictors of azimilide-associated torsades de pointes risk.

7.5.3 Atrial Repolarizing Delaying Agents. Experience with Vernakalant, a Drug that Blocks Multiple Cardiac Currents (Including the Atrial-Specific Repolarizing Current I_{Kur})

Vernakalant (RSD1235) is in clinical trials as a potential atrial antiarrhythmic drug. I_{Kur} (Kv1.5) is an ultrarapid delayed rectifier current that when blocked results in prolongation of the atrial effective refractory period. As Kv1.5 channel proteins are expressed predominantly in the atria, Kv1.5 blockers are expected to show no effect in ventricular tissue. The ultrarapid delayed potassium atrial rectifier current (I_{Kur}) is blocked by vernakalant, with other channels (I_{to}, I_{Nafast}, I_{NaL}, I_{Kr}, and I_{Ks}) also being affected to lesser extents. The block of fast inward sodium current by vernakalant is characterized by rapid offset kinetics, suggesting conduction slowing targeted to only more rapid heart rates (such as atrial flutter and fibrillation). In regard to antiarrhythmic drug classification, one might consider vernakalant as a "crossover drug" that mixes atrial selective repolarizing delaying activity (I_{Kur}) along with additional class III ion channel blocking activity. In randomized clinical trials, vernakalant has demonstrated efficacy at conversion of atrial fibrillation of short duration; in the ACT III study, the greatest conversion (71%) occurred with recent onset atrial fibrillation of less than 72 h [126]; lower conversion rates (9%) were reported for patients with atrial fibrillation duration greater than 7 days. The different conversion rates are consistent with a complex, dynamic electrophysiologic substrate after fibrillation onset (as has been described for animal models [104, 127, 128]), which represents a challenging "moving target" for atrial antiarrhythmic drugs afforded by atrial remodeling.

7.5.3.1 The Quest for Atrial Selective Ion Channel Blocking Drugs.
Several other atrial-selective targets have been identified, with greater or lesser selectivity for atrial channels. For example, AVE1008 affects I_{to}/I_{Kur} and has additional effects on I_{Kach} [129, 130]. Diphenyl-phosphine oxide (DPO) compounds, which may provide greater selectivity for block of I_{Kur} vs. I_{Kr} or I_{Ks} [131], have been shown to terminate atrial arrhythmia in a canine model of reentrant atrial flutter without affecting ventricular electrophysiology [132]. These findings support the advancement of more selective modulators of atrial refractoriness that block I_{Kur} in the search for safer (and more effective) atrial antiarrhythmic drugs. A recent *in silico* modeling study points toward the importance of the kinetics of I_{Kur} block in regard to the ability to delay atrial repolarization, and highlights the need to consider electrophysiologic differences across species when evaluating antiarrhythmic effects

of I_{Kur} blockers [133]. A more complete listing of new drugs targeting I_{Kur} can be found in a recent review by Ford and Milnes [134]. It remains to be demonstrated that inhibition of I_{Kur} is truly atrial selective and well tolerated clinically. A recent summary of more novel atrial selective ion channel approaches for the treatment of atrial fibrillation has recently been published [135].

7.5.3.2 Conclusions—Present-Day Safety Challenges in the Development of Novel Antiarrhythmic Drugs.

Present-day choices for antiarrhythmic drug therapy are often suboptimal in regard to providing adequate benefit (efficacy) as compared with potential (or realized) cardiac safety liabilities. For antiarrhythmic drugs targeting cardiac ion channels, concerns regarding efficacy and safety are often linked, as the therapeutic "window" for such drugs may be low because of potential untoward effects present in either atria or ventricles. This represents a primary difference when comparing safety pharmacology issues for antiarrhythmic versus noncardiovascular drugs, as secondary pharmacodynamic effects with off-target organs are typically of primary concern for the later group. Additionally, adverse effects on normal hearts may be quite different from those of hearts with structural disease, healing infarctions, or heart failure, and studies designed to evaluate efficacy may not be adequately powered to discern drug safety issues.

The various clinical trials, mechanistic rationales, and experimental approaches cited above provide an appreciation of the complexity of the therapeutic target, the dynamics of the cardiac electrophysiologic substrate, and the multiple (and often changing) roles an antiarrhythmic drug is expected to perform. In the case of ventricular proarrhythmia after myocardial infarction (the CAST study), the pharmacologic pursuit of the target (reduction of the trigger, namely ventricular ectopy) with three sodium channel blocking drugs affecting ventricular conduction was associated with adverse outcomes. The finding that Class I drugs increased arrhythmias and mortality eventually promoted the increased use of implantable cardiac defibrillators, along with an alternative pharmacologic strategy aimed at delaying repolarization. In the case of delayed repolarization with d,l-sotalol (the SWORD study), increased mortality in postinfarction patients with ventricular dysfunction (presumably due to proarrhythmic events) also points to a less than full understanding of the complexity of the electrophysiologic milieu. Amiodarone, an agent that blocks multiple cardiac ion channels and transporters with demonstrable antiarrhythmic efficacy, has not been shown to improve survival [136, 137]. The evolving story of ranolazine emphasizes the importance of considering the integrated systems response (effects on multiple ionic currents) when interpreting basic cellular electrophysiologic approaches and the context of overall cardiac safety. In terms of antiarrhythmic drug use after myocardial infarction, it seems that only chronic β-adrenergic receptor blockade is effective in reducing the incidence of sudden cardiac death, especially in patients with left ventricular dysfunction ([138, 139], see ref. 140 for a recent review of antiarrhythmic and antifibrillatory effects).

In the case of atrial antiarrhythmic drugs, preclinical studies again emphasize the importance of a dynamic, evolving electrophysiologic substrate in antiarrhythmic drug therapy. As a result of a changing substrate, different targets may be manifest at different times. Thus, it is questionable whether a single drug will be efficacious against most atrial proarrhythmia. Indeed, it is possible that a drug may be beneficial in an earlier setting and neutral (or potentially proarrhythmic) in a later setting. The limitations of preclinical arrhythmia models need to be recognized before cautiously moving to more complex situations in humans, and the characterization of cellular electrophysiologic effects of drugs on normal atrial myocardium represents a minimum evaluation of a drug's safety liabilities. Preclinical *in vivo* models used are, of necessity, complex and laborious, and typically are designed to demonstrate efficacy rather than safety. Only when results from clinical trials are subsequently compared and contrasted with preclinical findings can we guide and refine future antiarrhythmic model development. Such efforts will provide for more efficient future drug-discovery efforts and, most importantly, safe and efficacious antiarrhythmic drugs to meet the growing unmet medical needs.

REFERENCES

1. DiFrancesco, D., Borer, J.S. (2007). The funny current: Cellular basis for the control of heart rate. Drugs, 67, 15–24.

2. Schram, G., Pourrier, M., Melnyk, P., Nattel, S. (2002). Differential distribution of cardiac ion channel expression as a basis for regional specialization in electrical function. Circulation Research, 90, 939–950.

3. DiFrancesco, D. (1993). Pacemaker mechanisms in cardiac tissue. Annual Review of Physiology, 55, 455–472.

4. Savelieva, I., Camm, A.J. (2008). I_f inhibition with ivabradine: Electrophysiological effects and safety. Drug Safety, 31, 95–107.

5. Kendall, M.J., Lynch, K.P., Hjalmarson, A., Kjekshus, J. (1995). Beta-blockers and sudden cardiac death. Annuals of Internal Medicine, 123, 358–367.

6. Hjalmarson, A. (1997). Effects of beta blockade on sudden cardiac death during acute myocardial infarction and the postinfarction period. American Journal of Cardiology, 80, 35J–39J.

7. Amiodarone Trials Meta-Analysis Investigators. (1997). Effect of prophylactic amiodarone on mortality after acute myocardial infarction and in congestive heart failure: Meta-analysis of individual data from 6500 patients in randomised trials. Lancet, 350, 1417–1424.

8. Hancox, J.C., Mitcheson, J.S. (1997). Ion channel and exchange currents in single myocytes isolated from the rabbit atrioventricular node. Canadian Journal of Cardiology, 13, 1175–1182.

9. Hoffman, B.F., Moore, E.N., Stuckey, J.H., Cranefield, P.F. (1963). Functional properties of the atrioventricular conduction system. Circulation Research, 13, 308–28.

10. Delacretaz, F. (2006). Clinical practice: Supraventricular tachycardia. New England Journal of Medicine, 354, 1093–51.

11. Anugwom, C., Sulangi, S., Dachs, R. (2007). Adenosine vs. calcium channel blockers for supraventricular tachycardia. American Family Physician, 75, 1653–1654.

12. Adenosine. PDR. Product label.

13. Goldenberg, I., Moss, A.J., Zareba, W. (2006). QT interval: How to measure it and what is "normal". Journal Cardiovascular Electrophysiology, 17, 333–6.

14. Roden, D.M. (2008). Long-QT syndrome. New England Journal of Medicine, 358, 169–176.

15. Bjerregaard, P., Jahangir, A., Gussak, I. (2006). Targeted therapy for short QT syndrome. Expert Opinion on Therapeutic Targets, 10, 393–400.

16. Keating, M.T., Sanguinetti, M.C. (2001). Molecular and cellular mechanisms of cardiac arrhythmias. Cell, 104, 569–80.

17. Gussak, I., Brugada, P., Grugada, J., et al. (2000). Idiopathic short QT interval: A new clinical syndrome? Cardiology, 94, 99–102.

18. Cavero, I., Mestre, M., Guillon, J.M., Crumb, W. (2000). Drugs that prolong QT interval as an unwanted effect: Assessing their likelihood of inducing hazardous cardiac dysrhythmias. Expert Opinion of Pharmacotherapy, 1, 947–73.

19. Gintant, G.A., Su, Z., Martin, R., Cox, B.F. (2006). Utility of hERG assays as surrogate markers of delayed cardiac repolarization and QT safety. Toxicologic Pathology, 34, 81–90.

20. Sanguinetti, M.C., Tristani-Firouzi, M. (2006). hERG potassium channels and cardiac arrhythmia. Nature, 440, 463–9.

21. De Ponti, F., Poluzzi, E., Cavalli, A., Recanatini, M., Montanaro, N. (2002). Safety of non-antiarrhythmic drugs that prolong the QT interval or induce Torsade de Pointes. Drug Safety, 25, 263–86.

22. Mitcheson, J.S., Chen, J., Lin, M., Culberson, C., Sanguinetti, M.C. (2000). A structural basis for drug-induced long QT syndrome. Proceedings of the National Academy of Sciences USA, 97, 12329–33.

23. Mitcheson, J.S., Perry, M., Stansfeld, P., Sanguinetti, M.C., Witchel, H., Hancox, J. (2005). Structural determinants for high-affinity block of hERG potassium channels. Novartis Foundation Symposium, 266, 136–150.

24. Garberoglio, L., Giustetto, C., Wolpert, C., Gaita, F. (2007). Is acquired short QT due to digitalis intoxication responsible for malignant ventricular arrhythmias? Journal of Electrocardiology, 40, 43–46.

25. Hansen, R.S., Diness, T.G., Christ, T., Demnitz, J., Ravens, U., Olesen, S.P., Grunnet, M. (2006). Activation of human ether-a-go-go-related gene potassium channels by the diphenylurea 1,3-bis-(2-hydroxy-5-trifluoromethyl-phenyl)-urea (NS1643). Molecular Pharmacology, 69, 266–77.

26. Casis, O., Olesen, S.P., Sanguinetti, M.C. (2006). Mechanism of action of a novel human ether-a-go-go-related gene channel activator. Molecular Pharmacology, 69, 658–65.

27. Perry, M., Sachse, F.B., Sanguinetti, M.C. (2007). Structural basis of action for a human ether-a-go-go-related gene 1 potassium channel activator. PNAS, 104, 13827–32.

28. ICH S7A. (2000). Safety Pharmacology Studies for Human Pharmaceuticals. International Conference on Harmonisation of Technical Requirements for Registration of Pharmaceuticals for Human Use. Step 4. November.

29. Zhang, S., Zhou, Z., Gong, Q., Makielski, J.C., January, C.T. (1999). Mechanism of block and identification of the verapamil binding domain to HERG potassium channels. Circulation Research, 84, 989–998.

30. Fermini, B., Fossa, A.A. (2003). The impact of drug-induced QT interval prolongation on drug discovery and development. Nature Review Drug Discovery, 2, 439–447.

31. Singh, B.N. (1983). Amiodarone: Historical development and pharmacologic profile. American Heart Journal, 106, 788–97.

32. Rosenbaum, M.B., Chiale, P.A., Halpern, M.S., Nau, G.J., Przybylski, J., Levi, R.J., Lázzari, J.O., Elizari, M.V. (1976). Clinical efficacy of amiodarone as an antiarrhythmic agent. American Journal of Cardiology, 38, 934–44.

33. Singh, B.N. (2006). Amiodarone: A multifaceted antiarrhythmic drug. Current Cardiology Reports, 8, 349–55.

34. Dale, K.M., White, C.M. (2007). Dronedarone: An amiodarone analog for the treatment of atrial fibrillation and atrial flutter. Annals of Pharmacotherapy, 41, 599–605.

35. Hohnloser, S.H., Connolly, S.J., Crijns, H.J., Page, R.L., Seiz, W., Torp-Petersen, C. (2008). Rationale and design of ATHENA: A placebo-controlled, double-blind, parallel arm trial to assess the efficacy of dronedarone 400 mg bid for the prevention of cardiovascular Hospitalization or death from any cause in patients with atrial fibrillation/atrial flutter. Journal of Cardiovascular Electrophysiology, 19, 69–73.

36. Coletta, A.P., Cleland, J.G., Cullington, D., Clark, A.L. (2008). Clinical trials update from Heart Rhythm 2008 and Heart Failure 2008: ATHENA, URGENT, INH study, HEART and CK-1827452. European Journal of Heart Failure, 10, 917–20.

37. Cardiac Arrhythmia Suppression Trial (CAST) Investigators. (1989). Special report: Effect of encainide and flecainide on mortality in a randomized trial of arrhythmia suppression after myocardial infarction. New England Journal of Medicine, 321, 406–412.

38. Hine, L.K., Laird, N.M., Hewitt, P., Chalmers, T.C. (1989). Meta-analysis of empirical long-term antiarrhythmic therapy after myocardial infarction. JAMA, 262, 3037–40.

39. CAPS Investigators. (1988). Effects of encainide, flecainide, imipramine and moricizine on ventricular arrhythmias during the year after acute myocardial infarction: The CAPS. The Cardiac Arrhythmia Pilot Study (CAPS) investigators. American Journal of Cardiology, 61, 501–9.

40. Wyse, D.G., Morganroth, J., Ledingham, R., Denes, P., Hallstrom, A., Mitchell, L.B., Epstein, A.E., Woosley, R.L., Capone, R. (1994). New insights into the definition and meaning of proarrhythmia during initiation of antiarrhythmic drug therapy from the Cardiac Arrhythmia Suppression Trial and its pilot study. The CAST and CAPS Investigators. Journal of the American College of Cardiology, 23, 1130–40.

41. (1992). Effect of the antiarrhythmic agent moricizine on survival after myocardial infarction. The Cardiac Arrhythmia Suppression Trial II Investigators. New England Journal of Medicine, 327, 227–233.

42. Ehrlich, J.R., Biliczki, P., Hohnloser, S.H., Nattel, S. (2008). Atrial-selective approaches for the treatment of atrial fibrillation. Journal of the American College of Cardiology, 51, 787–92.

43. Bigger, J.T., Jr. (1990). Implications of the Cardiac Arrhythmia Suppression Trial for antiarrhythmic drug treatment. American Journal of Cardiology, 65, 3D–10D.

44. Anderson, J.L., Platia, E.V., Hallstrom, A., Henthorn, R.W., Buckingham, T.A., Carlson, M.D., Carson, P.E. (1994). Interaction of baseline characteristics with the hazard of encainide, flecainide, and moricizine therapy in patients with myocardial infarction. A possible explanation for increased mortality in the Cardiac Arrhythmia Suppression Trial (CAST). Circulation, 90, 2843–2852.

45. Cragun, K.T., Johnson, S.B., Packer, D.L. (1997). Beta-adrenergic augmentation of flecainide-induced conduction slowing in canine Purkinje fibers. Circulation, 96, 2701–2708.

46. Kou, W.H., Nelson, S.D., Lynch, J.J., Montgomery, D.G., DiCarlo, L., Lucchesi, B.R. (1987). Effect of flecainide acetate on prevention of electrical induction of ventricular tachycardia and occurrence of ischemic ventricular fibrillation during the early post-myocardial infarction period: evaluation in a conscious canine model of sudden death. Journal of the American College of Cardiology, 9, 359–365.

47. Lederman, S.N., Wenger, T.L., Bolster, D.E., Strauss, H.C. (1989). Effects of flecainide on occlusion and reperfusion arrhythmias in dogs. Journal of Cardiovascular Pharmacology, 13, 541–546.

48. Nattel, S. (1998). Experimental evidence for proarrhythmic mechanisms of antiarrhythmic drugs. Cardiovascular Research, 37, 567–577.

49. Coromilas, J., Saltman, A.E., Waldecker, B., Dillon, S.M., Wit, A.L. (1995). Electrophysiological effects of flecainide on anisotropic conduction and reentry in infarcted canine hearts. Circulation, 91, 2245–2263.

50. Nattel, S. (1999). The molecular and ionic specificity of antiarrhythmic drug actions. Journal of Cardiovascular Electrophysiology, 10, 272–282.

51. Weiss, J.N., Garfinkel, A., Karagueuzian, H.S., Qu, Z., Chen, P.S. (1999). Chaos and the transition to ventricular fibrillation: A new approach to antiarrhythmic drug evaluation. Circulation, 99, 2819–2826.

52. Weiss, J.N., Garfinkel, A., Chen, P.S. (2003). Novel approaches to identifying antiarrhythmic drugs. Trends in Cardiovascular Medicine, 13, 326–30.

53. Yap, Y.G., Duong, T., Bland, M., Malik, M., Torp-Pedersen, C., Køber, L., Connolly, S.J., Marchant, B., Camm, J. (2005). Temporal trends on the risk of arrhythmic vs. non-arrhythmic deaths in high-risk patients after myocardial infarction: A combined analysis from multicentre trials. European Heart Journal, 26, 1385–1393.

54. Adabag, A.S., Therneau, T.M., Gersh, B.J., Westgon, S.A., Roger, V.L. (2008). Sudden death after myocardial infarction. NEJM, 300, 2022–2029.

55. Pratt, C.M., Camm, A.J., Cooper, W., Friedman, P.L., MacNeil, D.J., Moulton, K.M., Pitt, B., Schwartz, P.J., Veltri, E.P., Waldo, A.L. (1998). Mortality in the Survival With ORal D-sotalol (SWORD) trial: Why did patients die? American Journal of Cardiology, 81, 869–876.

56. Doggrell, S.A., Brown, L. (2000). D-Sotalol: Death by the SWORD or deserving of further consideration for clinical use? Expert Opinion on Investigational Drugs, 9, 1625–1634.

57. Sicouri, S., Moro, S., Elizari, M.V. (1997). D-sotalol induces marked action potential prolongation and early afterdepolarizations in M but not empirical or endocardial cells of the canine ventricle. Journal of Cardiovascular Pharmacology and Therapeutics, 2, 27–38.

58. Thomsen, M.B., Verduyn, S.C., Stengl, M., Beekman, J.D., de Pater, G., van Opstal, J., Volders, P.G., Vos, M.A. (2004). Increased short-term variability of repolarization predicts d-sotalol-induced torsades de pointes in dogs. Circulation, 110, 2453–2459.

59. Jurkiewicz, N.K., Sanguinetti, M.C. (1993). Rate-dependent prolongation of cardiac action potentials by a methanesulfonanilide class III antiarrhythmic agent. Specific block of rapidly activating delayed rectifier K + current by dofetilide. Circulation Reseach, 72, 75–83.

60. Torp-Pedersen, C., Møller, M., Bloch-Thomsen, P.E., Køber, L., Sandøe, E., Egstrup, K., Agner, E., Carlsen, J., Videbaek, J., Marchant, B., Camm, A.J. (1999). Dofetilide in patients with congestive heart failure and left ventricular dysfunction. Danish Investigations of Arrhythmia and Mortality on Dofetilide Study Group. New England Journal of Medicine, 341, 857–865.

61. Køber, L., Bloch Thomsen, P.E., Møller, M., Torp-Pedersen, C., Carlsen, J., Sandøe, E., Egstrup, K., Agner, E., Videbaek, J., Marchant, B., Camm, A.J. (2000). Danish Investigations of Arrhythmia and Mortality on Dofetilide (DIAMOND) Study Group. Effect of dofetilide in patients with recent myocardial infarction and left-ventricular dysfunction: A randomised trial. Lancet, 356, 2052–2058.

62. Brendorp, B., Elming, H., Jun, L., Køber, L., Malik, M., Jensen, G.B., Torp-Pedersen, C., Group, D.S. (2001). QTc interval as a guide to select those patients with congestive heart failure and reduced left ventricular systolic function who will benefit from antiarrhythmic treatment with dofetilide. Circulation, 103, 1422–1427.

63. Brendorp, B., Elming, H., Jun, L., Køber, L., Torp-Pedersen, C. Diamond Study Group. (2003). The prognostic value of QTc interval and QT dispersion following myocardial infarction in patients treated with or without dofetilide. Clinical Cardiology, 26, 219–225.

64. Pedersen, H.S., Elming, H., Seibaek, M., Burchardt, H., Brendorp, B., Torp-Pedersen, C., Køber, L. (2007). DIAMOND Study Group. Risk factors and predictors of Torsade de pointes ventricular tachycardia in patients with left ventricular systolic dysfunction receiving Dofetilide. American Journal of Cardiology, 100, 876–880.

65. Elming, H., Brendorp, B., Pehrson, S., Pedersen, O.D., Køber, L., Torp-Petersen, C. (2004). A benefit-risk assessment of class III antiarrhythmic agents. Expert Opinion on Drug Safety, 3, 559–577.

66. Brendorp, B., Pedersen, O., Torp-Pedersen, C., Sahebzadah, N., Køber, L. (2002). A benefit-risk assessment of class III antiarrhythmic agents. Drug Safety, 25, 847–865.

67. Fenichel, R.R., Malik, M., Antzelevitch, C., Sanguinetti, M., Roden, D.M., Priori, S.G., Ruskin, J.N., Lipicky, R.J., Cantilena, L.R.. Independent Academic Task Force. (2004). Drug-induced torsades de pointes and implications for drug development. Journal of Cardiovascular Electrophysiology, 15, 475–95.

68. Roden, D.M., Kannankeril, P.J., Roden, D.M. (2007). Drug-induced long QT and torsade de pointes: Recent advances. Current Opinion on Cardiology, 22, 39–43.

69. Hii, J.T.Y., George Wyse, G., Gillis, A.M., Duff, H.J., Solylo, M.A., Mitchell, L.B. (1992). Precordial QT interval dispersion as a marker of torsade de pointes. Disparate effects of class 1a antiarrhythmic drugs and amiodarone. Circulation, 86, 1376–1382.

70. Yap, Y.G., Camm, A.J. (1999). Lessons from antiarrhythmic trials involving class III antiarrhythmic drugs. American Journal of Cardiology, 84, 83R–89R.

71. Naccarelli, G.V., Wolbrette, D.L., Dell'Orfano, J.T., Patel, H.M., Luck, J.C. (2000). Amiodarone: What have we learned from clinical trials? Clinical Cardiology, 23, 73–82.

72. Kamath, G.S., Mittal, S. (2008). The role of antiarrhythmic drug therapy for the prevention of sudden cardiac death. Progress in Cardiovascular Diseases, 50, 439–448.

73. Chaitman, B.R., Pepine, C.J., Parker, J.O., Skopal, J., Chumakova, G., Kuch, J., Wang, W., Skeeting, S.L., Wolff, A.A. (2004). Effects of ranolazine with atemolol, amlodipine, or diltiazem on exercise tolerance and angina frequency in patients with severe chronic angina: A randomized controlled trial. JAMA, 291, 309–316a.

74. Chaitman, B.R., Skeeting, S.L., Parker, J.O., Hanley, P., Meluzin, J., Kuch, J., Pepine, C.J., Wang, W., Nelson, J.J., Hebert, D.A., Wolff, A.A. (2004). Anti-ischemic effects and long-term survival during ranolazine monotherapy in patients with chronic severe angina. Journal of the American College of Cardiology, 43, 1375–1382.

75. Gintant, G.A., Datyner, N.B., Cohen, I.S. (1984). Slow inactivation of a tetrodotoxin-sensitive current in canine cardiac Purkinje fibers. Biophysical Journal, 45, 509–512.

76. Carmeliet, E. (1987). Slow inactivation of the sodium current in rabbit cardiac Purkinje fibres. Pflugers Archiv—European Journal of Physiology, 408, 18–26.

77. Patlak, J.B., Ortiz, M. (1995). Slow currents through single sodium channels of the adult rat heart. Journal of General Physiology, 86, 89–104.

78. Kiyosue, T., Arita, M. (1989). Late sodium current and its contribution to action potential configuration in guinea pig ventricular myocytes. Circulation Research, 64, 389–397.

79. Maltsev, V.A., Undrovinas, A. (2006). A multi-modal composition of the late Na + current in human ventricular cardiomyocytes. Cardiovascular Research, 69, 116–27.

80. Bennett, P.B., Yazawa, K., Makita, N., George, A.L. (1995). Molecular mechanism for an inherited cardiac arrhythmia. Nature, 376, 683–685.

81. Remme, C.A., Wilde, A.A., Bezzina, C.R. (2008). Cardiac sodium channel overlap syndromes: Different faces of SCN5A mutations. Trends in Cardiovascular Medicine, 8, 78–87.

82. Antzelevitch, C., Belardinelli, L., Zygmunt, A.C., Burashnikov, A., Di Diego, J.M., Fish, J.M., Cordeiro, J.M., Thomas, G. (2004). Electrophysiological effects of ranolazine, a novel antianginal agent with antiarrhythmic properties. Circulation, 110, 904–910.

83. Rajamani, S., Shryock, J.C., Belardinelli, L. (2008). Rapid kinetic interactions of ranolazine with HERG K + current. Journal of Cardiovascular Pharmacology, 51, 581–589.

84. Scirica, B.M., Morrow, D.A., Hod, H., Murphy, S.A., Belardinelli, L., Hedgepeth, C.M., Molhoek, P., Verheugt, F.W., Gersh, B.J., McCabe, C.H., Braunwald, E. (2007). Effect of ranolazine, an antianginal agent with novel electrophysiological properties, on the incidence of arrhythmias in patients with non ST-segment elevation acute coronary syndrome: results from the Metabolic Efficiency With Ranolazine for Less Ischemia in Non ST-Elevation Acute Coronary Syndrome Thrombolysis in Myocardial Infarction 36 (MERLIN-TIMI 36) randomized controlled trial. Circulation, 116, 1647–1652.

85. Nagatomo, T., January, C.T., Makielski, J.C. (2000). Preferential block of the late sodium current in the LQT-3 delta KPQ mutant by the class Ic antiarrhythmic drug flecainide. Molecular Pharmacology, 57, 101–107.

86. Faivre, J.-F., Forest, M.C., Gout, B., Bril, A. (1999). Electrophysiological characterization of BRL-32872 in canine Purkinje fiber and ventricular muscle. Effect on early after-depolarizations and repolarization dispersion. European Journal of Pharmacology, 383, 215–222.

87. Martin, R.L., McDermott, J.J., Salmen, H.J., Palmatier, J., Cox, B.F., Gintant, G.A. (2004). The Utility of hERG and repolarization assays in evaluating delayed cardiac repolarization: influence of multi-channel block. Journal of Cardiovascular Pharmacology, 43, 369–379.

88. Stork, D., Timin, E.N., Berjukow, S., Huber, C., Hohaus, A., Auer, M., Hering, S. (2007). State dependent dissociation of HERG channel inhibitors. British Journal of Pharmacology, 151, 1368–1376.

89. Gralinski, M.R., Black, S.C., Kilgore, K.S., Chou, A.Y., McCormack, J.G., Lucchesi, B.R. (1994). Cardioprotective effects of ranolazine (Rs-43285) in the isolated-perfused rabbit heart. Cardiovascular Research, 28, 1231–1237.

90. Wang, S.Y., Wang, G.K. (2003). Voltage-gated sodium channels as primary targets of diverse lipid-soluble neurotoxins. Cell Signal, 15, 151–159.

91. Miyamoto, S., Zhu, B.M., Aye, N.N., Hashimoto, K. (2001). Slowing Na+ channel inactivation prolongs QT interval and aggravates adrenaline-induced arrhythmias. Japan Journal of Pharmacology, 86, 114–119.

92. Song, Y., Shryock, J.C., Wu, L., Belardinelli, L. (2004). Antagonism by ranolazine of the pro-arrhythmic effects of increasing late I_{Na} in guinea-pig ventricular myocytes. Journal of Cardiovascular Pharmacology, 44, 192–199.

93. Ju, K., Saint, D.A., Gage, P.W. (1996). Hypoxia increases persistent sodium current in rat ventricular myocytes. Journal of Physiology, 497, 337–347.

94. Undrovinas, A.I., Fleidervish, I.A., Makielski, J.C. (1992). Inward sodium current at resting potentials in single cardiac myocytes induced by the ischemic metabolite lysophosphatidylcholine. Circulation Research, 71, 1231–1241.

95. Valdivia, C.R., Chu, W.W., Pu, J.L., Foell, J.D., Haworth, R.A., Wolff, M.R., Kamp, T.J., Makielski, J.C. (2005). Increased late sodium current in myocytes from a canine heart failure model and from failing human heart. Journal of Molecular Cell Cardiology, 38, 475–483.

96. Lacerda, A.E., Kuryshev, Y.A., Chen, Y., Renganathan, M., Eng, H., Danthi, S.J., Kramer, J.W., Yang, T., Brown, A.M. (2008). Alfuzosin delays cardiac repolarization by a novel mechanism. Journal of Pharmacology and Experimental Therapeutics, 324, 427–433.

97. Saint, D.A. (2008). The cardiac persistent sodium current: An appealing therapeutic target? British Journal of Pharmacology, 153, 1133–1142.

98. Maltsev, V.A., Undrovinas, A. (2008). Late sodium current in failing heart: Friend or foe? Progress in Biophysics and Molecular Biology, 96, 421–451.

99. Belardinelli, L., Shryock, J.C., Fraser, H. (2006). Inhibition of the late sodium current as a potential cardioprotective principle: Effects of the late sodium current inhibitor ranolazine. Heart, 92, iv6–iv14.

100. Moss, A.J., Zareba, W., Schwarz, K.Q., Rosero, S., McNitt, S., Robinson, J.L. (2008). Ranolazine shortens repolarization in patients with sustained inward sodium current due to type-3 long-QT syndrome. Journal of Cardiovascular Electrophysiology, 19, 1294–1295.

101. Windle, J.R., Geletka, R.C., Moss, A.J., Zareba, W., Atkins, D.L. (2001). Normalization of ventricular repolarization with flecainide in long QT syndrome patients with SCN5A: DeltaKPQ mutation. Annals of Noninvasive Electrocardiology, 6, 153–158.

102. Savelieva, I., Camm, J. (2008). Reviews. Update on atrial fibrillation: Part II. Clinical Cardiology, 31, 102–108.

103. Savelieva, I., Camm, J. (2008). Anti-arrhythmic drug therapy for atrial fibrillation: Current anti-arrhythmic drugs, investigational agents, and innovative approaches. Europace, 10, 647–665.

104. Wijffels, M.C., Kirchhof, C.J., Dorland, R., Allessie, M.A. (1995). Atrial fibrillation begets atrial fibrillation. A study in awake chronically instrumented goats. Circulation, 92, 1954–1968.

105. Casaclang-Verzosa, G., Gersh, B.J., Tsang, T.S. (2008). Structural and functional remodeling of the left atrium: clinical and therapeutic implications for atrial fibrillation. Journal of the American College of Cardiology, 51, 1–11.

106. Cohen, M., Naccarelli, G.V. (2008). Pathophysiology and disease progression of atrial fibrillation: Importance of achieving and maintaining sinus rhythm. Journal of Cardiovascular Electrophysiology, 9, 885–890.

107. Knackstedt, C., Gramley, F., Schimpf, T., Mischke, K., Zarse, M., Plisiene, J., Schmid, M., Lorenzen, J., Frechen, D., Neef, P., Hanrath, P., Kelm, M., Schauerte, P. (2008). Association of echocardiographic atrial size and atrial fibrosis in a sequential model of congestive heart failure and atrial fibrillation. Cardiovascular Pathology, 17, 318–324.

108. Laughlin, J.C., Kowey, P.R. (2008). Dronedarone. Journal of Cardiovascular Electrophysiology, 19, 1220–1226.

109. Wang, Z., Fermini, B., Nattel, S. (1993). Sustained depolarization-induced outward current in human atrial myocytes. Evidence for a novel delayed rectifier K+ current similar to Kv1.5 cloned channel currents. Circulation Research, 73, 1061–1076.

110. Ehrlich, J.R., Hoche, C., Coutu, P., et al. (2006). Properties of a time-dependent potassium current in pig atrium—evidence for a role of Kv1.5 in repolarization. Journal of Pharmacology and Experimental Therapeutics, 319, 898–906.

111. Dobrev, D., Friedrich, A., Voigt, N., Jost, N., Wettwer, E., Christ, T., Knaut, M., Ravens, U. (2005). The G protein-gated potassium current I(K,ACh) is constitutively active in patients with chronic atrial fibrillation. Circulation, 112, 3697–3706.

112. Naccarelli, G.V., Wolbrette, D.L., Samii, J., Banchs, J.E., Penny-Peterson, E., Stevenson, R., Gonzalez, M.D. (2008). Vernakalant: Pharmacology, electrophysiology, safety, and efficacy. Drugs of Today, 44, 325–329.

113. Pritchett, E.L.C., Kowey, P., Connolly, S., Page, R.L., Kerr, C., Wilkinson, W.E., for the A-Comet-1 Investigators. (2006). Antiarrhythmic efficacy of azimilide in patients with atrial fibrillation Maintenance of sinus rhythm after conversion to sinus rhythm. American Heart Journal, 151, 1043–1049.

114. Freeman, L.C., Kass, R.S. (1996). Dual action of the novel class III antiarrhythmic drug (NE-10064) on delayed potassium channel currents in the guinea pig ventricular and sinoatrial node cells. Journal of Pharmacology and Experimental Therapeutics, 276, 1149–1154.

115. Salata, J.J., Brooks, R.R. (1997). Pharmacology of azimilide dihydrochloride (NE-10064), a class III antiarrhythmic agent. Cardiovascular Drug Review, 15, 137–156.

116. Gintant, G.A. (1998). Azimilide causes reverse rate-dependent block while reducing both components of delayed-rectifier current in canine ventricular myocytes. Journal of Cardiovascular Pharmacology, 31, 945–953.

117. Dorian, P., Dunnmon, P., Elstun, L., Newman, D. (2002). The effect of isoproterenol on the Class III effect of azimilide in humans. Journal of Cardiovascular and Pharmacology Therapeutics, 7, 211–217.

118. Gintant, G.A. (1996). Two components of delayed rectifier current in canine atrium and ventricle. Does I_{Ks} play a role in the reverse rate dependence of class III agents? Circulation Research, 78, 26–37.

119. Bányász, T., Koncz, R., Fülöp, L., Szentandrássy, N., Magyar, J., Nánási, P.P. (2004). Profile of I(Ks) during the action potential questions the therapeutic value of I(Ks) blockade. Current Medicinal Chemistry, 11, 45–60.

120. Thomsen, M.B. (2007). Commentary. Double pharmacological challenge on repolarization opens new avenues for drug safety research. British Journal of Pharmacology, 151, 909–911.

121. Black, S.C., Butterfield, J.L., Lucchesi, B.R. (1993). Protection against programmed electrical stimulation-induced ventricular tachycardia and sudden cardiac death by NE-10064, a class III antiarrhythmic drug. Journal of Cardiovascular Pharmacology, 22, 810–818.

122. Nattel, S., Liu, L., St-Georges, D. (1998). Effects of the novel antiarrhythmic agent azimilide on experimental atrial fibrillation and atrial electrophysiologic properties. Cardiovascular Research, 37, 627–635.

123. Karam, R., Marcello, S., Brooks, R.R., Corey, A.E., Moore, A. (1998). Azimilide dihydrochloride, a novel antiarrhythmic agent. American Journal of Cardiology, 81, 40D–46D.

124. Lombardi, F., Borggrefe, M., Ruzyllo, W., Luderitz, B., for the A-Comet II Investigators. (2006). Azimilide vs. placebo and sotalol for persistent atrial fibrillation: The A_COMET-II (Azimilide-CardiOversion MaintEnance Trial-II) Trial. European Heart Journal, 27, 2224–2231.

125. Pratt, C.M., Al-Khalidi, H.R., Brum, J.M., Holroyde, M.J., Schwartz, P.J., Marcello, S.R., Borggrefe, M., Dorian, P., Camm, J., on behalf of the Azimilide Trials Investigators. (2006). Cumulative experience of azimilide-associated torsades de pointes ventricular tachycardia in the azimilide database. Journal of the American College of Cardiology, 48, 471–477.

126. Pratt, C., Roy, D., Juul-Møller, S., Torp-Pedersen, C., Toft, E., Wyse, D.G., Nielsen, T., Rasmussen, S.L., on behalf of the ACT III Investigators. (2006). Efficacy and tolerance of RSD1235 in the treatment of atrial fibrillation or atrial flutter: Results of a phase III, randomized, placebo-controlled, multicenter trial. Journal of the American College of Cardiology, 47, 10A.

127. Morillo, C.A., Klein, G.J., Jones, D.L., Guiraudon, C.M. (1995). Chronic rapid atrial pacing: Structural, functional, and electrophysiological characteristics of a new model of sustained atrial fibrillation. Circulation, 91, 1588–1599.

128. Wang, Liu, L., Feng J., Nattel, S. (1996). Regional and functional factors determining induction and maintenance of atrial fibrillation in dogs. American Journal of Physiology, 270, H148–58.

129. Gogelein, H., Brendel, J., Steinmeyer, K., et al. (2004). Effects of the atrial antiarrhythmic drug AVE0118 on cardiac ion channels. Naunyn Schmiedebergs Archives of Pharmacology, 370, 183–192.

130. Ehrlich, J.R., Cha, T.J., Zhang, L., Chartier, D., Villeneuve, L., Hebert, T.E., Nattel, S. (2004). Characterization of a hyperpolarization-activated time-dependent potassium current in canine cardiomyocytes from pulmonary vein myocardial sleeves and left atrium. Journal of Physiology, 557, 583–597.

131. Lagrutta, A., Fermini, B., Salata, J. (2004). Novel potent inhibitors of cloned Kv1.5 potassium channels and human IKur. FASEB. J, 18, A1282.

132. Stump, G.L., Wallace, A.A., Regan, C.P., Lynch, J.J., Jr. (2005). In vivo antiarrhythmic and cardiac electrophysiologic effects of a novel diphenylphosphine oxide IKur blocker (2-isopropyl-5-methylcyclohexyl) diphenylphosphine oxide. Journal of Pharmacology and Experimental Therapeutics, 315, 1362–1367.

133. Tsujimae, K., Murakami, S., Kurachi, Y. (2008). In silico study on the effects of IKur block kinetics on prolongation of human action potential after atrial fibrillation-induced electrical remodeling. Am J Physiol. Heart Circulation Physiology, 294, H793–800.

134. Ford, J.W., Milnes, J.T. (2008). New drugs targeting the cardiac ultra-rapid delayed-rectifier current (I Kur): Rationale, pharmacology and evidence for potential therapeutic value. Journal of Cardiovascular Pharmacology, 52, 105–120.

135. Ehrlich, J.R., Biliczki, P., Hohnloser, S.H., Nattel, S. (2008). Atrial-selective approaches for the treatment of atrial fibrillation. Journal of the American College of Cardiology, 51, 787–792.

136. Julian, D.G., Camm, A.J., Frangin, G., Janse, M.J., Munoz, A., Schwartz, P.J., Simon, P. (1997). Randomised trial of effect of amiodarone on mortality in patients with left-ventricular dysfunction after recent myocardial infarction: EMIAT. European Myocardial Infarct Amiodarone Trial Investigators. Lancet, 349, 667–674.

137. Cairns, J.A., Connolly, S.J., Roberts, R., Gent, M. (1997). Randomised trial of outcome after myocardial infarction in patients with frequent or repetitive ventricular premature depolarisations: CAMIAT. Canadian Amiodarone Myocardial Infarction Arrhythmia Trial Investigators. Lancet, 349, 675–682.

138. Gottlieb, S.S., McCarter, R.J., Vogel, R.A. (1998). Effect of beta-blockade on mortality among high-risk and low-risk patients after myocardial infarction. New England Journal of Medicine, 339, 489–497.

139. Janse, M.J. (2003). A brief history of sudden cardiac death and its therapy. Pharmacology Therapy, 100, 89–99.

140. Singh, B.N. (2005). β-Adrenergic blockers as antiarrhythmic and antifibrillatory compounds: An overview. Journal of Cardiovascular and Pharmacological Therapeutics, 10, S3–S14.

CHAPTER 8

Safety Pharmacology and Regulatory Issues in the Development of Antiarrhythmic Medications

ARMANDO LAGRUTTA and JOSEPH J. SALATA

8.1 INTRODUCTION

In this chapter, we examine the development of antiarrhythmic therapeutic agents from a safety pharmacology perspective. Safety pharmacology is concerned with adverse pharmacodynamic effects of a drug in the therapeutic or supratherapeutic range. In the case of antiarrhythmic agents, the major concern is, paradoxically, the risk of proarrhythmia. There is a physiological basis for this risk. The heart, with its electrical, mechanical, and hemodynamic properties, is an exquisitely synchronized, anatomically specialized organ. Perturbations to the natural order, even those carefully considered and modeled to be antiarrhythmic, may prove proarrhythmic. Proarrhythmia and antiarrhythmia are two sides of the same coin [1]. There is also a historical basis for the concern about proarrhythmia risk. In the late 1980s and 1990s, results from clinical trials of sodium channel blockers as antiarrhythmic agents revealed increased mortality when compared with placebo, despite significant suppression of premature ventricular contractions [2]. Separately, reports of case studies began to link the risk of torsades de pointes, which is a ventricular polymorphic arrhythmia, and ensuing ventricular fibrillation and death to drug action on a cardiac potassium ion channel not long before considered a reasonable candidate for antiarrhythmic therapy [3].

Here, we review physiological and historical considerations of proarrhythmia risks connected to antiarrhythmic drug development to frame a discussion about opportunities for antiarrhythmic drug development in the present regulatory environment. It should be stated at the outset that safety-minded, "regulatory" concepts and decisions have been proposed and embraced by everyone involved in the development of

Novel Therapeutic Targets for Antiarrhythmic Drugs, Edited by George Edward Billman
Copyright © 2010 John Wiley & Sons, Inc.

antiarrhythmic agents. These concepts include guidelines adopted in concert or separately by the pharmaceutical industry and regulatory agencies throughout the world. They also include recommendations adopted by medical associations, regarding clinical management of arrhythmias, patient risk stratification, and consideration of comorbidities and risk factors. Last but not least, in this examination, the term "regulatory" also includes authoritative opinions expressed in the published literature regarding practical drug development decisions, such as considerations about the design and conduct of randomized clinical trials. Increased awareness of safety concerns, combined with a better understanding of cardiovascular physiology and pathology, are leading to a more focused development of antiarrhythmic agents, side by side with increased exploration of novel avenues where the proarrhythmic risk is potentially lower, such as the prevention of arrhythmogenic remodeling [4].

8.2   BASIC PHYSIOLOGICAL CONSIDERATIONS

Approximately 25% of all cardiovascular-associated deaths, which is equivalent to 7% of all worldwide deaths, are ultimately connected to an arrhythmogenic basis disrupting the synchrony of cardiac sodium, potassium, and calcium ion fluxes [5]. Cardiac arrhythmias continue to be a huge clinical problem, in great part to the complexity of the disease. A basic triangle of factors play a role in their genesis: electrical instability, hemodynamic function, and ischemia, each presenting static and dynamic components [6].

Arrhythmias and their lethal consequences originate from the interplay of a receptive substrate and a transient initiating event or trigger [7, 8]. Mechanisms of cardiac arrhythmias are typically divided into two categories: enhanced or abnormal impulse formation and abnormal impulse conduction or propagation [9]. Enhanced normal automaticity and triggered activity are the best studied cellular mechanisms of abnormal impulse formation [10]. Reentry is a form of abnormal impulse conduction caused by reexcitation of a previously activated area of the heart [9] that depends on the balance between refractory and conduction properties [10]. It is the most commonly observed mechanism among clinical arrhythmias [6, 9, 11]. At the molecular level, impaired calcium cycling has been proposed to underlie arrhythmogenic impulse formation and propagation [12, 13]. Cellular events related to abnormal calcium handling have been implicated in both abnormal impulse formation and propagation [14–16]. Readers are referred to the chapters on basic cardiac electrophysiology and arrhythmia mechanisms for more detailed information on the physiological basis of arrhythmogenesis. Here, we review concepts that are directly pertinent to our safety-minded perspective, including the evolving understanding of antiarrhythmic agents.

8.2.1   Ion Channels and Arrhythmogenesis

The cardiac action potential, which is a representation of the changes in electrical potential differences across cardiac cell membranes as a function of time, is an ion-channel-driven process. At the body surface, the electrocardiogram (ECG) is a measurement of cardiac electrical activity, exhibiting a distinct pattern of waves, which are designated P, QRS, T, and sometimes U. These wave patterns correspond to the self-propagating wave of depolarizations and repolarizations from the sinoatrial node, which is the pacemaker region of the heart, through the atria, the atrioventricular node, and finally extending to the ventricles. The ECG has become an invaluable diagnostic tool of physiological and pathological activity. For example, abnormal elevation of the ST segment, abnormal lengthening of the QRS peak, and abnormal prolongation of the QT interval are useful clinical markers of arrhythmias.

Arrhythmia susceptibility at the molecular level is promoted by changes prolonging action potential duration and increasing intracellular calcium load, such as enhanced calcium current, reduced delayed rectifier potassium current, reduced transient outward potassium current, and reduced electrogenic sodium/potassium ATPase [17]. Arrhythmogenic triggers have been linked to abnormal calcium handling [18, 19].

The elucidation of monogenic inherited disorders linked to arrhythmias has provided insights into arrhythmogenic mechanisms. For instance, rare ion channelopathies involving the cardiac sodium channel gene have been linked to inherited arrhythmias, such as Brugada syndrome, sick sinus syndrome, and long QT syndrome. Similarly, mutations in the genes encoding subunits of the rapid and slow delayed rectifier cardiac potassium currents, I_{Kr} and I_{Ks}, have been linked to inherited long QT syndrome and short QT syndrome [20–25]. Pharmacological tools designed as antiarrhythmics have helped provide additional important details. One example is the pharmacological dissection of I_{Kr} and I_{Ks} in guinea pig ventricular myocytes, using the class III antiarrhythmic agent E-4031 [26]. That initial effort has led to an understanding of the complementary and somewhat overlapping properties of I_{Kr} and I_{Ks}, which are thought to form the basis for a ventricular repolarization reserve. Evidence linking arrhythmia risk factors with a reduction in this reserve has been presented [27].

At the cellular level, inhibition of I_{Kr} or I_{Ks} prolongs action potential duration (APD), a situation that can degenerate in afterdepolarizations, and particularly early afterdepolarizations (EADs), during the plateau phase of the cardiac action potential, when the cardiac cell membrane is vulnerable to minor alterations in the balance of inward and outward currents [13]. At the tissue level, a normal spatial dispersion of repolarization is imparted by slight differences in the complement of I_{Kr} and I_{Ks} currents across ventricular layers. Transmural dispersion of repolarization (TDR) across layers forming the ventricular wall has received much attention, because of its study in preclinical models [28–30], but analogous phenomena have been observed in atrial tissues also [31, 32]. An abnormal amplification of spatial dispersion is believed to be the substrate for arrhythmogenesis, at least for arrhythmias related to delayed ventricular repolarization [33]. Cases of the idiopathic ventricular fibrillation Brugada syndrome, which is diagnosed by ST segment elevation in the electrocardiogram and linked to loss of function in the SCN5A sodium channel gene, similarly implicate abnormal dispersion of repolarization. In these cases, disruptions, not in the major repolarizing event but in an early repolarizing event in epicardial cells, are proposed to alter the normal epicardial–endocardial electrical gradient [21, 34–36].

8.2.2 Antiarrhythmic Agents

Here, we summarize developments on the classification of antiarrhythmic agents proposed in the 1970s, its various revisions, and their critical review, based on previously published historical perspectives, reflective commentaries, and references therein [10, 37–46]. In the early 1970s, E.M. Vaughan Williams and B.N. Singh formulated a classification of mechanisms of action by antiarrhythmic drugs. A point made by these investigators is that their intent was to classify antiarrhythmic action and not the drugs themselves [38, 42–44, 47]. Grouping drugs by their dominant action followed closely a series of experimental studies of many structurally distinct compounds with discrete electrophysiological actions, including sodium channel blockers (class I action), β-adrenergic receptor blockers (class II action), drugs that selectively prolong cardiac repolarization (class III action), and calcium channel blockers (class IV action). Class I action was subclassified into Ia, Ib, and Ic groupings, based on clinical electrophysiological observations that were later connected biophysically to various modes of action on the open, closed and inactivated states of sodium channels [48–50]. Grouping drugs by their dominant action also led to the realization that many antiarrhythmic drugs in the clinic exerted a varying spectrum of actions with both beneficial and deleterious clinical effects. This uneasy understanding of benefit versus risk can be traced back to the 1920s, when mechanistic studies of quinidine on atrial fibrillation reported both its efficacy in restoring sinus rhythm and its proarrhythmic risk (reviewed in ref. 41).

The classification of antiarrhythmic actions in four admittedly disparate classes with regard to underlying mechanisms has been criticized as a hybrid, unsystematically based both on molecular targets and on mechanistic action, limited, and incomplete. In 1991, an alternative "framework" known as the Sicilian Gambit was proposed [51]. The point of departure for this framework was the complexity of drug action that, practically, prevents simple classification based on the most notable or dominant effect. The framework focuses on the molecular entities that underlie proarrhythmic substrates or triggers, and on the mechanisms responsible for arrhythmias, most notably the vulnerable parameters that may be more accessible to drug effects [51]. Since its initial proposal, the Sicilian Gambit has been revised, reviewed, and criticized [44, 45, 47, 52, 53]. The more recent revisions emphasize its pathophysiologic approach and its practical applications to develop novel antiarrhythmics [51, 54].

The Vaughan Williams classification is still predominantly used. The Sicilian Gambit framework can be practically viewed as an expansion, pointing to complexities beyond dominant antiarrhythmic action and primary molecular targets, and amenable to additional expansion. This is an important consideration, because our understanding of what constitutes an antiarrhythmic agent continues to evolve, based on the successes and disappointments of available therapies. Two cases in point, which are discussed below, are the transition from class I agents and focus on extinction of ectopic ventricular activity to class III agents and focus on prolongation of action potential duration, as well as the transition in targets, from molecules clearly implicated in cardiac electrical activity to molecules implicated in developing the proarrhythmic substrate. Insightful perspectives about the evolving understanding of antiarrhythmic agents have been presented [5, 6, 38, 40, 55–61].

8.3   HISTORICAL CONSIDERATIONS

Chronic pharmacological interventions on arrhythmias date back even earlier than the routine use of quinidine for atrial fibrillation early in the twentieth century. These interventions became widespread after sodium channel blockers were shown to virtually eliminate premature ventricular contractions (PVCs).* The correlation between sudden cardiac death and decreased PVCs, however, was not well studied, until the surprising findings of the Cardiac Arrhythmia Suppression Trial (CAST) in the late 1980s. This trial revealed that fleicainide and encainide, which are extremely effective agents in eliminating PVCs in postmyocardial infarction patients, paradoxically increased mortality compared with placebo, primarily because of an increased incidence of sudden cardiac death. Soon after these findings, mortality related to drug-acquired ventricular fibrillation was reported, implicating the inhibition of the ventricular I_{Kr} potassium channel and yet another class of antiarrhythmic agents. Almost 20 years later, the chronic use of antiarrhythmic drugs has been increasingly limited by the risk of proarrhythmia and the availability of highly effective nonpharmacological alternatives, particularly ablation and cardioverter defibrillators [10, 41].

8.3.1   CAST: Background, Clinical Findings, and Aftermath

The scientific efforts that fueled the initial characterization and classification of antiarrhythmic agents also fostered a line of reasoning regarding arrhythmogenesis that became known as the "electrical accident" hypothesis. This narrow view of arrhythmias proposed that PVCs initiated a chaotic disorganization of cardiac electrical activity degenerating in fibrillation and death. Accordingly, suppression of PVCs was proposed to prevent lethal sustained ventricular tachyarrhythmias, and early successes with the class Ia agent lidocaine led to widespread efforts for better "PVC killers," such as the class Ic agents flecainide and encainide (reviewed in ref. 55). Several clinical trials were completed to demonstrate that these agents reduced the frequency of PVCs in patients thought to be at risk of sudden cardiac death [62, 63], but none of the trials were large enough to determine the simpler but more fundamental question about reduction of sudden death. It was only after the drugs were already in the market that a large-scale, randomized controlled trial was proposed to determine effects of class Ic agents on mortality, and specifically on sudden cardiac death. The trial directly tested the hypothesis that the suppression of asymptomatic or mildly symptomatic PVCs in survivors of myocardial infarction

---

*A premature ventricular contraction (PVC), also known as a premature ventricular complex, ventricular premature contraction or complex (VPC), ventricular premature beat (VPB), or extrasystole, is a relatively common event where the heartbeat is initiated by the heart ventricles rather than by the sinoatrial node.

would decrease the number of deaths from ventricular arrhythmias and improve overall survival.

To evaluate the possibility of success of such a trial, a pilot trial was conducted, designated as the Cardiac Arrhythmia Pilot Study (CAPS). In this randomized, double-blind study, which started in September of 1982, one of four antiarrhythmic drugs (flecainide, encainide, moricizine, and imipramine) were compared with placebo in 502 patients with at least 10 PVCs/hour 6 to 60 days after acute myocardial infarction. Patients were followed for a year, and all death and cardiac arrest events were classified as cardiac arrhythmic, cardiac nonarrhythmic, or noncardiac. The sole purpose of CAPS was to test the feasibility of conducting a larger scale trial to test specifically the hypothesis that suppression of PVCs after acute myocardial infarction could improve survival [64–66]. Of the 502 patients, 108, 119, 56, 77, and 87 patients were assigned, respectively, to encainide, flecainide, imipramine, moricizine, and placebo at the end of dosing. A total of 55 patients (11%) withdrew or died in all treatment arms before the completion of dosing. As anticipated, there were no observed statistically significant differences in survival among any of the treatment groups, because the CAPS was not designed to have the statistical power to detect differences in survival [66].

CAST was initiated in August of 1986 to determine whether drug treatment of asymptomatic ventricular arrhythmias in postmyocardial infarction patients reduced the incidence of sudden cardiac death and total mortality. Patients with asymptomatic or mildly symptomatic ventricular arrhythmia (six or more PVCs per hour) after myocardial infarction were placed in one of three treatment groups (encainide, flecainide, or moricizine) or in a placebo group. By March 1989, 2309 patients had been recruited for the initial drug-titration phase of the study: 1727 (75%) had initial suppression of their arrhythmia through the use of one of the three study drugs and had been randomly assigned to receive active drug or placebo. During an average follow-up of 10 months, the patients treated with active drug had a higher rate of mortality from arrhythmia than the patients assigned to placebo. Encainide and flecainide accounted for the excess of deaths from arrhythmia and nonfatal cardiac arrests, in the following manner: 33 of 730 patients taking encainide or flecainide (4.5%), as opposed to 9 of 725 taking placebo (1.2%). These drugs also accounted for the higher total mortality (7.7% for drugs; 3.0% for placebo). Because of these results, the part of the trial involving encainide and flecainide was discontinued [2, 67].

Without a clear involvement of moricizine in excess mortality, a separate arm of the trial, comparing moricizine and placebo, was allowed to continue as CAST-II, with a modified protocol [68]. CAST-II was divided into two blinded, randomized phases: an early, 14-day exposure phase that evaluated the risk of starting treatment with moricizine after myocardial infarction (1325 patients), and a long-term phase that evaluated the effect of moricizine on survival after myocardial infarction in patients whose ventricular premature depolarizations were either adequately suppressed by moricizine (1155 patients) or only partially suppressed (219 patients). The trial was stopped early because the first 14-day period of treatment with moricizine after a myocardial infarction was associated with excess mortality (17 of 665 patients died or had cardiac arrests), as compared with no treatment or placebo (3 of 660 patients died or had cardiac arrests). Estimates of conditional power indicated that it was highly unlikely (less than 8 percent chance) that a survival benefit from moricizine could be observed if the trial were completed. At the completion of the long-term phase, 49 deaths or cardiac arrests occurred because of arrhythmias in patients assigned to moricizine, and 42 deaths occurred in patients assigned to placebo [69, 70].

In conclusion, the use of the antiarrhythmic agents flecainide, encainide, and moricizine to suppress asymptomatic or mildly symptomatic ventricular premature depolarizations to try to reduce mortality after myocardial infarction was shown to be not only ineffective but also harmful. In the aftermath of CAST and CAST II, many noteworthy editorials, reviews, and opinion articles were issued [71–75]. A particular focus of interest was the failure of PVC suppression as a surrogate end point for mortality, and a search for alternative prognostic and diagnostic measures, pursued in follow-up and sub-studies [76–79]. A separate focus of interest, alluded to in the previous section, was the class Ic antiarrhythmic action of the potent PVC suppressors responsible for the increased cardiac mortality. Scrutiny of this antiarrhythmic action, which is characterized by slow sodium channel blocking kinetics effecting slower ventricular action potential depolarization without a marked change in action potential duration, favored attention to theoretical considerations about ideal antiarrhythmic action. Ideal agents, as envisioned in a *modulated receptor* hypothesis, would be effective in terminating arrhythmias and would produce no adverse actions in the absence of arrhythmias. These considerations led to interest in class III agents that would prolong cardiac action potential in rate-dependent fashion based on use-dependent block characteristics [40, 54, 80–82].

Adverse clinical findings in the early 1990s, involving noncardiac drugs, presented new challenges, impacting particularly class III agents. A connection was made between excessive QT prolongation and drug-acquired cases of the polymorphic ventricular arrhythmia torsades de pointes. Consequent research implicated I_{Kr} and its molecular correlate (hERG channel; KCNH2 gene), a ventricular potassium channel actively considered at the time as a class III antiarrhythmic target, which prompted a reevaluation of all existing strategies for antiarrhythmic development. In addition, mortality trials on class III agents have been disappointing, in some cases, such as the SWORD trial of d-sotalol, showing evidence of increased risk compared with placebo [83]. In the next section, we turn our attention to these important topics.

8.3.2 Torsades de Pointes and hERG Channel Inhibition: Safety Pharmacology Concern with Critical Impact on Antiarrhythmic Development

The connection between abnormal prolongation of the QT interval and predisposition to torsades de pointes is well established [84], although the role of additional risk factors [85] and alternate measurements of proarrhythmic risk [13, 85–88] continue to be discussed. The genetic characterization of inherited forms of QT prolongation (long QT syndrome), implicating loss of function in I_{Kr} and I_{Ks}, and gain of function in the cardiac sodium channel, presented a challenge to antiarrhythmic development strategies based on action at these molecules [22, 25, 89, 90]. A more direct challenge arose based on clinical reports of drug-acquired torsades de pointes and ensuing mechanistic studies implicating primarily the hERG channel, which is a molecular correlate of I_{Kr}. [3, 24, 91–95].

The first notable examples of drugs removed from the market because of documented cases of torsades de pointes were the antihistamines terfenadine and astemizole, which are marketed as Seldane™ and Hismanal™, respectively. The proarrhythmic potential of these drugs is clearly caused by hERG inhibition resulting in long QT and precipitating into torsades de pointes. Both drugs inhibit the hERG channel potently at low nanomolar concentrations. Because of extensive first-pass metabolic transformation before entering the systemic circulation, the drugs do not normally accumulate to nanomolar levels in plasma, and the concentrations that inhibit hERG channels are deemed "supratherapeutic." Instances of drug-related torsades de pointes have been generally attributed to changes in the normal drug metabolism, such as the reported increase in unmetabolized terfenadine after concomitant ketoconazole administration [96]. In the case of astemizole and its first-pass metabolite, desmethylastemizole, proarrhythmic effects were correlated to "therapeutic" concentrations of the metabolite, similarly efficacious as the parent molecule. After close examination of hERG inhibition, it was found that desmethylastemizole inhibits hERG with nanomolar potency similar to astemizole [91, 92].

Since the 1990s, several other marketed drugs and many drug development programs have been affected adversely by the intricate connection between hERG channel block and torsades de pointes. Retrospectives and analyses have been published elsewhere [84, 85, 88, 95, 97–105]. Like the results of CAST only a few years before, these findings and their ripple effect throughout the pharmaceutical industry and regulatory agencies affected antiarrhythmic drug development [41, 106]. Yet, one should be reminded that, even before CAST, there was a sobering understanding about the unintended consequences of any pharmacological intervention aimed at cardiac rhythm control.

It is important to note that restrictive "black box" warnings had been issued in the United States for many antiarrhythmic agents in connection to CAST findings and class Ic-related mortality. This information has been reviewed in a comprehensive analysis of drugs approved in the years 1975–2000 [107]. Since the year 2000, new "black box" warnings have been issued for antiarrhythmic agents, either specifically related to QT prolongation or related to less well-defined proarrhythmic concerns. Table 8.1 presents a summary of "black box" labels and market withdrawals among antiarrhythmic agents. Other agents, like propafenone hydrochloride, have had their labels modified to include proarrhythmic effect warnings and contraindications. An independent assessment of the risk of torsades de pointes among marketed antiarrhythmic agents is also available from the Arizona Center for Education and Research on Therapeutics (CERT; see next section for additional information on this organization). Table 8.2 summarizes torsades de pointes risk information extracted from Arizona CERT drug lists, which was revised in March 2008.

Antiarrhythmic agents, as a therapeutic class, have been impacted by findings of drug-acquired QT prolongation; class III antiarrhythmic agents, especially those known to act by inhibiting the hERG channel, have been obviously affected. This

Table 8.1. Antiarrhythmic Drugs with a "Black Box" Warning

Drug Name	Warning
Disopyramide phosphate	Increased mortality with class Ic antiarrhythmics
Mexiletine hydrochloride	Increased mortality with class Ic antiarrhythmics
Flecainide acetate	Increased mortality with class Ic antiarrhythmics
Encainide hydrochloride[1]	Increased mortality in patients with asymptomatic ventricular arrhythmias
Propafene hydrochloride	Increased mortality with class Ic antiarrhythmics
Bepridil hydrochloride	Increased mortality with class Ic antiarrhythmics
Moricizine	Increased mortality with class Ic antiarrhythmics
Dofetilide	Ventricular arrhythmia, primarily TdP associated with QT prolongation
Ibutilide fumarate	Ventricular arrhythmia, primarily TdP[2] associated with QT prolongation
Sotalol hydrochloride	Restricted dose regiment because of a risk of ventricular arrhythmia, primarily TdP associated with QT prolongation
Amiodarone	Pulmonary toxicity, hepatic injury, and worsened arrhythmia

[1]Eventually withdrawn from the market for safety reasons.
[2]TdP: Torsades de Pointes.

safety concern, nevertheless, does not completely close the door on discovery and development efforts centering on the I_{Ks} (KCNQ1/KCNE1) channel [108] or even the hERG channel [109]. Rather, it presents challenges and opportunities. The main challenge is a clearer understanding of the fine balance constituting normal cardiac

Table 8.2. TdP Risk Associated with Antiarrhythmic Drugs (from Arizona CERT)

Torsade List[1]	
Amiodarone	Females > Males, TdP risk regarded as low
Disopyramide	Females > Males
Dofetilide	
Ibutilide	Females > Males
Procainamide	
Quinidine	Females > Males
Sotalol	Females > Males
Possible Torsade List[2]	
Flecainide	
Conditional Torsade List[3]	
Mexiletine	

[1]Drugs that are generally accepted by the QTdrugs.org Advisory Board of the Arizona CERT to have a risk of causing torsade de pointes.
[2]Drugs that, in some reports, have been associated with torsades de pointes and/or QT prolongation but at this time lack substantial evidence for causing torsades de pointes.
[3]Drugs that, in some reports, have been weakly associated with torsades de pointes and/or QT prolongation but that are unlikely to be a risk for torsades de pointes when used in usual recommended dosages and in patients without other risk factors.

repolarization and of proarrhythmic and antiarrhythmic disruptions to that balance. Testable hypotheses, like the amplification of spatial dispersion of repolarization [33], the role of a repolarization reserve [27], or a possible connection between proarrhythmic risk and state-dependent interactions between drug and channel target, present opportunities. Inherited proarrhythmic disorders provide additional opportunities, for example in the seemingly paradoxical proarrhythmic consequences of hERG-channel mediated long-QT and short-QT syndromes [110].

8.3.3   Recent Clinical Trials

We close this section on historical considerations with an overview of recent clinical trials to illustrate important safety-minded trends. These trials reflect the shift toward class III antiarrhythmic agents mentioned above. They also reflect a shift toward supraventricular arrhythmias, where conversion and maintenance of sinus rhythm is the overriding consideration, and mortality risk is not a major concern. Recent trials have also defined the therapeutic space for devices, such as implantable cardioverter defibrillators (ICDs). ICDs have been clearly effective in reducing mortality, leading to their widespread use, despite cost and quality of life considerations [111–114]. In this regard, recent clinical trials have explored adverse effects by inappropriate shocks [115] and mitigation of undesirable effects by antiarrhythmic drugs [116, 117].

Table 8.3 presents a representative, not exhaustive, list of antiarrhythmic clinical trials after CAST. Sotalol trials, testing effects of d,l-sotalol, with mixed class II and III action, showed modest reduction on mortality over placebo [118, 119], but when the pure class III effect was tested, on the SWORD trial using d-sotalol, a small risk increase was noted [83, 120, 121]. Amiodarone, which is categorized as a class III agent but is known to act by its effect on multiple cardiac ion channels, has shown modest and not completely reproducible success on patients with myocardial infarction (MI), ventricular arrhythmias or left ventricular dysfunction [122, 123]. Dronedarone, which is a derivative developed to remove extracardiac adverse effects of amiodarone, was initially tested on the ANDROMEDA trial, on high-risk patients with moderate-to-severe congestive heart failure and ventricular dysfunction. This trial was discontinued because of the potential excess risk of death in the dronedarone group [124]. It should be noted, however, that excess mortality in the dronedarone arm of ANDROMEDA has been qualified and recently questioned [125]. Trials with other class III agents, like the recent ALIVE trial, testing effects of azimilide, has shown no overall survival benefit on post-MI patients [126].

More recently, dronedarone has been clinically tested to treat supraventricular arrhythmias, such as atrial fibrillation. In these trials (EURIDIS and ADONIS), maintaining sinus rhythm and not reducing mortality risk was the overriding consideration, and dronedarone showed longer time to atrial fibrillation relapse than placebo [124]. Furthermore, preliminary results from the ATHENA trial [127], presented in abstract form, indicate that dronedarone reduced the incidence of the composite outcome of cardiovascular hospitalisation or death in patients with atrial fibrillation or flutter; 29% of patients had a history of heart failure compared with

Table 8.3. Recent Clinical Trials Involving Antiarrhythmic Drugs

Trial	Year	Patients (n)	Findings	Agent(s)
Sotalol	1982	1456	Reduced mortality risk (7.3% mortality vs. 8.9% in placebo)	Racemic mixture of D- and L-sotalol
SWORD	1996	3121	Increased mortality risk (5% mortality vs. 3.1% in placebo)	D-sotalol
EMIAT	1997	1486	Reduced arrhythmic but not overall mortality risk (7.2% mortality both groups)	Amiodarone
ALIVE	2004	3717	No overall benefit in post-MI patients	Azimilide
AVID	1997	1016	ICD: 25% mortality; antiarrhythmic: 36% at 3 years	Amiodarone or sotalol vs. ICDs
SHIELD	2004	633	Reduced incidence of ICD therapies	Azimilide in patients with ICDs
DIAMOND	2001	3028	59% vs. 34% cardioversion in 506/3028 AF patients	Dofetilide
ADONIS	2004	625	59% vs. 70% (placebo) rate of relapse of atrial arrhythmia	Dronedarone
CRAFT	2007	56	56% vs. 5% cardioversion (high dose vs. placebo)	Vernakalant (RSD1235)
BEAUTIFUL		10917	reduced secondary endpoints (hospital admission for fatal and non-fatal MI and coronary revascularization in high-rate subgroup)	Ivabradine

placebo [128]. These recent findings are being closely followed in light of prior findings in the ANDROMEDA trial [125].

Newer agents, such as dofetilide and vernakalant, have been developed and tested for the treatment of atrial fibrillation. Dofetilide is an I_{Kr} inhibitor, with known ventricular proarrhythmic liability and limited use. With appropriate considerations regarding dose and patient enrollment, as shown for example in the DIAMOND studies, dofetilide was proven to be more effective than placebo on patients with left ventricular dysfunction, converting to sinus rhythm and preventing atrial fibrillation relapse, while showing no differences in mortality risk in patients with MI or chronic heart failure (CHF). [129–131]. Vernakalant, which is an inhibitor of the atrial-specific I_{Kur} ultrarrapid potassium current and cardiac sodium current, was shown to be effective in stopping recent-onset atrial fibrillation in CRAFT, a phase II clinical trial [132], and more recently, in preliminary form, in the ACT I-III trials [125]. Ivabradine, an inhibitor of the I_f current in the sinoatrial node and indicated for rate control, was tested on a large-scale, randomized trial on high-risk populations with coronary artery disease and ventricular dysfunction. The drug was shown to be marginally effective, not on primary mortality outcomes but on related secondary outcomes, on a high-risk, predefined subpopulation of patients with heart rates higher than 70 beats per minute [133, 134]. The development of newer antiarrhythmic agents for atrial fibrillation is also worth noting in light of an ongoing discussion about the merits of rhythm control versus rate control for this therapeutic need. Readers are referred to other reviews and primary sources related to the Atrial Fibrillation Follow-up Investigation of Rhythm Management (AFFIRM) clinical trial, for additional information [135–137].

With regards to ICDs, cost and quality-of-life concerns notwithstanding, some experts have proposed their prophylactic implantation [138]. The MADDIT trial, comparing ICDs with "conventional therapy," gave the first indication on the effectiveness of ICDs on high-risk patients [139]. The AVID trial, comparing amiodarone or sotalol to ICDs, was designed to determine whether placement of an ICD or antiarrhythmic drug therapy resulted in longer survival in patients with life-threatening ventricular arrhythmias. The study was terminated prematurely because of a 26% to 31% reduction in mortality over 1 to 3 years with ICD therapy [111, 123, 140, 141]. With the increasingly prevalent use of ICDs, more recent clinical trials have explored mitigating action by antiarrhythmics, for example on refractory arrhythmias leading to frequent defibrillator shocks. One prominent example is the SHIELD trial, where azimilide was found to reduce electrical episodes triggering ICD shocks [116, 117].

8.4 OPPORTUNITIES FOR ANTIARRHYTHMIC DRUG DEVELOPMENT IN THE PRESENT REGULATORY ENVIRONMENT

In this section, we review the regulatory environment, focusing first on the International Conference on Harmonization of Technical Requirements for Registration of Pharmaceuticals for Human Use (ICH) and guidelines related to cardiac safety subsequently adopted directly by regulatory agencies in the United States, the European Union, and Japan. In second place, we review additional regulatory guidance relevant to antiarrhythmic drug development. In third place, we review guidelines for clinical management of arrhythmias, expert opinion on randomized clinical trials, and emerging considerations about genomic variability in the patient population. Together, these considerations address concerns about a heterogeneous, stratified patient population on which antiarrhythmic development is pursued. Finally, we mention what could be termed consortial efforts by academic, industry, and government scientists, impacting the regulatory environment.

With this information, and integrating the physiological and historical lessons from previous sections, we will describe where the opportunities exist and how they are being explored. The major lesson in this final section is the continuing evolution in our understanding of antiarrhythmic agents and the connection between opportunity and unmet medical need. In the years ahead, pharmacological interventions to prevent arrhythmias will continue to play an important role, but this role is expected to be increasingly focused. Taking into account the different mechanisms of arrhythmias, the improvements in risk classification, and the genetic diversity among the patient population, among other factors, notions of widely applicable blockbuster therapies seem unrealistic.

8.4.1 ICH—S7A and S7B; E14

The ICH was created in 1990 as a project uniting the regulatory agencies of Europe, Japan, and the United States with experts from the pharmaceutical industry in the three regions, to discuss scientific and technical aspects of product registration. The stated goal of the ICH is a more economical use of human, animal, and material resources, as well as the elimination of unnecessary delays in the global development and availability of new medicines, while maintaining safeguards on quality, safety, and efficacy, as well as regulatory obligations to protect public health [142]. In addition to the six permanent members, World Health Organization (WHO), European Free Trade Association (EFTA), and Canada (represented by Health Canada) have observer status. These non-voting members act as a link between the ICH and non-ICH countries and regions. In addition, the ICH Global Cooperation Group, a subcommittee of the ICH steering committee, is charged with greater global harmonization, by interaction with other regional harmonization initiatives, namely Asia-Pacific Economic Cooperation (APEC), Association of Southeast Asian Nations (ASEAN), Gulf Cooperation Countries (GCC), Pan American Network on Drug Regulatory Harmonization (PANDRH), and Southern African Development Community (SADC). These organizations have been invited to designate permanent representatives to the ICH Global Cooperation Group. Among the six ICH parties, the mechanism for harmonization is a stepwise process of consensus building on a draft guideline or recommendation, followed by the initiation of consultation and regulatory action within each of the three regions, arriving to a tripartite harmonized text. At the consultation step, feedback is received from regulatory organizations and industry associates, both within the ICH and outside. When a harmonized document is fully adopted, regulatory implementation according to normal mechanisms within each of the three regions ensues. ICH guidelines, which are categorized into quality, safety, efficacy, and multidisciplinary topics, move through the steps of harmonization and become instruments of useful discussion and debate until their eventual recognition as widely applied, enforceable standards and procedures throughout the pharmaceutical industry. Quality topics relate to chemical and pharmaceutical quality assurance; safety topics, to *in vitro* and *in vivo* preclinical studies; efficacy topics, to clinical studies in human subjects; and multidisciplinary topics, to cross-cutting issues not neatly defined as any of the other three categories. Figure 8.1 summarizes the ICH structure and the ICH guideline harmonization process. Readers are referred to the ICH website and related links for additional information [142].

The recognition of safety pharmacology as a discipline on its own right can be attributed, to a great extent, to the implementation in Europe, Japan, and the United States, of ICH guideline S7A, on Safety Pharmacology Studies for Human Pharmaceuticals. Since its adoption by regulatory agencies in 2000, safety pharmacology studies have been an important component of all regulatory submissions. These studies are defined in the S7A document as "those studies that investigate the potential undesirable pharmacodynamic effects of a substance on physiological functions in relation to exposure in the therapeutic range and above" [143]. The view of safety

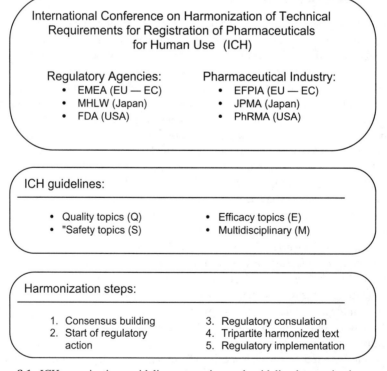

Figure 8.1. ICH organization, guideline categories, and guideline harmonization process.

pharmacology as a distinct scientific discipline integrating best practices from other disciplines is now well established, and it has been recently reviewed [144–149]. Here, we highlight details about the safety pharmacology guideline, its companion guideline ICH S7B, and the related efficacy guideline for clinical studies ICH E14. Table 8.4 summarizes these and other related guidelines.

The ICH S7A guideline recommends a core battery of *in vivo* observations, investigating the cardiovascular, respiratory, and nervous systems, preferably in non-anesthetized animals chronically instrumented for telemetry measurements. Core cardiovascular studies mentioned in the document include measurements of blood pressure, heart rate, and the electrocardiogram. Core respiratory measurements include respiratory rate and other measurements of respiratory function, such as tidal volume and hemoglobin oxygen saturation. Core nervous system measurements include motor activity, coordination, behavioral changes, sensory/motor reflex responses, and body temperature, using commonly accepted methodologies, such as the functional observation battery. S7A also mentions the possible need of follow-up studies within each of the core systems and supplemental studies on other systems. The document is not meant to be an exhaustive or prescriptive list of safety pharmacology studies. It is, rather, a reminder of the importance and usefulness of traditional pharmacology on well-accepted and tested animal models [143].

Table 8.4. ICH Guidelines Relevant to Antiarrhythmic Drug Development

ICH guideline	Harmonization step	Date
E6(R1): Good Clinical Practice	5	1996
E8: General Considerations for Clinical Trials	5	1997
M3: ICH Guideline on Non-Clinical Safety Studies for the Conduct of Human Clinical Trials for Pharmaceuticals	4	1997
M3(R1): Maintenance of the ICH Guideline on Non-Clinical Safety Studies for the Conduct of Human Clinical Trials for Pharmaceuticals [1]	5	2000
S7A: Safety Pharmacology Studies for Human Pharmaceuticals	5	2000
S7B: The Nonclinical Evaluation of the Potential for Delayed Ventricular Repolarization (QT Interval Prolongation) By Human Pharmaceuticals	5	2005
E14: The Clinical Evaluation of QT/QTc Interval Prolongation and Proarrhythmic Potential for Non-Antiarrhythmic Drugs	5	2005
E14: The Clinical Evaluation of QT/QTc Interval Prolongation and Proarrhythmic Potential for Non-Antiarrhythmic Drugs Questions & Answers	5	2008
M3(R2): Guidance on Nonclinical Safety Studies for the Conduct of Human Clinical Trials and Marketing Authorization for Pharmaceuticals [2]	2	2008

[1] Amended under the Maintenance process of the ICH.
[2] Additional harmonization on scope and duration of nonclinical safety studies.

The ICH S7B guideline on Safety Pharmacology Studies for Assessing the Potential for Delayed Ventricular Repolarization (QT interval prolongation) by Human Pharmaceuticals was approved for wide implementation in 2005. The important circumstances behind the drafting of this guideline were the withdrawal of four major drugs from the market (terfenadine, astemizole, grepafloxacin, and cisapride) in the 1990s, the imposition of availability restrictions on several others, and a general desire for an improvement in the preclinical determination of this risk for new investigational drugs. In 1997, the Committee for Proprietary Medicinal Products (CPMP; now CHMP, Committee on Medicinal Products for Human Use) of the EMEA, EU, issued a "points to consider" document outlining a number of recommendations for *in vitro* and *in vivo* safety studies to address the potential for QT prolongation [150], which was later harmonized in the ICH draft guideline. The prolongation of the QT interval in the electrocardiogram has been recognized as a useful marker for abnormal electrical activity, which may lead to ventricular fibrillation and cardiac death, despite caveats in its accurate prediction of the risk for torsades de pointes [13, 84, 86–88]. The finalized S7B guideline emphasizes *in vivo* studies of long QT prolongation in animal models and *in vitro* studies of IKr/hERG current, and it refers to an "integrated risk assessment" in general terms.

The ICH guideline E14 on Clinical Evaluation of QT/QTc Interval Prolongation and Proarrhythmic Potential for Non-Antiarrhythmic Drugs was also finalized in 2005. It outlines the conduct of a "thorough QT/QTc study" during clinical trials (QTc refers to the QT interval corrected for changes in heart rate). The underlying rationale behind this guideline is whether preclinical testing can sufficiently exclude a clinical risk for the prolongation of QT and proarrhythmia. ICH E14 views the conduct of the "thorough QT/QTc study" as a requirement of most clinical trials [151]. Implementation of the guideline has had great impact on all drug development programs, and it continues to generate discussion [152, 153]. As reviewed above, additional factors influence torsades de pointes risk. The incidence of a clinically identifiable risk is extremely low, and the number of subjects studied during clinical trials might not be sufficient to prognosticate risk. Another concern is the relevance of studying normal subjects, as opposed to a population with idiosyncratic predisposition for a long QT interval.

8.4.2 Additional Regulatory Guidance

Notably, the European Medicines Agency has issued fairly detailed guidance for the development of antiarrhythmics, either specifically or within the larger context of cardiovascular disease prevention. Noteworthy documents are summarized on Table 8.5. Readers are referred to the EMEA website for additional details. Here, we highlight the guidance on antiarrhythmics (1996) and its recent addendum on atrial fibrillation (2008). The first point made is that critical evaluation of efficacy and safety of antiarrhythmic agents is complicated by the following:

1. The drugs themselves, which differ in their mechanism of action, activity, cardiac, or extra-cardiac effects; kinetics; drug interactions; interactions with devices; and proarrhythmic effects

Table 8.5. EMEA Guidances Relevant to Antiarrhythmic Drug Development

Regulatory Guidance	Drug development stage	Date
Note for guidance on antiarrhythmics CPMP/EWP/ 237/95[1]	Clinical efficacy/safety	1996
Points to Consider: the Assessment of the Potential for QT Interval Prolongation by Non-Cardiovascular Medicinal Products[2]	Nonclinical/preclinical	1997
Points to Consider on Clinical Investigation of New Medicinal Products for the Treatment of Acute Coronary syndrome (ACS) without persistent ST-Segment Elevation	Clinical efficacy/safety	2000
Reflection Paper on Gender Differences in Cardiovascular Diseases CHMP/EWP/498145/06	Clinical efficacy/safety	2007[3]
Evaluation of Medicinal Products for Cardiovascular Disease Prevention CHMP/EWP/311890/07	Clinical efficacy/safety	2008[4]
Note for guidance on antiarrhytmics—addendum on atrial fibrillation CHMP/EWP/352438/08	Clinical efficacy/safety	2008[5]

[1]CPMP, Committee for Proprietary Medicinal Products; now CHMP, Committee on Medicinal Products for Human Use
[2]Replaced by ICH S7A and taken off EMEA website on May 18, 2006
[3]Released for consultation Dec 2006; deadline for comments Mar 2007
[4]Released for consultation Jul 2007; deadline for comments Jan 2008
[5]Released for consultation Jul 2008; deadline for comments Jan 2009

2. Heterogeneity in rhythm disorders, which differ in pathogenesis, origin, manifestations, duration, prognostic significance, stability of pathogenetic mechanisms, instability in clinical expression, and underlying and/or concomitant diseases

3. The aim of the treatment—to improve the patient's condition by diminishing disabling symptoms and/or increase life expectancy, and whether it is curative, prophylactic, or palliative.

With regard to clinical studies and methods to assess efficacy, one important consideration is the need for multiple lead ECG studies (at least the standard 12 lead ECG) and continuous long-term ECG recording, e.g., Holter monitoring, 24 h before and during therapy. The importance of survival studies in randomized clinical trials with a large number of patients is mandatory or desirable. To minimize risks, therapeutic clinical studies should be initiated in specialized hospitals under close surveillance by experienced cardiologists with broad experience in antiarrhythmic products.

The stated goal of the addendum on atrial fibrillation is to cover previously incomplete regulatory guidance. It begins with an assessment of antiarrhythmic development, noting the detrimental effects by class I and class III antiarrhythmics, the decline in the number of new drugs intended for the treatment of ventricular arrhythmias, and a shift in attention to areas like atrial fibrillation, because proarrhythmic effects seem to be less dominant in supraventricular arrhythmias. Regarding clinical trials, the assessment of a variety of outcomes in every trial is recommended, because of the complex consequences of atrial fibrillation. Primary efficacy, whether rhythm or rate control, should be the focus, but other measures of clinical benefit—symptomatic improvement, morbidity, and mortality—need to be assessed. If restoration of sinus rhythm is claimed, then successful conversion, i.e., termination of atrial fibrillation, should be the primary end point. If rate control is claimed, then resting heart rate and heart rate during moderate exercise are relevant efficacy measures. Symptoms and atrial fibrillation-related quality of life are considered secondary outcome parameters. Regarding patient selection, the type of atrial fibrillation should be documented as first detected, paroxysmal, persistent, and permanent, because the inherent risk for recurrent atrial fibrillation and atrial fibrillation-related complications is influenced by the patient characteristics. Study design requirements may vary, depending on the claimed indication.

The Food and Drug Administration (FDA) in the United States has not issued analogous guidance documents, except for its endorsement of ICH harmonized guidelines. More broadly, we can mention clinical/medical and procedural guidances on the conduct of clinical trials that are relevant to the development of antiarrhythmic agents. These documents are summarized on Table 8.6. Readers are referred to the original material, which is available at the FDA website.

8.4.3   Clinical Management Guidelines and Related Considerations About Patient Populations

Assigning the mortality risk of arrhythmias to the patient population at large is important, not only for clinical management but also for continuous improvement on clinical trial design. Stratification refers to the classification of patients in groups, as risk is assessed. In assessing risk, one must consider the mechanism of arrhythmia (for example, abnormal impulse formation versus abnormal impulse propagation), its site of origin (for example, ventricular versus supra-ventricular), and its etiology (for example, risk posed by ventricular tachycardia after prior myocardial infarction versus asymptomatic ventricular tachycardia). Existing methodologies to diagnose risk,

Table 8.6. FDA Guidances Relevant to Antiarrhythmic Drug Development

Regulatory Guidance	Drug development stage	Date
Guidance for Institutional Review Boards and Clinical Investigators	Information sheet guidances	1998
Guidance for Clinical Trial Sponsors On the Establishment and Operation of Clinical Trial Data Monitoring Committees	Clinical/medical	2006
Guidance for Industry and Review Staff Target Product Profile—A Strategic Development Process Tool	Procedural	2007

including ambulatory ECG recordings, invasive electrophysiologic study, signal-averaged ECG, echocardiography, heart rate variability, and T-wave alternans, have been reviewed [6, 122]. Refining risk stratification continues to be a priority, because the cumulative incidence of sudden death in the whole population remains large, as the majority of sudden deaths occur in low-risk segments of the population [154]. In this context, we discuss the following three concerns centered on assessing the risk of arrhythmia in the population at large: professional guidelines for the management of arrhythmia patients, considerations about design and interpretation of randomized clinical trials, and considerations about genetic determinants.

Professional organizations, such as the American College of Cardiology, the American Heart Association, and the European Society of Cardiology, have come together to issue guidelines for the management of patients with ventricular arrhythmias and the prevention of sudden cardiac death [155], management of patients with supraventricular arrhythmias [156], and management of patients with atrial fibrillation [157]. More recently, guidelines for device-based therapies of cardiac rhythm abnormalities have been issued [158]. These critical evaluations of diagnostic procedures and therapies to detect, manage, or prevent arrhythmias have helped define needs and opportunities in antiarrhythmic development, for example, improving risk stratification in patients with high risk of sudden cardiac death, where the conventional classification, based on left ventricular ejection fraction (LVEF) is inadequate (reviewed in ref. 122). One recent example of this refinement in risk stratification is a post-hoc analysis of the AVID study mentioned above, comparing ICDs with antiarrhythmic drugs. The initial results of the study relied on LVEF at 35% to stratify risk and enroll patients. The post-hoc analysis, using the baseline history of CHF as discriminator, established that the survival advantage with an ICD, as compared with antiarrhythmic drug therapy, is largely restricted to patients with a history of CHF [159]. Clearly, an inextricable connection exists between improvements in the classification and in the clinical trials where novel antiarrhythmic treatments are tested [160–162].

A comprehensive, critical examination of randomized clinical trials and the rigor necessary for their successful design, conduct, and interpretation, with particular relevance to antiarrhythmic development, has been offered [163–167]. The lessons derived center on the following issues: surrogate outcome measures, composite clinical end points, subgroups and treatment interactions, structural issues in the conduct of trials, bias minimization, monitoring, ethical mandates, negative trends, publication of negative trials, inferiority trials, confirmation trials, and specification of primary and secondary end points [163, 164]. Here, we review some of these lessons in detail.

Surrogate outcomes, which are measured instead of clinical outcomes, allow for shorter, less costly studies, with fewer subjects, and also for monitoring the effect of therapy on individual patients. Potential surrogates, however, need to predict the relevant clinical outcome, and fully or nearly capture the effect on clinical outcome. Looking back to CAST, one can reasonably recognize PVC suppression as a widely accepted, but not thoroughly validated, proposed surrogate for the clinical outcome of reduced cardiac mortality after myocardial infarction. The forward-looking challenge remains to ensure thorough validation of proposed surrogate outcome measures, and thoughtful proposals have been made in this regard [168].

Composite clinical end points, for example measurements of overall and cardiac arrhythmic mortality in CAPS and CAST, are highly valuable but pose problematic interpretation when elements of the composite seem to go in opposite directions. Assigning unequal weight to individual end points in composite measures is a good strategy to facilitate interpretation, but there is little agreement on objective criteria to achieve this task.

The evaluation of treatment effects in subgroups with the use of baseline variables is intuitively advocated to provide clinicians insights into the treatment of their individual patients. This lesson is related to the connection between clinical trials and patient management guidelines mentioned above. Advance subgroup analysis and independent confirmation of subgroup findings are recommended, along with a reminder that, in the absence of better risk stratification in populations, the best estimate of expected treatment effect continues to be the overall estimate.

Structural issues in the conduct of clinical trials refer to an organization that is by now well regulated, based on the National Institutes of Health clinical trial model. It includes the sponsoring agency, steering committee, data coordinating center, and data monitoring committee, along with the clinical centers and their institutional review boards. The industry-modified model for cardiovascular clinical trials with irreversible outcomes (mortality) preserves the independent input provided by the steering committee and data coordinating center, substitutes the industry sponsor acting in concert with the regulatory agency for the sponsoring agency, and includes an independent data monitoring committee.

Finally, lessons regarding negative trends address the monitoring of trends favoring the control or standard of care over the experimental intervention, as well as the timing of decisions based on monitored data. CAST is presented as an example where an unambiguous, statistically powered demonstration of an emerging negative trend was really necessary. The experimental intervention, based on class Ic antiarrhythmics, was already in widespread use at the start of the trial, and shortening the study, it is argued, could have led to ambiguous findings.

A proposed path forward for improved risk stratification of arrhythmia is a deeper understanding of genetic determinants within the population. An examination of polymorphisms in genes clearly implicated in inherited arrhythmias, such as the ion channel genes involved in long QT syndrome, has been recently reviewed within the context of sudden cardiac death. The examination covers rare variants in families with recognizable syndromes, rare variants in the general population not ascertained through affected families, and common variants in the general population. As sudden cardiac death pathways implicating structural heart disease are elucidated, the same approach is used to examine polymorphisms, particularly common ones, in additional candidate genes [169–172]. Recent clinical evidence on familial sudden death as an important risk factor for primary ventricular fibrillation [173], warrants this type of approach.

8.4.4 Consortia Efforts to Address Safety Concerns Related to Antiarrhythmic Drug Development

Consortia efforts share the collaborative emphasis among regulatory and drug development patterns described above for the ICH initiative. Their goal, however is more programmatic, to provide a necessary fundamental investment in evaluative sciences. The level of involvement by regulatory agencies and by academic institutions, as well as the scope of their programs, is variably defined in these organizations. Here, we highlight three of these consortia efforts, all within the United States: the Technical Committee on Cardiac Safety of International Life Sciences Institute (ILSI)/Health and Environmental Sciences Institute (HESI), the Arizona CERT, and the Cardiac Safety Research Consortium (CSRC). Each of these efforts explicitly claims a connection to the FDA's Critical Path Initiative. This initiative, which was launched in 2004, is the agency's plan to stimulate and facilitate a national effort to modernize the scientific process through which a potential human drug, biological product, or medical device is transformed from a discovery or "proof of concept" into a medical product [174]. With regard to the specific need for better antiarrhythmic agents, these efforts collectively aim to improve the understanding of drug-induced arrhythmias and proarrhythmic remodeling, and to expedite discovery of better arrhythmia predictors than those currently available. Readers are referred to the websites of the respective organizations for additional details and updates [175–177].

ILSI is a global network of scientists devoted to enhancing the scientific basis for public health decision making, and it was founded in 1978. HESI was established in 1989 as a global branch of ILSI to provide an international forum to advance the understanding of scientific issues related to human health, toxicology, risk assessment, and the environment. In 2002, HESI was recognized by the U.S. government as a publicly supported, tax-exempt organization, independently chartered from ILSI. HESI's scientific programs bring together scientists from around the world from academia, industry, and regulatory agencies and other governmental institutions to address and reach consensus on scientific questions that have the potential to be resolved through creative application of intellectual and financial resources. This "tripartite" approach forms the core of every HESI scientific endeavor. HESI is governed by a Board of Trustees composed of scientists from industry and the public sector, with the HESI Executive Director serving as an ex-officio member of the Board. The Board provides oversight to HESI's various activities and sets the policy that guides the functioning of the overall organization. Scientific programs are implemented by committees and subcommittees, led by their chairs and vice chairs, scientific advisors, and the HESI scientific and support staff. In the fall of 2008, the Technical Committee on Cardiac Safety was born out of the strategic reorganization of existing programs to coordinate and synergize the following projects already underway at HESI: the Biomarkers of Cardiac Toxicity Project (the Cardiac Troponins working group of the Biomarkers Technical Committee), the Proarrhythmia Models Project Committee, and the Predictive CV Genomics Project [176].

The Arizona CERT is an independent research and education center whose mission is to improve therapeutic outcomes and reduce adverse events caused by drug interactions and drugs that prolong the QT interval, especially those affecting women. The Arizona CERT is a program of the Critical Path Institute in collaboration with The University of Arizona College of Pharmacy. They are one of 15 national CERTs funded by the U.S. Agency for Healthcare Research and Quality (AHRQ), in consultation with the FDA, both under the U.S. Department of Health and Human Services. The Critical Path Institute, in turn, was established in 2005 as a publicly funded, independent nonprofit institute, unaffiliated with any single entity or interest group, created to support the FDA in its effort to implement the Critical Path Initiative, by developing innovative collaborative projects in research and education to enable the safe acceleration of medical product development. One prominent activity of the Arizona CERT is the management of QT Drug Lists for consumer and professional education, under the consultation of a QT drug lists advisory board [175]. Table 8.2, for example, was extracted from the QT drug Lists, grouped by risk of torsades de pointes, possible risk of torsades de pointes, and conditional risk of torsades de pointes.

The CSRC was launched in September 2006 as a public-private partnership between the FDA and Duke University's Clinical Research Institute (DCRI) to focus on cardiac safety and new medicinal product development. The consortium, involving industry, academics, and regulators, is particularly interested in bridging the gap between evaluative sciences and a fundamental understanding of cardiac disease, and in helping define a better balance between safety and efficacy. The CSRC defines itself as a first step in bringing together key constituencies to focus on cardiac safety issues during the drug development process. Using the principles of the Critical Path Initiative, the CSRC aims to focus on improving the evaluative sciences, specifically in relation to cardiac safety [177].

8.4.5 The Unmet Medical Need: Challenges and Opportunities

Amiodarone, despite its extracardiac adverse effects, exemplifies the limited success of antiarrhythmic pharmacological interventions, and the safety-minded shift in interest at the end of the last century, first from class I to class III antiarrhythmics, and then to a pragmatic focus on mixed ion channel mechanisms to provide added efficacy and/or safety [136, 178, 179]. Amiodarone also exemplifies a related transition, from applications in ventricular to supraventricular arrhythmias, and specifically atrial fibrillation. As discussed, this is primarily attributed to the space that ICDs have occupied in populations at higher risk of cardiac and overall mortality. Atrial fibrillation is the most common sustained arrhythmia, but its severity is generally attributed to cardiovascular comorbidities. Compelling review and commentary have been published, regarding novel targets and novel therapeutic agents for its treatment and cure [136, 178–180]. From the epidemiological perspective, ventricular fibrillation and sudden cardiac death, particularly low-incidence sudden death on a large low-risk population, are a greater concern [154, 169, 181].

One strategy being proposed and used to develop safer antiarrhythmic agents is mixed ion channel activity, to mitigate the risk of excessive action potential prolongation in the ventricle. The notion of multichannel block to provide additional cardiac safety and/or efficacy has been explicitly examined and reviewed [125, 182, 183]. Many agents of this type have been studied preclinically. Examples are BRL-32872 [184], KB-130015 [185], and SSR149744C [186, 187]. Ranolazine, with effects on the late I_{Na} and on I_{Kr}, is an antianginal agent that has shown promising, safe antiarrhythmic activity in recent clinical trials [188, 189]. A similar inhibition of late I_{Na} has been reported for vernalakant, generating interest in this action as a novel antiarrhythmic mechanism [190–192], but its role in the absence of multichannel activity remains unexplored.

In the case of atrial fibrillation, drugs targeted to atrial ion channels have been developed to restore and/or maintain sinus rhythm control without adverse ventricular arrhythmias. In addition to vernakalant, several other agents targeting I_{Kur} have been studied preclinically. Examples are AVE-0118 and related compounds [193, 194], NIP-141 [195], and DPO-1 [135, 196]. NIP-142, the free amine of NIP-141, was also found to target the acetylcholine-activated inward rectifier potassium current expressed in atria [197]. Tedisamil, which was recently reported to be clinical efficacious for atrial fibrillation but is not without ventricular tachycardia safety concerns [198], has been reported to act on multiple ventricular and atrial channels [199]. A separate strategy proposed to reduce risk of ventricular fibrillation has been the use of class III agents highly selective for I_{Ks} instead of I_{Kr}, with self-limiting effects on ventricular action potential prolongation [108]. Thus, strategies where I_{Kr} activity is either dialed out or mitigated empirically by multichannel block have been pursued.

An alternative, safety-minded approach to drugs targeting ion channels playing a primary role in normal cardiac rhythm is to design drugs somewhat removed from this process. Included in this category are drugs targeting the mechanoelectrical feedback that triggers arrhythmias [200], the intracellular calcium-handling machinery [12], and deficiencies in cell-to-cell coupling [201]. Rotigaptide (ZP-123; GAP-486) is the best known gap-junction agonist [202–204]. K201, which is known to exert multichannel block [205], has also been shown to be a ryanodine-receptor stabilizer [206]. Overall, its multiple effects are thought to provide effective regulation of intracellular calcium [207]. Included as well in the category of agents removed from primary role in cardiac rhythm are drugs targeting proarrhythmic remodeling of cardiac structure and function. Examples of this action, designated *upstream therapy* [4, 10], are angiotensin-converting-enzyme inhibitors or angiotensin-receptor blockers, as well as agents targeting oxidative stress and inflammation to prevent fibrosis and atrial structural remodeling leading to atrial fibrillation.

This brief overview of agents in the preclinical space or starting to move through clinical phases of development is not intended to be an exhaustive list of all the novel approaches to antiarrhythmic pharmacological therapy. Readers are referred to other published reviews and references therein [4, 5, 10, 170, 200, 208–210]. The take-home lesson, to those discerning the value of pharmacological intervention in the era of implantable cardioverter devices, is that opportunities exist, because devices have limitations and drawbacks, and because morbidity and mortality triggered by or related to arrhythmias continue to be major unmet medical problems [211, 212]. Combined with efforts to stratify proarrhythmic risk in the population at large, discussed above, a two-pronged approach has been recommended, "rediscovering" old drugs and discovering new ones to target processes leading to the arrhythmic state, as opposed to single, preconceived targets [5].

REFERENCES

1. Kowey, P.R., Yan, G.X. (2005). Proarrhythmias and antiarrhythmias: Two sides of the same coin. Heart Rhythm, 2, 957–959.
2. The Cardiac Arrhythmia Suppression Trial (CAST) Investigators (1989). Preliminary report: Effect of encainide and flecainide on mortality in a randomized trial of arrhythmia suppression after myocardial infarction. New England Journal of Medicine, 321, 406–412.
3. Sanguinetti, M.C., Jiang, C.G., Curran, M.E., Keating, M.T. (1995). A mechanistic link between an inherited and an acquired cardiac-arrhythmia - herg encodes the I-Kr potassium channel. Cell. 81, 299–307.
4. Nattel, S., Maguy, A., Le Bouter, S., Yeh, Y.H. (2007). Arrhythmogenic ion-channel remodeling in the heart: Heart failure, myocardial infarction, and atrial fibrillation. Physiological Reviews, 87, 425–456.
5. George, C.H., Barberini-Jammaers, S.R., Muller, C.T. (2008). Refocussing therapeutic strategies for cardiac arrhythmias: defining viable molecular targets to restore cardiac ion flux. Expert Opinion on Therapeutic Patents, 18, 1–19.
6. Wellens, H.J.J., Brugada, P. (1989). Treatment of cardiac-arrhythmias - when, how and where. Journal of the American College of Cardiology, 14, 1417–1428.
7. Zipes, D.P., Wellens, H.J.J. (1998). Sudden cardiac death. Circulation, 98, 2334–2351.
8. Lopshire, J.C., Zipes, D.P. (2006). Sudden cardiac death—Better understanding of risks, mechanisms, and treatment. Circulation, 114, 1134–1136.
9. Zipes, D.P., Wellens, H.J.J. (2000). What have we learned about cardiac arrhythmias? Circulation, 102, 52–57.
10. Nattel, S., Carlsson, L. (2006). Innovative approaches to anti-arrhythmic drug therapy. Nature Reviews Drug Discovery, 5, 1034–1049.
11. Antzelevitch, C. (2001). Basic mechanisms of reentrant arrhythmias. Current Opinion in Cardiology, 16, 1–7.
12. Laurita, K.R., Rosenbaum, D.S. (2008). Mechanisms and potential therapeutic targets for ventricular arrhythmias associated with impaired cardiac calcium cycling. Journal of Molecular and Cellular Cardiology, 44, 31–43.
13. Anderson, M.E. (2006). QT interval prolongation and arrhythmia: An unbreakable connection? Journal of Internal Medicine, 259, 81–90.
14. Boyden, P.A., ter Keurs, H.E.D.J. (2005). An intimate relationship - Ca2 + and cardiac ion channels. Circulation Research, 96, 393–394.
15. Ter Keurs, H.E.D.J., Boyden, P.A. (2007). Calcium and arrhythmogenesis. Physiological Reviews, 87, 457–506.
16. Ter Keurs, H.E.D.J., Shinozaki, T., Zhang, Y.M., Zhang, M.L., Wakayama, Y., Sugai, Y., Kagaya, Y., Miura, M., Boyden, P.A., Stuyvers, B.D.M., Landesberg, A. (2008). Sarcomere mechanics in uniform and non-uniform cardiac muscle: A link between pump function and arrhythmias. Progress in Biophysics & Molecular Biology, 97, 312–331.

17. Rubart, M., Zipes, D.P. (2005). Mechanisms of sudden cardiac death. Journal of Clinical Investigation, 115, 2305–2315.

18. January, C.T., Riddle, J.M., Salata, J.J. (1988). A model for early afterdepolarizations—induction with the Ca-2 + channel agonist bay-K-8644. Circulation Research, 62, 563–571.

19. Schlotthauer, K., Bers, D.M. (2000). Sarcoplasmic reticulum Ca2 + release causes myocyte depolarization—Underlying mechanism and threshold for triggered action potentials. Circulation Research, 87, 774–780.

20. Roberts, R. (2006). Genomics and cardiac arrhythmias. Journal of the American College of Cardiology, 47, 9–21.

21. Lehnart, S.E., Ackerman, M.J., Benson, W., Grant, A.O., Groft, S.C., January, C.T., Lathrop, D.A., Lederer, W.J., Makielski, J.C., Mohler, P.J., Moss, A., Nerbonne, J.M., Olson, T.M., Przywara, D.A., Towbin, J.A., Wang, L.H., Marks, A.R. (2007). Inherited arrhythmias—A national heart, lung, and blood institute and office of rare diseases workshop consensus report about the diagnosis, phenotyping, molecular mechanisms, and therapeutic approaches for primary cardiomyopathies of gene mutations affecting ion channel function. Circulation, 116, 2325–2345.

22. Splawski, I., Shen, J.X., Timothy, K.W., Lehmann, M.H., Priori, S., Robinson, J.L., Moss, A.J., Schwartz, P.J., Towbin, J.A., Vincent, G.M., Keating, M.T. (2000). Spectrum of mutations in long-QT syndrome genes KVLQT1, HERG, SCN5A, KCNE1, and KCNE2. Circulation, 102, 1178–1185.

23. Wang, Q., Curran, M.E., Splawski, I., Burn, T.C., Millholland, J.M., VanRaay, T.J., Shen, J., Timothy, K.W., Vincent, G.M., deJager, T., Schwartz, P.J., Towbin, J.A., Moss, A.J., Atkinson, D.L., Landes, G.M., Connors, T.D., Keating, M.T. (1996). Positional cloning of a novel potassium channel gene: KVLQT1 mutations cause cardiac arrhythmias. Nature Genetics, 12, 17–23.

24. Trudeau, M.C., Warmke, J.W., Ganetzky, B., Robertson, G.A. (1995). Herg, a human inward rectifier in the voltage-gated potassium channel family. Science, 269, 92–95.

25. Curran, M.E., Splawski, I., Timothy, K.W., Vincent, G.M., Green, E.D., Keating, M.T. (1995). A molecular-basis for cardiac-arrhythmia—Herg mutations cause long Qt syndrome. Cell, 80, 795–803.

26. Sanguinetti, M.C., Jurkiewicz, N.K. (1990). Two components of cardiac delayed rectifier K + current - differential sensitivity to block by class-III antiarrhythmic agents. Journal of General Physiology, 96, 195–215.

27. Roden, D.M. (2006). Long QT syndrome: reduced repolarization reserve and the genetic link. Journal of Internal Medicine, 259, 59–69.

28. Antzelevitch, C. (2005). Role of transmural dispersion of repolarization in the genesis of drug-induced torsades de pointes. Heart Rhythm, 2, S9–S15.

29. Antzelevitch, C., Oliva, A. (2006). Amplification of spatial dispersion of repolarization underlies sudden cardiac death associated with catecholaminergic polymorphic VT, long QT, short QT and Brugada syndromes. Journal of Internal Medicine, 259, 48–58.

30. Lankipalli, R.S., Zhu, T.G., Guo, D.L., Yan, G.X. (2005). Mechanisms underlying arrhythmogenesis in long QT syndrome. Journal of Electrocardiology, 38, 69–73.

31. Burashnikov, A., Mannava, S., Antzelevitch, C. (2004). Transmembrane action potential heterogeneity in the canine isolated arterially perfused right atrium: effect of I-Kr and I-Kur/I-to block. American Journal of Physiology Heart and Circulatory Physiology, 286, H2393–H2400.

32. Gong, D.M., Zhang, Y., Cai, B.Z., Meng, Q.X., Jiang, S.L., Li, X., Shan, L.C., Liu, Y.Y., Qiao, G.F., Lu, Y.J., Yang, B.F. (2008). Characterization and comparison of Na +, K + and Ca2 + currents between myocytes from human atrial right appendage and atrial septum. Cellular Physiology and Biochemistry, 21, 385–394.

33. Antzelevitch, C. (2007). Role of spatial dispersion of repolarization in inherited and acquired sudden cardiac death syndromes. American Journal of Physiology Heart and Circulatory Physiology, 293, H2024–H2038.

34. Shah, M., Akar, F.G., Tomaselli, G.F. (2005). Molecular basis of arrhythmias. Circulation, 112, 2517–2529.

35. Benito, B., Brugada, R., Brugada, J., Brugada, P. (2008). Brugada syndrome. Progress in Cardiovascular Diseases, 51, 1–22.

36. Kurita, T., Shimizu, W., Inagaki, M., Suyama, K., Taguchi, A., Satomi, K., Aihara, N., Kamakura, S., Kobayashi, J., Kosakai, Y. (2002). The electrophysiologic ST-segment elevation mechanism of in Brugada syndrome. Journal of the American College of Cardiology, 40, 330–334.

37. Singh, B.N. (1998). Antiarrhythmic drugs: A reorientation in light of recent developments in the control of disorders of rhythm. American Journal of Cardiology, 81, 3d–13d.

38. Singh, B.N. (1997). Controlling cardiac arrhythmias: An overview with a historical perspective. American Journal of Cardiology, 80, G4–G15.

39. Singh, B.N. (1993). Controlling cardiac-arrhythmias by lengthening repolarization—historical overview. American Journal of Cardiology, 72, F18–F24.

40. Nattel, S., Singh, B.N. (1999). Evolution, mechanisms, and classification of antiarrhythmic drugs: Focus on class III actions. American Journal of Cardiology, 84, 11r–19r.

41. Guerra, P.G., Talajic, M., Roy, D., Dubuc, M., Thibault, B., Nattel, S. (1998). Is there a future for antiarrhythmic drug therapy? Drugs, 56, 767–781.

42. Vaughan, W.E. (1984). A classification of antiarrhythmic actions reassessed after a decade of new drugs. Journal of Clinical Pharmacology, 24, 129–147.

43. Vaughan, W.E. (1992). The relevance of cellular to clinical electrophysiology in classifying antiarrhythmic actions. Journal of Cardiovascular Pharmacology, 20.

44. Vaughan, W.E. (1992). Classifying antiarrhythmic actions: By facts or speculation. Journal of Clinical Pharmacology, 32, 964–977.

45. Rosen, M.R. (2004). Principles of electropharmacology. In Electrophysiological Disorders of the Heart. 1st edition (Saksena, S., Camm, A.J., eds.). Elsevier, Philadelphia, PA.

46. Pugsley, M.K. (2002). Antiarrhythmic drug development: Historical review and future perspective. Drug Development Research, 55, 3–16.

47. Singh, B.K. (2004). Antiarrhythmic drugs. In Electrophysiological Disorders of the Heart. 1st edition (Saksena, S., Camm, A.J., eds.). Elsevier, Philadelphia, PA..

48. Hauswirth, O., Singh, B.N. (1978). Ionic mechanisms in heart-muscle in relation to the genesis and the pharmacological control of cardiac-arrhythmias. Pharmacological Reviews, 30, 5–63.

49. Campbell, T.J. (1983). Kinetics of onset of rate-dependent effects of class-I antiarrhythmic drugs are important in determining their effects on refractoriness in guinea-pig ventricle, and provide a theoretical basis for their subclassification. Cardiovascular Research, 17, 344–352.

50. Campbell, T.J. (1983). Resting and rate-dependent depression of maximum rate of depolarization (Vmax) in guinea-pig ventricular action-potentials by mexiletine, disopyramide, and encainide. Journal of Cardiovascular Pharmacology, 5, 291–296.

51. Task Force of the Working Group on Arrhythmias of the European Society of Cardiology (1991). The Sicilian gambit—a new approach to the classification of antiarrhythmic drugs based on their actions on arrhythmogenic mechanisms. Circulation, 84, 1831–1851.

52. Garratt, C.J., Griffith, M.J. (1996). The Sicilian gambit: An opening move that loses the game? European Heart Journal, 17, 341–343.

53. MacFadyen, R.J., Prasad, N. (1995). Clinical pharmacology and classification of antiarrhythmic drugs. British Journal of Hospital Medicine, 54, 515–519.

54. Members of the Sicilian Gambit. (1998). The search for novel antiarrhythmic strategies. European Heart Journal, 19, 1178–1196.

55. Nattel, S., Waters, D. (1990). What Is an antiarrhythmic drug—from clinical-trials to fundamental-concepts. American Journal of Cardiology, 66, 96–99.

56. Singh, B.N. (1990). Do antiarrhythmic drugs work—some reflections on the implications of the cardiac-arrhythmia suppression trial. Clinical Cardiology, 13, 725–728.

57. Singh, B.N., Kowey, P.R. (1995). Changing perspectives in cardiac-arrhythmia control—agents, techniques, goals, and outcomes—Introduction. Journal of Cardiovascular Electrophysiology, 6, 865–867.

58. Roden, D.M. (1996). Ionic mechanisms for prolongation of refractoriness and their proarrhythmic and antiarrhythmic correlates. American Journal of Cardiology, 78, 12–16.

59. Trybulski, E.J. (1997). Anti-arrhythmic agents. Expert Opinion on Therapeutic Patents, 7, 457–469.

60. Link, M.S., Homoud, M., Foote, C.B., Wang, P.J., Estes, N.A.M. (1996). Antiarrhythmic drug therapy for ventricular arrhythmia: Current perspectives. Journal of Cardiovascular Electrophysiology, 7, 653–670.

61. Ahmed, R., Singh, B.N. (1993). Antiarrhythmic drugs. Current Opinion in Cardiology, 8, 10–21.

62. Anderson, J.L., Stewart, J.R., Perry, B.A., Vanhamersveld, D.D., Johnson, T.A., Conard, G.J., Chang, S.F., Kvam, D.C., Pitt, B. (1981). Oral flecainide acetate for the treatment of ventricular arrhythmias. New England Journal of Medicine, 305, 473–477.

63. Dibianco, R., Fletcher, R.D., Cohen, A.I., Gottdiener, J.S., Singh, S.N., Katz, R.J., Bates, H.R., Sauerbrunn, B. (1982). Treatment of frequent ventricular arrhythmia with encainide—assessment using serial ambulatory electrocardiograms, intracardiac electrophysiologic studies, treadmill exercise tests, and radionuclide cineangiographic studies. Circulation, 65, 1134–1147.

64. The CAPS Investigators (1986). Effects of encainide, flecainide, imipramine and moricizine on ventricular arrhythmias during the year after acute myocardial-infarction. American Journal of Cardiology, 57, 91–95.

65. The CAPS Investigators (1988). Effects of encainide, flecainide, imipramine and moricizine on ventricular arrhythmias during the year after acute myocardial-infarction. American Journal of Cardiology, 61, 501–509.

66. Greene, H.L., Richardson, D.W., Barker, A.H., Roden, D.M., Capone, R.J., Echt, D.S., Friedman, L.M., Gillespie, M.J., Hallstrom, A.P., Verter, J. (1989). Classification of

deaths after myocardial-infarction as arrhythmic or nonarrhythmic (the cardiac-arrhythmia pilot-study). American Journal of Cardiology, 63, 1–6.

67. Echt, D.S., Liebson, P.R., Mitchell, L.B., Peters, R.W., Obiasmanno, D., Barker, A.H., Arensberg, D., Baker, A., Friedman, L., Greene, H.L., Huther, M.L., Richardson, D.W. (1991). Mortality and morbidity in patients receiving encainide, flecainide, or placebo—the cardiac-arrhythmia suppression trial. New England Journal of Medicine, 324, 781–788.

68. Bigger, J.T. (1990). The events surrounding the removal of encainide and flecainide from the cardiac-arrhythmia suppression trial (cast) and why cast is continuing with moricizine. Journal of the American College of Cardiology, 15, 243–245.

69. Greene, H.L., Roden, D.M., Katz, R.J., Woosley, R.L., Salerno, D.M., Henthorn, R.W. (1992). The cardiac-arrhythmia suppression trial - 1st Cast . . . Then Cast-II. Journal of the American College of Cardiology, 19, 894–898.

70. The Cardiac Arrhythmia Suppression Trial II Investigators. (1992). Effect of the antiarrhythmic agent moricizine on survival after myocardial infarction. New England Journal of Medicine, 327, 227–233.

71. Ruskin, J.N. (1989). The cardiac-arrhythmia suppression trial (Cast). New England Journal of Medicine, 321, 386–388.

72. Reiffel, J.A., Estes, N.A.M., Waldo, A.L., Prystowsky, E.N., Dibianco, R. (1994). A consensus report on antiarrhythmic drug-use. Clinical Cardiology, 17, 103–116.

73. Vlay, S.C. (1990). Lessons from the past and reflections on the cardiac-arrhythmia suppression trial. American Journal of Cardiology, 65, 112–113.

74. Morganroth, J., Bigger, J.T. (1990). Pharmacological management of ventricular arrhythmias after the cardiac-arrhythmia suppression trial. American Journal of Cardiology, 65, 1497–1503.

75. Pratt, C.M., Moye, L.A. (1990). The cardiac-arrhythmia suppression trial - background, interim results and implications. American Journal of Cardiology, 65, B20–B29.

76. Goldstein, S., Brooks, M.M., Ledingham, R., Kennedy, H.L., Epstein, A.E., Pawitan, Y., Bigger, J.T. (1995). Association between ease of suppression of ventricular arrhythmia and survival. Circulation, 91, 79–83.

77. el-Sherif, N., Denes, P., Katz, R., Capone, R., Mitchell, L.B., Carlson, M., Reynoldshaertle, R. (1995). Definition of the best prediction criteria of the time-domain signal-averaged electrocardiogram for serious arrhythmic events in the postinfarction period. Journal of the American College of Cardiology, 25, 908–914.

78. Anderson, J.L., Hallstrom, A., Platia, E.V., Carlson, M.D., Henthorn, R.W., Buckingham, T.A., Carson, P.E. (1994). Interaction of base-line characteristics and moricizine on risk of mortality after myocardial-infarction in the cardiac-arrhythmia suppression trial (cast). Circulation, 90, 280–280.

79. Anderson, J.L., Karagounis, L.A., Stein, K.M., Moreno, F.L., Ledingham, R., Hallstrom, A. (1997). Predictive value for future arrhythmic events of fractal dimension, a measure of time clustering of ventricular premature complexes, after myocardial infarction. Journal of the American College of Cardiology, 30, 226–232.

80. Hondeghem, L.M., Katzung, B.G. (1984). Antiarrhythmic agents—the modulated receptor mechanism of action of sodium and calcium channel-blocking drugs. Annual Review of Pharmacology and Toxicology, 24, 387–423.

81. Hondeghem, L.M. (1987). Antiarrhythmic agents—modulated receptor applications. Circulation, 75, 514–520.

82. Hondeghem, L.M., Snyders, D.J. (1990). Class-III antiarrhythmic agents have a lot of potential but a long way to go—reduced effectiveness and dangers of reverse use dependence. Circulation, 81, 686–690.

83. Doggrell, S.A., Brown, L. (2000). D-Sotalol: Death by the SWORD or deserving of further consideration for clinical use? Expert Opinion on Investigational Drugs, 9, 1625–1634.

84. Fenichel, R. (2004). Drug-induced Torsades de Pointes and implications for drug development. Journal of Cardiovascular Electrophysiology, 15, 475–495.

85. Kannankeril, P.J., Roden, D.M. (2007). Drug-induced long QT and torsade de pointes: recent advances. Current Opinion in Cardiology, 22, 39–43.

86. Antzelevitch, C. (2004). Arrhythmogenic mechanisms of QT prolonging drugs: Is QT prolongation really the problem? Journal of Electrocardiology, 37, 15–24.

87. Shah, R.R. (2005). Drug-induced QT dispersion: Does it predict the risk of Torsade de Pointes? Journal of Electrocardiology, 38, 10–18.

88. Thomsen, M.B., Matz, J., Volders, P.G.A., Vos, M.A. (2006). Assessing the proarrhythmic potential of drugs: Current status of models and surrogate parameters of torsades de pointes arrhythmias. Pharmacology & Therapeutics, 112, 150–170.

89. Chen, J., Zou, A.R., Splawski, I., Keating, M.T., Sanguinetti, M.C. (1999). Long QT syndrome-associated mutations in the Per-Arnt-Sim (PAS) domain of HERG potassium channels accelerate channel deactivation. Journal of Biological Chemistry, 274, 10113–10118.

90. Robertson, G.A. (2000). LQT2—Amplitude reduction and loss of selectivity in the tail that wags the HERG channel. Circulation Research, 86, 492–493.

91. Vorperian, V.R., Zhou, Z.F., Mohammad, S., Hoon, T.J., Studenik, C., January, C.T. (1996). Torsade de pointes with an antihistamine metabolite: Potassium channel blockade with desmethylastemizole. Journal of the American College of Cardiology, 28, 1556–1561.

92. Zhou, Z.F., Vorperian, V.R., Gong, Q.M., Zhang, S.T., January, C.T. (1999). Block of HERG potassium channels by the antihistamine astemizole and its metabolites desmethylastemizole and norastemizole. Journal of Cardiovascular Electrophysiology, 10, 836–843.

93. Mitcheson, J.S., Chen, J., Lin, M., Culberson, C., Sanguinetti, M.C. (2000). A structural basis for drug-induced long QT syndrome. Proceedings of the National Academy of Sciences USA, 97, 12329–12333.

94. Mitcheson, J.S., Chen, J., Sanguinetti, M.C. (2000). Trapping of a methanesulfonanilide by closure of the HERG potassium channel activation gate. Journal of General Physiology, 115, 229–239.

95. De Bruin, M.L., Pettersson, M., Meyboom, R.H.B., Hoes, A.W., Leufkens, H.G.M. (2005). Anti-HERG activity and the risk of drug-induced arrhythmias and sudden death. European Heart Journal, 26, 590–597.

96. Honig, P.K., Wortham, D.C., Zamani, K., Conner, D.P., Mullin, J.C., Cantilena, L.R. (1993). Terfenadine-ketoconazole interaction - pharmacokinetic and electrocardiographic consequences. JAMA, 269, 1513–1518.

97. Thomas, D., Karle, C.A., Kiehn, J. (2006). The cardiac hERG/I-Kr potassium channel as pharmacological target: Structure, function, regulation, and clinical applications. Current Pharmaceutical Design, 12, 2271–2283.

98. Lagrutta, A.A., Salata, J.J. (2006). Ion channel safety issues in drug development. In Voltage-Gated Ion Channels as Drug Targets (Triggle, D.J., Gopalakrishnan, M., Rampe, D., Zheng, W., eds.) Vol. 29. Wiley, New York.

99. Jamieson, C., Moir, E.M., Rankovic, Z., Wishart, G. (2006). Medicinal chemistry of hERG optimizations: Highlights and hang-ups. Journal of Medicinal Chemistry, 49, 5029–5046.

100. Cavero, I., Crumb, W. (2006). Moving towards better predictors of drug-induced Torsade de Pointes - 2-3 November 2005, Crystal City, Virginia, USA. Expert Opinion on Drug Safety, 5, 335–340.

101. Sanguinetti, M.C., Mitcheson, J.S. (2005). Predicting drug-hERG channel interactions that cause acquired long QT syndrome. *Trends in Pharmacological Sciences*, 26, 119–124.

102. Recanatini, M., Poluzzi, E., Masetti, M., Cavalli, A., De Ponti, F. (2005). QT prolongation through hERG K + channel blockade: Current knowledge and strategies for the early prediction during drug development. Medicinal Research Reviews, 25, 133–166.

103. Shah, R.R. (2004). Drug-induced QT interval prolongation: regulatory perspectives and drug development. Annals of Medicine, 36, 47–52.

104. Redfern, W.S., Carlsson, L., Davis, A.S., Lynch, W.G., MacKenzie, I., Palethorpe, S., Siegl, P.K.S., Strang, I., Sullivan, A.T., Wallis, R., Camm, A.J., Hammond, T.G. (2003). Relationships between preclinical cardiac electrophysiology, clinical QT interval prolongation and torsade de pointes for a broad range of drugs: Evidence for a provisional safety margin in drug development. Cardiovascular Research, 58, 32–45.

105. Lagrutta, A.A., Trepakova, E.S., Salata, J.J. (2008). The hERG channel and risk of drug-acquired cardiac arrhythmia: An overview. Current Topics in Medicinal Chemistry, 8, 1102–1112.

106. Roden, D.M. (1998). Taking the "idio" out of "idiosyncratic": Predicting torsades de pointes. PACE-Pacing and Clinical Electrophysiology, 21, 1029–1034.

107. Lasser, K.E., Allen, P.D., Woolhandler, S.J., Himmelstein, D.U., Wolfe, S.N., Bor, D.H. (2002). Timing of new black box warnings and withdrawals for prescription medications. JAMA, 287, 2215–2220.

108. Salata, J.J., Selnick, H.G., Lynch, J.J. (2004). Pharmacological modulation of I-Ks: Potential for antiarrhythmic therapy. Current Medicinal Chemistry, 11, 29–44.

109. Witchel, H.J. (2007). The hERG potassium channel as a therapeutic target. Expert Opinion on Therapeutic Targets, 11, 321–336.

110. Antzelevitch, C. (2005). Cardiac repolarization. The long and short of it. Europace, 7, S3–S9.

111. Cannom, D.S. (1998). A review of the implantable cardioverter defibrillator trials. Current Opinion in Cardiology, 13, 3–8.

112. Groeneveld, P.W., Matta, M.A., Suh, J.J., Heidenreich, P.A., Shea, J.A. (2006). Costs and quality-of-life effects of implantable cardioverter-defibrillators. American Journal of Cardiology, 98, 1409–1415.

113. Gehi, A.K., Mehta, D., Gomes, J.A. (2006). Evaluation and management of patients after implantable cardioverter-defibrillator shock. JAMA, 296, 2839–2847.

114. Higgins, S.L. (1999). Impact of the multicenter automatic defibrillator implantation trial on implantable cardioverter defibrillator indication trends. American Journal of Cardiology, 83, 79d–82d.

115. Daubert, J.P., Zareba, W., Cannom, D.S., McNitt, S., Rosero, S.Z., Wang, P., Schuger, C., Steinberg, J.S., Higgins, S.L., Wilber, D.J., Klein, H., Andrews, M.L., Hall, W.J., Moss, A.J., for the Madit II Investigators (2008). Inappropriate implantable cardioverter-defibrillator shocks in MADIT II. Journal of the American College of Cardiology, 51, 1357–1365.

116. Dorian, P., Al-Khalidi, H.R., Hohnloser, S.H., Brum, J.M., Dunnmon, P.M., Pratt, C.M., Holroyde, M.J., Kowey, P., on behalf of the SHIELD (SHock Inhibition Evaluation with AzimiLiDe) Investigators. (2008). Azimilide reduces emergency department visits and hospitalizations in patients with an implantable cardioverter-defibrillator in a placebo-controlled clinical trial. Journal of the American College of Cardiology, 52, 1076–1083.

117. Hohnloser, S.H., Al-Khalidi, H.R., Pratt, C.M., Brum, J.M., Tatla, D.S., Tchou, P., Dorian, P., on behalf of the SHock Inhibition Evaluation with AzimiLiDe (SHIELD) Investigators. (2006). Electrical storm in patients with an implantable defibrillator: incidence, features, and preventive therapy: Insights from a randomized trial. European Heart Journal, 27, 3027–3032.

118. Julian, D.G., Jackson, F.S., Prescott, R.J., Szekely, P. (1982). Controlled trial of sotalol for one year after myocardial-infarction. Lancet, 1, 1142–1147.

119. Julian, D.G., Jackson, F.S., Szekely, P., Prescott, R.J. (1983). A controlled trial of sotalol for 1 year after myocardial-infarction. Circulation, 67, 61–62.

120. Waldo, A.L., Camm, A.J., deRuyter, H., Friedman, P.L., MacNeil, D.J., Pauls, J.F., Pitt, B., Pratt, C.M., Schwartz, P.J., Veltri, E.P. (1996). Effect of d-sotalol on mortality in patients with left ventricular dysfunction after recent and remote myocardial infarction. Lancet, 348, 7–12.

121. Pratt, C.M., Camm, A.J., Cooper, W., Friedman, P.L., MacNeil, D., Moulton, K.M., Pitt, B., Schwartz, P.J., Veltri, E.P., Waldo, A.L., for the SWORD Investigators (1998). Mortality in the Survival With ORal D-sotalol (SWORD) trial: Why did patients die? American Journal of Cardiology, 81, 869–876.

122. Siddiqui, A., Kowey, P.R. (2006). Sudden death secondary to cardiac arrhythmias: mechanisms and treatment strategies. Current Opinion in Cardiology, 21, 517–525.

123. Naccarelli, G.V., Wolbrette, D.L., Patel, H.M., Luck, J.C. (2000). Amiodarone: Clinical trials. Current Opinion in Cardiology, 15, 64–72.

124. Tafreshi, M.J., Rowles, J. (2007). A review of the investigational antiarrhythmic agent dronedarone. Journal of Cardiovascular Pharmacology and Therapeutics, 12, 15–26.

125. Conway, E., Musco, S., Kowey, P.R. (2008). New horizons in antiarrhythmic therapy: Will novel agents overcome current deficits? American Journal of Cardiology, 102, 12h–19h.

126. Camm, A.J., Pratt, C.M., Schwartz, P.J., Al-Khalidi, H.R., Spyt, M.J., Holroyde, M.J., Karam, R., Sonnenblick, E.H., Brum, J.M.G., on Behalf of the AzimiLide post Infarct surVival Evaluation (ALIVE) Investigators. (2004). Mortality in patients after a recent myocardial infarction—a randomized, placebo-controlled trial of azimilide using heart rate variability for risk stratification. Circulation, 109, 990–996.

127. Hohnloser, S.H., Connolly, S.J., Crijns, H.J.G.M., Page, R.L., Seiz, W., Torp-Petersen, C. (2008). Rationale and design of ATHENA: A placebo-controlled, double-blind, parallel arm trial to assess the efficacy of dronedarone 400 g bid for the prevention of cardiovascular hospitalization or death from any cause in PatiENts with atrial fibrillation/atrial flutter. Journal of Cardiovascular Electrophysiology, 19, 69–73.

128. Coletta, A.P., Cleland, J.G.F., Cullington, D., Clark, A.L. (2008). Clinical trials update from Heart Rhythm 2008 and Heart Failure 2008: ATHENA, URGENT, INH study, HEART and CK-1827452. European Journal of Heart Failure, 10, 917–920.

129. Pedersen, O.D., Bagger, H., Keller, N., Marchant, B., Kober, L., Torp-Pedersen, C., for the Danish Investigations of Arrhythmia and Mortality ON Dofetilide Study Group (2001). 104, Efficacy of dofetilide in the treatment of atrial fibrillation-flutter in patients with reduced left ventricular function—A Danish Investigations of Arrhythmia and Mortality ON Dofetilide (DIAMOND) substudy. Circulation, 104, 292–296.

130. Falk, R.H., DeCara, J.M. (2000). Dofetilide: A new pure class III antiarrhythmic agent. American Heart Journal, 140, 697–706.

131. Mounsey, J.P., DiMarco, J.P. (2000). Dofetilide. Circulation, 102, 2665–2670.

132. Fedida, D. (2007). Vernakalant (RSD1235): A novel, atrial-selective antifibrillatory agent. Expert Opinion on Investigational Drugs, 16, 519–532.

133. Fox, K., Ford, I., Steg, P.G., Tendera, M., Ferrari, R., Investigators, B. (2008). Ivabradine for patients with stable coronary artery disease and left-ventricular systolic dysfunction (BEAUTIFUL): A randomised, double-blind, placebo-controlled trial. Lancet, 372, 807–816.

134. Fox, K., Recena, J.B., Garcia-Aranda, V.L., Valderrama, J.C., Alonso, L.F.I., Calvar, A.S.R., Aviles, F.F., Villa, F.P., Cortada, J.B., Alvarez, R.F., et al. (2008). The BEAUTIFUL study: Randomized trial of ivabradine in patients with stable coronary artery disease and left ventricular systolic dysfunction baseline characteristics of the study population. Cardiology, 110, 271–282.

135. Lagrutta, A., Wang, J.X., Fermini, B., Salata, J.J. (2006). Novel, potent inhibitors of human Kv1.5 K+ channels and ultrarapidly activating delayed rectifier potassium current. Journal of Pharmacology and Experimental Therapeutics, 317, 1054–1063.

136. Waldo, A.L. (2006). A perspective on antiarrhythmic drug therapy to treat atrial, fibrillation: There remains an unmet need. American Heart Journal, 151, 771–778.

137. Salam, A.M. (2003). Rate control versus rhythm control for the management of atrial fibrillation: the verdict of the AFFIRM trial. Expert Opinion on Investigational Drugs, 12, 1231–1237.

138. Brugada, P., Wellens, F., Andries, E. (1996). A prophylactic implantable cardioverter-defibrillator? American Journal of Cardiology, 78, 128–133.

139. Moss, A.J., Hall, W.J., Cannom, D.S., Daubert, J.P., Higgins, S.L., Klein, H., Levine, J. H., Saksena, S., Waldo, A.L., Wilber, D., Brown, M.W., Heo, M. (1996). Improved survival with an implanted defibrillator in patients with coronary disease at high risk for ventricular arrhythmia. New England Journal of Medicine, 335, 1933–1940.

140. The Antiarrhythmics versus Implantable Defibrillators (AVID) Investigators (1997). A comparison of antiarrhythmic-drug therapy with implantable defibrillators in patients resuscitated from near-fatal ventricular arrhythmias. New England Journal of Medicine, 337, 1576–1584.

141. Hallstrom, A.P., Anderson, J.L., Cobb, L.A., Friedman, P.L., Herre, J.M., Klein, R.C., McAnulty, J., Steinberg, J.S., for AVID Investigators (2000). Advantages and disadvantages of trial designs: A review of analysis methods for ICD studies. PACE, 23, 1029–1038.

142. International Conference on Harmonisation of Technical Requirements for Registration of Pharmaceuticals for Human Use (ICH). Available at http://www.ich.org.

143. (2001). Guidance for industry S7A. Safety pharmacology studies for human pharmaceuticals. Available at http://www.ich.org..

144. Kinter, L.B., Valentin, J.P. (2002). Safety pharmacology and risk assessment. Fundamental & Clinical Pharmacology, 16, 175–182.

145. Pugsley, M.K., Authier, S., Curtis, M.J. (2008). Principles of safety pharmacology. British Journal of Pharmacology, 154, 1382–1399.

146. Bass, A.S., Vargas, H.M., Kinter, L.B. (2004). Introduction to nonclinical safety pharmacology and the safety pharmacology society. Journal of Pharmacological and Toxicological Methods, 49, 141–144.

147. Safety Pharmacology Society. Mission statement. Available at http://www.safetypharmacology.org.

148. Valentin, J.P., Hammond, T.G. (2006). Safety pharmacology: Past, present, and future. In The Process of New Drug Discovery and Development 2nd editition. (Smith, C.G., O'Donnell, J.T., eds.). Informa Health Care, London, UK,.

149. Hock, F. (2006). Status of safety pharmacology and present guidelines In Drug Discovery and Evaluation: Safety and Pharmacokinetic Assays (Vogel, H.G., Hock, F.J., Maas, J., Mayer, D., eds.). Springer, Berlin, Germany.

150. Committee for Proprietary Medicinal Products (1997) Points to consider: The assessment of the potential for QT interval prolongation by non-cardiovascular medicinal products. Document no.: CPMP/986/96.

151. (2005). Guidance for industry E14 clinical evaluation of QT/QTc interval prolongation and proarrhythmic potential for non-antiarrhythmic drugs.

152. Hanton, G., Tilbury, L. (2006). Cardiac safety strategies - 25–26 October 2005, the Radisson SAS Hotel, Nice, France. Expert Opinion on Drug Safety, 5, 329–333.

153. Darpo, B., Nebout, T., Sager, P.T. (2006). Clinical evaluation of QT/QTc prolongation and proarrhythmic potential for nonantiarrhythmic drugs: The international conference on harmonization of technical requirements for registration of pharmaceuticals for human use E14 guideline. Journal of Clinical Pharmacology, 46, 498–507.

154. Huikuri, H.V., Castellanos, A., Myerburg, R.J. (2001). Medical progress: Sudden death due to cardiac arrhythmias. New England Journal of Medicine, 345, 1473–1482.

155. Zipes, D.P., Camm, A.J., Borggrefe, M., Buxton, A.E., Chaitman, B., Fromer, M., Gregoratos, G., Klein, G., Moss, A.J., Myerburg, R.J., et al. (2006). ACC/AHA/ESC 2006 guidelines for management of patients with ventricular arrhythmias and the prevention of sudden cardiac death-executive summary. European Heart Journal, 27, 2099–2140.

156. Blomstrom-Lundqvist, C., Scheinman, M.M., Aliot, E.M., Alpert, J.S., Calkins, H., Camm, A.J., Campbell, W.B., Haines, D.E., Kuck, K.H., Lerman, B.B., et al. (2003). ACC/AHA/ESC guidelines for the management of patients with supraventricular arrhythmias - executive summary—A report of the American College of Cardiology/ American Heart Association task force on practice guidelines and the European Society of Cardiology Committee for Practice Guidelines (Writing Committee to Develop Guidelines for the Management of Patients with Supraventricular Arrhythmias). European Heart Journal, 24, 1857–1897.

157. Fuster, V., Ryden, L.E., Cannom, D.S., Crijns, H.J., Curtis, A.B., Ellenbogen, K.A., Halperin, J.L., Le Heuzey, J.Y., Kay, G.N., Lowe, J.E., et al. (2006). ACC/AHA/ESC 2006 guidelines for the management of patients with atrial fibrillation - executive

summary—A report of the American College of Cardiology/American Heart Association Task Force on practice guidelines and the European Society of Cardiology Committee for Practice Guidelines (Writing Committee to Revise the 2001 Guidelines for the Management of Patients with Atrial Fibrillation) Developed in collaboration with the European Heart Rhythm Association and the Heart Rhythm Society. European Heart Journal, 27, 1979–2030.

158. Lewin, J.C., May, C., Bradfield, L., Stewart, M.D., Fobbs, K.N., Barrett, E.A., Wheeler, M.C., Whitman, G.R., Taubert, K.A. (2008). ACC/AHA/HRS 2008 guidelines for device-based therapy of cardiac rhythm abnormalities: Executive summary—a report of the American College of Cardiology/American Heart Association Task Force on practice guidelines (Writing committee to revise the ACC/AHA/NASPE 2002 guideline update for implantation of cardiac pacemakers and antiarrhythmia devices). Journal of the American College of Cardiology, 51, 2085–2105.

159. Brodsky, M.A., McAnulty, J., Zipes, D.P., Baessler, C., Hallstrom, A.P., The AVID Investigators (2006). A history of heart failure predicts arrhythmia treatment efficacy: Data from the Antiarrythmics versus Implantable Defibrillators (AVID) Study. American Heart Journal, 152, 724–730.

160. Welch, P.J., Page, R.L., Hamdan, M.H. (1999). Management of ventricular arrhythmias—a trial-based approach. Journal of the American College of Cardiology, 34, 621–630.

161. Bunch, T.J., Hohnloser, S.H., Gersh, B.J. (2007). Mechanisms of sudden cardiac death in myocardial infarction survivors—insights from the randomized trials of implantable cardioverter-defibrillators. Circulation, 115, 2451–2457.

162. Malik, M. (1997). Analysis of clinical follow-up databases: Risk stratification studies and prospective trial design. PACE-Pacing and Clinical Electrophysiology, 20, 2533–2544.

163. DeMets, D.L., Califf, R.M. (2002). Lessons learned from recent cardiovascular clinical trials: Part II. Circulation, 106, 880–886.

164. DeMets, D.L., Califf, R.M. (2002). Lessons learned from recent cardiovascular clinical trials: Part I. Circulation, 106, 746–751.

165. Califf, R.M., DeMets, D.L. (2002). Principles from clinical trials relevant to clinical practice: Part I. Circulation, 106, 1015–1021.

166. Califf, R.M., DeMets, D.L. (2002). Principles from clinical trials relevant to clinical practice: Part II. Circulation, 106, 1172–1175.

167. Califf, R.M. (2006). Clinical trials bureaucracy: Unintended consequences of well-intentioned policy. Clinical Trials, 3, 496–502.

168. Lassere, M.N. (2008). The Biomarker-Surrogacy Evaluation Schema: A review of the biomarker-surrogate literature and a proposal for a criterion-based, quantitative, multi-dimensional hierarchical levels of evidence schema for evaluating the status of biomarkers as surrogate endpoints. Statistical Methods in Medical Research, 17, 303–340.

169. Noseworthy, P.A., Newton-Cheh, C. (2008). Genetic determinants of sudden cardiac death. Circulation, 118, 1854–1863.

170. Knollmann, B.C., Roden, D.M. (2008). A genetic framework for improving arrhythmia therapy. Nature, 451, 929–936.

171. Makita, N., Behr, E., Shimizu, W., Horie, M., Sunami, A., Crotti, L., Schulze-Bahr, E., Fukuhara, S., Mochizuki, N., Makiyama, T., Itoh, H., Christiansen, M., McKeown, P., Miyamoto, K., Kamakura, S., Tsutsui, H., Schwartz, P.J., George, A.L., Roden, D.M.

(2008). The E1784K mutation in SCN5A is associated with mixed clinical phenotype of type 3 long QT syndrome. Journal of Clinical Investigation, 118, 2219–2229.

172. Gollob, M.H. (2006). Genetic profiling as a marker for risk of sudden cardiac death. Current Opinion in Cardiology, 21, 42–46.

173. Dekker, L.R.C., Bezzina, C.R., Henriques, J.P.S., Tanck, M.W., Koch, K.T., Alings, M.W., Arnold, A.E.R., de Boer, M.J., Gorgels, A.P.M., Michels, H.R., Verkerk, A., Verheugt, F.W.A., Zijlstra, F., Wilde, A.A.M. (2006). Familial sudden death is an important risk factor for primary ventricular fibrillation—a case-control study in acute myocardial infarction patients. Circulation, 114, 1140–1145.

174. FDA's Critical Path Initiative to New Medical Products. Available at http://www.fda.gov/oc/initiatives/criticalpath.

175. Arizona CERT (Center for Education and Research on Therapeutics). Available at http://www.azcert.org.

176. ILSI Health and Environmental Sciences Institute. Available at http://www.hesiglobal.org.

177. Cardiac Safety Research Consortium. Available at http://www.cardiac-safety.org.

178. Page, R.L. (2007). Medical management of atrial fibrillation: Future directions. Heart Rhythm, 4, S91–S94.

179. Patton, K.K., Page, R.L. (2007). Cardiovascular & renal—Pharmacological therapy of atrial fibrillation. Expert Opinion on Investigational Drugs, 16, 169–179.

180. Lagrutta, A., Kiss, L., Salata, J.J. (2008). Kv1.5 potassium channel inhibitors for the treatment and prevention of atrial fibrillation. In Ion Channels (Fermini, B., Priest, B.T., eds.), Vol.3, Springer, Berlin, Germany.

181. Myerburg, R.J., Mitrani, R., Interian, A., Castellanos, A. (1998). Interpretation of outcomes of antiarrhythmic clinical trials—Design features and population impact. Circulation, 97, 1514–1521.

182. Martin, R.L.M., Salmen, H.J., Palmatier, J., Cox, B.F., Gintant, G.A. (2004). The utility of hERG and repolarization assays in evaluating delayed cardiac repolarization: Influence of multi-channel block. Journal of Cardiovascular Pharmacology, 43, 369–379.

183. Sarraf, G.B., Walker, M.J.A. (2003). Tedisamil and lidocaine enhance each other's antiarrhythmic activity against ischaemia-induced arrhythmias in rats. British Journal of Pharmacology, 139, 1389–1398.

184. Karle, C.A., Thomas, D., Kiehn, J. (2002). The antiarrhythmic drug BRL-32872. Cardiovascular Drug Reviews, 20, 111–120.

185. Mubagwa, K.M.R., Viappiani, S., Gendviliene, V., Carlsson, B., Brandts, B. (2003). KB130015 a new amiodarone derivative with multiple effects on cardiac ion channels. Cardiovascular Drug Reviews, 21, 216–235.

186. Gautier, P.G.E., Djandjighian, L., Marion, A., Planchenault, J., Bernhart, C., Herbert, J.M., Nisato, D. (2004). In vivo and in vitro characterization of the novel antiarrhythmic agent SSR149744C—electrophysiological, anti-adrenergic, and anti-angiotensin II effects. Journal of Cardiovascular Pharmacology, 44, 244–257.

187. Gautier, P.S.M., Cosnier-Pucheu, S., Djandjighian, L., Roccon, A., Herbert, J.M., Nisato, D. (2005). In vivo and in vitro antiarrhythmic effects of SSR149744C in animal models of atrial fibrillation and ventricular arrhythmias. Journal of Cardiovascular Pharmacology, 45, 125–135.

188. Antzelevitch, C. (2008). Ranolazine: a new antiarrhythmic agent for patients with non-ST-segment elevation acute coronary syndromes? Nature Clinical Practice Cardiovascular Medicine, 5, 248–249.

189. Scirica, B.M., Morrow, D.A., Hod, H., Murphy, S.A., Belardinelli, L., Hedgepeth, C.M., Molhoek, P., Verheugt, F.W.A., Gersh, B.J., McCabe, C.H., Braunwald, E. (2007). Effect of ranolazine, an antianginal agent with novel electrophysiological properties, on the incidence of Arrhythmias in patients with Non-ST-Segment-Elevation acute coronary syndrome—Thrombolysis in myocardial infarction 36 (MERLIN-TIMI 36) Randomized controlled trial. Circulation, 116, 1647–1652.

190. Saint, D.A. (2008). The cardiac persistent sodium current: an appealing therapeutic target? British Journal of Pharmacology, 153, 1133–1142.

191. Makielski, J.C., Valdivia, C.R. (2006). Ranolazine and late cardiac sodium current—a therapeutic target for angina, arrhythmia and more? British Journal of Pharmacology, 148, 4–6.

192. Belardinelli, L., Shryock, J.C., Fraser, H. (2006). Inhibition of the late sodium current as a potential cardioprotective principle: effects of the late sodium current inhibitor ranolazine. Heart, 92, 6–14.

193. Wirth, K.J., Pachler, T., Rosenstein, B., Knobloch, K., Maier, T., Frenzel, J., Brendel, J., Busch, A.E., Bleich, M. (2003). Atrial effects of the novel K +-channel-blocker AVE0118 in anesthetized pigs. Cardiovascular Research, 60, 298–306.

194. Ehrlich, J.R., Ocholla, H., Ziemek, D., Rutten, H., Hohnloser, S.H., Gogelein, H. (2008). Characterization of human cardiac kv1.5 inhibition by the novel atria I-selective antiarrhythmic compound AVE1231. Journal of Cardiovascular Pharmacology, 51, 380–387.

195. Seki, A., Hagiwara, N., Kasanuki, H. (2002). Effects of NIP-141 on K currents in human atrial myocytes. Journal of Cardiovascular Pharmacology, 39, 29–38.

196. Stump, G.L., Wallace, A.A., Regan, C.P., Lynch, J.J. (2005). In vivo antiarrhythmic and cardiac electrophysiologic effects of a novel diphenylphosphine oxide I-Kur blocker (2-isopropyl-5-methylcyclohexyl) diphenylphosphine oxide. Journal of Pharmacology and Experimental Therapeutics, 315, 1362–1367.

197. Matsuda, T., Ito, M., Ishimaru, S., Tsuruoka, N., Saito, T., Iida-Tanaka, N., Hashimoto, N., Yamashita, T., Tsuruzoe, N., Tanaka, H., Shigenobu, K. (2006). Blockade by NIP-142, an antiarrhythmic agent, of carbachol-induced atrial action potential shortening and GIRK1/4 channel. Journal of Pharmacological Sciences, 101, 303–310.

198. Hohnloser, S.H., Dorian, P., Straub, M., Beckmann, K., Kowey, P. (2004). Safety and efficacy of intravenously administered tedisamil for rapid conversion of recent-onset atrial fibrillation or atrial flutter. Journal of the American College of Cardiology, 44, 99–104.

199. Freestone, B., Lip, G.Y.H. (2004). Tedisamil: a new novel antiarrhythmic. Expert Opinion on Investigational Drugs, 13, 151–160.

200. Kirchhof, P., Fortmuller, L., Waldeyer, C., Breithardt, G., Fabritz, L. (2008). Drugs that interact with cardiac electro-mechanics: Old and new targets for treatment. Progress in Biophysics & Molecular Biology, 97, 497–512.

201. Eloff, B.C., Gilat, E., Wan, X.P., Rosenbaum, D.S. (2003). Pharmacological modulation of cardiac gap junctions to enhance cardiac conduction—Evidence supporting a novel target for antiarrhythmic therapy. Circulation, 108, 3157–3163.

202. Wit, A.L., Duffy, H.S. (2008). Drug development for treatment of cardiac arrhythmias: targeting the gap junctions. American Journal of Physiology Heart and Circulatory Physiology, 294, H16–H18.

203. Kjolbye, A.L., Dikshteyn, M., Eloff, B.C., Deschenes, I., Rosenbaum, D.S. (2008). Maintenance of intercellular coupling by the antiarrhythmic peptide rotigaptide suppresses arrhythmogenic discordant alternans. American Journal of Physiology Heart and Circulatory Physiology, 294, H41–H49.

204. Kjolbye, A.L., Haugan, K., Hennan, J.K., Petersen, J.S. (2007). Pharmacological modulation of gap junction function with the novel compound rotigaptide: A promising new principle for prevention of arrhythmias. Basic & Clinical Pharmacology & Toxicology, 101, 215–230.

205. Hasumi, H., Matsuda, R., Shimamoto, K., Hata, Y., Kaneko, N. (2007). K201, a multichannel blocker, inhibits clofilium-induced torsades de pointes and attenuates an increase in repolarization. European Journal of Pharmacology, 555, 54–60.

206. Yamamoto, T., Yano, M., Xu, X.J., Uchinoumi, H., Tateishi, H., Mochizuki, M., Oda, T., Kobayashi, S., Ikemoto, N., Matsuzaki, M. (2008). Identification of target domains of the cardiac ryanodine receptor to correct channel disorder in failing hearts. Circulation, 117, 762–772.

207. Chen, Y.J., Chen, Y.C., Wongcharoen, W., Lin, C.I., Chen, S.A. (2008). Effect of K201, a novel antiarrhythmic drug on calcium handling and arrhythmogenic activity of pulmonary vein cardiomyocytes. British Journal of Pharmacology, 153, 915–925.

208. Ehrlich, J.R., Nattel, S., Hohnloser, S.H. (2007). Novel anti-arrhythmic drugs for atrial fibrillation management. Current Vascular Pharmacology, 5, 185–194.

209. George, C.H., Lai, F.A. (2007). Developing new anti-arrhythmics: Clues from the molecular basis of cardiac ryanodine receptor (RyR2) Ca2 + -release channel dysfunction. Current Pharmaceutical Design, 13, 3195–3211.

210. Wettwer, E., Christ, T., Dobrev, D., Ravens, U. (2007). Novel anti-arrhythmic agents for the treatment of atrial fibrillation. Current Opinion in Pharmacology, 7, 214–218.

211. Christ, T., Ravens, U. (2005). Do we need new antiarrhythmic compounds in the era of implantable cardiac devices and percutaneous ablation? Cardiovascular Research, 68, 341–343.

212. Levy, S. (2006). Do we need pharmacological therapy for atrial fibrillation in the ablation era? Journal of Interventional Cardiac Electrophysiology, 17, 189–194

CHAPTER 9

Ion Channel Remodeling and Arrhythmias

TAKESHI AIBA and GORDON F. TOMASELLI

9.1 INTRODUCTION

The normal electrical activation of the heart requires the precisely orchestrated activity of several ion channels and transporters and the orderly propagation of electrical impulses throughout the myocardium. Disruption of either ion channel functional expression or the cardiac architecture may result in potentially lethal heart rhythm disturbances. This chapter focuses on the molecular and cellular basis of excitability, conduction, and electrical recovery in the heart under normal and pathophysiological conditions with a focus on active membrane property remodeling in heart failure (HF) and cardiac resynchronization. Several excellent encyclopedic reviews of ion channel remodeling in a host of structural heart diseases have been published, and the interested reader is referred to these references [1, 2].

9.2 MOLECULAR AND CELLULAR BASIS OF CARDIAC EXCITABILITY

Ion channels and transporters are multisubunit protein complexes that perform the seemingly paradoxical task of mediating the exquisitely selective flux of millions of ions per second across cell membranes. In the past two decades, most of the relevant ion channel genes encoding the major or pore-forming (α) subunits and many of the ancillary (β) subunits corresponding to ionic currents in the heart have been cloned, sequenced, and functionally characterized. A growing number of inherited arrhythmias have been linked to mutations in ion channel subunit genes. We are just beginning to discover that subtle variations in gene sequences that occur in a significant

Novel Therapeutic Targets for Antiarrhythmic Drugs, Edited by George Edward Billman
Copyright © 2010 John Wiley & Sons, Inc.

proportion of the population (i.e., polymorphisms) may dramatically and lethally alter the response to drugs that act on ion channels [3, 4].

Myocardial cells have a characteristically long action potential (Figure 9.1); depolarizing currents, primarily sodium (Na^+) and calcium (Ca^{2+}), are responsible for the action potential (AP) upstroke and maintenance of the AP plateau, whereas repolarizing currents, primarily potassium, in concert with a reduction in depolarizing currents, are responsible for restoration of the resting membrane potential. Several electrogenic transporters contribute to the action potential profile; the magnitude and direction of the current depends on the transmembrane voltage and concentration gradient of the ions being transported.

9.3 HEART FAILURE—EPIDEMIOLOGY AND THE ARRHYTHMIA CONNECTION

Over 5 million Americans suffer from HF and more than 250,000 die annually. The incidence and prevalence has continued to increase with the aging of the U.S. population [5]. Neurohumoral blockade is the foundation of pharmacotherapy for HF, which delays but does not prevent mortality and has limited effectiveness in halting or reversing disease progression or preventing sudden death [5].

The failing heart is remodeled structurally, electrically, and metabolically. In an attempt to compensate for the reduction in cardiac function the sympathetic nervous system (SNS), renin-angiotensin-aldosterone system (RAAS), and other neurohumoral mechanisms are activated. Indeed, the understanding of the activation of such signaling systems in HF has led to the emergence of neurohormonal receptor blockers as mainstays of therapy. Ultimately, the changes in myocyte function and gene expression that initially maintain tissue perfusion prove to be maladaptive, predisposing to myocyte loss, ventricular chamber remodeling, and interstitial hyperplasia, resulting in a progressive reduction in force development and impairment of ventricular relaxation and potentially lethal alterations in cardiac electrophysiology. Indeed, abnormalities of atrial [6] and ventricular [7] electrophysiology in diseased human hearts have been recognized for more than four decades.

Remodeling of myocyte electrophysiology in HF is well described [1, 2, 8]. The hallmark signature of cells and tissues isolated from failing hearts independent of the etiology is AP prolongation [9, 10]. The AP prolongation is heterogeneous particularly across the ventricular wall, resulting in exaggeration of the physiological heterogeneity of electrical properties in the failing heart [11–14] (Figure 9.2). AP prolongation in HF is arrhythmogenic with frequent early afterdepolarizations (EADs) that are typically not observed in myocytes isolated from the non-failing (NF) hearts. Remarkably, cardiac resynchronization therapy (CRT) has the unique effect of regional shortening of the action potential duration (APD), reducing heterogeneity of repolarization and frequency of EADs in failing hearts with dyssynchronous contraction (DHF) [15] (Figure 9.3). We will include a description of the effects of CRT on the electrophysiology of DHF.

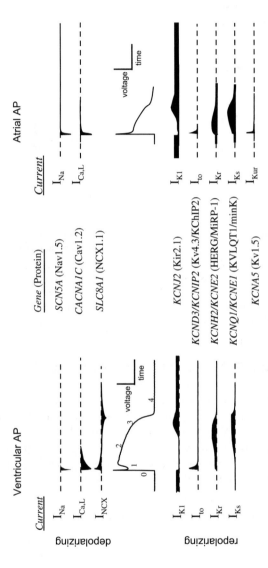

Figure 9.1. The inward and outward currents, pumps and exchangers that underlie the mammalian ventricular (left) and atrial (right) action potentials. A schematic of the time course of each current is shown, and the gene product that underlies the current is indicated.

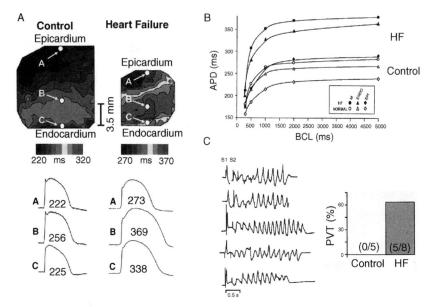

Figure 9.2. Heart Failure prolongs the AP and increases arrhythmia susceptibility **A. (Upper panel)** Representative APD contour maps recorded from the transmural surfaces of a control (left) and canine tachypacing HF wedge (right). APD was heterogeneously prolonged across all layers in HF. **(Lower panel)** Representative action potentials from subepicardial, midmyocardial, and subendocardial layers of the control and HF wedges. B. HF wedges exhibited a significant prolongation of APD in all layers of the myocardium, which was associated with a marked increase in arrhythmia inducibility (PVT%). **C.** with a single premature stimulus (modified from ref. 9). See color insert.

9.4 K$^+$ CHANNEL REMODELING IN HEART FAILURE

Downregulation of K$^+$ currents is the most consistent ionic current change in animal models [16–19] and human HF [10], K$^+$ current downregulation may promote ventricular tachycardia (VT)/ventricular fibrillation (VF) [19] either by direct prolongation of AP [14] in the voltage range at which I$_{Ca,L}$ reactivation occurs predisposing to the development of EADs [20] or by heterogeneously reducing repolarization reserve and promoting functional reentry [21].

9.4.1 Transient Outward Potassium Current (I$_{to}$)

Although expressed cardiac K$^+$ channels vary in different species, I$_{to}$ downregulation is the most consistent ionic current change in failing mammalian hearts [10, 16, 18, 19, 22–24]. However, the effect on ventricular repolarization is complex and species dependent [25].

I$_{to}$ activates shortly after the onset of the AP and is responsible for the early phase of repolarization (phase 1 notch of the AP) and setting the membrane potential at which the L-type Ca^{2+} current (I$_{Ca,L}$) reactivates. Because I$_{to}$ is an early transient current,

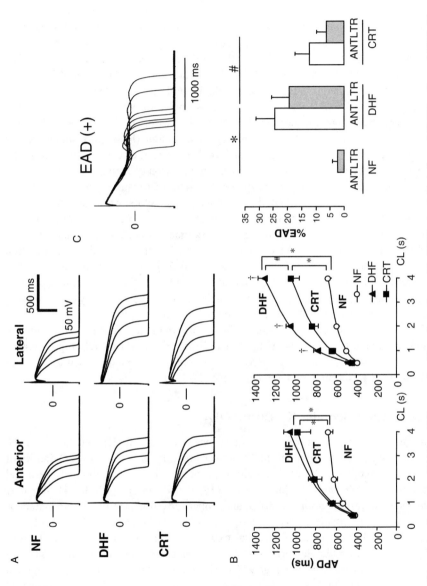

Figure 9.3. APD and development of EADs. APD were significantly prolonged in DHF especially in lateral (LTR) cells, and CRT abbreviated APD in LTR cells but not in anterior (ANT) cells. EADs were more frequent in DHF but partially reduced in CRT (modified from ref. 15).

it may not directly affect the ventricular APD in large mammalian hearts [13] as it does in rodent ventricles [26]. Interestingly, downregulation of I_{to} in cells isolated from terminally failing human hearts is not associated with a change in its voltage dependence or kinetics [10].

Kv4.3 is the gene that encodes the α subunit of cardiac I_{to} in large mammals [16]. Other accessory subunits may also participate in the formation of native I_{to} channels. For example, Kv4 subunits may form heteromeric complexes with a class of Kv-channel interacting proteins (KChIPs) [27, 28]. In the heart, KChIP2 along with at least two splice variants is expressed [29]. KChIP2 significantly modulates Kv4.3 function when expressed in heterologous systems [30, 31] and may impart Ca^{2+} sensitivity to the gating of Kv4.3 [32]. However, it remains uncertain whether KChIP2 or other accessory subunits, such as the potassium channel accessory protein (KChAP) [33–35] or the voltage-activated potassium channel beta subunit (Kvb) [36], merely act to increase the sarcolemmal expression of Kv4.3 or, in fact, directly participate in the formation, active phenotypic expression and modulation of native ventricular I_{to}.

The molecular mechanism of I_{to} downregulation in HF is likely to be multifactorial. For one, I_{to} is tightly regulated by neurohumoral factors, which are significantly altered in HF [37]. In addition, there is compelling evidence for a component of transcriptional regulation of I_{to} in HF. For example, reduced steady-state levels of Kv4 messenger RNA (mRNA) are highly correlated with functional downregulation of I_{to} in both humans [22, 38] and canines [15, 16, 39]. In a canine pacing model of HF, tachycardia downregulates I_{to} expression, with the Ca^{2+}/calmodulin-dependent protein kinase II (CaMKII) and calcineurin/NFAT systems playing key Ca^{2+}-sensing and signal-transducing roles in rate-dependent I_{to} control [40].

The downregulation of I_{to} is regionally uniform in the left ventricle and is unique among regulated K^+ currents in HF in that it is *not* reversed by CRT (Figure 9.4A). In parallel, Kv4.3 and KChIP2 mRNA and protein expression are downregulated in DHF without restoration by CRT (Figure 9.4D) [15].

9.4.2   Inward Rectifier K^+ Current (I_{K1})

Changes in other K^+ currents have also been reported in HF but not with the consistency of I_{to} downregulation. The inward rectifier K^+ current (Kir2 family of genes, I_{K1}) maintains the resting membrane potential and contributes to terminal repolarization (phase 3). Reduced inward I_{K1} density in HF [18, 38, 41, 42] may contribute to prolongation of APD and enhanced susceptibility to spontaneous membrane depolarizations including delayed afterdepolarizations (DADs) [41, 43].

Reported changes in I_{K1} functional expression are more variable than I_{to}. For example, in ventricular hypertrophy, I_{K1} has been reported to increase [44], decrease [45], and remain unchanged [46, 47]. Even within the same experimental model of HF induction (e.g., pacing tachycardia), inconsistencies have been observed across species: reduced I_{K1} density in canine [16, 42] but no change in rabbit [24]. In terminal human heart failure, I_{K1} is significantly reduced at negative voltages [10], but the underlying basis for such downregulation seems to be posttranscriptional in light of the absence of changes in the steady-state level of Kir2.1 mRNA [38]. Interestingly, a differential reduction in I_{K1} was noted between cells isolated from

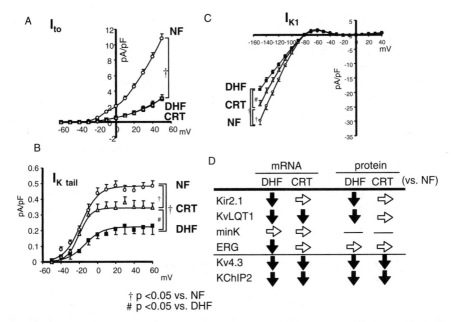

Figure 9.4. CRT partially reverses DHF-induced downregulation of I_{K1} and I_K but not I_{to}. A-C. DHF significantly reduces the inward rectifier I_{K1}, the delayed rectifier (I_K) and transient outward K^+ currents (I_{to}) in both ANT and LTR cells. CRT partially restores the DHF-induced reduction of I_{K1} and I_K, but not I_{to}, in both ANT and LTR cells. **D.** The current changes are generally consistent with changes in steady-state K^+ channel mRNA subunit and protein expression (modified from ref. 15).

failing hearts with dilated versus ischemic cardiomyopathy, with the former group exhibiting a lower whole-cell slope conductance at the reversal potential for K^+ than the latter [48].

The underlying molecular basis of I_{K1} downregulation in HF remains controversial in the absence of consistent changes in the expression of Kir2 family of genes. The specific subunit(s) that underlie I_{K1} vary as a function of the species and cardiac chamber, although Kir2.1 and 2.2 knockout twice [49] and Kir2.1 dominant negative overexpressing mice [50] exhibit prolonged APDs.

CRT even in the setting of continued HF partially restores I_{K1} density (Figure 9.4B) [15] and decreases membrane resistance and in the setting of improved Ca^{2+} handling in CRT (see below) may reduce the frequency of arrhythmogenic DADs. Kir2.1 mRNA and protein levels are partially restored by CRT in the canine model (Figure 9.4D) [15], suggesting that different mechanisms of regulation of current are operative in some animal models and human HF.

9.4.3 Delayed Rectifier K Currents (I_{Kr} and I_{Ks})

The delayed rectifier K^+ currents play a prominent role in the late phase of repolarization [51], therefore changes in either the slow (I_{Ks}) or fast (I_{Kr}) activating components of this current could contribute significantly to action potential prolongation in HF. Reduced I_K density, slower activation, and faster deactivation kinetics have been observed in hypertrophied feline ventricles [52]. In addition, downregulation of both I_{Kr} and I_{Ks} have been reported in a rabbit model of rapid ventricular pacing HF [19], whereas I_{Ks} but not I_{Kr} was downregulated in all layers of the left ventricular myocardium in a canine model of same tachy-pacing HF [42].

The molecular basis for I_K downregulation in HF remains controversial. We recently measured mRNA levels of the genes encoding the α subunits for the rapidly (hERG) and slowly (KvLQT1) activating components of I_K in normal and failing canine hearts and found no statistical difference [38]. Others have reported a decrease in hERG expression in human HF [53].

CRT partially restores DHF-induced downregulation of I_K density in both anterior and lateral LV myocytes (Figure 9.4C, D) without a significant change in mRNA or protein levels of KvLQT1 or minK compared with DHF, whereas ERG mRNA levels were partially restored by CRT in either the anterior or lateral left ventricular (LV) wall [15].

9.5 Ca^{2+} HANDLING AND ARRHYTHMIC RISK

Altered Ca^{2+} homeostasis underlies abnormalities in excitation-contraction coupling (ECC) and arrhythmic risk in HF. Intracellular $[Ca^{2+}]i$ and the AP are intricately linked by a variety of Ca^{2+}-mediated cell surface channels and transporters such as I_{Ca-L}, I_K, Ca^{2+}-activated Cl^- current and sodium–calcium exchanger current (NCX).

9.5.1 L-Type Ca^{2+} Current I_{Ca-L}

I_{Ca-L} density is unchanged or reduced in HF, the latter typically occurring in more advanced disease [1, 8, 54]. Remarkably, in human HF baseline, I_{Ca-L} density is consistently unchanged [55–58], although single-channel studies suggest a reduction in channel number with an increase in open probability perhaps because of altered phosphorylation or subunit composition [59, 60]. The molecular bases of changes in the density of I_{Ca-L} are incompletely understood, subunit mRNA expression in HF is variable [59, 61–63]. The complexity of the molecular basis of channel remodeling is highlighted by reports of isoform switching of both $\alpha1C$ [62, 64] and β subunits [65] in the failing heart.

In canine DHF model, are intraventricular regional changes in I_{Ca-L} are partially restored by CRT [15]. DHF produced a reduction peak I_{Ca-L} density and slowed current decay in myocytes isolated from the lateral LV wall. In contrast, the peak I_{Ca-L} density in anterior myocytes was increased compared with nonfailing controls; thus, DHF produced regional heterogeneity of current density and kinetics. CRT restored the peak current density but did not alter the I_{Ca-L} decay in the lateral cells, eliminating the anterior-lateral current density gradient [15] (Figure 9.5A).

9.5.2 Sarcoplasmic Reticulum Function

Heart failure is associated with major changes in intracellular and sarcoplasmic reticulum (SR) Ca^{2+} homeostasis [66]. The amplitude of the calcium transient

(CaT) and its rate of decay are reduced in intact preparations [67] and cells [68–70] isolated from failing ventricles. The SR Ca^{2+}-ATPase (SERCA2a), its inhibitor phospholamban (PLN) and NCX are primary mediators of Ca^{2+} removal from the cytoplasm. In HF, ventricular myocytes exhibit a greater reliance on NCX for removal of Ca^{2+} from the cytosol and an increase in NCX function [69, 71], which leads to defective SR Ca^{2+} loading. The enhanced NCX function in the failing heart, particularly in the setting of changes in intracellular [Na$^+$], contribute to the augmented transient inward current (I$_{ti}$) that underlies arrhythmogenic DADs [41].

Heart failure-associated changes in the function of the key Ca^{2+} release channel in the SR, the ryanodine receptor (RyR2) also contributes to defective SR loading

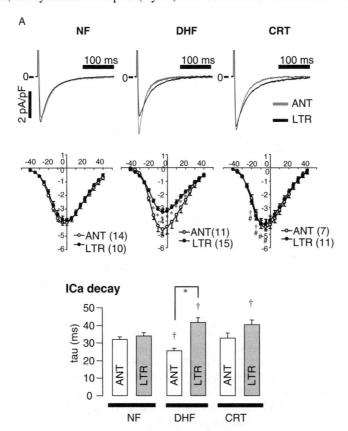

Figure 9.5. CRT restores DHF-induced regional differences in Ca^{2+} currents (I$_{Ca-L}$) and transients (CaT). **A**. In DHF, the peak I$_{Ca-L}$ density was smaller and the decay was slower in the LTR myocytes, whereas the peak current density was larger and decay was faster in the ANT myocytes. The reduced current density is observed over a wide range of activation voltages. CRT restored the the peak I$_{Ca-L}$ density in LTR cells, but the decay was still slow. **B**. Compared with the control, DHF significantly reduced the CaT amplitude and slowed the rate of decay of the transient most prominently in the LTR myocytes. CRT partially restored the CaT amplitude of LTR cells but did not significantly change the amplitude of ANT myocytes. However, it did hasten the slowed decay to nearly that of normal ANT control cells.

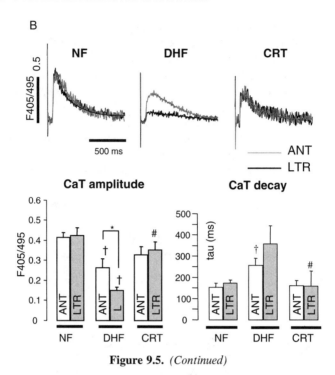

Figure 9.5. *(Continued)*

and excitation-contraction coupling. In failing hearts, the stoichiometry and function of the RyR2 macromolecular complex is altered [72]. Decreased levels of phosphatases (PP1 and PP2A) and hyperphosphorylation by protein kinase A (PKA) result in dissociation of the regulatory protein FKBP12.6 and channels with increased Ca^{2+} sensitivity resulting in an increase in open probability that produces a Ca^{2+} leak

Figure 9.6. Intracellular Ca^{2+} cycling and associated signaling pathways in cardiomyocytes. On a beat-by-beat basis, calcium transients (CaTs) are elicited by the influx of a small amount of Ca^{2+} through the I_{Ca-L} and the subsequent large-scale Ca^{2+} release from the SR through the RyR. During diastole, cytosolic Ca^{2+} is taken up into the SR by the PLN-regulated SERCA2a pump. β-AR–mediated PKA stimulation regulates this Ca^{2+} cycling by phosphorylating I_{Ca-L}, RyR, and phosphalamben (PLB). In normal hearts, sympathetic stimulation activates the $\beta1$-adrenergic receptor, which in turn stimulates the production of cAMP by adenylyl cyclase and thereby activates PKA. PKA phosphorylates PLN and RyR, both of which contribute to an increased intracellular CaT and enhanced cellular contractility. PP1 and PP2A regulate the dephosphorylation process of these Ca^{2+} regulatory proteins (RyR, PLN, and I_{Ca-L}). The PLN hypophosphorylation inhibits SERCA2a activity, which thereby decreases SR Ca^{2+} uptake. The increased Ca^{2+} level in the cytosol activates CaMKII, which affects the functions of RyR and PLB. The activation or deactivation of these molecules at a node in the signaling cascade affects beat-by-beat Ca^{2+} cycling, and such maneuvers have recently been highlighted as potential new therapeutic strategies against HF. Increased INCX, reduced IK1, and residual coupling to β-AR signaling may predispose to arrhythmogenic delayed after depolarization (DAD) [41].

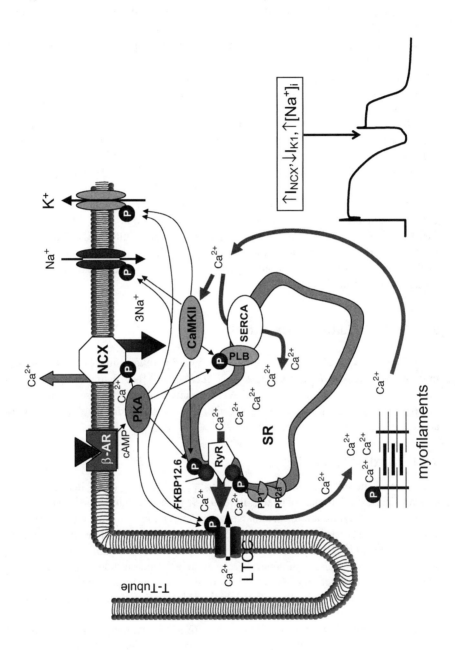

from the SR (Figure 9.6) [73, 74]. The enhanced Ca^{2+} sensitivity that causes the leak may increase the fractional release of Ca^{2+} during EC coupling so the effect on systolic function and the role of phosphorylation of RyR2 continues to be hotly debated [66, 73, 75–81]. However, it is likely that defects in RyR2 function contribute to the development of triggered arrhythmias in the failing heart, and as such they remain an attractive therapeutic target [82, 83]. Beta-adrenergic receptor blockers reverse PKA hyperphosphorylation of RyR2, restores the stoichiometry of the RyR2 macromolecular complex, and normalizes single-channel function in a canine model and human HF [74, 84].

Several studies have demonstrated reductions in SERCA2a and PLN mRNA, but fewer have shown a reduction in immunoreactive protein; however, reductions in PLN phosphorylation [85, 86] may result in enhanced inhibition of SERCA in HF. Increases in NCX mRNA and protein have been regularly observed in failing hearts [1, 8]. Levels of RyR mRNA and protein in HF are variable [87, 88].

Abnormal SR Ca^{2+} handling in DHF is also functionally restored by CRT [15, 89]. CRT dramatically increases the amplitude and hastens the decay kinetics of the CaT particularly in cells isolated from the lateral LV wall (Figure 9.5B). The reversal in SR function by CRT occurs without a change in mRNA or protein levels of PLN, SERCA2a, NCX, or RyR2 [15]; thus, these levels are likely to be the result of altered posttranslational modifications.

9.6   INTRACELLULAR [Na$^+$] IN HF

Intracellular $[Na^+]_i$ and Ca^{2+} handling are intimately linked and $[Na^+]_i$ is increased in failing ventricular myocytes [41, 90, 91]. Increases in $[Na^+]_i$ may be the result of diminished efflux by reduced Na^+/K^+ ATPase activity or an increase in Na^+ influx via I_{Na}, Na^+/H^+ exchanger, NCX, or other Na^+ cotransporters. We will briefly address changes in Na current and Na^+/K^+ ATPase.

9.6.1   Cardiac I$_{Na}$ in HF

A prominent increase in late Na^+ current (I_{Na-L}) and slowing of I_{Na} decay has been described in several models of heart failure [92–95]. The mechanism(s) of the increase in I_{Na-L} in heart failure are uncertain. No consistent changes in Na^+ channel subunit expression have been reported in HF [16, 39, 94]. But block of the late current inhibits oxidant-induced EADs and contractile dysfunction [96] and alterations in calmodulin kinase (CaMK) signaling influence I_{Na} decay and the magnitude of I_{Na-L} [97, 98], suggesting posttranslational modifications of the Na^+ current. A post translational mechanism is suggested by the inhibition of oxidant-induced EADs and contractile dysfunction by Na channel blockers [96] and slowing of the decay and an increase in the magnitude of INa-L by calmodulin kinase (CaMK). Oxidant stress and increased CaMKII activity are prominent in the failing heart. I_{Na} blockers have an infamous history in the treatment of cardiac arrhythmias with substantial proarrhythmic liability [99]; however, new strategies that target the late current may have more promise [100, 101].

9.6.2 Na$^+$/K$^+$ ATPase

The Na$^+$/K$^+$ ATPase, or Na$^+$ pump, is responsible for the establishment and maintenance of the major ionic gradients across the cell membrane and belongs to the widely distributed class of P-type ATPases that are responsible for transporting several cations. The Na$^+$/K$^+$ ATPase hydrolyzes a molecule of ATP to transport K$^+$ into the cell and Na$^+$ out with a stoichiometry of $2:3$, therefore generating a time-independent outward current.

The consensus of experimental data reveal that the expression and function of the Na$^+$/K$^+$ -ATPase are reduced in HF compared with control hearts [102–106]. The density as assessed by ^{3}[H]-ouabain binding of the Na$^+$/K$^+$ ATPase is decreased in HF. The decrease occurs without a significant impact on the inotropic effect of digitalis glycosides in human ventricular myocardium [107]. Decreased Na$^+$ pump function in HF has several consequences that might be relevant to production of arrhythmias. First, the reduction in the outward repolarizing current could prolong APD. Second, reduced pump function reduces Na$^+$ efflux and may increase intracellular $[Na^+]_i$. Finally, cells with less Na$^+$/K$^+$ -ATPase activity have greater difficulty handling changes in extracellular $[K^+]_o$. Low $[K^+]_o$ itself tends to inhibit the ATPase, whereas increases in $[K^+]_o$ would tend to be cleared less rapidly in the setting of relative pump inhibition.

The consequences of increased Na$^+$ influx or decreased efflux in HF, particularly in the setting of regionally variable lengthening of the APD, is heterogenous cytosolic Na$^+$ loading and subsequent activation of "reverse mode" NCX function. NCX functioning the reverse mode in response to increased $[Na^+]_i$ may be adaptive promoting an increase influx in activator Ca^{2+} (Figure 9.6). However, the slowed I_{Na} decay and increased I_{Na-L} may contribute to the regional AP prolongation and more frequent EADs in DHF (Figure 9.3).

9.7 GAP JUNCTIONS AND CONNEXINS

Gap junction channels are intercellular channel proteins that permit electrical and chemical communication between cells. These channels are major mediators of conduction in the heart. Mammalian gap junction channels or connexons are built by the oligomerization of a family of closely related genes encoding connexins (Cx) [108]. Connexins are integral membrane proteins consisting of four highly conserved membrane-spanning α-helices, two extracellular loops, and one intracellular loop. Three different Cx have been identified in the mammalian heart, Cx40, Cx43, and Cx45, which are named for their respective molecular masses.

Slowed intraventricular conduction is a prominent feature of HF and is associated with a reduction in the density, altered distribution, and posttranslational modification of the major cardiac gap junction protein (Cx43) [109]. Similar findings have been observed in hypertrophied and ischemic human ventricular myocardium. Cx43 is downregulated and redistributed from the intercalated disk to the entire cell border (lateralization) [110–114]; this pattern is observed in early cardiac development. We observe downregulation and lateralization of Cx43 in DHF [109] that is progressive with duration of tachypacing [115] and associated with conduction slowing. The mechanism of Cx43 downregulation is not completely understood but may involve altered RAAS signaling [116, 117] and changes in binding partners [118–120]. In the pacing tachycardia HF, Cx43 downregulation is associated with a reduction in Cx43 mRNA and may be regulated by a microRNA (miR-1) [121].

9.8 AUTONOMIC SIGNALING

The hemodynamic alterations resulting from impaired contractile performance in systolic HF activate the SNS and RAAS. Activation of the SNS increases heart rate and contractility and redistributes blood flow centrally by peripheral vasoconstriction. The RAAS activation similarly causes vasoconstriction and increases circulatory volume, allowing individuals to respond appropriately to physiological stress or exercise. Neurohumoral activation is initially adaptive, maintaining systolic function and vital organ perfusion, then ultimately leads to the progression of the heart failure phenotype. The combination of neurohumoral activation and mechanical stress activates signal transduction cascades that produce myocyte hypertrophy and result in the elaboration of trophic factors that increase the interstitial content of collagen, and they have profound effects on the electrophysiology of the failing heart.

Changes in adrenergic signaling in the failing heart are well characterized [122–124]. The β_1, β_2, and α_1 adrenergic receptors mediate the effects of increased catecholamines, both circulating epinephrine and norepinephrine that is released from cardiac nerve terminals in the heart. These receptor subtypes are coupled to different signaling systems. The β_1 and β_2 adrenergic receptors (β-ARs) are coupled by stimulatory G proteins to adenylyl cyclase; activation results in increased cellular levels of cyclic adenosine $3',5'$-monophosphate (cAMP), which may be local in the case of β_2 adrenergic receptors [125]. The α_1 receptor is coupled by a G protein to phospholipase C (PLC), which hydrolyzes inositol phospholipids increasing cellular inositol 1,4,5-trisphosphate (IP3) and diacylglycerol (DAG). Activation of the α-adrenergic receptor pathway initiates a cascade triggering cell growth and alters the intracellular Ca^{2+} load. The possible adverse consequences of increased Ca^{2+} load include the activation of phospholipases, proteases, and endonucleases, which culminate in cell necrosis or apoptosis and progression of the failing phenotype.

Chronic β-AR stimulation by catecholamines can be cardiotoxic, and multiple regulatory adjustments produce desensitization of downstream effector responses in the failing heart such as functional upregulation of inhibitory G proteins (G_i) and inhibitory regulators of G protein signaling (RGS). In human and animal models of chronic HF, the cardiac response to β-AR stimulation is blunted, and a positive correlation is found between increased plasma catecholamine levels and the degree of the diminution of the β-AR response [122, 126–129]. In most studies of end-stage human HF [122, 126, 128] and some failing animal models [129], the β_1-AR undergoes subtype-selective downregulation such that the proportions of β_1-:β_2-ARs are nearly equal in abundance [128, 130] compared with the dominance of the β_1-AR subtype in normal hearts [126]. In addition, the remaining β-ARs are significantly desensitized because of uncoupling of the receptors from their respective signaling pathways [131, 132].

The β-AR subtype signaling pathways may have markedly different chronic effects on growth and survival in the heart. The hypertrophic response, is manifested by the distinct phenotypes of transgenic mice overexpressing cardiac β_1- [133] versus β_2-ARs [134, 135]. Recent evidence also suggests that the β-AR subtypes even have opposing effects on apoptosis in cultured rat cardiomyocytes: β_1-adrenergic receptor stimulation induces apoptosis [136], whereas β_2-adrnergic receptor stimulation inhibits apoptosis [137].

In chronic HF in both humans [138–140] and animal models [129], a marked increase in G_i mRNA levels has been reported. Studies in rats and guinea pigs have shown that chronic infusion of catecholamines increases the expression of G_i [139, 141], in parallel, the overexpression of the human β_2-AR in transgenic mice was associated with enhanced G_i protein abundance [142].

Protein phosphorylation mediated by β-adrenergic receptor activation is decreased in the failing human heart [143, 144]. The PKA signaling pathway seems to be downregulated at several levels beyond the β-adrenergic receptor, with the functional implication of limiting PKA targeting to important subcellular locations such as the sarcolemma and the SR in the failing cardiac myocytes [145]. There is increasing evidence for local regulation of PKA activity by binding of PKA to A-kinase anchoring proteins (AKAPs) [146, 147]. Such compartmentalization of PKA in the human heart may be disrupted in HF as yet another mechanism of abnormal autonomic signaling in the failing heart [145].

Adrenergic signaling pathways affect the function of many ion channels and transporters. The net effect of β-adrenergic receptor stimulation is to shorten the ventricular APD because of an increase of I_K density [148], despite β_1-adrenergic receptor stimulation of depolarizing current through the L-type Ca channel. α_1-adrenergic receptor stimulation inhibits several K^+ currents in the mammalian heart, including I_{to}, I_{K1}, and I_K, with the net effect of prolonging APD [149]. In a rat HF model, the inotropic responses to β-adrenergic receptor stimulation and to direct stimulation of adenylyl cyclase, were diminished based on desensitization of the stimulatory side of the adenylyl cyclase signal transduction system [150]. In parallel, the responses to inhibitory receptors were augmented, leading to a pronounced G_i-mediated negative inotropic effect on failing heart muscle cells [150].

Interestingly, CRT produces a striking improvement in β-AR reserve in cells and tissues isolated from DHF. The effects were particularly prominent in myocytes isolated from the lateral wall of DHF hearts where isoproterenol augmentation of I_{Ca-L} density and CaT amplitude were nearly completely restored in myocytes from CRT hearts. The profoundly slowed CaT decay in DHF myocytes was dramatically hastened by CRT. This restoration is the result of augmentation of β_1-adrenergic receptor abundance and a reduction in Gαi (presumably via β_2-AR) signaling mediated by an increase in the inhibitory regulator of G protein signaling, RGS3, in CRT [151].

9.9 CALMODULIN KINASE

Calmodulin (CaM) is the most ubiquitous Ca^{2+} binding protein in mammalian cells. CaM is a vital signaling molecule that regulates the function of many proteins critical to cellular metabolism, Ca^{2+} transport, contraction, electrophysiology, gene expression, and cell proliferation [152]. Ca^{2+}/CaM-dependent protein kinase II (CaMKII) is the main target of CaM binding in the heart and is a multifunctional enzyme capable of phosphorylating several substrates, including K channels, ryanodine release (RyR), and PLN [152–154]. CaMKII activity is increased, possibly as a compensatory mechanism for altered Ca^{2+} homeostasis in both human [153] and animal models [155] of HF. However, the regional differences in Ca^{2+} homeostasis and associated regulatory proteins in DHF and their restoration by CRT have not been studied.

9.10 CONCLUSIONS

Structural remodeling and HF-induced changes in ionic currents and transporters and Ca^{2+} handling creates a highly susceptible substrate for both triggered and reentrant atrial and potentially lethal ventricular arrhythmias. Understanding remodeling of the diseased heart also creates opportunities for interventions to reduce structural changes and reduce arrhythmic risk. Remarkably, CRT produces both global and regional improvement in cardiac performance, Ca^{2+} handling, and reversal of many aspects of electrophysiological remodeling.

REFERENCES

1. Nattel, S., Magoy, A., LeBouter, S., Yeh, Y.H. (2007). Arrhythmogenic ion-channel remodeling in the heart: Heart failure, myocardial infarction, and atrial fibrillation. Physiology Review, 87, 425–456.

2. Nass, R.D., Aiba, T., Tomaselli, G.F., Akar, F.G. (2008). Mechanisms of disease: ion channel remodeling in the failing ventricle. Nature Clinical Practice. Cardiovascular Medicine, 5, 196–207.

3. Fitzgerald, P.T., Ackerman, M.J. (2005). Drug-induced torsades de pointes: The evolving role of pharmacogenetics. Heart Rhythm, 2, S30–37.

4. Darbar, D., Roden, D.M. (2006). Pharmacogenetics of antiarrhythmic therapy. Expert Opinion Pharmacotherapy, 7, 1583–1590.

5. Rosamond, W., Flegal, K., Friday, G., Furie, K., Go, A., Greenland, K., et al. (2007). Heart disease and stroke statistics—2007 update: A report from the American Heart Association Statistics Committee and Stroke Statistics Subcommittee. Circulation, 115, e69–171.

6. van Dam, R.T., Durrer, D. (1961). Excitability and electrical activity of human myocardial strips from the left atrial appendage in cases of rheumatic mitral stenosis. Circulation Research, 9, 509–514.

7. Trautwein, W., Kassebaum, D.G., Nelson, R.N., Hech, T.H.H. (1962). Electrophysiological study of human heart muscle. Circulation Research, 10, 306–312.

8. Tomaselli, G.F., Marban, E. (1999). Electrophysiological remodeling in hypertrophy and heart failure. Cardiovascular Research, 42, 270–283.

9. Akar, F.G., Rosenbaum, D.S. (2003). Transmural electrophysiological heterogeneities underlying arrhythmogenesis in heart failure. Circulation Research, 93, 638–645.

10. Beuckelmann, D.J., Näbäurer, M., Erdmann, E. (1993). Alterations of K+ currents in isolated human ventricular myocytes from patients with terminal heart failure. Circulation Research, 73, 379–385.

11. Fedida, D., Giles, W.R. (1991). Regional variations in action potentials and transient outward current in myocytes isolated from rabbit left ventricle. Journal of Physiology, 442, 191–209.

12. Antzelevitch, C., Sicouri, S., Litovsky, S.H., Lukas, A., Krishman, S.C., Di Diego, J.M., Gintant, G.A., Liv, D.W. (1991). Heterogeneity within the ventricular wall Electrophysiology and pharmacology of epicardial, endocardial, and M cells. Circulation Research, 69, 1427–1449.

13. Akar, F.G., Wu, R.C., Juang, G.J., Tian, Y., Burysek, M., Disilvestre, D., Xiong, W., Armoundas, A.A., Tomaselli, G.B. (2005). Molecular mechanisms underlying K+ current downregulation in canine tachycardia-induced heart failure. American Journal of Physiology Heart Circulation Physiology, 288, H2887–2896.

14. Akar, F.G., Rosenbaum, D.S. (2003). Transmural electrophysiological heterogeneities underlying arrhythmogenesis in heart failure. Circulation Research, 93, 638–645.

15. Aiba, T., Hesketh, G.G., Barth, A.S., Liu, T., Daya, S., Chakir, K., Dimaano, V.L., Abraham, T.P., O'Rourke, B., et al. (2009). Electrophysiological consequences of dyssynchronous heart failure and its restoration by resynchronization therapy. Circulation, 119, 1130–1220.

16. Kaab, S., Nuss, H.B., Chiamvimonvat, N., O'Rourke, B., Pal, P.H., Kass, D.A., Marban, E., Tomaselli, G.F. (1996). Ionic mechanism of action potential prolongation in ventricular myocytes from dogs with pacing-induced heart failure. Circulation Research, 78, 262–273.

17. Tomaselli, G.F., Zipes, D.P. (2004). What causes sudden death in heart failure? Circulation Research, 95, 754–763.

18. Rose, J., Armoundas, A.A., Tian, Y., Disilvestre, D., Burysek, M., Halperin, V., O'Rourke, B., Kass, D.A., Marban, E., Tomaselli, G.F. (2005). Molecular correlates of altered expression of potassium currents in failing rabbit myocardium. American Journal of Physiology Heart Circulation Physiology, 288, H2077–2087.

19. Tsuji, Y., Zicha, S., Qi, X.Y., Kodama, I., Nattel, S. (2006). Potassium channel subunit remodeling in rabbits exposed to long-term bradycardia or tachycardia: Discrete arrhythmogenic consequences related to differential delayed-rectifier changes. Circulation, 113, 345–355.

20. Aiba, T., Shimizu, W., Inagaki, M., Noda, T., Mivoshi, S., Ding, W.G., Zankov, D.P., Toyoda, F., Matsarra, H., et al. (2005). Cellular and ionic mechanism for drug-induced long QT syndrome and effectiveness of verapamil. Journal of the American College of Cardiology, 45, 300–307.

21. Roden, D.M., Spooner, P.M. (1999). Inherited long QT syndromes: A paradigm for understanding arrhythmogenesis. Journal of Cardiovascular Electrophysiology, 10, 1664–1683.

22. Nabauer, M., Backelmann, D.S., Erdmann, E. (1993). Characteristics of transient outward current in human ventricular myocytes from patients with terminal heart failure. Circulation Research, 73, 386–394.

23. Wettwer, E., Amos, G.J., Posival, H., Ravens, U. (1994). Transient outward current in human ventricular myocytes of subepicardial and subendocardial origin. Circulation Research, 75, 473–482.

24. Rozanski, G.J., Xu, Z., Whitney, R.I., Murakami, H., Zucker, I.H. (1997). Electrophysiology of rabbit ventricular myocytes following sustained rapid ventricular pacing. Journal of Molecular and Cellular Cardiology, 29, 721–732.

25. Greenstein, J.L., Wu, R., Po, S., Tomaselli, G.F., Winslow, R.L. (2000). Role of the calcium-independent transient outward current i(to1) in shaping action potential morphology and duration [In Process Citation]. Circulation Research, 87, 1026–1033.

26. Nerbonne, J.M. (2000). Molecular basis of functional voltage-gated K+ channel diversity in the mammalian myocardium. Journal of Physiology, 525, 285–298.

27. An, W.F., Bowlby, M.R., Betty, M., Cao, J., Ling, H.P., Mendoza, G., Hinson, J.W., et al. (2000). Modulation of A-type potassium channels by a family of calcium sensors. Nature, 403, 553–556.

28. Rosati, B., Pan, Z., Lypen, S., Wang, H.S., Cohen, I., Dixon, J.E., McKinnon, D. (2001). Regulation of KChIP2 potassium channel beta subunit gene expression underlies the gradient of transient outward current in canine and human ventricle. Journal of Physiology, 533, 119–125.

29. Deschenes, I., Disilvestre, D., Juang, G.J., Wu, R.C., An, W.F., Tomaselli, G.F. (2002). Regulation of Kv4.3 current by KChIP2 splice variants: A component of native cardiac I(to)? Circulation, 106, 423–429.

30. Deschenes, I., Tomaselli, G. (2002). Modulation of Kv4.3 current by accessory subunits. FEBS Letters, 528, 183.

31. Patel, S.P., Campbell, D.L., Strauss, H.C. (2002). Elucidating KChIP effects on Kv4.3 inactivation and recovery kinetics with a minimal KChIP2 isoform. Journal of Physiology, 545, 5–11.

32. Patel, S.P., Parai, R., Campbell, D.L. (2004). Regulation of Kv4.3 voltage-dependent gating kinetics by KChIP2 isoforms. Journal of Physiology, 557, 19–41.

33. Wible, B.A., Yang, Q., Kuryshev, Y.A., Accili, E.A., Brown, A.M. (1998). Cloning and expression of a novel K+ channel regulatory protein, KChAP. Journal of Biological Chemistry, 273, 11745–11751.

34. Kuryshev, Y.A., Gudz, T.I., Brown, A.M., Wible, B.A. (2000). KChAP as a chaperone for specific K(+) channels. American Journal of Physiology Cell Physiology, 278, C931–941.

35. Abriel, H., Motoike, H., Kass, R.S. (2000). KChAP: A novel chaperone for specific K(+) channels key to repolarization of the cardiac action potential. Focus on "KChAP as a chaperone for specific K(+) channels". American Journal of Physiology Cell Physiology, 278, C863–864.

36. Kuryshev, Y.A., Wible, B.A., Gudz, T.I., Ramirez, A.N., Brown, A.M. (2001). KChAP/Kvbeta1.2 interactions and their effects on cardiac Kv channel expression. American Journal of Physiology Cell Physiology, 281, C290–299.

37. Fedida, D., Braun, A.P., Giles, W.R. (1991). Alpha 1-adrenoceptors reduce background K+ current in rabbit ventricular myocytes. Journal of Physiology, 441, 673–684.

38. Kääb, S., Dixon, J., Duc, J., Ashen, D., Näbauer, M., Beuckelmann, D.J., Steinbeck, G., McKinnon, D., Tomaselli, G.F. (1998). Molecular basis of transient outward potassium current downregulation in human heart failure: A decrease in Kv4.3 mRNA correlates with a reduction in current density. Circulation, 98, 1383–1393.

39. Zicha, S., Xiao, L., Stafford, S., Cha, T.J., Han, W., Varro, A., Nattel, S. (2004). Transmural expression of transient outward potassium current subunits in normal and failing canine and human hearts. Journal of Physiology, 561, 735–748.

40. Xiao, L., Contu, P., Villenveve, L.R., Tadevosyan, A., Maguay, A., Le Bouter, S., Allen, B.G., Nattel, S. (2008). Mechanisms underlying rate-dependent remodeling of transient outward potassium current in canine ventricular myocytes. Circulation Research, 103, 733–742.

41. Pogwizd, S.M., Schlotthaver, K., Li, L., Yuan, W., Bers, D.M. (2001). Arrhythmogenesis and contractile dysfunction in heart failure: Roles of sodium-calcium exchange, inward rectifier potassium current, and residual beta-adrenergic responsiveness. Circulation Research, 88, 1159–1167.

42. Li, G.R., Lau, C.P., Durcharme, A., Tardif, J.C., Nattel, S. (2002). Transmural action potential and ionic current remodeling in ventricles of failing canine hearts. American Journal of Physiology Heart Circulation Physiology, 283, H1031–1041.

43. Nuss, H.B., Kaab, S., Kass, D.A., Tomaselli, G.F., Marban, E. (1999). Cellular basis of ventricular arrhythmias and abnormal automaticity in heart failure. American Journal of Physiology, 277, H80–91.

44. Kleiman, R.B., Houser, S.R. (1989). Outward currents in normal and hypertrophied feline ventricular myocytes. American Journal of Physiology, 256, H1450–H1461.

45. Brooksby, P., Levi, A.J., Jones, J.V. (1993). The electrophysiological characteristics of hypertrophied ventricular myocytes from the spontaneously hypertensive rat. Journal of Hypertension, 11, 611–622.

46. Ryder, K.O., Bryant, S.M., Hart, G. (1993). Membrane current changes in left ventricular myocytes isolated from guinea pigs after abdominal aortic coarctation. Cardiovascular Research, 27, 1278–1287.

47. Cerbai, E., Barbieri, M., Li, Q., Mugelli, A. (1994). Ionic basis of action potential prolongation of hypertrophied cardiac myocytes isolated from hypertensive rats of different ages. Cardiovascular Research, 28, 1180–1187.

48. Koumi, S., Backer, C.L., Arentzen, C.E. (1995). Characterization of inwardly rectifying K+ channel in human cardiac myocytes. Alterations in channel behavior in myocytes isolated from patients with idiopathic dilated cardiomyopathy. Circulation, 92, 164–174.

49. Zaritsky, J.J., Eckman, D.M., Wellman, G.C., Nelson, M.T., Schwarz, T.L. (2000). Targeted disruption of Kir2.1 and Kir2.2 genes reveals the essential role of the inwardly rectifying K(+) current in K(+)-mediated vasodilation. Circulation Research, 87, 160–166.

50. McLerie, M., Lopatin, A.N. (2003). Dominant-negative suppression of I(K1) in the mouse heart leads to altered cardiac excitability. Journal of Molecular and Cellular Cardiology, 35, 367–378.

51. Liu, D.W., Antzelevitch, C. (1995). Characteristics of the delayed rectifier current (IKr and IKs) in canine ventricular epicardial, midmyocardial, and endocardial myocytes. A weaker IKs contributes to the longer action potential of the M cell. Circulation Research, 76, 351–365.

52. Furukawa, T., Bassett, A.L., Furukawa, N., Kimura, S., Myerburg, S.J. (1993). The ionic mechanism of reperfusion-induced early after depolarizations in feline left ventricular hypertrophy. 91, 1521–1531.

53. Choy, A.-M., Kuperschmidt, S., Lang, C.C., Pierson, R.N., Roden, D.M. (1996). Regional expression of HERG and KvLQT1 in heart failure. Circulation, 94, 164.

54. Pitt, G.S., Dun, W., Boyden, P.A. (2006). Remodeled cardiac calcium channels. Journal of Molecular and Cellular Cardiology, 41, 373–388.

55. Beuckelmann, D.J., Erdmann, E. (1992). Ca(2+)-currents and intracellular [Ca2+]i-transients in single ventricular myocytes isolated from terminally failing human myocardium. Basic Research Cardiology, 87, 235–243.

56. Mewes, T., Ravens, U. (1994). L-type calcium currents of human myocytes from ventricle of non-failing and failing hearts and from atrium. Journal of Molecular and Cellular Cardiology, 26, 1307–1320.

57. Li, G.R., Lau, C.P., Leung, T.K., Nattel, S. (2004). Ionic current abnormalities associated with prolonged action potentials in cardiomyocytes from diseased human right ventricles. Heart Rhythm, 1, 460–468.

58. Chen, X., Piacentino, V., Furukawa, S., Goldman, B., Margulies, K.B., Houser, S.R. (2002). L-type Ca2+ channel density and regulation are altered in failing human ventricular myocytes and recover after support with mechanical assist devices. Circulation Research, 91, 517–524.

59. Schroeder, F., Handrock, R., Beuckelmann, D.J., Hirt, S., Hullin, R., Priebe, L., Schwinger, R.H., Weil, J., Herzig, S. (1998). Increased availability and open probability of single L-type calcium channels from failing compared with nonfailing human ventricle. Circulation, 98, 969–976.

60. Handrock, R., Schrocker, F., Hirt, S., Haverich, A., Mittmann, C., Herzig, S. (1998). Single-channel properties of L-type calcium channels from failing human ventricle. Cardiovascular Research, 37, 445–455.

61. Takahashi, T., Allen, P.D., Lacro, R.V., Marks, A.R., Dennis, A.R., Schoen, F.J., Grossman, W., Marsh, J.D., Izumo, S. (1992). Expression of dihydropyridine receptor (Ca2+ channel) and calsequestrin genes in the myocardium of patients with end-stage heart failure. Journal of Clinical Investigation, 90, 927–935.

62. Yang, Y., Chen, X., Margulies, K., Jeevanandam, V., Pollack, P., Bailey, B.A., Houser, S.R. (2000). L-type Ca2+ channel alpha 1c subunit isoform switching in failing human ventricular myocardium. Journal of Molecular and Cellular Cardiology, 32, 973–984.

63. Hullin, R., Asmus, F., Ludwig, A., Hevsel, J., Boekstegers, P. (1999). Subunit expression of the cardiac L-type calcium channel is differentially regulated in diastolic heart failure of the cardiac allograft. Circulation, 100, 155–163.

64. Gidh-Jain, M., Huang, B., Jain, P., Battula, V., el-Sherif, N. (1995). Reemergence of the fetal pattern of L-type calcium channel gene expression in non infarcted myocardium during left ventricular remodeling. Biochemical & Biophysical Research Communications, 216, 892–897.

65. Hullin, R., Khan, I.F., Wirtz, S., Mohacsi, P., Varadi, G., Schwartz, A., Herzig, S. (2003). Cardiac L-type calcium channel beta-subunits expressed in human heart have differential effects on single channel characteristics. Journal of Biological Chemistry, 278, 21623–21630.

66. Bers, D.M. (2006). Altered cardiac myocyte Ca regulation in heart failure. Physiology, 21, 380–387.

67. Gwathmey, J.K., Copelas, L., MacKinnon, R., Schoen, F.J., Feldman, M.D., Grossman, W., Morgan, J.P. (1987). Abnormal intracellular calcium handling in myocardium from patients with end-stage heart failure. Circulation Research, 61, 70–76.

68. Pogwizd, S.M., Qi, M., Yuan, W., Samarel, A.M., Bers, D.M. (1999). Upregulation of Na(+)/Ca(2+) exchanger expression and function in an arrhythmogenic rabbit model of heart failure. Circulation Research, 85, 1009–1019.

69. O'Rourke, B., Kass, D.A., Tomaselli, G.F., Kaab, S., Tunin, R., Marban, E. (1999). Mechanisms of altered excitation-contraction coupling in canine tachycardia-induced heart failure, I: experimental studies. Circulation Research, 84, 562–570.

70. McIntosh, M.A., Cobbe, S.M., Smith, G.C. (2000). Heterogeneous changes in action potential and intracellular Ca2+ in left ventricular myocyte sub-types from rabbits with heart failure. Cardiovascular Research., 45, 397–409.

71. Hobai, I.A., O'Rourke, B. (2000). Enhanced Ca(2+)-activated Na(+)-Ca(2+) exchange activity in canine pacing-induced heart failure. Circulation Reserach, 87, 690–698.

72. Yano, M., Ikeda, Y., Matsuzaki, M. (2005). Altered intracellular Ca2+ handling in heart failure. Journal of Clinical Investigation, 115, 556–564.

73. Marx, S.O., Reiken, S., Hisamatsu, Y., Jayaraman, T., Burkhoff, D., Rosemblit, N., Marks, A.R. (2000). PKA phosphorylation dissociates FKBP12.6 from the calcium release channel (ryanodine receptor): Defective regulation in failing hearts. Cell, 101, 365–376.

74. Reiken, S., Gaburjakova, M., Guatimosim, S., Gomez, A.M., D'Armiento, J., Burkhoff, D., Wang, J., Vassort, G., Lederer, W.J., Marks, A.R. (2003). Protein kinase A phosphorylation of the cardiac calcium release channel (ryanodine receptor) in normal and failing hearts. Role of phosphatases and response to isoproterenol. Journal of Biological Chemistry, 278, 444–453.

75. Belevych, A., Kubalova, Z., Terentyev, D., Hamlin, R.L., Carnes, C.A., Gyorke, S. (2007). Enhanced ryanodine receptor-mediated calcium leak determines reduced sarcoplasmic reticulum calcium content in chronic canine heart failure. Biophysics Journal, 93, 4083–4092.

76. Wehrens, X.H., Lehnart, S.E., Reiken, S., Vest, J.A., Wronska, A., Marks, A.R. (2006). Ryanodine receptor/calcium release channel PKA phosphorylation: a critical mediator of heart failure progression. Proceedings of the National Academy of Sciences USA, 103, 511–518.

77. Huang, F., Shan, J., Reiken, S., Wehrens, X.H., Marks, A.R. (2006). Analysis of calstabin2 (FKBP12.6)-ryanodine receptor interactions: rescue of heart failure by calstabin2 in mice. Proceedings of the National Academy of Sciences USA, 103, 3456–3461.

78. Venetucci, L.A., Trafford, A.W., O'Neil, S.C., Eisner, D.A. (2008). The sarcoplasmic reticulum and arrhythmogenic calcium release. Cardiovascular Research, 77, 285–292.

79. Jiang, M.T., Lokuta, A.J., Farrell, E.F., Wolff, M.R., Haworth, R.A., Valdivia, N.H. (2002). Abnormal Ca2+ release, but normal ryanodine receptors, in canine and human heart failure. Circulation Research, 91, 1015–1022.

80. Shannon, T.R., Pogwizd, J.M., Bers, D.M. (2003). Elevated sarcoplasmic reticulum Ca2+ leak in intact ventricular myocytes from rabbits in heart failure. Circulation Research, 93, 592–594.

81. Piacentino, V., 3rd, Weber, C.R., Chen, X., Weisser-Thomas, J., Margoilies, K.B., Bers, D.M., Houser, S.R. (2003). Cellular basis of abnormal calcium transients of failing human ventricular myocytes. Circulation Research, 92, 651–658.

82. Yano, M., Kobayashi, S., Kohno, M., Doi, M., Tokuhisa, T., Okuda, S., Suetsugu, M., Hisaoka, T., Obayashi, M., Ohkusa, T., et al. (2003). FKBP12.6-mediated stabilization of calcium-release channel (ryanodine receptor) as a novel therapeutic strategy against heart failure. Circulation, 107, 477–484.

83. Wehrens, X.H., Lehnart, S.E., Reiken, S.R., Deng, S.X., Vest, J.A., Cervantes, D., Coromilas, J., Landry, D.W., Marks, A.R. (2004). Protection from cardiac arrhythmia through ryanodine receptor-stabilizing protein calstabin2. Science, 304, 292–296.

84. Reiken, S., Gaburjakova, M., Gaburjakova, J., He, K.L., Prieto, A., Becker, E., Yi, G.H., Wang, J., Burkhoff, D., Marks, A.R. (2001). beta-adrenergic receptor blockers restore cardiac calcium release channel (ryanodine receptor) structure and function in heart failure. Circulation, 104, 2843–2848.

85. Schwinger, R.H., Munch, G., Bolck, B., Karczewski, P., Krause, E.G., Erdmann, E. (1999). Reduced Ca(2+)-sensitivity of SERCA 2a in failing human myocardium due to reduced serin-16 phospholamban phosphorylation. Journal Molecular and Cellular Cardiology, 31, 479–491.

86. Dash, R., Kadambi, V., Schmidt, A.G., Tepe, N.M., Biniakiewicz, D., Gerst, M.J., Canning, A.M., Abraham, W.T., Hoit, B.D., Liggett, S.B. (2001). Interactions between phospholamban and beta-adrenergic drive may lead to cardiomyopathy and early mortality. Circulation, 103, 889–896.

87. Meyer, M., Schillinger, W., Pieske, B., Holubarsch, C., Heilmann, C., Posival, H., Kuwajima, G., Mikoshiba, K. (1995). Alterations of sarcoplasmic reticulum proteins in failing human dilated cardiomyopathy. Circulation, 92, 778–784.

88. Go, L.O., Moschella, M.C., Watras, J., Handa, K.K., Fyfe, B.S., Marks, A.R. (1995). Differential regulation of two types of intracellular calcium release channels during end-stage heart failure. Journal of Clinical Investigation, 95, 888–894.

89. Nishijima, Y., Sridhar, A., Viatchenko-Karpinski, S., Shaw, C., Bonagura, J.D., Abraham, W.T., Joshi, M.S., Bauer, J.A., Hamlin, R.L., Györke, S., et al. (2007). Chronic cardiac resynchronization therapy and reverse ventricular remodeling in a model of nonischemic cardiomyopathy. Life Science, 81, 1152–1159.

90. Pieske, B., Maier, L.S., Piacentino, V., Weisser, J., Hassenfuss, G., Houser, S. (2002). Rate dependence of [Na+]i and contractility in nonfailing and failing human myocardium. Circulation, 106, 447–453.

91. Despa, S., Islam, M.A., Weber, C.R., Pogwizd, S.M., Bers, D.M. (2002). Intracellular Na(+) concentration is elevated in heart failure but Na/K pump function is unchanged. Circulation, 105, 2543–2548.

92. Undrovinas, A.I., Maltsev, V.A., Sabbah, H.N. (1999). Repolarization abnormalities in cardiomyocytes of dogs with chronic heart failure: Role of sustained inward current. Cellular and Molecular Life Science, 55, 494–505.

93. Maltsev, V.A., Silverman, N., Sabbah, H.N., Undrovinas, A.I. (2007). Chronic heart failure slows late sodium current in human and canine ventricular myocytes: Implications for repolarization variability. European Journal of Heart Failure, 9, 219–227.

94. Valdivia, C.R., Chu, W.W., Pu, J., Foell, J.D., Haworth, R.A., Wolff, M.R., Kamp, T.J., Makielski, J.C. (2005). Increased late sodium current in myocytes from a canine heart failure model and from failing human heart. Journal of Molecular and Cellular Cardiology, 38, 475–483.

95. Pu, J., Boyden, P.A. (1997). Alterations of Na+ currents in myocytes from epicardial border zone of the infarcted heart. A possible ionic mechanism for reduced excitability and postrepolarization refractoriness. Circulation Research, 81, 110–119.

96. Song, Y., Shryock, J.C., Wagner, S., Maier, L.S., Belardinelli, L. (2006). Blocking late sodium current reduces hydrogen peroxide-induced arrhythmogenic activity and

contractile dysfunction. Journal of Pharmacological and Experimental Therapeutics, 318, 214–222.

97. Deschenes, I., Neyroud, N., DiSilvestre, D., Marbun, E., Yue, D.T., Tomaselli, G.F. (2002). Isoform-specific modulation of voltage-gated Na(+) channels by calmodulin. Circulation Research, 90, E49–57.

98. Wagner, S., Dybkova, N., Rasenack, E.C., Jacobshagen, C., Fabritz, C., Kirchof, P., Maier, S.K., Zhang, T., Hasenfuss, G., Brown, J.H., et al. (2006). Ca2+/calmodulin-dependent protein kinase II regulates cardiac Na+ channels. Journal of Clinical Investigation, 116, 3127–3138.

99. Echt, D.S., Liebson, P.R., Mitchell, L.B., Peters, R.W., Obias-Manno, D., Barker, A.H., Arensberg, D., Baker, A., Friedman, L., Greene, H.L. (1991). Mortality and morbidity in patients receiving encainide, flecainide, or placebo. The Cardiac Arrhythmia Suppression Trial. New England Journal of Medicine, 324, 781–788.

100. Makielski, J.C., Valdivia, C.R. (2006). Ranolazine and late cardiac sodium current—a therapeutic target for angina, arrhythmia and more? British Journal of Pharmacology, 148, 4–6.

101. Sossalla, S., Wagner, S., Rasenack, E.C., Ruff, H., Weber, S.L., Schöndube, F.A., Tirilomis, T., Tenderich, G., Hasenfuss, G., Belardinelli, L., et al. (2008). Ranolazine improves diastolic dysfunction in isolated myocardium from failing human hearts—role of late sodium current and intracellular ion accumulation. Journal of Molecular and Cellular Cardiology, 45, 32–43.

102. Houser, S.R., Freeman, A.R., Jaeger, J.M., Breisch, E.A., Coulson, R.L., Carey, R., Spann, J.F. (1981). Resting potential changes associated with Na-K pump in failing heart muscle. American Journal of Physiology, 240, H168–176.

103. Dhalla, N.S., Dixon, I.M., Ropp, H., Barwinsky, J. (1991). Experimental congestive heart failure due to myocardial infarction: Sarcolemmal receptors and cation transporters. Basic Research Cardiology, 86, 13–23.

104. Kjeldsen, K., Bierregaard, P., Richter, E.A., Thomsen, P.A., Nørgaard, A. (1988). Na+, K+-ATPase concentration in rodent and human heart and skeletal muscle: Apparent relation to muscle performance. Cardiovascular Research, 22, 95–100.

105. Spinale, F.G., Clayton, C., Tanaka, R., Fulbright, B.M., Mukherjee, R., Schulte, B.A., Crawford, F.A., Zile, M.R. (1992). Myocardial Na+,K(+)-ATPase in tachy-cardia induced cardiomyopathy. Journal of Molecular and Cellular Cardiology, 24, 277–294.

106. Zahler, R., Gilmore-Herbert, M., Sun, W., Benz, E.J. (1996). Na, K-ATPase isoform gene expression in normal and hypertrophied dog heart. Basic Research Cardiology, 91, 256–266.

107. Schwinger, R.H., Bohm, M., Erdmann, E. (1990). Effectiveness of cardiac glycosides in human myocardium with and without "downregulated" beta-adrenoceptors. Journal of Cardiovascular Pharmacology, 15, 692–697.

108. Saffitz, J.E., Schuessler, R.B., Yamada, K.A. (1999). Mechanisms of remodeling of gap junction distributions and the development of anatomic substrates of arrhythmias. Cardiovascular Research, 42, 309–317.

109. Akar, F.G., Spragy, D.D., Tunin, R.S., Kass, D.A., Tomaselli, G.F. (2004). Mechanisms underlying conduction slowing and arrhythmogenesis in nonischemic dilated cardiomy-opathy. Circulation Research, 95, 717–725.

110. Kalcheva, N., Qu, J., Sandeep, N., Garcia, L., Zhang, J., Wang, Z., Lampe, P.D., Suadicini, S.O., Spray, D.C., Fishman, G.I. (2007). Gap junction remodeling and cardiac arrhythmogenesis in a murine model of oculodentodigital dysplasia. Proceedings of the National Academy of Sciences USA, 104, 20512–20516.

111. Peters, N.S., Green, C.R., Pode-Wilson, P.A., Severs, N.J. (1993). Reduced content of connexin43 gap junctions in ventricular myocardium from hypertrophied and ischemic human hearts. Circulation, 88, 864–875.

112. Kostin, S., Dannmer, S., Hein, S., Klovekorn, W.P., Baver, E.P., Schaper, J. (2004). Connexin 43 expression and distribution in compensated and decompensated cardiac hypertrophy in patients with aortic stenosis. Cardiovascular Research, 62, 426–436.

113. Cabo, C., Yao, J., Boyden, P.A., Chen, S., Hussain, W., Duffy, H.S., Ciaccio, E.J., Peter, N.S., Wit, A.L. (2006). Heterogeneous gap junction remodeling in reentrant circuits in the epicardial border zone of the healing canine infarct. Cardiovascular Research, 72, 241–249.

114. Sato, T., Ohkusa, T., Honjo, H., Suzuki, S., Yoshida, M.A., Ishiguro, Y.S., Nakagawa, H., Yamazaki, M., Yano, M., Kodama, I., et al. (2008). Altered expression of connexin43 contributes to the arrhythmogenic substrate during the development of heart failure in cardiomyopathic hamster. American Journal of Physiology Heart Circulation Physiology, 294, H1164–1173.

115. Akar, F.G., Nass, R.D., Hahn, S., Cingolani, E., Shah, M., Hesketh, G.G., DiSilverstre, D., Tunin, R.S., Kass, D.A., Tomaselli, G.F. (2007). Dynamic changes in conduction velocity and gap junction properties during development of pacing-induced heart failure. American Journal of Physiology Heart Circulation Physiology, 293, H1223–1230.

116. Emdad, L., Uzzaman, M., Takagishi, Y., Honjo, H., Uchida, T., Severs, N.J., Kodama, I., Murata, Y. (2001). Gap junction remodeling in hypertrophied left ventricles of aortic-banded rats: prevention by angiotensin II type 1 receptor blockade. Journal of Molecular and Cellular Cardiology, 33, 219–231.

117. Yoshioka, J., Prince, R.N., Huang, H., Perkins, S.B., Cruz, F.B., MacGilivray, C., Lauffenberger, D.A., Lee, R.T. (2005). Cardiomyocyte hypertrophy and degradation of connexin43 through spatially restricted autocrine/paracrine heparin-binding EGF. Proceedings of the National Academy of Sciences USA, 102, 10622–10627.

118. Barker, R.J., Price, R.L., Goordie, R.G. (2002). Increased association of ZO-1 with connexin43 during remodeling of cardiac gap junctions. Circulation Research, 90, 317–324.

119. Shaw, R.M., Fay, A.J., Puthenveedu, M.A., von Zastrow, M., Jan, Y.N., Jan, L.Y. (2007). Microtubule plus-end-tracking proteins target gap junctions directly from the cell interior to adherens junctions. Cell, 128, 547–560.

120. Li, J., Patel, V.V., Kosteskii, I., Xiong, Y., Chu, A.F., Jacobson, J.T., Yu, C., Morley, G.E., Molkentin, J.D., Radice, G.L. (2005). Cardiac-specific loss of N-cadherin leads to alteration in connexins with conduction slowing and arrhythmogenesis. Circulation Research, 97, 474–481.

121. Yang, B., Lin, H., Xiao, J., Lu, Y., Lua, X., Li, B., Zhang, Y., Xu, C., Bai, Y., Wang, H., et al. (2007). The muscle-specific microRNA miR-1 regulates cardiac arrhythmogenic potential by targeting GJA1 and KCNJ2. Nature Medicine, 13, 486–491.

122. Bristow, M.R., Ginsburg, R., Minobe, W., Cubicciotti, R.S., Sageman, W.S., Lurie, K., Billingham, M.E., Harrison, D.C., Stinson, E.B. (1982). Decreased catecholamine sensitivity and beta-adrenergic-receptor density in failing human hearts. New England Journal of Medicine, 307, 205–211.

123. Bohm, M., Flesch, M., Schnabel, P. (1997). Beta-adrenergic signal transduction in the failing and hypertrophied myocardium. Journal of Molecular Medicine, 75, 842–848.

124. Bristow, M.R., Minobe, W.A., Raynolds, M.V., Port, J.D., Rasmussen, R., Ray, P.E., Feldman, A.M. (1993). Reduced beta 1 receptor messenger RNA abundance in the failing human heart. Journal of Clinical Investigation, 92, 2737–2745.

125. Zhou, Y.Y., Cheng, H., Bogdanov, K.Y., Hohl, C., Altschuld, R., Lakatta, E.G., Xiao, R.P. (1997). Localized cAMP-dependent signaling mediates beta 2-adrenergic modulation of cardiac excitation-contraction coupling. American Journal Physiology, 273, H1611–1618.

126. Bristow, M.R., Ginsburg, R., Umans, V., Fowler, M., Minobe, W., Rasmussen, R., Zera, P., Menlove, R., Shah, P., Jamieson, S., et al. (1986). Beta 1- and beta 2-adrenergic-receptor subpopulations in nonfailing and failing human ventricular myocardium: Coupling of both receptor subtypes to muscle contraction and selective beta 1-receptor down-regulation in heart failure. Circulation Research, 59, 297–309.

127. Bristow, M.R., Hershberger, R.E., Port, J.D., Gilbert, E.M., Sandoval, A., Rasmussen, R., Cates, A.E., Feldman, A.M. (1990). Beta-adrenergic pathways in nonfailing and failing human ventricular myocardium. Circulation, 82, I12–I25.

128. Brodde, O.E. (1991). Beta 1- and beta 2-adrenoceptors in the human heart: Properties, function, and alterations in chronic heart failure. Pharmacology Review, 43, 203–242.

129. Kiuchi, K., Shannon, R.P., Komamura, K., Cohen, D.J., Bianchi, C., Homcy, C.J., Vatner, S.F., Vatner, D.E. (1993). Myocardial beta-adrenergic receptor function during the development of pacing-induced heart failure. Journal of Clinical Investigation, 91, 907–914.

130. Brodde, O.E. (1988). The functional importance of beta 1 and beta 2 adrenoceptors in the human heart. American Journal of Cardiology, 62, 24C–29C.

131. Bristow, M.R., Hershberger, R.E., Port, J.D., Minobe, W., Rasnwssen, R. (1989). Beta 1- and beta 2-adrenergic receptor-mediated adenylate cyclase stimulation in nonfailing and failing human ventricular myocardium. Molecular Pharmacology, 35, 295–303.

132. Bristow, M.R., Anderson, F.L., Port, J.D., Skerl, L., Hershberger, R.E., Larrabee, P., O'Connell, J.B., Renlund, D.G., Volkman, K., Murray, J., et al. (1991). Differences in beta-adrenergic neuroeffector mechanisms in ischemic versus idiopathic dilated cardiomyopathy. Circulation, 84, 1024–1039.

133. Engelhardt, S., Hein, L., Wiesmann, F., Lohse, M.J. (1999). Progressive hypertrophy and heart failure in beta1-adrenergic receptor transgenic mice. Proceedings of the National Academy of Sciences USA, 96, 7059–7064.

134. Milano, C.A., Allen, L.F., Rockman, H.A., Dolber, P.C., McMinn, T.R., Chien, K.R., Johnson, T.D., Bond, R.A., Lefkowitz, R.J. (1994). Enhanced myocardial function in transgenic mice overexpressing the beta 2-adrenergic receptor. Science, 264, 582–586.

135. Xiao, R.P., Cheng, H., Zhou, Y.Y., Kuschel, M., Lakatta, E.G. (1999). Recent advances in cardiac beta(2)-adrenergic signal transduction. Circulation Research, 85, 1092–1100.

136. Communal, C., Singh, K., Pimental, D.R., Colocci, W.S. (1998). Norepinephrine stimulates apoptosis in adult rat ventricular myocytes by activation of the beta-adrenergic pathway. Circulation, 98, 1329–1334.

137. Chesley, A., Lundberg, M.S., Asai, T., Xiao, R.P., Ohtani, S., Lakatta, E.G., Crow, M.T. (2000). The beta(2)-adrenergic receptor delivers an antiapoptotic signal to cardiac myocytes through G(i)-dependent coupling to phosphatidylinositol 3'-kinase. Circulation Research, 87, 1172–1179.

138. Bohm, M., Eschenhagen, T., Gierschik, P., Larisch, K., Lensche, H., Mende, U., Schmitz, W., Schnabel, P., Scholz, H., Steinfath, M., et al. (1994). Radioimmunochemical quantification of Gi alpha in right and left ventricles from patients with ischaemic and dilated cardiomyopathy and predominant left ventricular failure. Journal of Molecular and Cellular Cardiology, 26, 133–149.

139. Eschenhagen, T., Mende, U., Nose, M., Schmitz, W., Scholz, H., Haverich, A., Hirt, S., Doring, V., Kalmar, P., Hoppner, W., et al. (1992). Increased messenger RNA level of the inhibitory G-protein alpha subunit Gialpha-2 in human end-stage heart failure. Circulation Research, 70, 688–696.

140. Feldman, A.M., Cates, A.E., Veazey, W.B., Hershberger, R.E., Bristow, M.R., Baughman, K.L., Baumgartner, W.A., Van Dop, C. (1988). Increase of the 40,000-mol wt pertussis toxin substrate (G protein) in the failing human heart. Journal of Clinical Investigation, 82, 189–197.

141. Mende, U., Eschenhagen, T., Geertz, B., Schmitz, W., Scholz, H., Schulte, E.J., Sempell, R., Steinfath, M. (1992). Isoprenaline-induced increase in the 40/41 kDa pertussis toxin substrates and functional consequences on contractile response in rat heart. Naunyn Schmiedebergs Archives of Pharmacology, 345, 44–50.

142. Xiao, R.P., Avdonin, P., Zhou, Y.Y., Cheng, H., Akhter, S.A., Eschenhagen, T., Lefkowitz, R.J., Koch, W.J., Lakatta, E.G. (1999). Coupling of beta2-adrenoceptor to Gi proteins and its physiological relevance in murine cardiac myocytes. Circulation Research, 84, 43–52.

143. Bodor, G.S., Oakeley, A.E., Allen, P.D., Crimmins, D.L., Lacknson, J.H., Anderson, P.A. (1997). Troponin I phosphorylation in the normal and failing adult human heart. Circulation, 96, 1495–1500.

144. Zakhary, D.R., Moravec, C.S., Stewart, R.W., Bond, M. (1999). Protein kinase A (PKA)-dependent troponin-I phosphorylation and PKA regulatory subunits are decreased in human dilated cardiomyopathy. Circulation, 99, 505–510.

145. Zakhary, D.R., Moravec, C.S., Bond, M. (2000). Regulation of PKA binding to AKAPs in the heart: Alterations in human heart failure. Circulation, 101, 1459–1464.

146. Dell'Acqua, M.L., Scott, J.D. (1997). Protein kinase A anchoring. Journal of Biological Chemistry, 272, 12881–12884.

147. Huang, L.J., Durick, K., Weiner, J.A., Chun, J., Taylor, S.S. (1997). Identification of a novel protein kinase A anchoring protein that binds both type I and type II regulatory subunits. Journal of Biological Chemistry, 272, 8057–8064.

148. Hartzell, H.C., Duchatelle-Gourdon, I. (1993). Regulation of the cardiac delayed rectifier K current by neurotransmitters and magnesium. Cardiovascular Drugs Theraphy, 7, 547–554.

149. Fedida, D., Bruan, A.P., Giles, W.R. (1993). Alpha 1-adrenoceptors in myocardium: Functional aspects and transmembrane signaling mechanisms. Physiology Review, 73, 469–487.

150. Borst, M.M., Szalai, P., Herzog, N., Kubler, W., Strasser, R.H. (1999). Transregulation of adenylyl-cyclase-coupled inhibitory receptors in heart failure enhances anti-adrenergic effects on adult rat cardiomyocytes. Cardiovascular Research, 44, 113–120.

151. Chakir, K., Daya, S.K., Aiba, T., Tunin, R.S., Dimaano, V.L., Abraham, T.P., Jaegves-Robinson, K.M., Pacak, K., Zho, W.Z. (2009). Mechanisms of enhanced beta-adrenergic reserve from cardiac resynchronization therapy. Circulation, 119, 1231–1240.

152. Zhang, T., Brown, J.H. (2004). Role of Ca2+/calmodulin-dependent protein kinase II in cardiac hypertrophy and heart failure. Cardiovascular Research, 63, 476–486.

153. Kirchhefer, U., Schmitz, W., Scholz, H., Neumann, J. (1999). Activity of cAMP-dependent protein kinase and Ca2+/calmodulin-dependent protein kinase in failing and nonfailing human hearts. Cardiovascular Research, 42, 254–261.

154. Maier, L.S., Bers, D.M. (2007). Role of Ca2+/calmodulin-dependent protein kinase (CaMK) in excitation-contraction coupling in the heart. Cardiovascular Research, 73, 631–640.

155. Netticadan, T., Tensah, R.M., Kawabata, K., Dhalla, N.S. (2000). Sarcoplasmic reticulum Ca(2+)/Calmodulin-dependent protein kinase is altered in heart failure. Circulation Research, 86, 596–605.

CHAPTER 10

Redox Modification of Ryanodine Receptors in Cardiac Arrhythmia And Failure: A Potential Therapeutic Target

ANDRIY E. BELEVYCH, DMITRY TERENTYEV, and SANDOR GYÖRKE

10.1 INTRODUCTION

Sudden cardiac death (SCD) from sustained ventricular arrhythmias (ventricular tachycardia or ventricular fibrillation) continues to be a major cause of mortality [1]. Most incidents of SCD are associated with electrical and mechanical cardiac remodeling that occurs in response to stress, such as myocardial infarction (MI) or chronic hypertension, and they form a substrate for the development of heart failure (HF) [2]. Abnormal intracellular Ca^{2+} handling, and in particular the defective ryanodine receptor (RyR) function, has been consistently implicated in the pathogenesis of cardiac disease, including HF and SCD.

The cardiac RyR2 is an intracellular Ca^{2+} release channel that is localized in the membrane of the sarcoplasmic reticulum (SR) and provides Ca^{2+} required for contractile activation of the heart [3]. Composed of four homologous subunits $\sim$500 kDa each, the RyR2 channels are the largest ion channels known. In addition, the RyR2 interacts with several proteins, which include FKBP12.6, triadin, junctin, and calsequestrin (CASQ2), forming a supramolecular molecular complex that extends from the cytosolic to the luminal side of the SR membrane [4].

Abnormal RyR2 function has been linked to several cardiac diseases, including congenital and acquired cardiac arrhythmias and HF [5–7]. The underpinning causes of certain familial arrhythmias, such as catecholaminergic polymorphic tachycardia (CPVT), have been successfully traced to specific mutations in genes encoding for the cardiac RyR2 and CASQ2 [8]. These genetic conditions, although relatively rare, have provided valuable insights into the relationship between abnormal RyR2

Novel Therapeutic Targets for Antiarrhythmic Drugs, Edited by George Edward Billman
Copyright © 2010 John Wiley & Sons, Inc.

behavior and cardiac disease. The mechanisms of the more common acquired forms of Ca^{2+}-dependent arrhythmia, including those that occur after myocardial infarction and accompany heart failure, remain less clearly understood. In recent years, considerable attention has been devoted to the possibility that arrhythmogenic derangements of RyR2s result from abnormal RyR2 phosphorylation by protein kinase A (PKA) and altered association with FKBP12.6 [9]. These proposed mechanisms continue to be a subject of intense debate and have been reviewed elsewhere [5, 7, 10]. Evidence is accumulating for an alternative possibility according to which posttranslational modification of RyR2 by reactive oxygen species (ROS) accounts for, or contributes to, abnormal RyR2 function in both cardiac arrhythmia and failure. In this chapter, we review the evidence for the link between abnormal RyR2 function and cardiac arrhythmia with a specific focus on the role of RyR2 redox modifications in arrhythmogenesis, and we consider abnormal RyR2 redox modification as a potential therapeutic target.

10.2   ACTIVATION AND DEACTIVATION OF RYANODINE RECEPTORS DURING NORMAL EXCITATION-CONTRACTION COUPLING

Preceding each heartbeat, Ca^{2+} entry through the L-type voltage-dependent Ca^{2+} channels of the sarcolemmal (I_{Ca}) during the plateau phase of the cardiac action potential (AP) triggers the release of Ca^{2+} from the SR through RyR2s; this process is known as Ca^{2+}-induced Ca^{2+} release (CICR) [4]. Calcium released from the SR causes activation of the contractile filaments, myocyte shortening, and contraction of the cardiac muscle, thus accounting for cardiac systole. The amount of Ca^{2+} released from the SR is a principal determinant of cardiac contractility and depends on I_{Ca} amplitude, SR Ca^{2+} content, and the functional state of RyR2s. For the heart to relax (diastole), SR Ca^{2+} release must stop and the Ca^{2+} translocated to the cytosol must be resequestered into the SR by the adenosine triphosphate (ATP) dependent SR Ca^{2+} pump, SERCA2a. The deactivation of RyR2s by reduced intra-SR $[Ca^{2+}]_{SR}$ that follows SR Ca^{2+} release plays a key role in timely termination of CICR [11]. It also accounts for the temporary refractoriness, or functional silencing of Ca^{2+} signaling, that sets in after each release to prevent Ca^{2+} release in the diastolic phase. On the other hand, at levels above normal (Ca^{2+} overload), SR luminal Ca^{2+} exerts a stimulatory influence on RyR2 function, which results in "spontaneous" SR Ca^{2+} release. This mechanism plays an important role in cardiac disease (see below). The control of RyR2 by luminal Ca^{2+} seems to be mediated by the SR luminal Ca^{2+} binding protein CASQ2, which inhibits RyR2 activity at low $[Ca^{2+}]$ in the partially depleted SR but relives this inhibition at elevated $[Ca^{2+}]_{SR}$ [11]. In addition to cytosolic and luminal Ca^{2+} and CASQ2, RyR2s are controlled by a number of effector molecules, including Mg^{2+}, ATP, and calmodulin, as well as signaling pathways such as phosphorylation and redox modification [3]. Normally, these multiple mechanisms work in synergy to sustain ordered, stable Ca^{2+} cycling and contractility over a broad range of physiological conditions.

10.3 DEFECTIVE RYANODINE RECEPTOR FUNCTION IS LINKED TO PROARRHYTHMIC DELAYED AFTERDEPOLARIZATIONS AND CALCIUM ALTERNANS

Abnormal RyR2-mediated SR Ca^{2+} release has been implicated in several different cardiac disease states that range from triggered and reentrant arrhythmias to HF [6]. Under various pathological conditions, SR Ca^{2+} release occurs spontaneously, rather than as a part of excitation-contraction coupling, causing inappropriately timed Ca^{2+} releases and contractions. The propensity of the SR Ca^{2+} stores to discharge spontaneously reflects the self-perpetuating (positive feedback) nature of CICR in which Ca^{2+} release from the SR tends to cause more release. Spontaneous discharges of SR Ca^{2+} stores occur when $[Ca^{2+}]_{SR}$ reaches a certain threshold level; this behavior is attributable to the stimulatory effects of luminal Ca^{2+} on RyR2s [11, 12]. Spontaneous Ca^{2+} release takes the form of self-propagating waves of CICR. These waves originate locally as spontaneous local release events, which are known as Ca^{2+} sparks, and then spread through the cell via diffusion-coupled CICR [13]. The role of luminal Ca^{2+} is to sensitize the RyR2s to activation by cytosolic Ca^{2+}, such that Ca^{2+} released from one release site can active SR Ca^{2+} release in the neighboring site [11]. Ca^{2+} waves are arrhythmogenic. They activate Ca^{2+}-dependent depolarizing membrane currents, which are mediated mainly by the electrogenic Na^+/Ca^{2+} exchanger (NCX1), thereby causing oscillations of the membrane potential known as delayed afterdepolarizations (DADs) [14]. DADs activate ectopic action potentials, which in turn can then initiate tachyarrhythmias.

Abnormal control of RyR2s can also give rise to instabilities of SR Ca^{2+} release, which is known as Ca^{2+} alternans [15, 16]. Alternans occurs when excessive, uncontrollable release during the first release cycle exhausts the SR Ca^{2+} store. As a result, the SR remains underfilled and only can release small amounts of Ca^{2+} during the next release cycle. This leads to beat-to-beat variations in Ca^{2+} transient amplitude and hence in the the action potential duration (APD). As in the case of DADs, the influence of the Ca^{2+} transient on APD can be attributed to the effects on Ca^{2+} dependent currents, such as the NCX1 current and I_{Ca} on the cell membrane potential [15]. For example, large Ca^{2+} transients can cause a prolongation of the action potential by stimulating the depolarizing NCX1 current during the action potential plateau (concordant electrical and mechanical activity). The large Ca^{2+} transient can also reduce the APD via Ca^{2+}-dependent inactivation of I_{Ca} (discordant electrical and mechanical activity). When APD alternans occurs in opposite phases in different regions of the heart (spatially discordant alternans), repolarization gradients arise, which can produce conduction block and form a substrate for reentrant excitation [15, 16].

Given the fact that similar alterations of RyR2 function (e.g., modification by ROS) can result in either DADs or alternans, it is interesting to consider the relationships between these apparently different proarrhythmic phenomena (See Figure 10.1). The specific reasons as to why in some cases abnormal RyR2 function results in DADs whereas in others in alternans is currently unknown. Both phenomena are linked to tachycardia, but it is unclear whether different windows of heart rates exist for each. It

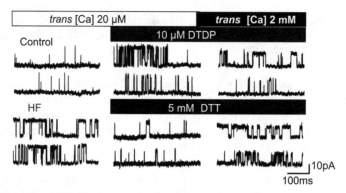

Figure 10.1. Effects of oxidizing and reducing reagents on activity of RyRs from control and failing hearts. Representative recordings of single RyR2 channels from control and HF samples (top and bottom recordings) at low and high *trans* $[Ca^{2+}]$ and in the presence of either DTDP (10 μM) or DTT (5 mM) as indicated. Single-channel activities were recorded in 350 mM symmetrical CsCH3SO3 solutions at 40 mV. Channel openings are shown as upward deflections from the closed level.

is likely that other factors besides RyR2s alterations, such as differences in SERCA activity, contribute to or account for these different arrhythmic phenotypes. For example, DADs are known to be greatly promoted by β-adrenergic receptor stimulation, which accelerates SR Ca^{2+} reuptake. It can be speculated that DADS (and the underlying spontaneous releases) occur when $[Ca^{2+}]_{SR}$ is restored sufficiently fast to reach the threshold for spontaneous release before the arrival of the next stimulus. With alternans, however, the uptake is not sufficiently fast to attain this $[Ca^{2+}]_{SR}$ threshold, and the beat-to-beat variations in $[Ca^{2+}]_{SR}$ give rise to beat-to-beat variations in the cytosolic Ca^{2+} transients.

10.4 GENETIC AND ACQUIRED DEFECTS IN RYANODINE RECEPTORS

Mechanistically, abnormal SR Ca^{2+} release can occur for several different reasons with RyR2 playing either primary or secondary role. Primary defects that involve intrinsic changes in the RyR2 complex can be either genetic, as in the case of CPVT linked to mutations in RyR2 and CASQ2, or acquired caused by posttranslational modifications of RyR2 by phosphorylation or oxidation. In other cases, abnormal Ca^{2+} signaling can occur as a result of intrinsically normal RyR2s behaving abnormally because of changes in intracellular milieu (e.g., Ca^{2+} overload).

Excess intracellular Ca^{2+} (i.e., Ca^{2+} overload) is a feature characteristic of various pathological states (such as metabolic inhibition, ischemia/reperfusion, and digitalis poisoning) and is a well-established cause of arrhythmia. Calcium overload is associated with triggered afterdepolarizations that can initiate sustained tachyarrhythmias [14, 17]. In settings of Ca^{2+} overload, abnormal RyR2 behavior is secondary to the elevation of the SR Ca^{2+} content, which results in the sensitization of RyR2s and inappropriately timed diastolic Ca^{2+} release. For example, in case of digoxin-induced arrhythmia, increased accumulation of intracellular $[Na^+]$ (caused by the inhibition of Na^+/K^+-ATPase) results in reduced NCX1-mediated Ca^{2+} extrusion and hence increased accumulation of Ca^{2+} in the SR. Elevated intra-SR $[Ca^{2+}]$ stimulates RyR2 activity, leading to spontaneous Ca^{2+} release and DADs [14]. Changes in APD could contribute to arrhythmogenesis (long QT syndrome) through a similar mechanism that involves elevated SR Ca^{2+} load secondary to increased Ca^{2+} entry during the prolonged action potential plateau [18].

CPVT, which is caused by mutations in RyR2 and CASQ2, is a clear case of arrhythmia with primary involvement of the RyR2 complex [8]. In CPVT, spontaneous Ca^{2+} release and DADs can occur without Ca^{2+} overload and even under conditions of reduced SR Ca^{2+} content [8, 19]. This arrhythmogenic Ca^{2+} release at reduced SR Ca^{2+} loads results from an enhanced responsiveness of RyR2s to luminal Ca^{2+}, which effectively lowers the $[Ca^{2+}]_{SR}$ threshold for activation of spontaneous Ca^{2+} release. In other words, sensitization to luminal Ca^{2+} produces a Ca^{2+} overload-like condition that promotes spontaneous Ca^{2+} release not as a result of $[Ca^{2+}]_{SR}$ becoming abnormally high, but rather because of lowering of the $[Ca^{2+}]_{SR}$ threshold for spontaneous Ca^{2+} release below normal baseline level ("perceived" Ca^{2+} overload [19]).

A similar mechanism may underlie triggered arrhythmia in other disease states, which include heart failure and postmyocardial infarction hearts, in which SR Ca^{2+} release regulation is compromised because of acquired rather than genetic modifications of components of the RyR2 channel complex.

10.5 EFFECTS OF THIOL-MODIFYING AGENTS ON RYANODINE RECEPTORS

Ryanodine receptor channels are subject to modifications by oxidizing and reducing agents that can interact with thiol-containing cysteine residues of the channel protein [20, 21]. The cardiac RyR2 contains approximately 90 cysteines per subunit, and approximately 20 of them are in reduced state [21]. These free cysteines are targets for several types of redox modifications, which include disulfide cross-linking, S-nitrosylation, and S-glutathionylation.

Different classes of oxidizing agents have been shown to increase RyR2 activity and stimulate SR Ca^{2+} release [22–24]. In terms of effects on RyR2 gating behavior, oxidation has been shown to increase the sensitivity of the channel to Ca^{2+} activation, whereas S-glutathionylation has been shown to decrease the sensitivity of the channel to inhibition by Mg^{2+} [25]. We recently demonstrated [26] that oxidation also altered the luminal Ca^{2+}-dependency of RyR2s by reducing the ability of the channel to decrease its activity in response to lowering luminal Ca^{2+} (See Figure 10.2). As discussed above, luminal Ca^{2+}-dependent deactivation contributes to termination of CICR and the prevention of diastolic SR Ca^{2+} release. Therefore, oxidation would be expected to increase diastolic release, which indeed seems to occur in a healed myocardial infarction model of SCD and HF (see below).

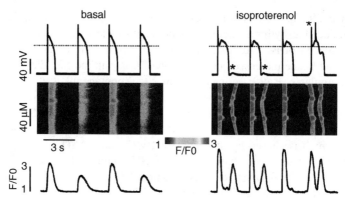

Figure 10.2. Two proarrhythmic phenotypes in HF: Calcium and action potential alternans (left) and DADs caused by spontaneous Ca^{2+} releases (right). Representative recordings of membrane potential with corresponding line-scan images and temporal profiles of Fluo-3 fluorescence in HF myocyte recorded in the absence (left panel) and in the presence (right panel) of 100 nM isoproterenol, a β-adrenergic receptor agonist. *Delayed afterdepolarizations. Dashed line marks 0 mV. See color insert.

Although most studies report that oxidation tends to increase ryanodine receptor activity, there is also evidence that prolonged exposure to high doses of oxidizing agents, after an initial stimulation of activity, can cause irreversible inactivation of ryanodine receptors [20]. These different actions of ryanodine receptors likely reflect the involvement of different cysteine residues under different oxidizing conditions. The role of specific cysteine residues in RyR2 redox modifications remains to be defined. It has been shown that redox modification involves only 12 of the total 100 cysteines on skeletal muscle ryanodine receptors [27]. Although some of these cysteines are non-specific targets for different redox agents, other sites are exclusively S-nitrosylated (Cys-1040 and Cys-1303) or S-glutathionylated (Cys-1591 and Cys-3193).

Endogenous oxidizing agents (ROS) are continuously generated in the heart and are likely to exert tonic influences on intracellular targets including SR Ca^{2+} release and might be involved in coupling Ca^{2+} signaling to cardiac metabolic activities [23].

10.6 REACTIVE OXYGEN SPECIES PRODUCTION AND OXIDATIVE STRESS IN CARDIAC DISEASE

ROS production has been shown to increase in various pathological settings, such as ischemia-reperfusion, postmyocardial infarction, cardiac remodeling, and heart failure [28, 29]. The main sources of ROS in the heart include the mitochondrial respiratory chain, xanthine oxidase (XO), and Nicotinamide adenine dinucleotide phosphate (NADPH) oxidase [29, 30]. These pathways lead to increased generation of the superoxide anion, a major precursor of reactive oxygen species. Additionally oxidative stress can lead to further ROS production by uncoupled NO synthase (NOS), secondary to the oxidation of the NOS cofactor BH4. Excessive ROS production by mitochondria [31, 32] and xanthine oxidase [33] has been shown in animal models of cardiac disease and in human HF. Recent evidence also points to NADPH oxidase as an important player in ROS signaling during disease states, such as tachycardia, postmyocardial infarction, cardiac remodeling, and HF [34]. The production of ROS is countered by several enzyme mechanisms [29, 30]. These mechanisms include superoxide dismutase (SOD), catalase, and glutathione peroxidase. Superoxide dismutase converts mitochondrially produced superoxide to H_2O_2, which is broken down by catalase and glutathione peroxidase to water. In HF, these antioxidant defense mechanisms are weakened, which contributes to increased oxidative stress [35]. Thus, in general, oxidative stress is caused by an imbalance between the activities of endogenous pro-oxidative and antioxidant enzymes.

10.7 REDOX MODIFICATION OF RYANODINE RECEPTORS IN CARDIAC ARRHYTHMIA AND HEART FAILURE

Altered redox balance and redox-mediated changes in Ca^{2+} handling are increasingly recognized as important pathogenic factors in different cardiac diseases, which include both ischemic and nonischemic disease processes [20, 36]. These disease states are accompanied by increased production of ROS, elevated oxidative stress, and protein oxidation [28, 29, 37]. RyR2 oxidation was specifically reported in several animal models, including pacing induced HF, chronic HF, and healed myocardial infarction sudden cardiac death [26, 38, 39]. Additionally, increased glutationylation of RyR2 has been shown during tachycardia [40].

Recently, we studied the role of redox modification if RyR2 in arrhythmogenesis using a canine postinfarction model of SCD and sustained ventricular fibrillation (VF) [26]. We found that left ventricular wedge preparations from VF dogs were more susceptible to AP alternans. Additionally, the frequency-dependence of Ca^{2+} alternans was shifted toward slower rates in myocytes isolated from VF dogs relative to controls. In both groups of cells, cytosolic Ca^{2+} transients ($[Ca^{2+}]c$) alternated in phase with changes in diastolic Ca^{2+} in sarcoplasmic reticulum ($[Ca^{2+}]_{SR}$), but the dependence of $[Ca^{2+}]c$ amplitude on $[Ca^{2+}]_{SR}$ was steeper in VF cells. Abnormal RyR2 function in VF cells was indicated by increased fractional Ca^{2+} release for a given amplitude of Ca^{2+} current and by elevated diastolic RyR2-mediated SR Ca^{2+} leak.

The steepness of the relationship between SR Ca^{2+} content and SR Ca^{2+} release is thought to be an important factor in the development of alternans [15, 41]. The steepness of this relationship is derived from the combination of stimulatory effects of luminal Ca^{2+} on RyR2 function and the presence of the positive feedback loop inherent to CICR. With a steep Ca^{2+} release-$[Ca^{2+}]_{SR}$ relationship, small differences in $[Ca^{2+}]_{SR}$ would be expected to lead to substantial differences in the amplitude of Ca^{2+} transients, i.e., alternans. In fact, we observed these differences in VF myocytes (see Figure 10.3). Treatment of VF myocytes with reducing agents, such as mercapto-propionylglycine (MPG), normalized parameters of Ca^{2+} handling

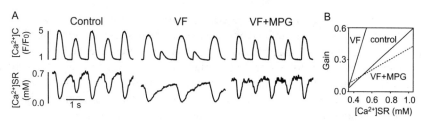

Figure 10.3. A reducing agent improves parameters calcium release in cardiac myocytes from susceptible to VF animal. **A,** Representative line-scan images and temporal profiles of Rhod-2 and Fluo-5N fluorescence recorded in voltage-clamped control cell and VF cells in the absence and presence of $750\,\mu M$ MPG. **B,** Dependence of the SR Ca^{2+} release gain function ($[Ca^{2+}]_c$ amplitude/density of peak Ca^{2+} current) on $[Ca^{2+}]SR$ measured for control cells and for VF cells in the absence and presence of MPG.

including the steepness of the Ca^{2+} release load relationship and shifted the threshold of Ca^{2+} alternans to higher frequencies. Therefore, these data suggested that redox modulation of RyR2s promotes the generation of Ca^{2+} alternans by enhancing the steepness of the Ca^{2+} release-load relationship and could thereby provide a substrate for ventricular fibrillation.

In several disease conditions, including acute ischemia and HF, alternans are thought to be caused by slowed Ca^{2+} cycling because of inhibition of sarcoendoplasmic reticulum Ca^{2+}-ATPase (SERCA) [15]. The effect of slowed Ca^{2+} uptake would be to decrease Ca^{2+} cycling such that normal Ca^{2+} release from the SR can be obtained only on alternating beats. However, in our postinfarction model of SCD, we did not find alterations in SR Ca^{2+} uptake rate [26].

Recently, we found evidence of oxidative stress and qualitatively similar alterations in RyR2 behavior in a nonischemic, chronic heart failure model [39]. Chronic heart failure also increased RyR2 activity and SR Ca^{2+} leak. However, the redox-induced changes in RyR2s in heart failure were substantially more severe than was observed in the canine postinfarction model of SCD; the result was diminished myocyte SR Ca^{2+} content and SR Ca^{2+} release characteristic of heart disease.

As mentioned above, three types of reversible redox modifications have been described for the RyR2 channel, including S-nitrosylation, S-glutathionylation, and disulfide oxidation. Application of modification-specific reducing agents revealed that thiol oxidation is the prevailing type of modification of RyR2 in HF, whereas S-nitrosylation and S-glutathionylation do not seem to play a role.

10.8 THERAPEUTIC POTENTIAL OF NORMALIZING RYANODINE RECEPTOR FUNCTION

Because enhanced SR Ca^{2+} leak through RyR2s is linked to HF and Ca^{2+}-dependent arrhythmia, pharmacologically "sealing" the leak has been considered as strategy for treating these disease states [42, 43]. An important issue is the selectivity of the ryanodine receptor modulator; the agent should be developed with a greater affinity/

sensitivity for cardiac as opposed to RyRs located in skeletal muscle and in the brain. Additionally, implementing this therapy could be challenging because of the nature of Ca^{2+} cycling in the heart. For example, inhibition of RyR2s may fix the diastolic leak, but it has the potential to compromise systolic function. Therefore, targeting the underpinning causes of altered RyR2 function rather than simply inhibiting the RyR2 channel seems to be a more promising approach for treating RyR2-linked cardiac diseases. Currently, several such strategies are emerging based on specific mechanisms proposed to underlie dysregulation of RyR2s in cardiac disease, which include abnormal PKA phosphorylation and altered redox modification.

JTV519 (K201) is a multichannel blocker with reported beneficial effects in both HF and arrhythmia [14, 44]. This drug is a 1,4 benzothiazepine and, thus, a L-type Ca^{2+} channel blocker, with multiple additional targets including PKC, mitochondrial K^+ channels, and RyR2. It has been suggested that JTV519 improves Ca^{2+} handling in both HF and CPVT by stabilizing binding of FKBP12.6 to RyR2, thereby reducing the RyR2-mediated SR Ca^{2+} leak [42, 45]. However, this proposed mode of action for JTV519 has been questioned [10, 46]. Although most studies agree that JTV519 improves cardiac function in HF [10], its beneficial effects in Ca^{2+}-dependent arrhythmia reported in earlier studies are not supported by more recent investigations [47]. This could be an indication that the beneficial effects of JTV519 on cardiac function in HF may involve targets other than the RyR2. The development of new derivatives with more specific effects on RyR2 is under way [48]. Studying the effects of these agents may clarify the mechanisms of action of this class of compounds, which may eventually lead to the development of pharmacologically optimized drugs.

Given the established role of RyR2 redox modifications in HF and arrhythmia, preventing or reversing these reactions seems to be a reasonable strategy to treat Ca^{2+}-dependent arrhythmia and HF. Many studies demonstrated the ability of antioxidants to improve cardiac performance in animal models of HF [49]. Despite these promising findings, a recent clinical trial evaluating the potential benefits of inhibition of xanthine oxidase in patients with HF was not successful [50]. It is unclear to what extent this lack of positive outcome is caused by the particular antioxidants used. Xanthine oxidase is only one reported source of ROS implicated in HF, and targeting it may not be sufficient to achieve a substantial reduction of ROS in relevant subcellular domains to attain the desired therapeutic effects.

Interestingly, the notion that targeting RyR2 redox modification may be beneficial is supported by the effects of some successful drugs that are already in clinical use. For example, the beneficial effects of the nonspecific β-adrenergic receptor blocker, carvedilol, in patients with heart failure could reflect, at least in part, the antioxidant actions of this agent on RyR2 oxidation (i.e., reversing this oxidation) [38]. In a similar manner, statins are a novel class of drugs that have favorable effects in patents with arrhythmia and HF [51]. These agents also have been shown to inhibit NADPH oxidase activation secondary to inhibition of small GTAases such as Rac [52]. NADPH oxidase, which is a reported source of increased ROS in various cardiac disease states [30], has been shown to colocalize with RyR2s in the SR [53]. These findings support the hypothesis that the beneficial effects of statins could result from decreased oxidation of SR Ca^{2+} handling proteins, including the RyR2. Clearly, more studies are required to provide a better understanding of the specific redox pathway abnormalities and the affected Ca^{2+} signaling mechanisms that involved in cardiac disease. Once these abnormalities have been identified, then it may be possible to develop new therapeutic strategies designed to restore normal redox and calcium signaling.

REFERENCES

1. Zheng, Z.J., Croft, J.B. Giles, W.H., Mensah, G.A. (2001). Sudden cardiac death in the United States, 1989 to 1998. Circulation, 104, 2158–2163.

2. Solomon, S.D., Zelenkofske, S., McMurray, J.J., Finn, P.V., Velazquez, E., Ertl, G., Harsanyi, A., Rouleau, J.L., Maggioni, A., Kober, L., White, H., Van de Werf, F., Pieper, K., Califf, R.M., Pfeffer, M.A. (2005). Sudden death in patients with myocardial infarction and left ventricular dysfunction, heart failure, or both. New England Journal of Medicine, 352, 2581–2588.

3. Fill, M., Copello, J.A. (2002). Ryanodine receptor calcium release channels. Physiological Reviews, 82, 893–922.

4. Bers, D.M. (2002). Cardiac excitation-contraction coupling. Nature, 415, 198–205.

5. Wehrens, X.H., Lehnart, S.E., Marks, A.R. (2005). Intracellular calcium release and cardiac disease. Annual Review of Physiology, 67, 69–98.

6. Gyorke, S., Carnes, C. (2008). Dysregulated sarcoplasmic reticulum calcium release: Potential pharmacological target in cardiac disease. Pharmacology and Therapeutics, 119, 340–354.

7. Yano, M., Yamamoto, T., Ikeda, Y., Matsuzaki, M. (2006). Mechanisms of disease: Ryanodine receptor defects in heart failure and fatal arrhythmia. Nature Clinical Practice Cardiovascular Medicine, 3, 43–52.

8. Gyorke, S. (2009). Molecular basis of catecholaminergic polymorphic ventricular tachycardia. Heart Rhythm, 6, 123–129.

9. Wehrens, X.H., Lehnart, S.E., Huang, F., Vest, J.A., Reiken, S.R., Mohler, P.J., Sun, J., Guatimosim, S., Song, L.S., Rosemblit, N., et al. (2003). FKBP12.6 deficiency and defective calcium release channel (ryanodine receptor) function linked to exercise-induced sudden cardiac death. Cell, 113, 829–840.

10. George, C.H., Jundi, H., Thomas, N.L., Fry, D.L., Lai, F.A. (2007). Ryanodine receptors and ventricular arrhythmias: emerging trends in mutations, mechanisms and therapies. Journal of Molecular and Cellular Cardiology, 42, 34–50.

11. Gyorke, S., Terentyev, D. (2008). Modulation of ryanodine receptor by luminal calcium and accessory proteins in health and cardiac disease. Cardiovascular Research, 77, 245–255.

12. Venetucci, L.A., Trafford, A.W., O'Neill, S.C., Eisner, D.A. (2008). The sarcoplasmic reticulum and arrhythmogenic calcium release. Cardiovascular Research, 77, 285–292.

13. Cheng, H., Lederer, W.J. (2008). Calcium sparks. Physiological Reviews, 88, 1491–1545.

14. Ter Keurs, H.E., Boyden, P.A. (2007). Calcium and arrhythmogenesis. Physiological Reviews, 87, 457–506.

15. Weiss, J.N., Karma, A., Shiferaw, Y., Chen, P.S., Garfinkel, A., Qu, Z. (2006). From pulsus to pulseless: The saga of cardiac alternans. Circulation Research, 98, 1244–1253.

16. Laurita, K.R., Rosenbaum, D.S. (2008). Mechanisms and potential therapeutic targets for ventricular arrhythmias associated with impaired cardiac calcium cycling. Journal of Molecular and Cellular Cardiology, 44, 31–43.

17. Pogwizd, S.M., Bers, D.M. (2004). Cellular basis of triggered arrhythmias in heart failure. Trends in Cardiovascular Medicine, 14, 61–66.

18. Huffaker, R., Lamp, S.T., Weiss, J.N., Kogan, B. (2004). Intracellular calcium cycling, early afterdepolarizations, and reentry in simulated long QT syndrome. Heart Rhythm, 1, 441–448.

19. Gyorke, S., Hagen, B.M., Terentyev, D., Lederer, W.J. (2007). Chain-reaction Ca^{2+} signaling in the heart. Journal of Clinical Investigation, 117, 1758–1762.

20. Hidalgo, C., Donoso, P. (2008). Crosstalk between calcium and redox signaling: From molecular mechanisms to health implications. Antioxidants and Redox Signaling, 10, 1275–1312.

21. Xu, L., Eu, J.P., Meissner, G., Stamler, J.S. (1998). Activation of the cardiac calcium release channel (ryanodine receptor) by poly-S-nitrosylation. Science, 279, 234–237.

22. Meissner, G. (2002). Regulation of mammalian ryanodine receptors. Frontiers in Bioscience, 7, d2072–2080.

23. Hidalgo, C., Aracena, P., Sanchez, G., Donoso, P. (2002). Redox regulation of calcium release in skeletal and cardiac muscle. Biological Research, 35, 183–193.

24. Zima, A.V., Blatter, L.A. (2006). Redox regulation of cardiac calcium channels and transporters. Cardiovascular Research, 71, 310–321.

25. Donoso, P., Aracena, P., Hidalgo, C. (2000). Sulfhydryl oxidation overrides Mg^{2+} inhibition of calcium-induced calcium release in skeletal muscle triads. Biophysical Journal, 79, 279–286.

26. Belevych, A.E., Terentyev, D., Viatchenko-Karpinski, S., Terentyeva, R., Sridhar, A., Nishijima, Y., Wilson, L.D., Cardounel, A.J., Laurita, K.R., Carnes, C.A., Billman, G.E., Gyorke, S. (2009). Redox modification of ryanodine receptors underlies calcium alternans in a canine model of sudden cardiac death. Cardiovascular Research 10.1093/cvr/cvp246.

27. Aracena-Parks, P., Goonasekera, S.A., Gilman, C.P., Dirksen, R.T., Hidalgo, C., Hamilton, S.L. (2006). Identification of cysteines involved in S-nitrosylation, S-glutathionylation, and oxidation to disulfides in ryanodine receptor type 1. Journal of Biological Chemistry, 281, 40354–40368.

28. Sawyer, D.B., Siwik, D.A., Xiao, L., Pimentel, D.R., Singh, K., Colucci, W.S. (2002). Role of oxidative stress in myocardial hypertrophy and failure. Journal of Molecular and Cellular Cardiology, 34, 379–388.

29. Giordano, F.J. (2005). Oxygen, oxidative stress, hypoxia, and heart failure. Journal of Clinical Investigation, 115, 500–508.

30. Seddon, M., Looi, Y.H., Shah, A.M. (2007). Oxidative stress and redox signalling in cardiac hypertrophy and heart failure. Heart, 93, 903–907.

31. Ide, T., Tsutsui, H., Hayashidani, S., Kang, D., Suematsu, N., Nakamura, K., Utsumi, H., Hamasaki, N., Takeshita, A. (2001). Mitochondrial DNA damage and dysfunction associated with oxidative stress in failing hearts after myocardial infarction. Circulation Research, 88, 529–535.

32. Redout, E.M., Wagner, M.J., Zuidwijk, M.J., Boer, C., Musters, R.J., van Hardeveld, C., Paulus, W.J., Simonides, W.S. (2007). Right-ventricular failure is associated with

increased mitochondrial complex II activity and production of reactive oxygen species. Cardiovascular Research, 75, 770–781.

33. Berry, C.E., Hare, J.M. (2004). Xanthine oxidoreductase and cardiovascular disease: molecular mechanisms and pathophysiological implications. Journal of Physiology, 555, 589–606.

34. Murdoch, C.E., Zhang, M., Cave, A.C., Shah, A.M. (2006). NADPH oxidase-dependent redox signalling in cardiac hypertrophy, remodelling and failure. Cardiovascular Research, 71, 208–215.

35. Dhalla, N.S., Temsah, R.M., Netticadan, T. (2000). Role of oxidative stress in cardiovascular diseases. Journal of Hypertension, 18, 655–673.

36. Dhalla, N.S., Temsah, R.M. (2001). Sarcoplasmic reticulum and cardiac oxidative stress: an emerging target for heart disease. Expert Opinion on Therapeutic Targets, 5, 205–217.

37. Cesselli, D., Jakoniuk, I., Barlucchi, L., Beltrami, A.P., Hintze, T.H., Nadal-Ginard, B., Kajstura, J., Leri, A., Anversa, P. (2001). Oxidative stress-mediated cardiac cell death is a major determinant of ventricular dysfunction and failure in dog dilated cardiomyopathy. Circulation Research, 89, 279–286.

38. Mochizuki, M., Yano, M., Oda, T., Tateishi, H., Kobayashi, S., Yamamoto, T., Ikeda, Y., Ohkusa, T., Ikemoto, N., Matsuzaki, M. (2007). Scavenging free radicals by low-dose carvedilol prevents redox-dependent Ca^{2+} leak via stabilization of ryanodine receptor in heart failure. Journal of the American College of Cardiology, 49, 1722–1732.

39. Terentyev, D., Gyorke, I., Belevych, A.E., Terentyeva, R., Sridhar, A., Nishijima, Y., de Blanco, E.C., Khanna, S., Sen, C.K., Cardounel, A.J. et al. (2008). Redox modification of ryanodine receptors contributes to sarcoplasmic reticulum Ca^{2+} leak in chronic heart failure. Circulation Research, 103, 1466–1472.

40. Sanchez, G., Pedrozo, Z., Domenech, R.J., Hidalgo, C., Donoso, P. (2005). Tachycardia increases NADPH oxidase activity and RyR2 S-glutathionylation in ventricular muscle. Journal of Molecular and Cellular Cardiology, 39, 982–991.

41. Eisner, D.A., Li, Y., O'Neill, S.C. (2006). Alternans of intracellular calcium: Mechanism and significance. Heart Rhythm, 3, 743–745.

42. Wehrens, X.H., Marks, A.R. (2004). Novel therapeutic approaches for heart failure by normalizing calcium cycling. Nature Review Drug Discovery, 3, 565–573.

43. Yano, M. (2008). Ryanodine receptor as a new therapeutic target of heart failure and lethal arrhythmia. Circulation Journal, 72, 509–514.

44. Antoons, G., Oros, A., Bito, V., Sipido, K.R., Vos, M.A. (2007). Cellular basis for triggered ventricular arrhythmias that occur in the setting of compensated hypertrophy and heart failure: Considerations for diagnosis and treatment. Journal of Electrocardiology, 40, S8–14.

45. Yano, M., Ikeda, Y., Matsuzaki, M. (2005). Altered intracellular Ca^{2+} handling in heart failure. Journal of Clinical Investigation, 115, 556–564.

46. Hunt, D.J., Jones, P.P., Wang, R., Chen, W., Bolstad, J., Chen, K., Shimoni, Y., Chen, S.R. (2007). K201 (JTV519) suppresses spontaneous Ca^{2+} release and [3H]ryanodine binding to RyR2 irrespective of FKBP12.6 association. Biochemical Journal, 404, 431–438.

47. Liu, N., Colombi, B., Memmi, M., Zissimopoulos, S., Rizzi, N., Negri, S., Imbriani, M., Napolitano, C., Lai, F.A., Priori, S.G. (2006). Arrhythmogenesis in catecholaminergic polymorphic ventricular tachycardia: Insights from a RyR2 R4496C knock-in mouse model. Circulation Research, 99, 292–298.

48. Lehnart, S.E., Wehrens, X.H., Marks, A.R. (2005). Defective ryanodine receptor inter-domain interactions may contribute to intracellular Ca^{2+} leak: A novel therapeutic target in heart failure. Circulation, 111, 3342–3346.

49. Pacher, P., Nivorozhkin, A., Szabo, C. (2006). Therapeutic effects of xanthine oxidase inhibitors: Renaissance half a century after the discovery of allopurinol. Pharmacological Reviews, 58, 87–114.

50. Hare, J.M., Mangal, B., Brown, J., Fisher, C., Jr., Freudenberger, R., Colucci, W.S., Mann, D.L., Liu, P., Givertz, M.M., Schwarz, R.P. (2008). Impact of oxypurinol in patients with symptomatic heart failure. Results of the OPT-CHF study. Journal of the American College of Cardiology, 51, 2301–2309.

51. Mitchell, L.B. (2008). Role of drug therapy for sustained ventricular tachyarrhythmias. Cardiology Clinics, 26, 405–418, vi.

52. Mital, S., Liao, J.K. (2004). Statins and the myocardium. Seminars in Vascular Medicine, 4, 377–384.

53. Hidalgo, C., Sanchez, G., Barrientos, G., Aracena-Parks, P. (2006). A transverse tubule NADPH oxidase activity stimulates calcium release from isolated triads via ryanodine receptor type 1 S -glutathionylation. Journal of Biological Chemistry, 281, 26473–26482.

■■■■■ CHAPTER 11

Targeting Na^+/Ca^{2+} Exchange as an Antiarrhythmic Strategy

GUDRUN ANTOONS, RIK WILLEMS, and KARIN R. SIPIDO

11.1 INTRODUCTION

In the early 1990s, the major advances and new insights in ion channel structure and function led to an intense program of drug development with high selectivity for specific ion channels. A landmark paper, which was the result of a task force with leaders in the field from basic to clinical electrophysiology, identified the specific targets for different types of arrhythmias according to their mechanism [1]. In more recent years, the enthusiasm for drug therapy for ventricular arrhythmias has waned because of life-threatening side effects of antiarrhythmic therapy [2, 3] and disappointing clinical results compared with the success of implantable defibrillators [4]. In other areas, such as atrial fibrillation, ion channels remain targets of interest. The identification of specific targets, such as the ultra-rapid delayed rectifier I_{Kur}, was a major step forward and additional development is ongoing (for review, see ref. 5).

Device therapy for life-threatening ventricular arrhythmias, however, cannot be considered a final answer. There is a significant negative impact on the quality of life if repeated interventions for ventricular arrhythmia are necessary [6, 7]. Although drug therapy can decrease this risk significantly [8], the high upfront costs of device therapy represent another problem. The cost effectiveness is highly dependent on accurate risk stratification for sudden cardiac death and on identification of the patients that will benefit most [9]. Although these problems are not necessarily solved by new drug development, drug therapy could help those patients that either do not qualify device therapy or for whom the benefit of device therapy is uncertain. Alternatively, drug therapy could serve as adjuncts to device therapy.

The possibility of targeting calcium (Ca^{2+}) handling in arrhythmias was already outlined in the Sicilian Gambit [1]. Ca^{2+} channel blockers are part of the classic battery of available antiarrhythmic drugs but have been most frequently used for their

Novel Therapeutic Targets for Antiarrhythmic Drugs, Edited by George Edward Billman
Copyright © 2010 John Wiley & Sons, Inc.

effects on sinus node (pacemaker) rate and atrioventricular node conduction. Attempts to modify Ca^{2+} handling through other pathways were hampered by the lack of available drugs or by the complexity of the drug effects [10]. The development of suitable drugs that block Na$^+$/Ca^{2+} exchange (NCX) has now opened a new field of research. In this chapter, we review the rationale for targeting NCX, the arrhythmias that may benefit from such a block, the experience so far, and the outlook for further development.

11.2 WHY TARGET NCX IN ARRHYTHMIAS?

The Na$^+$/Ca^{2+} exchanger is an essential regulator of Ca^{2+} balance in the cardiac myocyte (Figure 11.1) [12, 13]. It exchanges three Na$^+$ ions for one divalent Ca^{2+} ion and thus generates a net charge of 1 on each transport cycle. When Ca^{2+} leaves the cell (forward mode), the current is inward, whereas when Ca^{2+} enters the cell (the so-called reverse mode), the current is outward. As for any ionic current, the driving force, i.e., the difference between the membrane potential and the equilibrium potential of the channel (in this case the transporter), determines the sign and amplitude of the current. What distinguishes the NCX current from a classic ion channel current is that, during a single cardiac cycle, major changes in Ca^{2+} concentration shift the reversal potential (E$_{NCX}$). The transient rise in Ca^{2+} during excitation-contraction coupling because of Ca^{2+} release from the sarcoplasmic reticulum (SR) makes the E$_{NCX}$ more positive and drives an inward current. This Ca^{2+} efflux out of the cell is essential to balance the Ca^{2+} influx that occurred through the L-type Ca^{2+} channel, I$_{CaL}$. A similar shift of E$_{NCX}$ during spontaneous SR Ca^{2+} release occurring at the resting membrane potential is responsible for the activation of the inward current that leads to membrane depolarization and delayed afterdepolarizations (DADs) [14]. Any factor that reduces Ca^{2+} efflux will lead to a net gain of Ca^{2+} for the cell that usually results in a higher content of Ca^{2+} in the SR. Conversely, an increase of Ca^{2+} efflux will deplete the cell of Ca^{2+} and reduce the SR Ca^{2+} content. It is to be noted that this will lead to a new steady state, and at that time, on a single-cycle basis, the balance between Ca^{2+} influx via L-type channels and efflux via NCX will remain the same [15].

Short-lived increases in Na$^+$ with Na$^+$ channel activation may enhance the brief Ca^{2+} entry via NCX immediately following depolarization, but this has been very difficult to quantify [16]. The effect of changes in Na$^+$ concentration on a longer term, such as the increase in cellular Na$^+$ with Na$^+$/K$^+$ pump block, during ischemia/reperfusion or in heart failure is well established. These long-term changes lead to a small left-ward shift of E$_{NCX}$ and a new equilibrium resulting in an enhanced SR Ca^{2+} load.

The contribution of the NCX current to the time course of the action potential is less well defined than it is for other ionic currents. The lack of fast and selective blockers of the NCX current have, to date, prevented the direct measurement of the ion flow in an action potential clamp experiment, as can be done, for example, for K$^+$ currents [17]. The time course of the NCX current has been derived from experiments that indirectly affected the current, such as changes in Ca^{2+}, complemented by theoretical

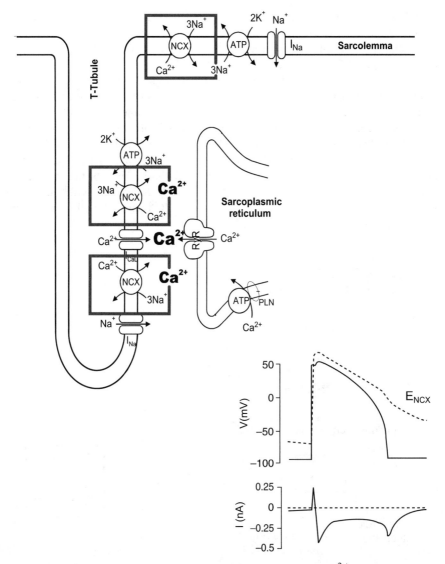

Figure 11.1. Schematic illustration of a ventricular myocyte and Ca^{2+} handling proteins involved in excitation-contraction coupling. The Na^{+}/Ca^{2+} exchanger, NCX, modulates Ca^{2+} balance of the cell, by extruding one Ca^{2+} ion in exchange for three Na^{+} ions operating in the forward mode or bringing Ca^{2+} into the cell and removing Na^{+} through the reverse mode. The mode of the exchanger depends on the driving force and reversal potential, E_{NCX}, which is dynamically changing during a single cardiac cycle. The inset shows calculated changes in E_{NCX} (dashed line) and NCX current (lower trace) during an action potential in a guinea pig ventricular myocyte. Reproduced from ref. 11.

modeling [18, 19]. Such studies have emphasized that the changes in NCX current are driven by the ion concentration directly beneath the membrane, which may differ considerably from what is observed during measurements of the bulk cytosolic concentrations of Ca^{2+} (or Na$^+$).

The available evidence indicates that, in physiological conditions, the current is briefly outward at the start of the action potential and then becomes an inward current with variable amplitude, depending on the time course of the Ca^{2+} transient in relation to the membrane potential (Figure 11.1 insert). A disease will affect this relationship. For example, on the one hand in heart failure, the higher Na$^+$ will prolong the duration of Ca^{2+} influx and hence the outward current [20], which may lead to action potential shortening. On the other hand, during conditions of high Ca^{2+} load and Ca^{2+} influx, as with adrenergic stimulation, the Ca^{2+} efflux mode and inward NCX current will increase and lead to an action potential prolongation.

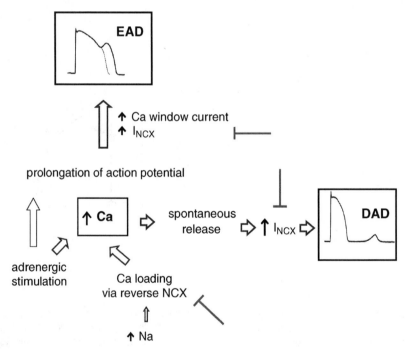

Figure 11.2. Calcium-dependent mechanisms of afterdepolarizations and interference with NCX blockers as antiarrhythmic strategy. Increasing the Ca^{2+} load of the cell with adrenergic stimulation, or under conditions of Na$^+$ overload, triggers afterdepolarizations: directly, through spontaneous diastolic release producing Ca^{2+} waves, inward Na$^+$/Ca^{2+} exchange current, I_{NCX}, and DADs; indirectly, through dynamic modulation of calcium-dependent currents (L-type Ca^{2+} channels and I_{NCX}) and action potential duration providing a favorable setting for EADs. The levels at which NCX blockers may interfere to prevent afterdepolarizations are indicated by red arrows. Modified after ref. 22.

Thus, we can summarize how NCX can contribute to arrhythmogenesis. In the presence of high Na^+, it is Ca^{2+} influx via NCX in reverse mode that leads to the cellular Ca^{2+} load. Consequent spontaneous Ca^{2+} release from the SR (potentially facilitated by other causes, see below) induces an inward NCX current that is responsible for membrane depolarization. When this occurs at the resting membrane potential, it induces a DAD that can trigger an action potential. This is the cellular mechanism underlying triggered arrhythmias. Enhanced Ca^{2+} efflux during the action potential can lead to action potential prolongation and can help set the stage for early afterdepolarizations (EADs). This is a less recognized condition where NCX contributes to proarrhythmia. With spontaneous release during the action potential plateau, the current can actually be responsible for the EAD [21]. EADs are unlikely to trigger an action potential, but with long action potentials and the temporal and spatial variability enhanced by the presence of EADs, local reentry can trigger an extrasystole, and dispersion of action potential duration can then contribute to reentry arrhythmias.

The different cellular mechanisms are highlighted in Figure 11.2.

11.3   WHEN DO WE SEE TRIGGERED ARRHYTHMIAS?

The triggered arrhythmias ascribed to spontaneous SR Ca^{2+} release were studied in detail many years ago in the context of digitalis intoxication [14]. These studies can be considered as examples of reverse translational research where a bedside problem studied at the bench led to fundamental insights into molecular mechanisms. Fortunately, digitalis intoxication is currently a rare event. However, arrhythmias observed during ischemia/reperfusion actually represent a similar phenomenon, since they result from an increase in Na. Although these arrhythmias are rarely life threatening, the Ca^{2+} influx with reverse mode NCX also contributes to the reperfusion damage and additional loss of viable tissue. This is one of the main reasons why NCX inhibition has been tried as a protective strategy during reperfusion [23].

In the laboratory, excessive catecholamine stimulation can lead to triggered arrhythmias that are driven by DADs and NCX currents, but adrenergic stimulation rarely does so in healthy people. However, in individuals with genetic mutations in the SR Ca^{2+} release channel (ryanodine receptors [RyRs]) or the SR Ca^{2+} binding protein calsequestrin (CSQ), adrenergic stimulation can facilitate the opening of the RyR, thereby provoking DADs and triggered arrhythmias. This condition is known as catecholaminergic polymorphic ventricular tachycardia (CPVT). These life-threatening arrhythmias are rare but are of particular importance because they affect patients often at young age [24, 25].

Conditions that prolong the action potential and incidence of EADs can also lead to polymorphic ventricular tachycardia or torsades de pointes. Typical examples are again genetic mutations in K^+ or Na^+ channels, as in the congenital long QT syndromes (LQTS1-3) [26]. The role of NCX in this type of arrhythmia is less well studied but may be important for LQTS3. Increased Na^+ influx may promote Ca^{2+} influx via NCX and thereby facilitate the arrhythmias [27]. It is also striking that the occurrence of arrhythmias in these patients is related to exercise (KVLQT1 mutations), emotional stress (hERG mutations), or sudden arousal (SCN5A mutations), conditions that all provoke a surge of catecholamines. Acquired long QT caused by the loss of K$^+$ currents, either through disease (see below) or related to drugs that block hERG channels, theoretically fall in the same category.

A major subgroup of the population with sudden cardiac death is heart failure patients. The type of life-threatening arrhythmias occurring in heart failure is actually not studied that extensively, but an earlier study suggested that triggered arrhythmias indeed played a major role [28]. From the cellular point of view on Ca^{2+} handling, this may at first glance seem surprising because the archetypical Ca^{2+} transient of a human myocyte from a patient with end-stage heart failure has a small amplitude, and SR Ca^{2+} content is low [29, 30]. In the presence of catecholamines, however, DADs and EADs are readily observed [31, 32]. Other elements that would favor DADs is the loss of a stabilizing I$_{K1}$ current and an increase in NCX current density that would enhance the depolarizing force for a given instance of spontaneous Ca^{2+} release [33, 34]. Finally, the increased phosphorylation of RyR may on the one hand contribute to depletion of the SR Ca^{2+}, but, on the other hand, it may facilitate spontaneous Ca^{2+} release by lowering the threshold for release when the Ca^{2+} content increases [35]. Loss of repolarizing K$^+$ currents also contributes to the prolongation of the action potential [36, 37], another typical finding in heart failure, and it may thereby set the stage for EADs, partially supported by NCX.

In summary, triggered arrhythmias as occurring in many congenital arrhythmias but also in ischemia-reperfusion and in heart failure, particularly under adrenergic stimulation, could potentially benefit from NCX inhibition.

11.4   WHAT DRUGS ARE AVAILABLE?

The NCX has long been an orphan in pharmacology, and tools that were available to researchers to study NCX had poor selectivity (e.g., amiloride), were toxic agents (e.g., Ni^{2+}), or were manipulations of ion concentrations; none of these interventions were directly suited for application in human pathology. The first major breakthrough was the KB-R7943 compound. What was particularly exciting about this drug was the possibility that it would affect differentially the forward and the reverse mode of the Na$^+$/Ca^{2+} exchanger; this property is called mode selectivity [38]. When tested in cellular systems, either a heterologous NCX expressing cell line or cardiac myocytes, the Kd of the drug for inhibition of reverse mode was much lower than the Kd for inhibition of the forward mode. However, this observation was not confirmed when the drug was tested in a single experimental recording of NCX that simultaneously evaluated the forward and the reverse mode [39]. A more recent derivative of the same family, SEA-0400 [38] (Figure 11.3) has shown better mode selectivity than KB-R7943. In a giant patch, excised from oocytes expressing NCX, it can be observed in panel A that the block of the reverse mode, elicited by increasing Na$^+$ to 100 mM on the cytosolic side, is much more pronounced than inhibition of the forward mode, which is elicited by increasing Ca^{2+} from 1 to 10 µM on the cytosolic side. This difference is statistically significant, as shown in panel B. Yet, from a biophysical

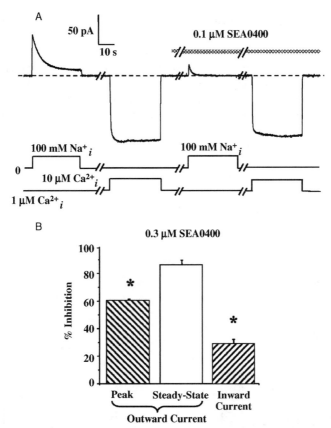

Figure 11.3. Unidirectional block of NCX current by SEA-0400. **A,** Typical Na^+/Ca^{2+} exchange currents from an excised membrane patch from a *X. laevis* oocyte expressing the cardiac Na/Ca exchanger, NCX1.1. The pipette contained 2 mM Ca^{2+} and 100 mM Na^+. Outward currents were activated by applying 100 mM Na^+ to the cytosolic surface of the patch in the continuous presence of 1 μM regulatory $[Ca^{2+}]_i$. Inward currents were activated by applying 100 mM Li^+ and 10 μM Ca^{2+} to the cytosolic surface of the patch. Currents are shown before and after (~1 min) the addition of 0.1 μM SEA0400. **B,** Pooled data illustrating the inhibitory effects of 0.3 μM SEA0400 on outward (peak and steady state) and inward Na^+/Ca^{2+} exchange currents (mean ± S.E., five patches; $^*P < 0.01$). Reproduced from ref. 40.

point of view, it is extremely difficult to conceive that one mode would be blocked more than the other [12]. In voltage-clamp experiments where the NCX current was activated by gradually changing the membrane potential while keeping Na^+ and Ca^{2+} concentrations constant, there was no evidence for mode dependence [41, 42]. The most likely explanation is that the drug binding and/or action would be facilitated in the presence of high Na^+ on the cytosolic side. In the presence of a constant drug concentration, this would then lead to a higher degree of block when conditions changed and reverse mode would be favored, as for example, during ischemia-reperfusion. Although not a true mode selectivity, this is an attractive property for a NCX blocker.

The different members of the class of compounds started by KB-R7943 are shown in Figure 11.4. These compounds exhibit different selectivity and potency for the block of NCX over other ion channels and transporters. SEA-0400 is ≈ 10-fold more potent than KB-R7943 with IC$_{50}$ values between 30 and 300 nM for SEA0400, and between 0.25 and 5 µM for KB-R7943 when NCX is measured as a voltage-dependent current in myocytes [41, 42], (for a review, see ref. 43). Both drugs have additional

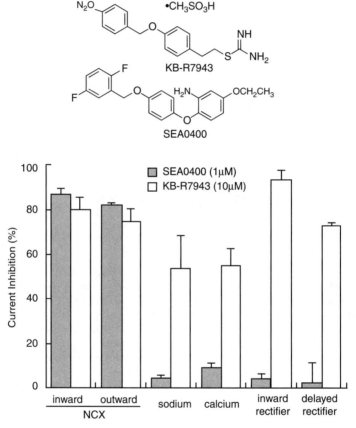

Figure 11.4. *Upper panel,* Chemical structure of members of a new class of NCX inhibitors sharing a common benzyloxyphenyl structure. *Lower panel,* Effects of SEA0400 and KB-R7943 on myocardial ionic currents in guinea pig ventricular myocytes. The inward and outward NCX currents were measured at −80 mV and + 30 mV, respectively; Na$^+$ current at −20 mV; L-type Ca^{2+} current at + 10 mV; inward rectifying potassium current, I$_{K1}$, at −60 mV and delayed rectifier potassium current, I$_{Kr}$, as the tail current on repolarization to −30 mV from + 50 mV. Inhibition of current amplitudes in the presence of SEA0400 (1 µM) and KB-R7943 (10 µM) were expressed as percentages of the value in the absence of compounds. Reproduced from ref. 41.

effects on I_{CaL} and block the channel with equal potency (IC_{50} values of 3.2 and 3.6 μM as reported by ref. 44). This finding suggests that, for a same degree of NCX inhibition, KB-R7943 causes a greater block of I_{CaL}, as illustrated in Figure 11.4 B, and is thus a less selective drug than SEA-0400 [41]. At the IC_{50} for NCX, SEA-0400 has virtually no effects on K^+ channels. SN-6 has a selectivity profile resembling that of SEA-0400 but has a higher potency [45]. It should be noted that all of these compounds block NCX in many tissues. Research is ongoing to identify tissue-specific block, e.g., in the brain [46].

11.5   EXPERIENCE WITH NCX INHIBITORS

The new generation of NCX blockers, with KB-R7943 as the prototype followed by SEA-0400, has been most extensively tested against arrhythmias where the arrhythmogenic mechanism directly involves the exchanger as the principle pathway for loading the cell with Ca^{2+}. This is the case for conditions of Na^+ overload as with digitalis and ischemia/reperfusion arrhythmias. At the onset, it was thought that the drugs being tested were more selective for reverse mode of the NCX, which would make these compounds a prime choice against these arrhythmias. More recently, NCX has been explored as a possible target in arrhythmias other than those related to the classic conditions of Na^+ and Ca^{2+} overload but still related to abnormal spontaneous Ca^{2+} release and DADs, e.g., adrenergic stimulation. The rationale here also considers the forward mode block of these compounds, which would reduce the inward current for a given Ca^{2+} wave and thereby prevent DADs. In a similar manner, reducing the NCX current that accompanies the "normal" Ca^{2+} release from the SR during an action potential would strengthen the repolarization reserve of the cell and provide less conditioning current for reactivation of I_{CaL}. This will minimize the likelihood for EADs, at least under certain conditions (Figure 11.1). An overview of studies using KB-R7943 and/or SEA-0400 testing the antiarrhythmic potential of NCX blockers is listed in Table 11.1 and briefly discussed.

A first set of data examines arrhythmias that are induced by digitalis or related compounds (ouabain and strophantidin). Cardiac glycosides block the Na^+/K^+ pump and induce a gradual rise of Na^+ and subsequently Ca^{2+} through activation of reverse NCX. This eventually causes Ca^{2+} overload, which is typically associated with spontaneous Ca^{2+} oscillations, DADs, and extrasystolic beats. In the case of digitalis, NCX blockers directly target the pathway responsible for excessive Ca^{2+} loading. This result could explain the more or less consistent efficiency against this type of arrhythmias in cardiac cells and tissues (Table 11.1 and references therein). Figure 11.5 illustrates the suppression of the irregular contractile activity and Ca^{2+} transients reflecting arrhythmias in a cellular experiment [53]. However, one study reported proarrhythmic effects with KB-R7943 when the heart was additionally challenged by rapid pacing. Even in the absence of ouabain, higher heart rates were sufficient for NCX blockers to be proarrhythmic [50, 68]. Another study did not confirm this observation [69]. These findings emphasize the delicate balance between the benefits of reducing Ca^{2+} influx during reverse mode (and concomitant block

Table 11.1. Effects of NCX blockers in models of arrhythmia

		Species	Intervention	Agent	Dose	Arrhythmia	Remarks	Ref
1. Digitalis intoxication	In vivo	Dog	Ouabain	KB-R	5 mg/kg	=	No effect on extrasystoles	47
		Dog	Digitalis	SEA	3 mg/kg	↓	↓ Extrasystolic activity; atrioventricular block and cardiac standstill in 2/8 dogs	48
		Guinea pig	Ouabain	KB-R	1 and 3 mg/kg	↓	↑ Threshold dose of ouabain to induce PVB, VT, VF and cardiac arrest	49
	Tissue cells	Guinea pig Atrial strips	Ouabain	KB-R	30 μmol/L	↓ (at 1Hz)	Prevents arrhythmogenic contractions;	50
		Guinea pig Atria	Ouabain	KB-R	10-30 μmol/L	↓	pro-arrhythmic at higher frequency (≥ 2Hz), also in the absence of ouabain	49
		Rabbit PV	Ouabain/spontaneous	KB-R	30 μmol/L	↓	↓ Ionotropic/tonotropic effects and arrhythmogenic contractions in spontaneously beating atria	51
		Guinea pig PM	Ouabain	SEA	1 μmol/L	↓	↓ Firing rates and ouabain-induced DADs	52
		Rat VM	Strophantidin	KB-R	5 μmol/L	↓	↓ Incidence arrhythmogenic contractions	53, 54
		Dog Purkinje	Strophantin	SEA	1 μmol/L	↓	↓ Ca oscillations and arrhythmogenic contractions ↓ DAD amplitude; no effect on I_{CaL} in dog VM	55

2. Ischemia/ reperfusion	*In vivo*	Dog	Coronary ligation	SEA	5 and 10 mg/kg	=	No effect on premature ectopic beats and VF incidence	48
		Dog	Coronary occlusion	KB-R	0.3-10 mg/kg	=	No effect on extrasystoles and survival	49
		Rat	Coronary occlusion	SEA	0.3-1 mg/kg	→	↓ VF incidence and mortality	56
		Rat	Coronary occlusion	KB-R	1.25 mg/kg	=	No effect on PVB, VT, VF incidence	57
	Intact heart	Rabbit	Global I/R	KB-R	3 μmol/L	→	↓ VT and VF incidence	58
		Rat	Coronary ligation	KB-R	1 and 10 μmol/L	→	Concentration-dependent ↓ VF incidence	59
		Rat	Global I/R	KB-R	1 nmol/L	→	↓ VF duration after reperfusion; drug sensitivity is strain dependent	60
		Rat	Global I/R	SEA	1 μmol/L	←	↑ VF incidence and duration; 60–65% block of inward and outward I_{NCX} in rat VM	61
	Tissue cells	Rat VM	Anoxia induced	KB-R	10 μmol/L	→	↓ Spontaneous Ca^{2+} oscillations after reperfusion	62
		Guinea pig PM	Hypoxia induced	KB-R	10 μmol/L	→	↓ Arrhythmogenic electrical and contractile activity	63
		Guinea pig PM	Hypoxia induced	KB-R	10 μmol/L	→	↓ Incidence, duration and amplitude of arrhythmogenic contractions	54
		Guinea pig VM	Simulated ischemia	KB-R	0.1-1 μmol/L	→	↓ I_{TI} and aftercontractions amplitude and incidence no effect at higher doses (0.5–1 μM)	64

(continued)

Table 11.1. (*Continued*)

	Species		Intervention	Agent	Dose	Arrhythmia	Remarks	Ref
3. Abnormal Na channel activity (LQT3)	Guinea pig	*In vivo*	Aconitine induced	KB-R	1 and 30 mg/kg	↓	↓ Duration PVB and VT	65
				SEA	10 mg/kg	=	KB-R (10 µmol/L) but not SEA (100 µmol/L) suppressed aconitine-induced DAD in single myocytes	
	Rabbit	*Intact heart*	Veratridine induced	SEA	1 µmol/L	→	↓ EADs and TdP incidence	66
Other								
LQT syndrome	Rabbit	*Intact heart*	Sotalol induced	SEA	1 µmol/L	→	↓ EADs and TdP incidence	66
	Dog PM	*Tissue/cells*	Dofetilide + $BaCl_2$	SEA	1 µmol/L	→	↓ EAD amplitude	55
							No effect on I_{CaL} in dog VM	
Atrial fibrillation	Dog	*In vivo*	Acute AF induced by rapid pacing	KB-R	5 mg/kg	→	Prolongs refractory period in atria (not in ventricle) peak plasma concentration was 30 nmol/L; in atrial cells, 15 nmol/L caused 60% block of reverse, and no effect on forward NCX	67
Rapid pacing	Dog	*In vivo*	Rapid pacing	KB-R	2 mg/kg	↑	Induces alternans, EADs, and VT at a CL of 300 ms	
	Rat	*Intact heart*	Rapid pacing/ adrenergic stimulation/ low K^+	SEA	3 µmol/L	→	Abolishes DADs, but not spontaneous Ca^{2+} waves	

Abbreviations: PVB, premature ventricular beats; VT, ventricular tachycardia; VF, ventricular fibrillation; TdP, torsades de pointes arrhythmias; AF, atrial fibrillation; I_{TI}, transient inward current; CL, cycle length; I/R, ischemia/reperfusion; PV, pulmonary veins; PM, papillary muscle; VM, ventricular myocytes.

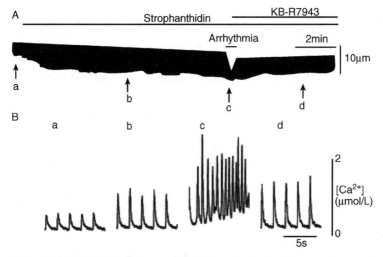

Figure 11.5. KB-R7943 blocks strophanthidin-induced arrhythmia but not inotropy. **A**, Continuous recording of twitch cell shortening from a typical experiment in a rat ventricular myocyte, with 50 μmol/L strophanthidin and 5 μmol/L KB-R7943 added as indicated by bars. **B**, Calcium transients recorded during control perfusion (a), 5 min after starting strophanthidin perfusion (b), when arrhythmia appeared (11 min, indicated by bar; c), and 3 min after addition of KB-R7943 (d). Reproduced from ref. 47.

of I_{CaL}) and the risk of Ca^{2+} overload by inhibiting the pathway for Ca^{2+} removal; the adverse effects of NCX block will be most pronounced when imposing additional Ca^{2+} loads on the cell, as with high heart rates, when the cell has less capacity to store excessive Ca^{2+}. In the intact animal, SEA-0400 seemed to be more efficient than KB-R7943 [47, 48]. As pointed out earlier, digitalis intoxication is a rare event, and the clinical relevance of these studies may therefore be limited. These data do, however, provide proof of concept for testing NCX block as an antiarrhythmic strategy in more complex settings of ischemia/reperfusion that share a common mechanism with digitalis.

An acute ischemic event causes imbalance and redistribution of ions across the sarcolemma [70]. Typical changes are a drop of pH, net cellular loss of K^+ and depolarization, and accumulation of Na^+. The latter is caused by an increased Na^+ leak and a less efficient Na^+/K^+ pump for Na^+ removal; high Na^+ drives the exchanger in its reverse mode loading the cell with Ca^{2+}. This observation is exaggerated during reperfusion, when there is a large gradient for the Na^+/H^+ exchanger to extrude protons, which imposes additional Na^+ and Ca^{2+} loads on the cell. During this phase, the heart is particularly vulnerable for developing arrhythmias, and the putative mechanism is the same as proposed for digitalis. Excessive Ca^{2+} also causes cell death and myocardial damage, and the interest for using NCX blockers was initially focused on protecting the heart from injury. These studies documented that KB-R7943 and SEA-0400 prevented excessive Ca^{2+} accumulation during an ischemic event, limited myocardial injury, and improved recovery of contractile function after reperfusion (e.g., [62, 71]). The cardioprotective effects are highly reproducible and in line with the observations in the NCX KO mouse [72]. Studies that addressed NCX block in the context of reperfusion arrhythmias are summarized in Table 11.1 and include cellular, multicellular, and *in vivo* studies. NCX blockers reduce spontaneous Ca^{2+} oscillations typically observed during reperfusion and, overall, have antiarrhythmic effects in experimental models of global ischemia. The efficiency seems to be strain dependent [60], and the concentration of the drug is an important factor: protection was lost at higher concentrations [64]. In the intact animal, where ischemia is induced by ligation or occlusion of the coronary arteries and more closely mimics the clinical situation, results with NCX blockers are somewhat disappointing. In the dog, NCX blockers failed to reduce the incidence of ventricular fibrillation and sudden death after ischemia/reperfusion [47, 48]. Only one study that was performed in rats reported beneficial effects of SEA-0400, but not of KB-R7943, on ischemia/reperfusion arrhythmias [56, 57].

NCX inhibition has also been tested in arrhythmias associated with LQTS3. This congenital arrhythmic disease is a combination of abnormally delayed and slow repolarization and Na$^+$ accumulation caused by gain-of-function mutations in the Na$^+$ channel. Increased Na$^+$ channel activity produces a sustained inward current that prolongs action potential duration and facilitates EADs; it also provides a pathway for increased Na$^+$ influx and subsequent Ca^{2+} accumulation [27]. Thus, theoretically, NCX inhibition is an attractive strategy in LQT3: 1) reducing reverse mode would prevent Ca^{2+} overload due to net Na$^+$ gain and 2) reducing forward mode would provide less inward current for a given amount of SR Ca^{2+} release, spontaneous or triggered, during an action potential. This mechanism may be of particular relevance when adrenergic drive to the heart has increased. To our knowledge, to date, only two studies have tried NCX blockers against pharmacological models of LQT3, yielding inconsistent results. In isolated rabbit hearts, SEA-0400 shortened the action potential and lowered torsades de pointes incidence (Figure 11.6, top panel) [66]. In an earlier study in guinea pigs that compared the more selective SEA-0400 with KB-R7943, SEA-0400 had no effect on DADs and arrhythmias, whereas KB-R7943 was antiarrhythmic [65]. This was supported by modeling studies, showing that a 90% inhibition of NCX actually enhances arrhythmogenic activity caused by increased Na$^+$ channel opening. The authors concluded that the antiarrhythmic effect of KB-R7943 must be explained by mechanisms other than NCX inhibition, possibly through off-target effects on other ion channels, with I$_{CaL}$ and I$_{Na}$ being the most likely candidates because inhibition of these ion channels would reduce the Ca^{2+} gain of the cell.

Interestingly, in the study by Milberg et al. [66], SEA-0400 was also tested against arrhythmias induced by sotalol, an I$_{Kr}$ blocker, mimicking LQT2S, and completely suppressed torsades de pointes episodes (Figure 11.6, lower panel). These effects were explained by inhibition of forward mode of the NCX, based on the observations of action potential shortening and reduced dispersion of repolarization. These findings were confirmed by cellular studies where SEA-0400 lowered the amplitude of EADs that were induced by I$_K$ block [55]. In atria, NCX block with KB-R7943 has opposite effects: it prolongs repolarization and prevents shortening of the refractory

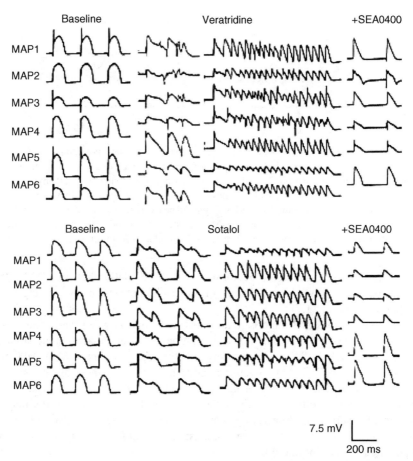

Figure 11.6. SEA0400 suppresses EAD and torsades de pointes induced by the Na channel opener veratridine (upper panel) and sotalol, a selective I_{Kr} blocker (lower panel) during bradycardia (AV block) and hypokalemia in the isolated Langendorff-perfused rabbit heart. Monophasic action potentials, MAP1-6, were simultaneously recorded using catheters that were placed at different regions of the heart. Reproduced from ref. 66.

period during acute fibrillation induced by rapid pacing [67]. This property may be an advantage for preventing atrial fibrillation. The mechanism by which KB-R7943 selectively prolongs refractoriness in the atria and not in the ventricles is unknown. An attractive explanation would be that KB-R7943 has additional (yet unknown) effects on ion currents that are specifically expressed in the atria, like I_{Kur} or acetylcholine-dependent K^+ currents.

The most recent data on NCX inhibition were obtained in the intact guinea pig heart using dual-view and rapid-scanning confocal microscopy that allows simultaneous measurement of fluorescence Ca^{2+} and membrane potential in cells of the subepicardial layer. Fujiwara et al. [69] could confirm experimentally a mechanistic link among intracellular Ca^{2+} waves, membrane oscillations, and extrasystoles in the

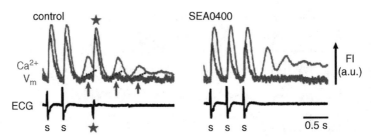

Figure 11.7. Effects of SEA-0400 on calcium waves, membrane potential, and triggered activity in the intact rat heart. *Left*, Example of fluorescence signals for [Ca^{2+}]$_i$ (fluo-4, red trace) and membrane potential V$_m$ (RH237, green traces) in a subepicardial myocyte in a Langendorff-perfused rat heart, with simultaneous ECG recording after pacing under low K (2.4 mmol/L) and isoproterenol (3 nmol/L). Triggered beats are indicated by stars, DADs by red arrows; S below ECG denotes pacing. *Right*, DADs and triggered activity are abolished by SEA0400, whereas [Ca^{2+}]$_i$ oscillations remains. Reproduced from ref. 69.

intact heart. This study nicely demonstrated that SEA0400 abolishes DADs that accompany Ca^{2+} waves by inhibiting inward NCX but without preventing Ca^{2+} oscillations (Figure 11.7).

The above summary should be interpreted with caution when the data are used to support or refute the potential of NCX inhibition as an antiarrhythmic strategy. SEA-0400 and KB-R7943 are not entirely selective agents, although SEA-0400 may be more so than KB-R7943. Given the additional effects of these agents on other cardiac ion currents, in particular Ca^{2+} channels, the observed beneficial effects could be related to either or both of these targets. However, the results may be interpreted to support multitargeting as antiarrhythmic strategy. The data obtained in these studies thus remain of value and interest in the evaluation of this new category of potential antiarrhythmic drugs.

11.6 CAVEAT—THE CONSEQUENCES ON CA^{2+} HANDLING

NCX is a major determinant of cellular Ca^{2+} homeostasis. The selective inhibition of NCX therefore will alter Ca^{2+} balance. Considering that in physiological conditions the net movement of Ca^{2+} by NCX is outward to provide Ca^{2+} efflux, inhibition can therefore be expected to raise the cellular Ca^{2+} load. With a full block, the remaining Ca^{2+} transport capacity for removal of Ca^{2+} from the cell is indeed low, as it is restricted to the plasma membrane calcium ATPase (PMCA). Experiments performed in completely Na$^+$-free conditions, therefore, often lead to cellular Ca^{2+} overload unless the Ca^{2+} influx is kept low (e.g., by low frequency stimulation) [73]. The ultimate example of full block of NCX is represented by the cardiac-specific NCX knockout mouse. Much to the surprise of cardiac cell physiologists, these mice seemed to be normal [74]. Cardiac myocytes had near-normal Ca^{2+} transients, although the absence of the NCX current was confirmed in voltage-clamp recording.

The explanation is a pronounced reduction of Ca^{2+} influx through I_{CaL} with an increase in gain of SR Ca^{2+} release [75]. This lesson can perhaps be applied to pharmacology and to drug development. These mice indeed have advantages in conditions where NCX contributes to pathology, and they seem to be more resistant to ischemia-reperfusion [72].

The concept that NCX inhibition would reduce Ca^{2+} efflux was the motivation to examine the effect of the NCX inhibitory peptide, XIP, in cardiac myocytes from dogs with heart failure, as NCX was thought to be responsible for loss of Ca^{2+} and reduced SR Ca^{2+} load in heart failure [76]. Indeed, these experiments showed a beneficial effect with an increase in SR Ca^{2+} load and Ca^{2+} release. Remarkably, the rate of relaxation was not reduced, presumably because of a shift toward more SR Ca^{2+} uptake. The concept was not pursued further, because XIP had to be administered into the myocytes via a patch pipette.

Initially, the first generation of small molecule NCX inhibitors discussed above was not extensively studied with regard to the effects on Ca^{2+} handling, but newer reports are emerging. In the mouse, the increase of $[Ca^{2+}]_i$ transient amplitude was reported [77] with a rather high dose of 10 µmol/L of SEA-0400, and this also induced an increase in resting Ca^{2+}. In the dog, only a minor effect on $[Ca^{2+}]_i$ transients was observed, possibly because of the concomitant block of I_{CaL} [44, 78]. Recently, we extensively investigated the effects of SEA-0400 in normal healthy and in diseased cardiac myocytes from pig and mouse [79]. Figure 11.8(A, B) confirms that, with a constant concentration of intracellular Na^+, the inhibition of reverse and forward mode is equal. Figure 11.8(C) illustrates how SEA-0400 reduces the arrhythmogenic current evoked by Ca^{2+} release from the SR during Ca^{2+} overload, which is here mimicked by a brief pulse of caffeine. This then predicts that the result of partial inhibition of NCX will lead to a net gain of Ca^{2+} in cardiac myocytes. Figure 11.9 shows the increase in the amplitude of the Ca^{2+} transient evoked during depolarizing steps. The increase present at all potentials, indicating that it results from a net gain of Ca^{2+} in the SR and is not related to a difference in the trigger for release. This gain of SR Ca^{2+} content is confirmed from measurement of the Ca^{2+} extruded after releasing all Ca^{2+} stored in the SR (right panel). Diastolic Ca^{2+} also increased and the rate of relaxation decreased.

As mentioned, the different compounds have a variable degree of Ca^{2+} channel block. Figure 11.10 illustrates that Ca^{2+} channel block is indeed present and inherent to the compound, but it is also accentuated by the effects on Ca^{2+} handling because of NCX block. The left panel shows a block of around 25% in the absence of NCX and with Ca^{2+} buffering; the block is independent of the frequency of stimulation. The right panel shows that the block is more pronounced when there is a concomitant block of NCX and that the reduction of Ca^{2+} current increases with higher frequencies of stimulation. This effect can be related to the increase of Ca^{2+} with NCX block; this increase is more pronounced when diastolic intervals get shorter.

We next examined whether in heart failure the net gain of Ca^{2+} could be an interesting side effect and lead to positive inotropy. We used two well-established

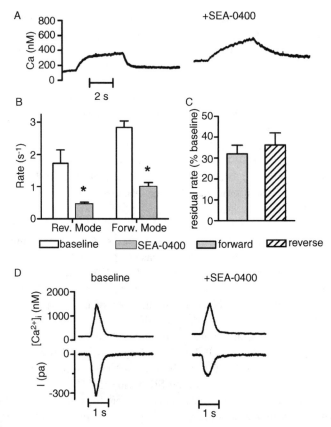

Figure 11.8. Block of calcium fluxes through NCX by SEA-0400 in single myocytes. **A**, [Ca^{2+}]$_i$ transients during a 5-s depolarizing step from –40 to +60 mV in the presence of nifedipine, ryanodine, and thapsigargin; Ca^{2+} influx and Ca^{2+} efflux rates were measured by exponential fitting. **B**, Mean rate constants of forward and reverse mode and inhibition by SEA-0400 (n = 8). **C**, Residual fraction of the forward and reverse mode rate. **D**, SEA-0400 reduces inward NCX current (lower trace) activated upon Ca^{2+} release from the SR (upper trace) with a short (300 ms) application of 10 mmol/L caffeine. Modified after 79.

models of heart failure in mice. In the MLP$^{-/-}$ with dilated cardiomyopathy, SEA-0400 failed to increase the amplitude of contraction, but it had a positive effect in myocytes from hypertrophic remodeling after aortic constriction. In both cases, the effect was less pronounced than in healthy myocytes.

All the above data indicate that we have to be well aware of the effect on NCX inhibition on Ca^{2+} handling through its direct effects and, consequently, on accentuated L-type Ca^{2+} channel block. This may be advantageous in heart failure, but with caution, and it may differ in different types of heart failure. The concomitant L-type Ca^{2+} channel block may not be a disadvantage and, rather, might help to mitigate effects on Ca^{2+} handling. It is reminiscent of the "adaptation" in the NCX KO mouse.

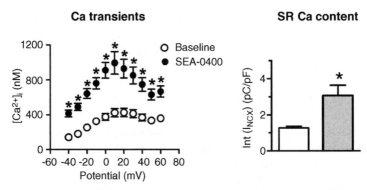

Figure 11.9. Increase in $[Ca^{2+}]_i$ with SEA-0400 in pig myocytes. *Left*, Peak $[Ca^{2+}]_i$ and voltage dependence during depolarizing steps to different voltages under baseline and with SEA-0400 ($n = 14$). *Right*, Increase in SR Ca^{2+} content calculated from integrated inward I_{NCX} during a 10-s application of 10 mmol/L caffeine before and after SEA-0400 ($n = 9$, $*P < 0.05$).

11.7 NEED FOR MORE DEVELOPMENT

The current data only open the field. The drugs tested, to date, may have therapeutic potential, but many questions remain to be answered. The current data by no means indicate that pure and selective NCX inhibition is a good treatment strategy, but these data also do not refute the concept, simply because this strategy has not been fully

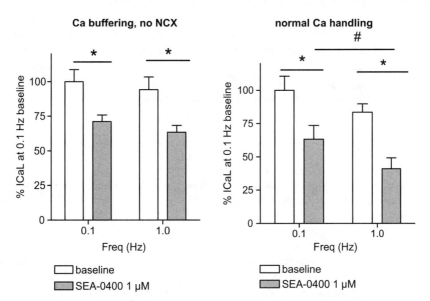

Figure 11.10. Effects of Ca^{2+} on L-type calcium channel block by SEA-0400. Amplitude of I_{CaL} as a percentage of maximal current measured during depolarizing steps from -40 mV to $+10$ mV at 0.1 Hz or 1 Hz, before and after SEA-0400, in calcium-buffered myocytes and no NCX (*left panel*), and in nonbuffered cells with normal Ca^{2+} and NCX function (*right panel*).

tested. It is unclear currently what contribution the Ca^{2+} channel block has on the beneficial effects that have been observed. Partial inhibition of NCX leading to a net gain of Ca^{2+} is not a desirable side effect, unless this Ca^{2+} gain is beneficial in heart failure. Concomitant Ca^{2+} channel block may mitigate this effect. It is striking that a reduction of Ca^{2+} current is also observed in the NCX KO mouse, although it should be noted that, in the mouse, the loss of Ca^{2+} current is larger than what is observed with the current NCX inhibitors.

Recent history has shown that drugs with multiple targets, such as amiodarone and dronedarone, can have a good therapeutic profile [80, 81]. This may be related to the fact that arrhythmias also have multiple mechanisms. Within the Ca^{2+} handling field, alternative transporters, most notably the ryanodine receptor, are being targeted to reduce arrhythmias [82]. One must be cautioned that the suppression of NCX in conditions of Ca^{2+} overload is likely to increase cellular Ca^{2+} load. However, this may not create problems if the cellular increase of Ca^{2+} is well sequestered into the SR. However, if unchecked, Ca^{2+} waves could lead to cell damage. Evidence hints that increasing SR Ca^{2+} pump activity may also prove to be a valuable strategy [83]. A broader strategy of reducing Ca^{2+}-triggered arrhythmias may involve combining multiple targets.

Testing in relevant animal models is an absolute requirement for several reasons. First, the mode of action must be tested in diseased hearts and for different mechanisms of arrhythmias. Second, so far we have not truly considered that NCX inhibition is not restricted to the heart. NCX inhibitors may lower blood pressure [48]. This integrated response will need to be considered in an eventual therapeutic strategy.

In conclusion, NCX inhibition is a novel treatment strategy that is distinct from earlier ion channel blockers, which merits additional exploration. There are indications that this approach has considerable therapeutic potential for the management of arrhythmias, but many potential pitfalls or limitations need to be investigated carefully. An interactive translational approach that requires close collaboration among basic research, industry, and the clinic is needed.

REFERENCES

1. Members of the Sicilan Gambit. (2001). New approaches to antiarrhythmic therapy: Emerging therapeutic applications of the cell biology of cardiac arrhythmias. Cardiovascular Research, 52, 345–360.

2. The CAST Investigators. (1989). Preliminary report: Effect of encainide and flecainide on mortality in a randomized trial of arrhythmia suppression after myocardial infarction. The Cardiac Arrhythmia Suppression Trial (CAST) Investigators. New England Journal of Medicine, 321, 406–412.

3. Boriani, G., Lubinski, A., Capucci, A., Niederle, P., Kornacewicz-Jack, Z., Wnuk-Wojnar, A.M., Borggrefe, M., Brachmann, J., Biffi, M., Butrous, G.S., (2001). A multicentre, double-blind randomized crossover comparative study on the efficacy and safety of dofetilide vs sotalol in patients with inducible sustained ventricular tachycardia and ischaemic heart disease. European Heart Journal, 22, 2180–2191.

4. Bardy, G.H., Lee, K.L., Mark, D.B., Poole, J.E., Packer, D.L., Boineau, R., Domanski, M., Troutman, C., Anderson, J., Johnson, G., et al. (2005). Amiodarone or an implantable cardioverter-defibrillator for congestive heart failure. New England Journal of Medicine, 352, 225–237.

5. Ehrlich, J.R., (2008). Inward rectifier potassium currents as a target for atrial fibrillation therapy. Journal of Cardiovascular Pharmacology, 52, 129–135.

6. Schron, E.B., Exner, D.V., Yao, Q., Jenkins, L.S., Steinberg, J.S., Cook, J.R., Kutalek, S.P., Friedman, P.L., Bubien, R.S., Page, R.L., et al. (2002). Quality of life in the antiarrhythmics versus implantable defibrillators trial: Impact of therapy and influence of adverse symptoms and defibrillator shocks. Circulation, 105, 589–594.

7. Passman, R., Subacius, H., Ruo, B., Schaechter, A., Howard, A., Sears, S.F., Kadish, A., (2007). Implantable cardioverter defibrillators and quality of life: Results from the defibrillators in nonischemic cardiomyopathy treatment evaluation study. Archives of Internal Medicine, 167, 2226–2232.

8. Connolly, S.J., Dorian, P., Roberts, R.S., Gent, M., Bailin, S., Fain, E.S., Thorpe, K., Champagne, J., Talajic, M., Coutu, B., et al. (2006). Comparison of beta-blockers, amiodarone plus beta-blockers, or sotalol for prevention of shocks from implantable cardioverter defibrillators: The OPTIC Study: A randomized trial. JAMA, 295, 165–171.

9. Sanders, G.D., Hlatky, M.A., Owens, D.K., (2005). Cost-effectiveness of implantable cardioverter-defibrillators. New England Journal of Medicine, 353, 1471–1480.

10. Ver Donck, L., Borgers, M., Verdonck, F., (1993). Inhibition of sodium and calcium overload pathology in the myocardium: A new cytoprotective principle. Cardiovascular Research, 27, 349–357.

11. Janvier, N.C., Boyett, M.R., (1996). The role of Na-Ca exchange current in the cardiac action potential. Cardiovascular Research, 32, 69–84.

12. Blaustein, M.P., Lederer, W.J., (1999). Sodium/calcium exchange: Its physiological implications. Physiological Reviews, 79, 763–854.

13. Egger, M., Niggli, E., (1999). Regulatory function of Na-Ca exchange in the heart: Milestones and outlook. Journal of Membrane Biology, 168, 107–130.

14. Ferrier, G.R., Saunders, J.H., Mendez, C., (1973). A cellular mechanism for the generation of ventricular arrhythmias by acetylstrophanthidin. Circulation Research, 32, 600–609.

15. Eisner, D.A., Trafford, A.W., Diaz, M.E., Overend, C.L., O'Neill, S.C., (1998). The control of Ca release from the cardiac sarcoplasmic reticulum: Regulation versus autoregulation. Cardiovascular Research, 38, 589–604.

16. Weber, C.R., Ginsburg, K.S., Bers, D.M., (2003). Cardiac submembrane [Na +] transients sensed by Na + -Ca2 + exchange current. Circulation Research, 92, 950–952.

17. Rocchetti, M., Besana, A., Gurrola, G.B., Possani, L.D., Zaza, A., (2001). Rate dependency of delayed rectifier currents during the guinea-pig ventricular action potential. Journal of Physiology, 534, 721–732.

18. Weber, C.R., Piacentino, V., Ginsburg, K.S., Houser, S.R., Bers, D.M., (2002). Na(+)-Ca(2 +) exchange current and submembrane [Ca(2 +)] during the cardiac action potential. Circulation Research, 90, 182–189.

19. Egan, T.M., Noble, D., Noble, S.J., Powell, T., Spindler, A.J., Twist, V.W., (1989). Sodium-calcium exchange during the action potential in guinea-pig ventricular cells. Journal of Physiology, 411, 639–661.

20. Armoundas, A.A., Hobai, I.A., Tomaselli, G.F., Winslow, R.L., O'Rourke, B., (2003). Role of sodium-calcium exchanger in modulating the action potential of ventricular myocytes from normal and failing hearts. Circulation Research, 93, 46–53.

21. Volders, P.G., Vos, M.A., Szabo, B., Sipido, K.R., de Groot, S.H., Gorgels, A.P., Wellens, H.J., Lazzara, R., (2000). Progress in the understanding of cardiac early afterdepolarizations and torsades de pointes: Time to revise current concepts. Cardiovascular Research, 46, 376–392.

22. Antoons, G., Sipido, K.R., (2008). Targeting calcium handling in arrhythmias. Europace, 10, 1364–1369.

23. Rodriguez-Sinovas, A., Abdallah, Y., Piper, H.M., Garcia-Dorado, D., (2007). Reperfusion injury as a therapeutic challenge in patients with acute myocardial infarction. Heart Failure Reviews, 12, 207–216.

24. Napolitano, C., Priori, S.G., (2007). Diagnosis and treatment of catecholaminergic polymorphic ventricular tachycardia. Heart Rhythm, 4, 675–678.

25. Liu, N., Priori, S.G., (2008). Disruption of calcium homeostasis and arrhythmogenesis induced by mutations in the cardiac ryanodine receptor and calsequestrin. Cardiovascular Research, 77, 293–301.

26. Clancy, C.E., Kass, R.S., (2005). Inherited and acquired vulnerability to ventricular arrhythmias: cardiac Na + and K + channels. Physiology Reviews, 85, 33–47.

27. Zaza, A., Belardinelli, L., Shryock, J.C., (2008). Pathophysiology and pharmacology of the cardiac "late sodium current". Pharmacology Therapeutics, 119, 326–339.

28. Pogwizd, S.M., McKenzie, J.P., Cain, M.E., (1998). Mechanisms underlying spontaneous and induced ventricular arrhythmias in patients with idiopathic dilated cardiomyopathy. Circulation, 98, 2404–2414.

29. Beuckelmann, D.J., Nabauer, M., Erdmann, E., (1992). Intracellular calcium handling in isolated ventricular myocytes from patients with terminal heart failure. Circulation, 85, 1046–1055.

30. Piacentino, V. III, Weber, C.R., Chen, X., Weisser-Thomas, J., Margulies, K.B., Bers, D.M., Houser, S.R., (2003). Cellular basis of abnormal calcium transients of failing human ventricular myocytes. Circulation Research, 92, 651–658.

31. Veldkamp, M.W., Verkerk, A.O., van Ginneken, A.C., Baartscheer, A., Schumacher, C., de Jonge, N., de Bakker, J.M., Opthof, T., (2001). Norepinephrine induces action potential prolongation and early afterdepolarizations in ventricular myocytes isolated from human end-stage failing hearts. European Heart Journal, 22, 955–963.

32. Verkerk, A.O., Veldkamp, M.W., Baartscheer, A., Schumacher, C.A., Klopping, C., van Ginneken, A.C., Ravesloot, J.H., (2001). Ionic mechanism of delayed afterdepolarizations in ventricular cells isolated from human end-stage failing hearts. Circulation, 104, 2728–2733.

33. Pogwizd, S.M., Schlotthauer, K., Li, L., Yuan, W., Bers, D.M., (2001). Arrhythmogenesis and contractile dysfunction in heart failure: Roles of sodium-calcium exchange, inward rectifier potassium current, and residual ß-adrenergic responsiveness. Circulation Research, 88, 1159–1167.

34. Fauconnier, J., Lacampagne, A., Rauzier, J.M., Vassort, G., Richard, S., (2005). Ca2 + -dependent reduction of IK1 in rat ventricular cells: A novel paradigm for arrhythmia in heart failure? Cardiovascular Research, 68, 204–212.

35. Marx, S.O., Reiken, S., Hisamatsu, Y., Jayaraman, T., Burkhoff, D., Rosemblit, N., Marks, A.R., (2000). PKA phosphorylation dissociates FKBP12.6 from the calcium release channel (ryanodine receptor): defective regulation in failing hearts. Cell, 101, 365–376.

36. Tomaselli, G.F., Beuckelmann, D.J., Calkins, H.G., Berger, R.D., Kessler, P.D., Lawrence, J.H., Kass, D., Feldman, A.M., Marban, E., (1994). Sudden cardiac death in heart failure. The role of abnormal repolarization. Circulation, 90, 2534–2539.

37. Nattel, S., Maguy, A., Le Bouter, S., Yeh, Y.H., (2007). Arrhythmogenic ion-channel remodeling in the heart: Heart failure, myocardial infarction, and atrial fibrillation. Physiology Reviews, 87, 425–456.

38. Iwamoto, T., Watano, T., Shigekawa, M., (1996). A novel isothiourea derivative selectively inhibits the reverse mode of Na^+/Ca^{2+} exchange in cells expressing NCX1. Journal of Biological Chemistry, 271, 22391–22397.

39. Kimura, J., Watano, T., Kawahara, M., Sakai, E., Yatabe, J., (1999). Direction-independent block of bi-directional Na^+/Ca^{2+} exchange current by KB-R7943 in guinea-pig cardiac myocytes. Britsh Journal of Pharmacology, 128, 969–974.

40. Lee, C., Visen, N.S., Dhalla, N.S., Le, H.D., Isaac, M., Choptiany, P., Gross, G., Omelchenko, A., Matsuda, T., Baba, A., et al. (2004). Inhibitory profile of SEA0400 [2-[4-[(2,5-difluorophenyl)methoxy]phenoxy]-5-ethoxyaniline] assessed on the cardiac $Na+-Ca2+$ exchanger, NCX1.1. J Pharmacol Exp Ther, 311, 748–757.

41. Tanaka, H., Nishimaru, K., Aikawa, T., Hirayama, W., Tanaka, Y., Shigenobu, K., (2002). Effect of SEA0400, a novel inhibitor of sodium-calcium exchanger, on myocardial ionic currents. British Journal of Pharmacology, 135, 1096–1100.

42. Farkas, A.S., Acsai, K., Nagy, N., Toth, A., Fulop, F., Seprenyi, G., Birinyi, P., Nanasi, P.P., Forster, T., Csanady, M., Papp, et al. (2008). $Na(+)/Ca(2+)$ exchanger inhibition exerts a positive inotropic effect in the rat heart, but fails to influence the contractility of the rabbit heart. British Journal of Pharmacology, 154, 93–104.

43. Iwamoto, T., (2007). $Na+/Ca2+$ exchange as a drug target-insights from molecular pharmacology and genetic engineering. Sodium-calcium exchange and the plasma membrane $Ca2+$-Atpase in cell function. Fifth International Conference, 1099, 516–528.

44. Birinyi, P., Acsai, K., Banyasz, T., Toth, A., Horvath, B., Virag, L., Szentandrassy, N., Magyar, J., Varro, A., Fulop, F., et al. (2005). Effects of SEA0400 and KB-R7943 on Na^+/Ca^{2+} exchange current and L-type Ca^{2+} current in canine ventricular cardiomyocytes. Naunyn Schmiedebergs Archives of Pharmacology, 372, 63–70.

45. Niu, C.F., Watanabe, Y., Ono, K., Iwamoto, T., Yamashita, K., Satoh, H., Urushida, T., Hayashi, H., Kimura, J., (2007). Characterization of SN-6, a novel $Na+/Ca2+$ exchange inhibitor in guinea pig cardiac ventricular myocytes. European Journal of Pharmacology, 573, 161–169.

46. Annunziato, L., Pignataro, G., Di Renzo, G.F., (2004). Pharmacology of brain $Na+/Ca2+$ exchanger: From molecular biology to therapeutic perspectives. Pharmacological Reviews, 56, 633–654.

47. Miyamoto, S., Zhu, B.M., Kamiya, K., Nagasawa, Y., Hashimoto, K., (2002). KB-R7943, a $Na+/Ca2+$ exchange inhibitor, does not suppress ischemia/reperfusion arrhythmias nor digitalis arrhythmias in dogs. Japan Journal of Pharmacology, 90, 229–235.

48. Nagasawa, Y., Zhu, B.M., Chen, J., Kamiya, K., Miyamoto, S., Hashimoto, K., (2005). Effects of SEA0400, a $Na+/Ca2+$ exchange inhibitor, on ventricular arrhythmias in the *in vivo* dogs. European Journal of Pharmacology, 506, 249–255.

49. Watano, T., Harada, Y., Harada, K., Nishimura, N., (1999). Effect of Na$^+$/Ca^{2+} exchange inhibitor, KB-R7943 on ouabain-induced arrhythmias in guinea-pigs. British Journal of Pharmacology, 127, 1846–1850.

50. Shpak, B., Gofman, Y., Shpak, C., Hiller, R., Boyman, L., Khananshvili, D., (2006). Effects of purified endogenous inhibitor of the Na+/Ca2+ exchanger on ouabain-induced arrhythmias in the atria and ventricle strips of guinea pig. European Journal of Pharmacology, 553, 196–204.

51. Wongcharoen, W., Chen, Y.C., Chen, Y.J., Chang, C.M., Yeh, H.I., Lin, C.I., Chen, S.A., (2006). Effects of a Na+/Ca2+ exchanger inhibitor on pulmonary vein electrical activity and ouabain-induced arrhythmogenicity. Cardiovascular Research, 70, 497–508.

52. Tanaka, H., Shimada, H., Namekata, I., Kawanishi, T., Iida-Tanaka, N., Shigenobu, K., (2007). Involvement of the Na+/Ca2+ exchanger in ouabain-induced inotropy and arrhythmogenesis in guinea-pig myocardium as revealed by SEA0400. Journal of Pharmacological Sciences, 103, 241–246.

53. Satoh, H., Ginsburg, K.S., Qing, K., Terada, H., Hayashi, H., Bers, D.M., (2000). KB-R7943 block of Ca^{2+} influx via Na$^+$/Ca^{2+} exchange does not alter twitches or glycoside inotropy but prevents Ca^{2+} overload in rat ventricular myocytes. Circulation, 101, 1441–1446.

54. Satoh, H., Mukai, M., Urushida, T., Katoh, H., Terada, H., Hayashi, H., (2003). Importance of Ca2+ influx by Na+/Ca2+ exchange under normal and sodium-loaded conditions in mammalian ventricles. Molecular and Cellular Biochemistry, 242, 11–17.

55. Nagy, Z.A., Virag, L., Toth, A., Biliczki, P., Acsai, K., Banyasz, T., Nanasi, P., Papp, J.G., Varro, A., (2004). Selective inhibition of sodium-calcium exchanger by SEA-0400 decreases early and delayed afterdepolarization in canine heart. British Journal of Pharmacology, 143, 827–831.

56. Takahashi, K., Takahashi, T., Suzuki, T., Onishi, M., Tanaka, Y., Hamano-Takahashi, A., Ota, T., Kameo, K., Matsuda, T., Baba, A., (2003). Protective effects of SEA0400, a novel and selective inhibitor of the Na+/Ca2+ exchanger, on myocardial ischemia-reperfusion injuries. European Journal of Pharmacology, 458, 155–162.

57. Lu, H.R., Yang, P., Remeysen, P., Saels, A., Dai, D.Z., De Clerck, F., (1999). Ischemia/reperfusion-induced arrhythmias in anaesthetized rats: a role of Na+ and Ca2+ influx. European Journal of Pharmacology, 365, 233–239.

58. Elias, C.L., Lukas, A., Shurraw, S., Scott, J., Omelchenko, A., Gross, G.J., Hnatowich, M., Hryshko, L.V., (2001). Inhibition of Na+/Ca2+ exchange by KB-R7943: Transport mode selectivity and antiarrhythmic consequences. American Journal of Physiology Heart Circulation Physiology, 281, H1334–H1345.

59. Woodcock, E.A., Arthur, J.F., Harrison, S.N., Gao, X.M., Du, X.J., (2001). Reperfusion-induced Ins(1,4,5)P-3 generation and arrhythmogenesis require activation of the Na+/Ca2+ exchanger. Journal of Molecular and Cellular Cardiology, 33, 1861–1869.

60. Yamamura, K., Tani, M., Hasegawa, H., Gen, W., (2001). Very low dose of the Na(+)/Ca(2+) exchange inhibitor, KB-R7943, protects ischemic reperfused aged Fischer 344 rat hearts: Considerable strain difference in the sensitivity to KB-R7943. Cardiovascular Research, 52, 397–406.

61. Feng, N.C., Satoh, H., Urushida, T., Katoh, H., Terada, H., Watanabe, Y., Hayashi, H., (2006). A selective inhibitor of Na+/Ca2+ exchanger, SEA0400, preserves cardiac function and high-energy phosphates against ischemia/reperfusion injury. Journal of Cardiovascular Pharmacology, 47, 263–270.

62. Schafer, C., Ladilov, Y., Inserte, J., Schafer, M., Haffner, S., Garcia-Dorado, D., Piper, H.M., (2001). Role of the reverse mode of the Na + /Ca2 + exchanger in reoxygenation-induced cardiomyocyte injury. Cardiovascular Research, 51, 241–250.

63. Mukai, M., Terada, H., Sugiyama, S., Satoh, H., Hayashi, H., (2000). Effects of a selective inhibitor of Na + /Ca2 + exchange, KB-R7943, on reoxygenation-induced injuries in guinea pig papillary muscles. Journal of Cardiovascular Pharmacology, 35, 121–128.

64. MacDonald, A.C., Howlett, S.E., (2008). Differential effects of the sodium calcium exchange inhibitor, KB-R7943, on ischemia and reperfusion injury in isolated guinea pig ventricular myocytes. European Journal of Pharmacology, 580, 214–223.

65. Amran, M.S., Hashimoto, K., Homma, N., (2004). Effects of sodium-calcium exchange inhibitors, KB-R7943 and SEA0400, on aconitine-induced arrhythmias in guinea pigs in vivo, in vitro, and in computer simulation studies. Journal of Pharmacological and Experimental Therapeutics, 310, 83–89.

66. Milberg, P., Pott, C., Fink, M., Frommeyer, G., Matsuda, T., Baba, A., Osada, N., Breithardt, G., Noble, D., Eckardt, L., (2008). Inhibition of the Na + /Ca2 + exchanger suppresses torsades de pointes in an intact heart model of long QT syndrome-2 and long QT syndrome-3. Heart Rhythm, 5, 1444–1452.

67. Miyata, A., Zipes, D.P., Hall, S., Rubart, M., (2002). Kb-R7943 prevents acute, atrial fibrillation-induced shortening of atrial refractoriness in anesthetized dogs. Circulation, 106, 1410–1419.

68. Shinada, T., Hirayama, Y., Maruyama, M., Ohara, T., Yashima, M., Kobayashi, Y., Atarashi, H., Takano, T., (2005). Inhibition of the reverse mode of the Na + /Ca2 + exchange by KB-R7943 augments arrhythmogenicity in the canine heart during rapid heart rates. Journal of Electrocardiology, 38, 218–225.

69. Fujiwara, K., Tanaka, H., Mani, H., Nakagami, T., Takamatsu, T., (2008). Burst emergence of intracellular Ca2 + waves evokes arrhythmogenic oscillatory depolarization via the Na + -Ca2 + exchanger: Simultaneous confocal recording of membrane potential and intracellular Ca2 + in the heart. Circulation Research, 103, 509–518.

70. Carmeliet, E., (1999). Cardiac ionic currents and acute ischemia: From channels to arrhythmias. Physiological Reviews, 79, 917–1017.

71. Ladilov, Y., Haffner, S., Balser-Schafer, C., Maxeiner, H., Piper, H.M., (1999). Cardio-protective effects of KB-R7943: A novel inhibitor of the reverse mode of Na + /Ca2 + exchanger. American Journal of Physiology, 276, H1868–H1876.

72. Imahashi, K., Pott, C., Goldhaber, J.I., Steenbergen, C., Philipson, K.D., Murphy, E., (2005). Cardiac-specific ablation of the Na^+-Ca^{2+} exchanger confers protection against ischemia/reperfusion injury. Circulation Research, 97, 916–921.

73. Sipido, K.R., Callewaert, G., Carmeliet, E., (1995). Inhibition and rapid recovery of I_{Ca} during calcium release from the sarcoplasmic reticulum in guinea-pig ventricular myocytes. Circulation Research, 76, 102–109.

74. Henderson, S.A., Goldhaber, J.I., So, J.M., Han, T., Motter, C., Ngo, A., Chantawansri, C., Ritter, M.R., Friedlander, M., Nicoll, D.A., et al. (2004). Functional adult myocardium in the absence of Na^+-Ca^{2+} exchange: Cardiac-specific knockout of NCX1. Circulation Research, 95, 604–611.

75. Pott, C., Philipson, K.D., Goldhaber, J.I., (2005). Excitation-contraction coupling in Na^+-Ca^{2+} exchanger knockout mice: Reduced transsarcolemmal Ca^{2+} flux. Circulation Research, 97, 1288–1295.

76. Hobai, I.A., Maack, C., O'Rourke, B., (2004). Partial inhibition of sodium/calcium exchange restores cellular calcium handling in canine heart failure. Circulation Research, 95, 292–299.

77. Tanaka, H., Namekata, I., Takeda, K., Kazama, A., Shimizu, Y., Moriwaki, R., Hirayama, W., Sato, A., Kawanishi, T., Shigenobu, K., (2005). Unique excitation-contraction characteristics of mouse myocardium as revealed by SEA0400, a specific inhibitor of Na$^+$-Ca^{2+} exchanger. Naunyn Schmiedebergs Archives of Pharmacology, 371, 526–534.

78. Birinyi, P., Toth, A., Jona, I., Acsai, K., Almassy, J., Nagy, N., Prorok, J., Gherasim, I., Papp, Z., Hertelendi, Z., et al. (2008). The Na + /Ca2 + exchange blocker SEA0400 fails to enhance cytosolic Ca2 + transient and contractility in canine ventricular cardiomyocytes. Cardiovascular Research, 78, 476–484.

79. Ozdemir, S., Bito, V., Holemans, P., Vinet, L., Mercadier, J.J., Varro, A., Sipido, K.R., (2008). Pharmacological inhibition of na/ca exchange results in increased cellular Ca2 + load attributable to the predominance of forward mode block. Circulation Research, 102, 1398–1405.

80. Roy, D., Talajic, M., Dorian, P., Connolly, S., Eisenberg, M.J., Green, M., Kus, T., Lambert, J., Dubuc, M., Gagne, P., et al. (2000). Amiodarone to prevent recurrence of atrial fibrillation. Canadian Trial of Atrial Fibrillation Investigators. New England Journal of Medicine, 342, 913–920.

81. Singh, B.N., Connolly, S.J., Crijns, H.J., Roy, D., Kowey, P.R., Capucci, A., Radzik, D., Aliot, E.M., Hohnloser, S.H., (2007). Dronedarone for maintenance of sinus rhythm in atrial fibrillation or flutter. New England Journal of Medicine, 357, 987–999.

82. Lehnart, S.E., Wehrens, X.H., Laitinen, P.J., Reiken, S.R., Deng, S.X., Cheng, Z., Landry, D.W., Kontula, K., Swan, H., Marks, A.R., (2004). Sudden death in familial polymorphic ventricular tachycardia associated with calcium release channel (ryanodine receptor) leak. Circulation, 109, 3208–3214.

83. O'Neill, S.C., Miller, L., Hinch, R., Eisner, D.A., (2004). Interplay between SERCA and sarcolemmal Ca2 + efflux pathways controls spontaneous release of Ca2 + from the sarcoplasmic reticulum in rat ventricular myocytes. Journal of Physiology, 559, 121–128.

CHAPTER 12

Calcium/Calmodulin-Dependent Protein Kinase II (CaMKII)—Modulation of Ion Currents and Potential Role for Arrhythmias

DR. LARS S. MAIER

12.1 INTRODUCTION

The Ca^{2+}/calmodulin-dependent protein kinase II (CaMKII), which was identified more than 20 years ago, is the CaMK isoform predominantly found in the heart. Cardiac myocytes signaling during excitation-contraction coupling (ECC) is described by the increase in intracellular Ca^{2+} concentration ($[Ca^{2+}]_i$) during an action potential (AP). In consequence, CaMKII is activated, thereby phosphorylating several important Ca^{2+}-handling proteins with multiple functional consequences for cardiac myocytes. CaMKII activity and expression are reported to be increased in cardiac hypertrophy, in human heart failure, as well as in many animal models for cardiac diseases. Specific CaMKII overexpression in the hearts of animals and in isolated myocytes can exert distinct and novel effects on ECC.

The cardiac AP is regulated by the meticulous interplay of several sarcolemmal ion channels, of which Ca^{2+}, Na^+, and K^+ channels play an outstanding role. Although tiny alterations in channel function may result in little altered ion fluxes, this can have a great impact on AP characteristics and, thus, ECC. Increases in AP duration resulting in instability of the membrane potential at positive voltages can lead to early afterdepolarizations (EADs), but delayed afterdepolarizations (DADs) *in vitro* may serve as triggers for atrial or ventricular tachyarrhythmias even *in vivo*. During the last decade, several novel arrhythmic mechanisms for both triggered activity as well as reentry have been identified. Some of them are even associated with novel clinical entities of arrhythmia syndromes [e.g., Brugada syndrome and long QT syndrome

Novel Therapeutic Targets for Antiarrhythmic Drugs, Edited by George Edward Billman
Copyright © 2010 John Wiley & Sons, Inc.

(LQTS)]. Central to many of these mechanisms is an altered sarcolemmal Na^+ channel function, but how Na^+ channel activation and inactivation are regulated is still not completely understood. Previously, calmodulin (CaM) was shown to modulate cardiac Na^+ channels *in vitro*; however, whether Na^+ channels are regulated by CaMKII was unknown until recently. In contrast, it is well known that sarcolemmal L-type Ca^{2+} channels (LTCC) are regulated by several intracellular ions and proteins, such as Ca^{2+} itself, CaM, and CaMKII.

In this chapter, important aspects of the role of CaMKII in ECC and its role for arrhythmias are summarized with an emphasis on recent novel findings.

12.2   EVOLVING ROLE OF Ca^{2+}/CaMKII IN THE HEART

Intracellular Ca^{2+} ions translate electrical signals into mechanical activity of the heart leading to the shortening of the myocytes and the contraction of the whole heart known as ECC. Various transporters, pumps, and ion channels [sarcolemmal as well as in the sarcoplasmic reticulum (SR)] are involved in these intracellular Ca^{2+} fluxes. Several of these Ca^{2+} handling proteins, but also additional Ca^{2+}-activated intracellular proteins, contribute to the fine tuning of ECC.

One of the many Ca^{2+}-activated intracellular proteins is the second messenger CaMK, of which CaMKII is the predominant cardiac isoform [1–3]. After activation, CaMKII phosphorylates several Ca^{2+}-handling proteins, including SR Ca^{2+} release channels or ryanodine receptors (RyR2), phospholamban (PLB), and LTCC with multiple functional consequences [4, 5]. Novel data suggest that also sarcolemmal Na^+ and K^+ channels are regulated by CaMKII, thus influencing ECC via electrophysiological effects on AP characteristics.

About 10 years ago, it was described for the first time that CaMKII expression and activity are increased in the myocardium of patients with end-stage heart failure [6, 7]. Since then, and because of the relevance for pathophysiological conditions such as cardiac hypertrophy and heart failure, many original articles and reviews have been published describing the role of CaMKII for cardiac disease with a recent special review focus on "Calmodulin and Ca^{2+}/calmodulin kinases in the heart—Physiology and pathophysiology" in *Cardiovascular Research* [8–13]. In addition, a transatlantic network was established to understand CaMKII regulation, defining the role of "upstream" CaMKII effectors and "downstream" CaMKII molecular targets with the goal of developing a novel generation of highly specific therapies for heart failure and arrhythmias funded by the Leduqc Foundation (www.camk2.org).

12.3   ACTIVATION OF CaMKII

CaMKII is a serine/threonine protein kinase that phosphorylates many intracellular proteins in response to elevated $[Ca^{2+}]_i$ on a beat-to-beat basis [1–3, 5]. There are four different CaMKII genes (α, β, γ, and δ), with the δ isoform being predominant in the heart [3, 4, 8]. In addition, distinct splice variants have different subcellular

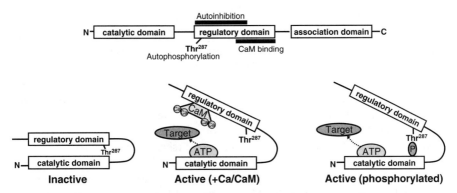

Figure 12.1. Domain layout of CaMKII. The three main domains of the CaMKII monomer are indicated in cartoon and linear layout (top). Lower panels show activation of CaMKII by Ca/CaM binding to the regulatory domain and subsequent autophosphorylation at Thr287 (or Thr-286 depending of the specific isoform). Ca/CaM binding is sufficient to activate CaMKII so the active site (ATP) can interact with phosphorylation target proteins. Subsequent autophosphorylation makes CaMKII active (20–80%) even after Ca/CaM dissociates (adapted from ref. 4).

localizations, with δ_B being compartmentalized to the nucleus and with δ_C being the cytosolic isoform [14].

The multimeric CaMKII holoenzyme consists of homomultimers or heteromultimers of a few (approximately 6–12) kinase subunits forming a wheel-like structure [3–5]. Each CaMKII monomer contains an aminoterminal catalytic domain, a regulatory domain with partially overlapping autoinhibitory and CaM binding regions, and a carboxyterminal association domain responsible for oligomerization [3, 4]. The autoinhibitory region close to the active site of the catalytic domain sterically blocks access to substrates (see Figure 12.1). When $[Ca^{2+}]_i$ increases (i.e., during systole), intracellular CaM binds its four Ca^{2+} ions [15]. The Ca^{2+}/CaM complex attaches to the regulatory domain of CaMKII and displaces the autoinhibitory domain on CaMKII, thereby activating the enzyme (half maximal activation at $[Ca^{2+}]_i$ of ~500–1000 nM). In addition, CaMKII can lock itself into an activated state after autophosphorylation of Thr-287 (or Thr-286, depending of the specific isoform) on the autoinhibitory segment [3, 8]. Autophosphorylation is not essential for CaMKII activity, but it does have important consequences, i.e., by increasing the affinity of the Ca^{2+}/CaM-kinase complex, thereby trapping Ca^{2+}/CaM on the autophosphorylated subunit [16]. Even when $[Ca^{2+}]_i$ declines to resting levels during diastole (i.e., about 100 nM), CaM is still trapped for several seconds. As a result, the kinase retains close to fully active as long as CaM is trapped, regardless of the $[Ca^{2+}]_i$ level. Interestingly, autophosphorylation significantly disrupts autoinhibition, such that even after Ca^{2+}/CaM has dissociated from the autonomous state, CaMKII remains partially active (about 20–80%) [17–19]. For complete inactivation to occur, autophosphorylated CaMKII must be dephosphorylated by protein phosphatases (e.g., PP1, PP2A, and PP2C) [8].

In contrast to the mode of CaMKII activation described above, it has been shown recently that CaMKII may be also activate Ca^{2+} independently by methionine oxidation [20]. These authors showed that CaMKII is activated by angiotensin-II–induced oxidation, leading to apoptosis in cardiomyocytes both *in vitro* and *in vivo*. CaMKII oxidation is reversed by methionine sulfoxide reductase A (MsrA) whereas MsrA-/- mice show exaggerated CaMKII oxidation and myocardial apoptosis, impaired cardiac function, and increased mortality after myocardial infarction [20]. However, it is still unclear under what exact pathophysiological conditions CaMKII activity increases, because we recently showed in a preliminary study that CaMKII activity indeed increases under conditions of increased afterload (banding mouse model) but not at all when preload was increased (shunt mouse model [21]).

Various CaMKII inhibitors were used in the past in myocytes, including the organic inhibitors KN-62 and KN-93 (whereas KN-92 is the inactive analogue of KN-93), which competitively inhibit CaM binding to CaMKII [4]. Of note, some of these agents seem to have direct effects on some ion channel (e.g., LTCC) [22], which seem independent of CaMKII actions [23, 24]. In contrast, the peptide inhibitors auto-camtide-2 related inhibitory peptide (AIP, a nonphosphorylatable, competitive substrate for autophosphorylation of CaMKII), and autocamtide-2 inhibitory peptide (AC3-I) are not thought to affect ion channels [25, 26].

12.4   ROLE OF CaMKII IN ECC

Without a doubt, Ca^{2+} clearly is the central regulator of ECC (see Figure 12.2). During a cardiac AP, Ca^{2+} enters the cell mainly through voltage-dependent LTCC, triggering subsequent Ca^{2+} release from the SR via RyR2, which is a process termed Ca^{2+} induced Ca^{2+}-release [27]. The resulting increase in $[Ca^{2+}]_i$ causes Ca^{2+} binding to troponin C, which activates the myofilaments leading to contraction during systole. Diastolic relaxation occurs when Ca^{2+} dissociates from troponin C and is removed from the cytoplasm. The SR Ca^{2+}-ATPase (SERCA2a) and the sarcolemmal Na^+/Ca^{2+}-exchanger (NCX) are the main mechanisms for Ca^{2+} removal in the heart [28].

About 25 LTCC proteins and 100 RyR2 proteins are colocalized forming a local SR Ca^{2+} release unit called a junction or couplon [29]. This local functional unit can be monitored by confocal microscopy measuring elementary Ca^{2+} release events from the SR (so-called Ca^{2+} sparks) occurring spontaneously in resting cardiac myocytes and summating during normal Ca^{2+} transients in ECC. Of pathophysiological relevance is a CaMKII-dependent high-frequency Ca^{2+} sparks responsible for the Ca^{2+} leak from the SR and decreased SR Ca^{2+} load when CaMKII activity is increased [9]. This is interesting because under normal physiological conditions, Ca^{2+} spark frequency depends critically on SR Ca^{2+} load and follows a linear correlation (load-leak relation) [30].

There is convincing evidence that fluctuations in $[Ca^{2+}]_i$ modify the activity of ion channels and transporters via CaMKII [4]. The integrative responses of these downstream messengers of Ca^{2+} giving a feedback on the ion channels and transporters that regulate $[Ca^{2+}]_i$ serve to tune ECC finely. As an example, CaMKII can modulate ECC by phosphorylating several important Ca^{2+}-handling proteins in the heart in response to Ca^{2+} signals, including RyR2, PLB, and LTCC with significant functional consequences [4, 31–34]. These proteins are involved in Ca^{2+}

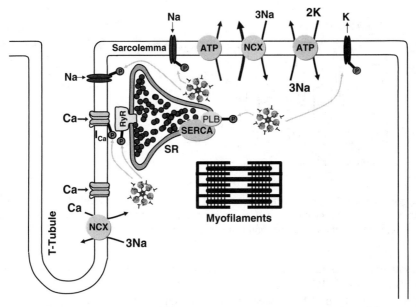

Figure 12.2. Effects of CaMKIIδ_C on ECC. CaMKII phosphorylates several Ca^{2+}-handling proteins, including PLB, SR Ca^{2+} release channels (RyR), and L-type Ca^{2+} channels responsible for Ca^{2+} influx (I_{Ca}). In addition, Na^+ channels and K^+ channels are also regulated by CaMKII. During the AP, Ca^{2+} enters the cell via L-type Ca^{2+} channels and reverse-mode of the NCX (left), thereby triggering Ca^{2+} release through RyR from the SR (filled with Ca^{2+}, red dots). This Ca^{2+} then activates the myofilaments during systole leading to contraction. During diastole, Ca^{2+} is taken up back into the SR by the SERCA and is transported outside the cells mainly by NCX, leading to relaxation. PLB inhibits SERCA when PLB is dephosphorylated. (adapted from ref. 9).

influx, SR Ca^{2+} release, and SR Ca^{2+} uptake with their specific role in ECC being discussed below. In addition, novel findings of CaMKII-dependent regulation of cardiac Na^+ and K^+ channels are presented in the subsequent paragraphs.

12.4.1 Ca^{2+} Influx and I_{Ca} Facilitation

Voltage-gated LTCC ($Ca_v1.2$) are modulated by CaMKII, thereby increasing Ca^{2+} current (I_{Ca}). This is most clearly viewed as a positive staircase of I_{Ca} with repeated depolarizations, a process termed Ca^{2+}-dependent I_{Ca} facilitation [35, 36]. Several groups demonstrated that Ca^{2+}-dependent I_{Ca} facilitation is mediated by CaMKII-dependent processes [37–40]. CaMKII is believed to tether to the pore forming α_{1C} subunit of the LTCC and to phosphorylate the α_{1C} subunit at both amino and carboxyl tails [41]. However, it was recently reported that CaMKII also seems to phosphorylate a site on the β_{2a}-subunit (Thr-498), which may be involved in I_{Ca} facilitation [12, 42]. At the single-channel level, this CaMKII-dependent I_{Ca} facilitation is manifested as longer single channel openings [43]. By overexpressing CaMKIIδ_C in transgenic mouse myocytes as well as in adenovirus-mediated rabbit myocytes, I_{Ca} amplitude

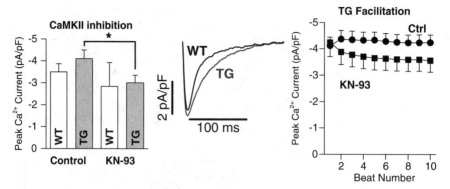

Figure 12.3. CaMKII-dependent regulation of Ca^{2+} current. Transgenic CaMKIIδ_C overexpression resulted in an increase in Ca^{2+} current, which could be reversed using KN-93 (left). Ca^{2+} current facilitation can be inhibited using KN-93 (right; adapted from ref. 44).

was increased and inactivation was slowed [44, 45]. I_{Ca} amplitude could be reduced back to control levels by blocking CaMKII (see Figure 12.3). Interestingly, enhanced open probability of LTCC because of increased CaMKII activity contributes to afterdepolarizations and to the increased propensity for arrhythmias in CaMKIV transgenic mice that also showed increased CaMKII activity [46].

In human heart failure where CaMKII expression and activity was reported to be increased [6, 7], ventricular myocytes have LTCC with enhanced opening probability [47], which may contribute to cardiac arrhythmias in heart failure. In line with this, it was recently shown that Timothy syndrome is a disease of excessive cellular Ca^{2+} entry and life-threatening arrhythmias caused by a mutation in the primary cardiac LTCC with increased CaMKII activity and a proarrhythmic phenotype that included AP prolongation, increased I_{Ca} facilitation, and afterdepolarizations. Intracellular dialysis of a CaMKII inhibitory peptide reversed increases in I_{Ca} facilitation, normalized the AP, and prevented afterdepolarizations [48].

12.4.2 SR Ca^{2+} Release and SR Ca Leak

RyR2 activity is also affected by CaMKII. Initially, it was reported that CaMKII phosphorylates RyR2 at one site (i.e., Ser-2809) activating SR Ca^{2+} release [31]. However, others showed that there may be at least four additional CaMKII phosphorylation sites on RyR2 [49]. The specific effects of CaMKII on RyR2 remained controversial. CaMKII either increased or decreased RyR2 open probability [31, 32, 50]. In intact cardiac myocytes, endogenous CaMKII increased the amount of SR Ca^{2+} release for a given SR Ca^{2+} content and I_{Ca} trigger in an elegant *in vivo* study [23]. This conclusion is also consistent with observations that protein phosphatases (PP1 and PP2A) can reduce RyR2 activity for a given I_{Ca} and SR Ca^{2+} load, and conversely that phosphatase inhibitors enhance it [51]. However, other studies found opposite results suggesting that CaMKII negatively regulates SR Ca^{2+} release [52, 53]. Unfortunately, in the previous report, no SR Ca^{2+} content was measured, whereas in the latter study species differences may have contributed to the divergent results.

New evidence was provided in isolated cardiomyocytes showing that CaMKII indeed is directly associated with RyR2: Transgenic CaMKIIδ_C overexpression increases fractional SR Ca^{2+} release during ECC and spontaneous SR Ca^{2+} release (i.e., Ca^{2+} spark frequency) for a given SR Ca^{2+} load ([44, 54–56]; see Figure 12.4). These results were confirmed by acute CaMKIIδ_C overexpression through adenovirus-mediated gene transfer in rabbit myocytes and direct application of pre-activated CaMKII to permeabilized mouse myocytes [45, 57]. Similarly, in rabbit hearts the

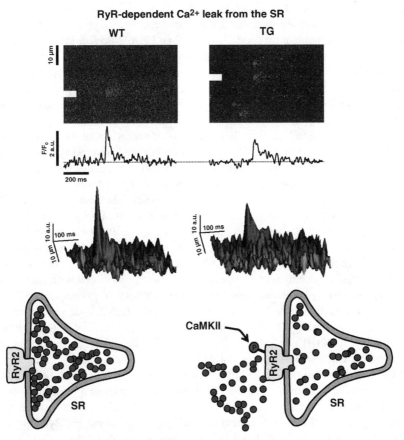

Figure 12.4. Increased SR Ca^{2+} leak caused by increased elementary SR Ca^{2+} release events (Ca^{2+} sparks). Original confocal images showing significantly increased Ca^{2+} spark frequency in CaMKIIδ_C transgenic mouse myocytes leading to a CaMKII-dependent diastolic SR Ca^{2+} leak. This leak is significantly (about four times) higher in TG than in WT. In contrast, CaMKII inhibition using KN-93 decreases Ca spark frequency back to control levels. An explanation for this increased Ca spark frequency most likely is the CaMKII-dependent hyperphosphorylation of SR Ca^{2+} release channels (RyR2; adapted from ref. 44). See color insert.

CaMKII peptide inhibitor AIP depresses Ca^{2+} spark frequency and ryanodine binding to RyR2, indicating that CaMKII activates RyR2 [56]. It was also shown that CaMKII-dependent RyR2 phosphorylation increases RyR2 open probability using single-channel measurements and that CaMKII-dependent RyR2 phosphorylation may be at Ser-2815, rather than Ser-2809 [55]. Whether CaMKII phosphorylates RyR2 at Ser-2809 is now controversial [as is the role of protein kinase A (PKA)-dependent phosphorylation and subsequent FKBP12.6 dissociation] [58]. However, in a series of recent reports, the role of PKA-dependent RyR2 phosphorylation was challenged. Curran et al. [59] showed that β-adrenergic stimulation using isoproterenol dramatically increases SR Ca^{2+} leak, whereas CaMKII inhibition (but not PKA inhibition) decreases SR Ca^{2+} leak. In addition, bypassing PKA activation using forskolin did not increase SR Ca^{2+} leak showing that β-adrenergic effects on RyR2 and SR Ca^{2+} leak may be mainly dependent on CaMKII rather than PKA. Two similar studies investigating the effects of β-adrenergic stimulation on RyR2 phosphorylation (but also PLB phosphorylation) support the prominent role of CaMKII [60, 61]. Interestingly, the recently described cAMP binding protein Epac, which was shown to phosphorylate the CaMKII site on RyR2, may be a potential link between cAMP and CaMKII-dependent signaling pathways [62].

In a rabbit heart failure model, it was shown recently that there is increased CaMKII expression, more CaMKII is autophosphorylated, and more of this CaMKII is associated with RyR2 [63]. There were also less phosphatases associated with RyR2, and RyR2 was more heavily phosphorylated [64]. Moreover, the enhanced diastolic SR Ca leak could be reversed by CaMKII inhibition but not by PKA inhibition [63, 65]. This CaMKII-dependent enhancement of SR Ca^{2+} leak in heart failure may contribute to both the diminished SR Ca^{2+} content characteristic of this disease as well as diastolic SR Ca^{2+} release, which can activate transient inward Na^+/Ca^{2+} exchange current resulting in arrhythmias. Indeed, CaMKII inhibition increases SR Ca^{2+} content [63]. Interestingly, this is associated with only modest inotropy most likely because although CaMKII inhibition limits diastolic SR Ca^{2+} leak thus enhancing SR Ca^{2+} content, it also prevents CaMKII-dependent stimulation of ECC at the RyR2, such that there is lower fractional SR Ca^{2+} release. In summary, CaMKII can enhance RyR2 activation during ECC, thus influencing fractional SR Ca^{2+} release during systole but also spontaneous SR Ca^{2+} release (i.e., SR Ca^{2+} leak) during diastole, when it may unload Ca^{2+} from the SR and also contribute to arrhythmias as we and others have shown in preliminary results recently [66, 67].

In addition, novel data suggest that CaMKII activation of mutant RyR2 promotes ectopic activity and atrial fibrillation in a transgenic mouse model [68]. These authors also found that inhibiting CaMKII using KN-93 may prevent SR Ca^{2+} leak through RyR2 and thus atrial fibrillation.

12.4.3 SR Ca^{2+} Uptake, FDAR, Acidosis

In its unphosphorylated form, PLB is an endogenous inhibitor of SERCA2a [69]. After phosphorylation of PLB, SERCA2a activity and thus SR Ca^{2+} uptake are enhanced. PLB is phosphorylated by PKA (Ser-16) and CaMKII (Thr-17) [69, 70]. Bassani et al. [71] initially showed that CaMKII enhances SR Ca^{2+} uptake. These authors speculated that CaMKII-dependent PLB phosphorylation might be responsible for the frequency-dependent acceleration of relaxation (FDAR) of twitches and SR Ca^{2+} uptake typically observed when increasing stimulation rate. In a different study, it was shown that a frequency-dependent increase in PLB Thr-17 phosphorylation occurs in rat myocytes (independent of Ser-16 phosphorylation) and that the level of Thr-17 phosphorylation correlated directly with the rate of relaxation [72].

FDAR is an important intrinsic mechanism to allow faster relaxation (and diastolic filling of the heart) when the heart rate is increased. FDAR also manifests as the slowing of twitch relaxation as time between beats is prolonged (i.e., at post-rest contractions) [73]. An attractive hypothesis was that FDAR might be because by enhanced SR Ca^{2+} uptake via CaMKII-dependent PLB phosphorylation (with rest leading to PLB dephosphorylation). However, we found that FDAR is still prominent in PLB-deficient (PLB-KO) mice [74]. Also, the time course of FDAR development is much faster during changes in frequency than that of PLB phosphorylation, and in atria of transgenic mice overexpressing the CaMKII inhibition protein AC3-I no difference in FDAR was observed as compared with control mice [75–77]. Moreover, in an elegant study by Varian and Janssen [78] it was proposed that troponin I and myosin light chain-2 phosphorylation may be critically involved in FDAR leading to decreased myofilament Ca^{2+} sensitivity at higher frequencies [78]. Thus, CaMKII-dependent PLB phosphorylation might contribute to FDAR, but it is unlikely to be the sole mechanism for FDAR. These observations are also supported by the fact that FDAR can be suppressed by CaMKII inhibitors in some reports, whereas other reports could not detect FDAR inhibition [71, 72, 74, 75, 79–82].

During acidosis, (i.e., when lowering extracellular pH from 7.4 below 7.0), after an initial depression of Ca^{2+} transients and contractility, there is a slow but progressive increase in Ca^{2+} transient amplitudes causing a partial recovery of contractions [83]. Interestingly, this recovery can be prevented by CaMKII inhibition, and it was proposed that CaMKII-dependent PLB phosphorylation may be responsible for the faster $[Ca^{2+}]_i$ decline and recovery of contractions that partially overcomes the direct inhibitory effect of acidosis [83–85]. We previously confirmed that PLB and CaMKII were both required for the recovery of Ca^{2+} transients and contraction during acidosis in mouse myocytes [86]. Indeed, recovery was prevented in myocytes from PLB-KO versus wild-type (WT) mice. In line, inhibition of CaMKII completely abolished recovery in WT mice, but it was without effect in PLB-KO mice [86]. Moreover, recent results show that acute overexpression of $CaMKII\delta_C$ in rabbit (as well as mouse) myocytes for 24 h using adenovirus-mediated gene transfer even improves recovery during late acidosis, with increased twitch shortening, $[Ca^{2+}]_i$ transient amplitude, and accelerated Ca^{2+} decline. This was accompanied by an increased SR Ca^{2+} content during late acidosis pointing to the relevance of CaMKII relevance for SR Ca^{2+} loading during acidosis [87]. Thus, CaMKII-dependent enhancement of SR Ca^{2+} uptake during acidosis may reflect an important physiological function.

Interestingly, it was shown recently that the heart when returning to normal pH after acidosis, similar to reperfusion after ischemia, is prone to arrhythmias because of a CaMKII-dependent mechanism on RyR2 [88]. These authors showed that ectopic activity was triggered by membrane depolarizations (delayed afterdepolarizations) primarily occurring in epicardium, which were prevented by KN-93.

12.4.4 Na$^+$ Channels

In addition to LTCC, CaMKII may also target cardiac Na$^+$ channels [89, 90]. Tan et al. [91] first reported a CaM-dependent regulation of cardiac voltage-gated Na$^+$ channels. The authors showed that Ca^{2+}/CaM bind to an IQ motif at the carboxyl-tail of the α-subunit. This interaction specifically altered Na$^+$ channel-gating properties. The accumulation of intermediate inactivation was enhanced consistent with a reduced channel function (loss of function). The Ca^{2+}-dependent regulation of Na$^+$ current (I$_{Na}$) may thus modulate excitability as a feedback mechanism during ECC.

Cardiac voltage-gated Na$^+$ channels are crucially involved in the shaping of the action potential as well as in the conduction of electrical activity across the myocardium. The typical fast upstroke ($\sim$200–300 V/s) of the action potential from a membrane potential of -85 mV to $+30$ mV is completely attributable to the Na$^+$ current (phase 0 of the action potential). The Na$^+$ channel—a glycosylated protein with a molecular mass of $\sim$260 kDa—is a member of an ion channel superfamily that includes voltage-gated K$^+$ and Ca^{2+}, as well as cyclic-nucleotide-gated channels. Their structure shares similarities with the other members of the superfamily (see Figure 12.5): Like voltage-gated Ca^{2+} channels, it consists of various subunits with the α-subunit required for function. The isoform Nav1.5 (SCN5A) of the α-subunit is the predominant isoform in the heart. However, other isoforms such as Nav1.1, Nav1.3, and Nav1.6, which were mainly expressed in the brain, were recently found in the heart. These isoforms seem to be localized in the transverse tubules, whereas cardiac Nav1.5 was preferentially localized in intercalated disks [92]. The cardiac α-subunit consists of four homologous domains (I-IV), with each domain containing six transmembrane segments (S1-S6). The central pore is formed by the four domains with the S5 and S6 transmembrane segments as putative pore center, which confer selectivity and conductance [73]. The linkers between each fifth and sixth segment, which are also called the P (pore) segments, determine the Na$^+$ selectivity of the pore relative to Ca^{2+} by a factor of $>$1000:1 or even higher [73]. The fourth transmembrane segment in each domain (S4) is covered with 4–8 positively charged residues that thereby serve as voltage sensors. Its orientation within the membrane field allows it to move outward in response to depolarization, resulting in the opening of the channel [73].

At resting membrane potentials (-80 to -90 mV), cardiac Na$^+$ channels are typically in closed-available resting states. During depolarization, the channels quickly activate. In the process of channel activation, each of the four S4 segments physically traverses the membrane; however, the extent of movement is unequally distributed among them. Conformational changes that are not fully understood then

Na⁺ channel

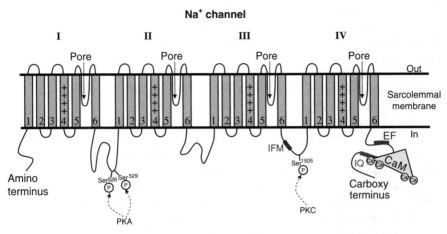

Figure 12.5. Structure of the cardiac Na$^+$ channel Nav1.5 (SCN5A). The Na$^+$ channel has four domains (I-IV), each of which has six homologous repeating transmembrane regions (S1-S6) and a pore loop. A repeating positively charged gating region in each S4 is indicated by $+ + + +$. Other noted sites are 1) PKA and PKC phosphorylation sites, 2) site implicated possibly in fast inactivation (inactivation gate; IFM), and 3) IQ motif at the carboxy terminus, which is the site of possible Ca/CaM binding. Of note: The Ca^{2+} channel has a similar topology (adapted from 73).

lead to the opening of the channel. Subsequent to channel activation, the channels enter inactivated states that are nonconducting for Na$^+$ ions. In this state, the channels are refractory to immediate depolarization, requiring time for recovery at resting membrane potentials to be available for a subsequent depolarization.

For Na$^+$ channel inactivation, a set of multiple processes seems to occur, each of which is distinguishable by its recovery kinetic at strongly negative potentials. The traditional "fast" inactivation is initiated over tens of milliseconds, whereas "intermediate" or "slow" inactivation processes occur with a much slower kinetic in the range of hundreds of milliseconds or tens of seconds, respectively [73]. Fast inactivation is at least partly mediated by the cytoplasmic linker between domains III and IV [93]. It is often recognized as a hinged lid covering the channel pore (inactivation gate). Consistent with this hypothesis, the treatment with internal proteases disrupts the fast inactivation process [93]. However, mutations in regions distinct from the cytoplasmic linker could also affect fast inactivation, thereby questioning the importance of this linker. Peptide-binding studies suggest that instead of being a lid for the pore, the linker may rather bind to a site on the channel that allosterically regulates pore closure using hydrophobic interactions [94]. In this respect, a region in the linker consisting of only the three hydrophobic amino acids isoleucine, phenylalanine, and methionine (IFM region, amino acids 1484–1486) seems to be involved. As has been shown recently, the interaction of the III-IV linker with the carboxyl terminus is required for stabilization of the closed gate [95]. A detailed analysis of the carboxyl terminus revealed that only the proximal part of this tail is organized as α-helical structure (6 helices), whereas the distal part seems to be little structured [96]. Interestingly, this helical structure shares striking similarities to the N-terminal domain of calmodulin. Disruption of the distal component did not affect channel gating. In contrast, truncation of the sixth helix (H6) containing a concentration of positively charged residues along with the distal C-terminus (S1885stop mutant) had profound effects on channel inactivation. The channel availability was shifted in the hyperpolarizing direction, and a 10-fold increase was observed in the percentage of channels that fail to inactivate. The authors suggested electrostatic interaction with other regions of the channel. These interactions are distinct from the hydrophobic interactions thought to be involved in the IFM-motif binding to the C-terminus [96]. The process of fast inactivation may be far more complex and involve more structural domains than originally thought.

In line with this, the structural determinants of intermediate and slow inactivation are even more difficult to localize. Mutations scattered widely throughout the channel could affect these processes. To reverse the different states of inactivation, repolarization of variable duration is required. Activation and inactivation are functionally coupled. It has been shown that a naturally occurring mutation in the S4 segment of domain IV (R1623Q) known to activate the channel also results in slowed inactivation [97]. Therefore, it seems that the S4 segments are the voltage sensors for both activation and inactivation, and the movement of these segments with voltage is a prerequisite for physiological inactivation.

An ultra-slow (or late) component of Na^+ current inactivation (several hundreds of milliseconds) named $I_{Na,late}$ was recently described, which may contribute to EADs and DADs and might even play a role for arrhythmias in heart failure [98]. Interestingly, a novel drug named ranolazine [99–102] can be used to inhibit $I_{Na,late}$ specifically.

Auxiliary β-subunits are important modulators of Na^+ channel gating and expression. They are of $\sim 20\,kDa$ molecular mass, and they contain a small carboxy-terminal cytoplasmic domain, a single membrane-spanning segment, and a large amino-terminal extracellular domain. The $\beta1$-subunit is widely expressed in the heart and encoded by a single gene (SCN1B) [103]. In contrast to brain and skeletal muscle where the association of both subunits increases current density, activation and inactivation gating, and the consequences of noncovalent association in the heart are controversially discussed [104, 105]. An α-β interaction has been suggested to be important for the maturation of Na channels from immature slow gating to mature rapid gating [106].

The regulation of the Na^+ channels by protein kinases is isoform specific. The cardiac isoform has two serine residues (Ser526 and Ser529) in the I-II cytoplasmic linker, which are shown to be subject to phosphorylation by cyclic adenosine 3′,5′-monophosphate (cAMP)-dependent PKA (β-adrenergic receptor stimulation, see Figure 12.5) [107]. After phosphorylation by PKA, Na channel gating remains unchanged, but whole-cell conductance increases [108]. Single-channel experiments revealed that the resulting increase in whole cell conductance is neither caused by increased single channel amplitude nor by altered mean open or closed times, but it is caused by an increase in the number of functional channels [109]. Substantial evidence indicates that this effect results from enhanced trafficking of Na^+ channels to the plasma membrane [110]. However, β-adrenergic receptor modulation of the cardiac Na$^+$ channel may be more complex and is not fully understood. It has been shown previously that the β-adrenergic receptor effects on Na$^+$ channels are at least partly directly mediated by G-protein stimulatory α subunit (Gsα) without the apparent involvement of PKA [109]. Also, some authors have found effects of upstream mediators of the β-adrenergic receptor cascade on gating that are in conflict with the hypothesis that PKA-dependent phosphorylation activates the Na current. These authors showed a cAMP-dependent shift in the steady-state availability into the hyperpolarizing direction, which is consistent with a reduced function [111].

For the cardiac isoform, it is unequivocally accepted that phosphorylation of a serine residue in the III-IV linker (Ser1505) by protein kinase C (PKC) results in a reduced maximal conductance as well as an enhanced inactivation with a shift of the steady-state availability into the hyperpolarizing direction [112]. Furthermore, PKC-dependent phosphorylation of the cardiac Na$^+$ channel is at least partially responsible for the modulatory action of lysophosphatidylcholine, which has been implicated in the arrhythmogenesis during ischemia [113]. Surprisingly, PKA and PKC modulate Na$^+$ channels divergently.

Most importantly, Na$^+$ channel activity may be also regulated by CaMKII, as these channels are multiprotein regulatory complexes [114, 115]. The first evidence for CaMK-dependent regulation of cardiac Na$^+$ channels was by Deschênes et al. [116]. These authors showed that the CaMK-inhibitor KN-93 slowed current decay, which is consistent with an inhibition of fast inactivation. Additionally, the steady-state voltage dependence of inactivation was shifted in the depolarizing direction resulting in an increased channel availability. Entry into the intermediate inactivated state was also slowed, whereas the recovery from inactivation was hastened. This was consistent with a CaMK-dependent loss-of-function effect similar to the above described CaM-dependent effects on Na$^+$ channel gating [91]. However, KN-92 (the inactive analoge of the CaMKII inhibitor KN-93) also had effects on Na$^+$ channel gating, and the specific CaMKII-inhibitor AIP did not seem to affect the Na$^+$ current. Therefore, the authors concluded that a kinase other than CaMKII might modulate Na$^+$ channels (suggesting CaMKIV). However, the expression levels of this kinase in the heart are low [117].

We recently examined Na$^+$ channel gating in rabbit myocytes overexpressing CaMKIIδ$_C$. CaMKIIδ$_C$ overexpression resulted in a leftward-shift in the steady-state voltage dependence of inactivation (see Figure 12.6A). The development of inter-mediate inactivation was enhanced and recovery from inactivation was prolonged (loss of function). All effects were reversible with CaMKII-inhibition using either KN-93 or AIP. In contrast, increased persistent I_{Na} or $I_{Na,late}$ was found (gain of function; see Figure 12.6B), thereby contributing to increased intracellular Na$^+$ accumulation and AP prolongation. These effects argue for specific CaMKII-dependent modulation of Na$^+$ channels. Moreover, we also found a direct association of CaMKII with the Na$^+$ channel and phosphorylation of Na$^+$ channels by CaMKII [89].

This new evidence for additional CaMKII-dependent effects besides other well-known effects on Ca^{2+}-handling proteins may be especially of pathophysiological

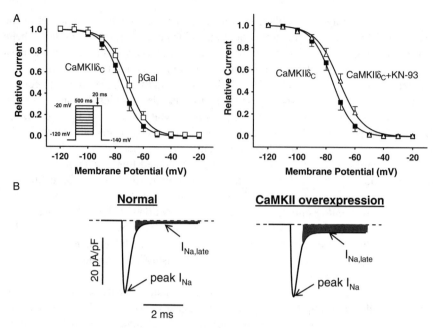

Figure 12.6. A: CaMKII-dependent regulation of Na$^+$ current. Adenovirus-mediated CaMKIIδ_C overexpression resulted in a significant leftward-shift in the steady-state voltage dependence of inactivation (availability) as compared with the control group with β-galactosidase (βGal) expression (left). This reduced availability could be reversed to control values in the presence of CaMKII inhibition using KN-93 (right; adapted from ref. 89) and AIP (data not shown). **B:** Increased persistent or late Na current (I$_{Na,late}$) in myocytes overexpressing CaMKII (adapted from ref. 89).

importance, because the upregulation of CaMKII activity and expression seem to be typical of cardiomyopathy from diverse causes in patients and animal models [6, 7, 44, 63, 118]. Furthermore, transgenic mice overexpressing CaMKIIδ_C develop heart failure and die early [54], which may be associated with ventricular arrhythmias that can be elicited in these mice [89]. Altered Na$^+$ channel function may therefore be associated with these arrhythmogenic processes. Interestingly, CaMKII inhibition can prevent myocardial remodeling after myocardial infarction or excessive β-adrenergic receptor stimulation [119].

Several human cardiac Na$^+$ channel mutations have been linked to either Brugada or LQT3 syndromes with life-threatening arrhythmias [114]. One such human mutation (Asp insertion at 1795 in the C-terminus, 1795InsD), shows simultaneous LQT3-like and Brugada-like phenotypes in the same individuals [120]. Remarkably, Na$^+$ channels bearing this mutation expressed in mammalian cells exhibit the same phenotype that we found for CaMKII-modified normal Na$^+$ channel above [89, 120, 121]. At low-stimulation frequencies, the impaired inactivation and I$_{Na,late}$ can cause AP prolongation consistent with LQT3 syndrome. However, at higher heart rates, incomplete I_{Na} recovery and limited I_{Na} availability shorten action potential duration, slow propagation, and increase dispersion of repolarization similarly found for Brugada syndrome. The intriguing thing is that CaMKII-dependent I_{Na} modulation caused by upregulated CaMKII could constitute a common acquired form of arrhythmia, in otherwise normal Na^+ channels (without 1795InsD mutation). Such an acquired Na^+ channel dysfunction may contribute to arrhythmias under conditions when CaMKII effects are enhanced, as in heart failure. Interestingly, CaMKII has already been linked causally to arrhythmias in a mouse model of cardiac hypertrophy and failure by Anderson's group [46, 119]. In addition, recent experimental data and simulated data suggest that CaMKII inhibition may be of relevance as a possible antiarrhythmic intervention [122, 123].

12.4.5 K$^+$ Channels

CaMKII may also regulate transient outward K^+ current (I_{to}) in human atrial myocytes from hearts with chronic atrial fibrillation [124]. These authors showed that CaMKII regulates I_{to} and CaMKII inhibition results in faster I_{to} inactivation. It was even speculated that K^+ channels or associated regulatory proteins must be in a certain state of phosphorylation to be available for cumulative inactivation resulting in a CaMKII-dependent "memory effect" [125]. Similarly, CaMKII was shown to regulate Kv4.2 and Kv4.3 in neuronal cells, and these two channels are known to contribute to cardiac I_{to} [126, 127]. The initial evidence for a CaMKII-dependent regulation of $I_{to,fast}$ in the myocardium came from human atrial myocytes showing that CaMKII inhibition accelerated $I_{to,fast}$ inactivation, whereas okadaic acid (phosphatase inhibitor) had opposite effects [125]. Similar results were obtained from rat ventricular myocytes recently [128] and in heterologous expression of KV4.2/KV4.3 [127, 128]. Even evidence suggest that CaMKII directly phosphorylates Kv4.3 at Ser-550, thereby prolonging open-state inactivation and accelerating the rate of recovery from inactivation [127]. CaMKII-dependent regulation of I_{to} is interesting because in heart failure, $I_{to,fast}$ mainly mediated by Kv4.2/3 is functionally reduced and expression of the channel proteins is lower [73]. A recent study suggests that I_{to} channels are a functional reservoir of CaMKII and that downregulation of I_{to} results in an increase in CaMKII activity leading to hypertrophy and heart failure. In line with this, the authors found that overexpression of the I_{to} channel Kv4.3 significantly reduced the autonomous CaMKII activity without changing the total CaMKII expression [129]. Similarly, it was also shown recently that inhibition of CaMKII with KN93 prevented I_{to} downregulation following sustained tachycardia *in vivo* [130]. In preliminary studies in myocytes acutely overexpressing CaMKIIδ_C, we find CaMKII-dependent enhancement of I_{to} consistent with increased Kv1.4 function and consequent APD shortening [131]. However, it was also reported that chronic CaMKII inhibition shortens AP because of upregulation of $I_{to,fast}$ and the inward rectifier current I_{K1} [132], suggesting that CaMKII overexpression would increase AP as also shown by chronic CaMKII overexpression [44]. Indeed, more studies need to be performed to elucidate the role of CaMK-dependent K^+ channel regulation.

12.5 ROLE OF CaMKII FOR ARRHYTHMIAS

Several animal models have linked increased CaMKII expression with arrhythmias *in vivo* (see Figure 12.7) [24, 26, 46, 89, 133].

Arrhythmia mechanisms *in vitro* are thought to be important as initiating mechanisms for focal arrhythmias and for initiating impulses *in vivo* that lead to arrhythmias sustained by reentrant circuits, such as ventricular tachycardia in post myocardial infarction border zone scar areas [134, 135]. These triggers are caused by increased net inward current and have been differentiated between EADs and DADs. EADs occur early relative to the completion of AP repolarization mostly during the AP plateau or during the early phases of AP resolution (so-called phase II and III) and are most often associated with repetitive LTCC openings [136] and increased $I_{Na,late}$ [99, 100, 102]. Signaling events that favor so-called mode 2 gating are associated with generation of EADs [137, 138]. Under some experimental conditions, EADs are independent of the release of intracellular Ca^{2+} stores [139], but it was shown that blocking SR Ca^{2+} cycling prevents the development of EADs and

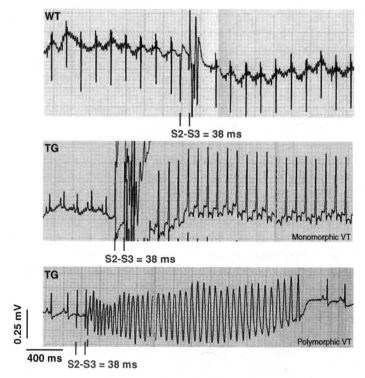

Figure 12.7. Arrhythmias in CaMKIIδ_C-transgenic mice with original ECG-traces during programmed electrical stimulation *in vivo*. In WT, two consecutive premature beats (S2-S3, coupling interval 38 ms) did not induce arrhythmias (above). In contrast, in two different TG mice, the same protocol induced monomorphic (middle) or polymorphic VT (below; adapted from ref. 89).

arrhythmias [26, 140]. One possible reason for the blockade of EADs and arrhythmias by inhibitors of SR Ca^{2+} cycling is that SR Ca^{2+} release is the predominant source of Ca^{2+} for CaMKII activation [141]. CaMKII inhibitory drugs or dialysis of highly specific CaMKII inhibitory peptides effectively inhibit EAD formation and arrhythmias even without shortening AP or QT intervals [26, 142, 143].

DADs are named because they take place after repolarization of the AP to baseline. These afterdepolarizations are mainly linked to conditions that favor the SR Ca^{2+} overload. A common example of a circumstance favoring DADs occurs during digitalis toxicity [73], where Ca^{2+} loading occurs because of poisoning of the Na^+ gradient across the cell membrane and secondary reduction in the ability of the electrogenic NCX to clear cytoplasmic Ca^{2+} to the extracellular space during its forward mode of operation [144]. CaMKII inhibition leads to a reduction in SR Ca^{2+} content, at least in structurally normal myocardium [119], and this is one potential mechanism for CaMKII inhibition reducing DADs [145]. However, DADs can occur simultaneously with AP prolongation and EADs [146] so that CaMKII could contribute to SR Ca^{2+} overload through enhanced cellular Ca^{2+} entry (e.g., by way of LTCC during EADs) [141]. These studies show that Ca^{2+} loading during a prolonged AP can overload the SR with Ca^{2+} and produce DADs. Although many inward currents have been considered as candidates responsible for the generation of DADs, most data point to the NCX as the source of inward current for DADs [144, 145]. Cellular arrhythmia triggers are a plausible initiating mechanism for arrhythmias, but in contrast to macro reentrant circuits, which are relatively easy to measure in an integrated preparation such as a whole heart or even a patient, it is not possible to directly measure cellular afterdepolarizations in situ. Some studies in patients have pointed to a potential role for initiation of reentrant arrhythmias by highly focal triggers that are consistent with initiation by earlier DADs [134, 135, 147]. Furthermore, it is well accepted that conditions such as excessive QT interval prolongation and Ca^{2+} overload are associated with both afterdepolarizations and with enhanced susceptibility to arrhythmias in patients. In this regard, a rabbit model of excessive QT interval prolongation and torsades de pointes shows that CaM or CaMKII inhibitors can prevent arrhythmias, suppress prominent secondary U waves that are linked to afterdepolarizations, and prevent arrhythmias without shortening the QT interval [142, 143]. These same conditions suppress EADs in cellular and isolated heart studies.

Taken together, these findings show that CaMKII can facilitate EADs and DADs, and it can plausibly link these afterdepolarizations to arrhythmias in animal models. Additional studies and possibly newer "mapping" techniques applicable to patients will be necessary before afterdepolarizations are definitively linked to arrhythmias in patients. Until then, also mathematical models will help understand the role of CaMKII for ECC and arrhythmias in heart disease [122, 123, 148].

12.6 SUMMARY

CaMKII in the heart has gained tremendous attention over the last few years. Its involvement at multiple levels in ECC and arrhythmogenesis indicate that it is an important protein for cellular signaling and regulation in the heart. Moreover, because CaMKII expression and activation may be elevated in important pathophysiological situations (e.g., heart failure and hypertrophy), investigating CaMKII regulation in the heart will help to understand the pathophysiology of the heart and may identify new modalities of treatment for arrhythmias in heart failure.

ACKNOWLEDGMENTS

This work is supported by grants from the German Research Foundation (Deutsche Forschungsgemeinschaft; DFG) through a Heisenberg-grant (MA 1982/4-1), a grant for a Clinical Research group KFO155 (MA 1982/2-1), and a Hengstberger grant by the German Cardiac Society to (D.G.K.). This work was also supported in part by the Fondation Leducq Award to the Alliance for Calmodulin Kinase Signaling in Heart Disease.

REFERENCES

1. Kennedy, M.B., Greengard, P. (1981). Two calcium/calmodulin-dependent protein kinases, which are highly concentrated in brain, phosphorylate protein I at distinct sites. Proceedings of the National Academy of Sciences USA, 78, 1293–1297.

2. Jett, M.F., Schworer, C.M., Bass, M., Soderling, T.R. (1987). Identification of membrane-bound calcium, calmodulin-dependent protein kinase II in canine heart. Archives of Biochemistry and Biophysics, 255, 354–360.

3. Braun, A.P., Schulman, H. (2005). The multifunctional calcium/calmodulin-dependent protein kinase: from form to function. Annual Review of Physiology, 57, 417–445.

4. Maier, L.S., Bers, D.M. (2002). Calcium, calmodulin, and calcium-calmodulin kinase II: Heartbeat to heartbeat and beyond. Journal of Molecular Cell Cardiology, 34, 919–939.

5. Hook, S.S., Means, A.R. (2001). Ca^{2+}/CaM-dependent kinases: From activation to function. Annual Review of Pharmacology and Toxicology, 41, 471–505.

6. Kirchhefer, U., Schmitz, W., Scholz, H., Neumann, J. (1999). Activity of cAMP-dependent protein kinase and Ca^{2+}/calmodulin-dependent protein kinase in failing and nonfailing human hearts. Cardiovascular Research, 42, 254–261.

7. Hoch, B., Meyer, R., Hetzer, R., Krause, E.G., Karczewski, P. (1999). Identification and expression of delta-isoforms of the multifunctional Ca^{2+}/calmodulin-dependent protein kinase in failing and nonfailing human myocardium. Circulation Research, 84, 713–721.

8. Zhang, T., Brown, J.H. (2004). Role of Ca^{2+}/calmodulin-dependent protein kinase II in cardiac hypertrophy and heart failure. Cardiovascular Research, 63, 476–486.

9. Maier, L.S., Bers, D.M. (2007). Role of Ca^{2+}/calmodulin-dependent protein kinase (CaMK) in excitation-contraction coupling in the heart. Cardiovascular Research, 73, 631–640.

10. Pitt, G.S. (2007). Calmodulin and CaMKII as molecular switches for cardiac ion channels. Cardiovascular Research, 73, 641–647.

11. Mattiazzi, A., Vittone, L., Mundiña-Weilenmann, C. (2007). Ca^{2+}/calmodulin-dependent protein kinase: A key component in the contractile recovery from acidosis. Cardiovascular Research, 73, 648–656.

12. Anderson, M.E. (2007). Multiple downstream proarrhythmic targets for calmodulin kinase II: Moving beyond an ion channel-centric focus. Cardiovascular Research, 73, 657–666.

13. McKinsey, T.A. (2007). Derepression of pathological cardiac genes by members of the CaM kinase superfamily. Cardiovascular Research, 73, 667–677.

14. Edman, C.F., Schulman, H. (1994). Identification and characterization of δ_B-CaM kinase and δ_C-CaM kinase from rat heart, two new multifunctional Ca/calmodulin-dependent protein kinase isoforms. Biochimica et Biophysica Acta, 1221, 89–101.

15. Maier, L.S., Ziolo, M.T., Bossuyt, J., Persechini, A., Mestril, R., Bers, D.M. (2006). Dynamic changes in free Ca-calmodulin levels in adult cardiac myocytes. Journal of Molecular and Cellular Cardiology, 41, 451–458.

16. Meyer, T., Hanson, P.I., Stryer, L., Schulman, H. (1992). Calmodulin trapping by calcium-calmodulin-dependent protein kinase. Science, 256, 1199–1202.

17. Lai, Y., Nairn, A.C., Greengard, P. (1986). Autophosphorylation reversibly regulates the Ca/calmodulin-dependent protein kinase II. Proceedings of the National Academy of Sciences USA, 83, 4253–4257.

18. Lou, L.L., Lloyd, S.J., Schulman, H. (1986). Activation of the multifunctional Ca/calmodulin-dependent protein kinase by autophosphorylation: ATP modulates production of an autonomous enzyme. Proceedings of the National Academy of Sciences USA, 83, 9497–9501.

19. Schworer, C.M., Colbran, R.J., Soderling, T.R. (1986). Reversible generation of a Ca-independent form of Ca (calmodulin)-dependent protein kinase II by an autophosphorylation mechanism. Journal of Biological Chemistry, 261, 8581–8584.

20. Erickson, J.R., Joiner, M.L., Guan, X., Kutschke, W., Yang, J., Oddis, C.V., Bartlett, R.K., Lowe, J.S., O'Donnell, S.E., Aykin-Burns, N., Zimmerman, M.C., Zimmerman, K., Ham, A.J., Weiss, R.M., Spitz, D.R., Shea, M.A., Colbran, R.J., Mohler, P.J., Anderson, M.E. (2008). A dynamic pathway for calcium-independent activation of CaMKII by methionine oxidation. Cell, 133, 462–474.

21. Rokita, A.G., Unsöld, B., Teucher, N., Schmidt, K., Sowa, T., Hünlich, M., Dybkova, N., Neef, S., Wagner, S., Maier, L.S. (2007). Differential regulation of Ca/calmodulin-dependent protein kinase II (CaMKII) in cardiac hypertrophy in the mouse: Pressure overload versus volume overload. Circulation, 116, 154–155.

22. Gao, L., Blair, L.A., Marshall, J. (2006). CaMKII-independent effects of KN93 and its inactive analog KN92: Reversible inhibition of L-type calcium channels. Biochemical and Biophysical Research Communications, 345, 1606–1610.

23. Li, L., Satoh, H., Ginsburg, K.S., Bers, D.M. (1997). The effect of Ca-calmodulin-dependent protein kinase II on cardiac excitation-contraction coupling in ferret ventricular myocytes. Journal of Physiology, 501, 17–32.

24. Anderson, M.E., Braun, A.P., Wu, Y., Lu, T., Wu, Y., Schulman, H., Sung, R.J. (1998). KN-93, an inhibitor of multifunctional Ca^{++}/calmodulin-dependent protein kinase, decreases early afterdepolarizations in rabbit heart. Journal of Pharmacology and Experimental Therapeutics, 287, 996–1006.

25. Ishida, A., Kameshita, I., Okuno, S., Kitani, T., Fujisawa, H. (1995). A novel specific and potent inhibitor of calmodulin-dependent protein kinase II. Biochemical and Biophysical Research Communications, 212, 806–812.

26. Wu, Y., MxacMillan, L.B., McxNeill, R.B., Colbran, R.J., Anderson, M.E. (1999). CaM kinase augments cardiac L-type Ca^{2+} current: A cellular mechanism for long Q-T arrhythmias. American Journal of Physiology, 276, H2168–H2178.

27. Fabiato, A. (1983). Calcium-induced release of calcium from the cardiac sarcoplasmic reticulum. American Journal of Physiology, 245, C1–C14.

28. Bers, D.M. (2002). Cardiac excitation-contraction coupling. Nature, 415, 198–205.

29. Bers, D.M., Guo, T. (2005). Calcium signaling in cardiac ventricular myocytes. Annals of the NY Academy of Sciences, 1047, 86–98.

30. Shannon, T.R., Ginsburg, K.S., Bers, D.M. (2002). Quantitative assessment of the SR Ca^{2+} leak-load relationship. Circulation Research, 91, 594–600.

31. Witcher, D.R., Kovacs, R.J., Schulman, H., Cefali, D.C., Jones, L.R. (1991). Unique phosphorylation site on the cardiac ryanodine receptor regulates calcium channel activity. Journal of Biological Chemistry, 266, 11144–11152.

32. Hain, J., Onoue, H., Mayrleitner, M., Fleischer, S., Schindler, H. (1995). Phosphorylation modulates the function of the calcium release channel of sarcoplasmic reticulum from cardiac muscle. Journal of Biological Chemistry, 270, 2074–2081.

33. Davis, B.A., Schwartz, A., Samaha, F.J., Kranias, E.G. (1983). Regulation of cardiac sarcoplasmic reticulum calcium transport by calcium-calmodulin-dependent phosphorylation. Journal of Biological Chemistry, 258, 13587–13591.

34. Simmerman, H.K.B., Collins, J.H., Theibert, J.L., Wegener, A.D., Jones, L.R. (1986). Sequence analysis of PLB: Identification of phosphorylation sites and two major structural domains. Journal of Biological Chemistry, 261, 13333–13341.

35. Lee, K.S. (1987). Potentiation of the calcium-channel currents of internally perfused mammalian heart cells by repetitive depolarization. Proceedings of the National Academy of Sciences USA, 84, 3941–3945.

36. Hryshko, L.V., Bers, D.M. (1990). Ca current facilitation during post-rest recovery depends on Ca entry. American Journal of Physiology, 259, H951–H961.

37. Anderson, M.E., Braun, A.P., Schulman, H., Premack, B.A. (1994). Multifunctional Ca/calmodulin-dependent protein kinase mediates Ca-induced enhancement of the L-type Ca current in rabbit ventricular myocytes. Circulation Research, 75, 854–861.

38. Xiao, R.P., Cheng, H., Lederer, W.J., Suzuki, T., Lakatta, E.G. (1994). Dual regulation of Ca/calmodulin kinase II activity by membrane voltage and by calcium influx. Proceedings of the National Academy of Sciences USA, 91, 9659–9663.

39. Yuan, W., Bers, D.M. (1994). Ca-dependent facilitation of cardiac Ca current is due to Ca-calmodulin dependent protein kinase. American Journal of Physiology, 267, H982–H993.

40. Nie, H.G., Hao, L.Y., Xu, J.J., Minobe, E., Kameyama, A., Kameyama, M. (2007). Distinct roles of CaM and Ca^{2+}/CaM-dependent protein kinase II in Ca^{2+}-dependent facilitation and inactivation of cardiac L-type Ca^{2+} channels. Journal of Physiological Sciences, 57, 167–173.

41. Hudmon, A., Schulman, H., Kim, J., Maltez, J.M., Tsien, R.W., Pitt, G.S. (2005). CaMKII tethers to L-type Ca^{2+} channels, establishing a local and dedicated integrator of Ca^{2+} signals for facilitation. Journal of Cellular Biology, 171, 537–547.

42. Grueter, C.E., Abiria, S.A., Dzhura, I., Wu, Y., Ham, A.J.L., Mohler, P.J., Anderson, M. E., Colbran, R.J. (2006). L-type Ca^{2+} channel facilitation mediated by phosphorylation of the β subunit by CaMKII. Molecular Cell, 23, 641–650.

43. Dzhura, I., Wu, Y., Colbran, R.J., Balser, J.R., Anderson, M.E. (2000). Calmodulin kinase determines calcium-dependent facilitation of L-type calcium channels. Nature Cell Biology, 2, 173–177.

44. Maier, L.S., Zhang, T., Chen, L., DeSantiago, J., Heller Brown, J., Bers, D.M. (2003). Transgenic CaMKIIδ_C overexpression uniquely alters cardiac myocyte Ca^{2+} handling: Reduced SR Ca^{2+} load and activated SR Ca^{2+} release. Circulation Research, 92, 904–911.

45. Kohlhaas, M., Zhang, T., Seidler, T., Zibrova, D., Dybkova, N., Steen, A., Wagner, S., Chen, L., Heller Brown, J., Bers, D.M., Maier, L.S. (2006). Increased sarcoplasmic reticulum calcium leak but unaltered contractility by acute CaMKII overexpression in isolated rabbit cardiac myocytes. Circulation Research, 98, 235–244.

46. Wu, Y., Temple, J., Zhang, R., Dzhura, I., Zhang, W., Trimble, R., Roden, D.M., Passier, R., Olson, E.N., Colbran, R.J., Anderson, M.E. (2002). Calmodulin kinase II and arrhythmias in a mouse model of cardiac hypertrophy. Circulation, 106, 1288–1293.

47. Schröder, F., Handrock, R., Beuckelmann, D.J., Hirt, S., Hullin, R., Priebe, L., Schwinger, R.H., Weil, J., Herzig, S. (1998). Increased availability and open probability of single L-type calcium channels from failing compared with nonfailing human ventricle. Circulation, 98, 969–976.

48. Thiel, W.H., Chen, B., Hund, T.J., Koval, O.M., Purohit, A., Song, L.S., Mohler, J.P., Anderson, M.E. (2008). Proarrhythmic defects in Timothy Syndrome require calmodulin kinase II. Circulation, 118, 2225–2234.

49. Rodriguez, P., Bhogal, M.S., Coyler, J. (2003). Stoichiometric phosphorylation of cardiac ryanodine receptor on serine-2809 by calmodulin-dependent kinase II and protein kinase A. Journal of Biological Chemistry, 278, 38593–38600.

50. Lokuta, A.J, Rogers, T.B., Lederer, W.J., Valdivia, H.H. (1997). Modulation of cardiac ryanodine receptors of swine and rabbit by a phosphorylation-deposphorylation mechanism. Journal of Physiology, 487, 609–622.

51. duBell, W.H., Lederer, W.J., Rogers, T.B. (1996). Dynamic modulation of excitation-contraction coupling by protein phosphatase in rat ventricular myocytes. Journal of Physiology, 493, 793–800.

52. Wu, Y., Colbran, R.J., Anderson, M.E. (2001). Calmodulin kinase is a molecular switch for cardiac excitation-contraction coupling. Proceedings of the National Academy of Sciences USA, 98, 2877–2881.

53. Yang, D., Zhu, W.Z., Xiao, B., Brochet, D.X., Chen, S.R., Lakatta, E.G., Xiao, R.P., Cheng, H. (2007). Ca^{2+}/calmodulin kinase II-dependent phosphorylation of ryanodine receptors suppresses Ca^{2+} sparks and Ca^{2+} waves in cardiac myocytes. Circulation Research, 100, 399–407.

54. Zhang, T., Maier, L.S., Dalton, N.D., Miyamoto, S., Ross, J. Jr., Bers, D.M., Heller Brown, J. (2003). The δ_C isoform of CaMKII is activated in cardiac hypertrophy and induces dilated cardiomyopathy and heart failure. Circulation Research, 92, 912–919.

55. Wehrens, X.H., Lehnart, S.E., Reiken, S.R., Marks, A.R. (2004). Ca^{2+}/calmodulin-dependent protein kinase II phosphorylation regulates the cardiac ryanodine receptor. Circulation Research, 94, e61–e70.

56. Currie, S., Loughrey, C.M., Craig, M.A., Smith, G.L. (2004). Calcium/calmodulin-dependent protein kinase IIδ associates with the ryanodine receptor complex and regulates channel function in rabbit heart. Biochemical Journal, 377, 357–366.

57. Guo, T., Zhang, T., Mestril, R., Bers, D.M. (2006). Ca/calmodulin-dependent protein kinase II phosphorylation of ryanodine receptor does affect calcium sparks in mouse ventricular myocytes. Circulation Research, 99, 398–406.

58. Bers, D.M., Eisner, D.A., Valdivia, H.H. (2003). Sarcoplasmic reticulum Ca and heart failure: Roles of diastolic leak and Ca transport. Circulation Research, 93, 487–490.

59. Curran, J., Hinton, M.J., Rios, E., Bers, D.M., Shannon, T.R. (2007). Beta-adrenergic enhancement of sarcoplasmic reticulum calcium leak in cardiac myocytes is mediated by calcium/calmodulin-dependent protein kinase. Circulation Research, 100, 391–398.

60. Ferrero, P., Said, M., Sanchez, G., Vittone, L., Valverde, C., Donoso, P., Mattiazzi, A., Mundiña-Weilenmann, C. (2007). Ca^{2+}/calmodulin kinase II increases ryanodine binding and Ca^{2+}-induced sarcoplasmic reticulum Ca^{2+} release kinetics during beta-adrenergic stimulation. Journal of Molecular and Cellular Cardiology, 43, 281–291.

61. Wang, W., Zhu, W., Wang, S., Yang, D., Crow, M.T., Xiao, R.P., Chen, H. (2004). Sustained β_1-adrenergic stimulation modulates cardiac contractility by Ca^{2+}/calmodulin kinase signaling pathway. Circulation Research, 95, 798–806.

62. Pereira, L., Metrich, M., Fernandez-Velasco, M., Lucas, A., Leroy, J., Perrier, R., Morel, E., Fischmeister, R., Richard, S., Benitah, J.P., Lezoualch, F., Gomez, A.M. (2007). Epac modulates Ca^{2+} spark by Ca^{2+}/calmodulin kinase signaling pathway in rat cardiac myocytes. Journal Physiology, 583, 685–694.

63. Ai, X., Curran, J.W., Shannon, T.R., Bers, D.M., Pogwizd, S.M. (2005). Ca^{2+}-calmodulin-dependent protein kinase modulates RyR2 phosphorylation and SR Ca^{2+} leak in a rabbit heart failure. Circulation Research, 97, 1314–1322.

64. Marx, S.O., Reiken, S., Hisamatsu, Y., Jayaraman, T., Burkhoff, D., Rosemblit, N., Marks, A.R. (2000). PKA phosphorylation dissociates FKBP12.6 from the calcium release channel: Defective regulation in failing hearts. Cell, 101, 365–376.

65. Shannon, T.R., Pogwizd, S.M., Bers, D.M. (2003). Elevated sarcoplasmic reticulum Ca leak in intact ventricular myocytes from rabbits in heart failure. Circulation Research, 93, 592–594.

66. Sag, C.M., Wadsack, D.P., Khabbazzadeh, S., Abesser, M., Grefe, C., Neef, S., Maier, S.K.G., Maier, L.S.(2009). CaMKII contributes to cardiac arrhythmogenesis in transgenic CaMKIIdeltaC mice having heart failure. Circulation Heart Failure. July 31 [Epub ahead of print].

67. Høydal, M.A., Stølen, T.O., Heller Brown, J., Maier, L.S., Smith, G.L., Wisløff, U. (2008). Endurance training abolish arrhythmogenic Ca^{2+} leak in cardiomyocytes from mice with transgenic overexpression of CaMKIIδ$_C$. Circulation, 118, 526

68. Chelu, M.G., Sood, S., Wang, S., Sarma, S., van Oort, R.J., Skapura, D.G., Anderson, M.E., Dobrev, D., Valderrabano, M., Wehrens, X.H. (2008). Calmodulin kinase II activation of mutant ryanodine channels promotes ectopic activity and atrial fibrillation. Circulation, 118, 437

69. Brittsan, A.G., Kranias, E.G. (2000). Phospholamban and cardiac contractile function. Journal of Molecular Cellular Cardiology, 32, 2131–2139.

70. Simmerman, H.K.B., Collins, J.H., Theibert, J.L., Wegener, A.D., Jones, L.R. (1986). Sequence analysis of PLB: Identification of phosphorylation sites and two major structural domains. Journal of Biological Chemistry, 261, 13333–13341.

71. Bassani, R.A., Mattiazzi, A., Bers, D.M. (1995). CaMKII is responsible for activity-dependent acceleration of relaxation in rat ventricular myocytes. American Journal of Physiology, 268, H703–H712.

72. Hagemann, D., Kuschel, M., Kuramochi, T., Zhu, W., Cheng, H., Xiao, R.P. (2000). Frequency-encoding Thr17 phospholamban phosphorylation is independent of Ser16 phosphorylation in cardiac myocytes. Journal of Biological Chemistry, 275, 22532–22536.

73. Bers, D.M. (2001). Excitation-Contraction Coupling and Cardiac Contractile Force. 2nd edition.) Kluwer Academic Publishers, Dordrecht, The Netherlands.

74. DeSantiago, J., Maier, L.S., Bers, D.M. (2002). Frequency-dependent acceleration of relaxation in the heart depends on CaMKII, but not phospholamban. Journal of Molecular Cellular Cardiology, 34, 975–984.

75. Valverde, C.A., Mundiña-Weilenmann, C., Said, M., Ferrero, P., Vittone, L., Salas, M., Palomeque, J., Petroff, M.V., Mattiazzi, A. (2005). Frequency-dependent acceleration of relaxation in mammalian heart: A property not relying on phospholamban and SERCA2a phosphorylation. Journal of Physiology, 562, 801–813.

76. Huke, S., Bers, D.M. (2007). Temporal dissociation of frequency-dependent acceleration of relaxation and protein phosphorylation by CaMKII. Journal of Molecular and Cellular Cardiology, 42, 590–599.

77. Grimm, M., El-Armouche, A., Zhang, R., Anderson, M.E., Eschenhagen, T. (2007). Reduced contractile response to alpha1-adrenergic stimulation in atria from mice with chronic cardiac calmodulin kinase II inhibition. Journal of Molecular and Cellular Cardiology, 42, 643–652.

78. Varian, K.D., Janssen, P.M.L. (2007). Frequency-dependent acceleration of relaxation involves decreased myofilament calcium sensitivity. ASP Heart Circulation Physiology, 292, H2212–H2219.

79. Li, L., Chu, G., Kranias, E.G., Bers, D.M. (1998). Cardiac myocyte calcium transport in phospholamban knockout mouse: relaxation and endogenous CaMKII effects. American Journal of Physiology, 274, H1335–H1347.

80. Hussain, M., Drago, G.A., Colyer, J., Orchard, C.H. (1997). Rate-dependent abbreviation of Ca^{2+} transient in rat heart is independent of phospholamban phosphorylation. American Journal of Physiology, 273, H695–H706.

81. Kassiri, Z., Myers, R., Kaprielian, R., Banijamali, H.S., Backx, P.H. (2000). Rate-dependent changes of twitch force duration in rat cardiac trabeculae: a property of the contractile system. Journal of Physiology, 524, 221–231.

82. Layland, J., Kentish, J.C. (1999). Positive force- and $[Ca^{2+}]_i$-frequency relationships in rat ventricular trabeculae at physiological frequencies. American Journal of Physiology, 276, H9–H18.

83. Nomura, N., Satoh, H., Terada, H., Matsunaga, M., Watanabe, H., Hayashi, H. (2002). CaMKII-dependent reactivation of SR Ca^{2+} uptake and contractile recovery during intracellular acidosis. American Journal of Physiology, 283, H193–H203.

84. Komukai, K., Pascarel, C., Orchard, C.H. (2001). Compensatory role of CaMKII on I_{Ca} and SR function during acidosis in rat ventricular myocytes. Pflügers Archive, 442, 353–361.

85. Mundiña-Weilenmann, C., Ferrero, P., Said, M., Vittone, L., Kranias, E.G., Mattiazzi, A. (2005). Role of phosphorylation of Thr (17) residue of phospholamban in mechanical recovery during hypercapnic acidosis. Cardiovascular Research, 66, 114–122.

86. DeSantiago, J., Maier, L.S., Bers, D.M. (2004). Phospholamban is required for CaMKII-dependent recovery of Ca transients and SR Ca reuptake during acidosis in cardiac myocytes. Journal of Molecular and Cellular Cardiology, 36, 67–74.

87. Sag, C.M., Dybkova, N., Neef, S., Maier, L.S. (2007). Effects on recovery during acidosis in cardiac myocytes overexpressing CaMKII. Journal of Molecular and Cellular Cardiology, 43, 696–709.

88. Said, M., Becerra, R., Palomeque, J., Rinaldi, G., Kaetzel, M.A., Diaz-Sylvester, P.L., Copello, J.A., Dedman, J.R., Mundiña-Weilenmann, C., Vittone, L., Mattiazzi, A. (2008). Increased intracellular Ca^{2+} and SR Ca^{2+} load contribute to arrhythmias after acidosis in rat heart. Role of Ca^{2+}/calmodulin-dependent protein kinase II. American Journal of Physiology Heart Circulatory Physiology, 295, H1669–H1683.

89. Wagner, S., Dybkova, N., Rasenack, E.C.L., Jacobshagen, C., Fabritz, L., Kirchhof, P., Maier, S.K., Zhang, T., Hasenfuss, G., Heller Brown, J., Bers, D.M., Maier, L.S. (2006). Ca/calmodulin-dependent protein kinase II regulates cardiac Na channels. Journal of Clinical Investigation, 116, 3127–3138.

90. Maltsev, V.A., Reznikov, V., Undrovinas, N.A., Sabbah, H.N., Undrovinas, A. (2008). Modulation of late sodium current by Ca^{2+}, calmodulin, and CaMKII in normal and failing dog cardiomyocytes: Similarities and differences. American Journal of Physiology Heart Circulation Physiology, 294, H1597–H1608.

91. Tan, H., Kupershmidt, S., Zhang, R., Stepanovic, S., Roden, D., Wilde, A., Anderson, M.E., Balser, J.R. (2002). A calcium sensor in the sodium channel modulates cardiac excitability. Nature, 415, 442–447.

92. Maier, S.K.G., Westenbroek, R.E., Schenkman, K.A., Feigl, E.O., Scheuer, T., Catterall, W.A. (2002). An unexpected role for brain-type sodium channels in coupling of cell surface depolarization to contraction in the heart. PNAS, 99, 4073–4078.

93. Stühmer, W., Conti, F., Suzuki, H., Wang, X.D., Noda, M., Yahagi, N., Kubo, H., Numa, S. (1989). Structural parts involved in activation and inactivation of the sodium channel. Nature, 339, 597–603.

94. Tang, L., Kallen, R., Horn, R. (1996). Role of an S4-S5 linker in sodium channel inactivation probed by mutagenesis and a peptide blocker. Journal of General Physiology, 108, 89–104.

95. Motoike, H.K., Liu, H., Glaaser, I.W., Yang, A.-S., Tateyama, M., Kass, R.S. (2004). The Na^+ channel inactivation gate is a molecular complex: A novel role of the COOH-terminal domain. Journal of General Physiology, 123, 155–165.

96. Cormier, J.W., Rivolta, I., Tateyama, M., Yang, A.S., Kass, R.S. (2002). Secondary structure of the human cardiac Na^+ channel C terminus. Evidence for a role of helical structures in modulation of channel inactivation, Journal of Biological Chemistry, 277, 9233–9241.

97. Kambouris, N.G., Nuss, H.B., Johns, D.C., Tomaselli, G.F., Marban, E., Balser, J.R. (1998). Phenotypic characterization of a novel long-QT syndrome mutation (R1623Q) in the cardiac sodium channel. Circulation, 97, 640–644.

98. Maltsev, V.A., Sabbah, H.N., Higgins, R.S.D., Silverman, N., Lesch, M., Undrovinas, A.I. (1998). Novel, ultraslow inactivating sodium current in human ventricular cardio-myocytes. Circulation, 98, 2545–2552.

99. Hale, S.L., Shryock, J.C., Belardinelli, L., Sweeney, M., Kloner, R.A. (2008). Late sodium current inhibition as a new cardioprotective approach. Journal of Molecular and Cellular Cardiology, 44, 954–967.

100. Hasenfuss, G., Maier, L.S. (2008). Mechanism of action of the new anti-ischemia drug ranolazine. Clinical Research Cardiology, 97, 222–226.

101. Sossalla, S.R., Rasenack, E.C.L., Wagner, S., Ruff, H., Hasenfuss, G., Belardinelli, L., Maier, L.S. (2008). Inhibition of late sodium current by ranolazine reduces diastolic dysfunction in human heart failure. Journal of Molecular and Cellular Cardiology, 45, 32–43.

102. Song, Y., Shryock, J.C., Wagner, S., Maier, L.S., Belardinelli, L. (2006). Blocking late sodium current reduces hydrogen peroxide-induced arrhythmogenic activity and contractile dysfunction. Journal of Pharmacological and Experimental Therapeutics, 318, 214–222.

103. Makita, N., Bennett, P. Jr., George, A. Jr. (1994). Voltage-gated Na^+ channel $\beta 1$ subunit mRNA expressed in adult human skeletal muscle, heart, and brain is encoded by a single gene. Journal of Biological Chemistry, 269, 7571–7578.

104. Nuss, H., Chiamvimonvat, N., Perez-Garcia, M., Tomaselli, G., Marban, E. (1995). Functional association of the $\beta 1$ subunit with human cardiac (hH1) and rat skeletal muscle ($\mu 1$) sodium channel α subunits expressed in Xenopus oocytes. Journal of General Physiology, 106, 1171–1191.

105. Qu, Y., Isom, L.L., Westenbroek, R.E., Rogers, J.C., Tanada, T.N., McCormick, K.A., Scheuer, T., Catterall, W.A. (1995). Modulation of cardiac Na^+ channel expression in Xenopus oocytes by $\beta 1$ subunits. Journal of Biological Chemistry, 270, 25696–25701.

106. Kupershmidt, S., Yang, T., Roden, D.M. (1998). Modulation of cardiac Na^+ current phenotype by $\beta 1$-subunit expression. Circulation Research, 83, 441–447.

107. Murphy, B.J., Rogers, J., Perdichizzi, A.P., Colvin, A.A., Catterall, W.A. (1996). cAMP-dependent phosphorylation of two sites in the alpha subunit of the cardiac sodium channel. Journal of Biological Chemistry, 271, 28837–28843.

108. Frohnwieser, B., Chen, L., Schreibmayer, W., Kallen, R. (1997). Modulation of the human cardiac sodium channel alpha-subunit by cAMP-dependent protein kinase and the responsible sequence domain. Journal of Physiology, 498, 309–318.

109. Lu, T., Lee, H.-C., Kabat, J.A., Shibata, E.F. (1999). Modulation of rat cardiac sodium channel by the stimulatory G protein α subunit. Journal of Physiology, 518, 371–384.

110. Zhou, J., Yi, J., Hu, N., George, A.L. Jr., Murray, K.T. (2000). Activation of protein kinase A modulates trafficking of the human cardiac sodium channel in Xenopus oocytes. Circulation Research, 87, 33–38.

111. Ono, K., Kiyosue, T., Arita, M. (1989). Isoproterenol, DBcAMP, and forskolin inhibit cardiac sodium current. American Journal of Physiology Cellular Physiology, 256, C1131–C1137.

112. Qu, Y., Rogers, J., Tanada, T., Catterall, W., Scheuer, T. (1996). Phosphorylation of S1505 in the cardiac Na^+ channel inactivation gate is required for modulation by protein kinase C. Journal of General Physiology, 108, 375–379.

113. Watson, C.L., Gold, M.R. (1997). Lysophosphatidylcholine modulates cardiac I_{Na} via multiple protein kinase pathways. Circulation Research, 81, 387–395.

114. Viswanathan, P.C., Balser, J.R. (2004). Inherited sodium channelopathies a continuum of channel dysfunction. Trends in Cardiovascular Medicine, 14, 28–35.

115. Abriel, H., Kass, R.S. (2005). Regulation of the voltage-gated cardiac sodium channel $Nav_{1.5}$ by interacting proteins. Trends in Cardiovascular Medicine, 15, 35–40.

116. Deschênes, I., Neyroud, N., DiSilvestre, D., Marbán, E., Yue, D.T., Tomaselli, G.F. (2002). Isoform-specific modulation of voltage-gated Na^+ channels by calmodulin. Circulation Research, 90, e49–e57.

117. Colomer, J.M., Mao, L., Rockman, H.A., Means, A.R. (2003). Pressure overload selectively up-regulates Ca^{2+}/calmodulin-dependent protein kinase II *in vivo*. Molecular Endocrinology, 17, 183–192.

118. Currie, S., Smith, G.L. (1999). Calcium/calmodulin-dependent protein kinase II activity is increased in sarcoplasmic reticulum from coronary artery ligated rabbit hearts. FEBS Letters, 459, 244–248.

119. Zhang, R., Khoo, M.S., Wu, Y., Yang, Y., Grueter, C.E., Ni, G., Price, E.E. Jr., Thiel, W., Guatimosim, S., Song, L.S., Madu, E.C., Shah, A.N., Vishnivetskaya, T.A., Atkinson, J.B., Gurevich, V.V., Salama, G., Lederer, W.J., Colbran, R.J., Anderson, M.E. (2005). Calmodulin kinase II inhibition protects against structural heart disease. Nature Medicine, 11, 409–417.

120. Veldkamp, M.W., Viswanathan, P.C., Bezzina, C., Baartscheer, A., Wilde, A.A.M., Balser, J.R. (2000). Two distinct congenital arrhythmias evoked by a multidysfunctional Na^+ channel. Circulation Research, 86, e91–e97.

121. Bezzina, C., Veldkamp, M.W., van Den Berg, M.P., Postma, A.V., Rook, M.B., Viersma, J.W., van Langen, I.M., Tan-Sindhunata, G., Bink-Boelkens, M.T., van Der Hout, A.H., Mannens, M.M., Wilde, A.A. (1999). A single Na^+ channel mutation causing both long-QT and Brugada syndromes. Circulation Research, 85, 1206–1213.

122. Livshitz, L.M., Rudy, Y. (2007). Regulation of Ca^{2+} and electrical alternans in cardiac myocytes: Role of CaMKII and repolarizing currents. American Journal of Physiology Heart Circulation Physiology, 292, H2854–H2866.

123. Grandi, E., Puglisi, J.L., Wagner, S., Maier, L.S., Severi, S., Bers, D.M. (2007). Simulation of Ca/calmodulin-dependent protein kinase II on rabbit ventricular myocyte ion currents and action potentials. Biophysical Journal, 93, 3835–3847.

124. Tessier, S., Karczewski, P., Krause, E.G., Pansard, Y., Acar, C., Lang-Lazdunski, M., Mercadier, J.J., Hatem, S.N. (1999). Regulation of the transient outward K^+ current by Ca^{2+}/calmodulin-dependent protein kinases II in human atrial myocytes. Circulation Research, 85, 810–819.

125. Tessier, S., Godreau, D., Vranckx, R., Lang-Lazdunski, L., Mercadier, J.J., Hatem, S.N. (2001). Cumulative inactivation of the outward potassium current: A likely mechanism underlying electrical memory in human atrial myocytes. Journal of Molecular and Cellular Cardiology, 33, 755–767.

126. Varga, A.W., Yuan, L.L., Anderson, A.E., Schrader, L.A., Wu, G.Y., Gatchel, J.R., Johnston, D., Sweatt, J.D. (2004). Calcium-calmodulin-dependent kinase II modulates Kv4.2 channel expression and upregulates neuronal A-type potassium currents. Journal of Neuroscience, 24, 3643–3654.

127. Sergeant, G.P., Ohya, S., Reihill, J.A., Perrino, B.A., Amberg, G.C., Imaizumi, Y., Horowitz, B., Sanders, K.M., Koh, S.D. (2005). Regulation of Kv4.3 currents by Ca^{2+}/calmodulin-dependent protein kinase II. American Journal of Physiology Cell Physiology, 288, C304–C313.

128. Colinas, O., Gallego, M., Setien, R., Lopez-Lopez, J.R., Perez-Garcia, M.T., Casis, O. (2006). Differential modulation of KV4.2 and KV4.3 channels by calmodulin-dependent

protein kinase II in rat cardiac myocytes. American Journal of Physiology Heart Circulation Physiology, 291, H1978–H1987.

129. Keskanokwong, T., Cheng, J., Wang, Y. (2008). The CaMKII-I_{to} channel functional unit in cardiomyocytes. Circulation, 118, 346

130. Xiao, L., Coutu, P., Villeneuve, L.R., Tadevosyan, A., Maguy, A., Le Bouter, S., Allen, B.G., Nattel, S. (2008). Mechanisms underlying rate-dependent remodeling of transient outward potassium current in canine ventricular myocytes. Circulation Research, 103, 733–742.

131. Wagner, S., Hacker, E., Grandi, E., Weber, S.L., Dybkova, N., Sossalla, S., Sowa, T., Bers, D.M., Maier, L.S. (2009). Ca/calmodulin kinase II differentially modulates potassium currents. Circulation Arrhythmia Electrophysiology, 2, 285–294.

132. Li, J., Marionneau, C., Zhang, R., Shah, V., Hell, J.W., Nerbonne, J.M., Anderson, M.E. (2006). Calmodulin kinase II inhibition shortens action potential duration by upregulation of K^+ currents. Circulation Research, 99, 1092–1099.

133. Khoo, M.S., Li, J., Singh, M.V., Yang, Y., Kannankeril, P., Wu, Y., Grueter, C.E., Guan, X., Oddis, C.V., Zhang, R., Mendes, L., Ni, G., Madu, E.C., Yang, J., Bass, M., Gomez, R.J., Wadzinski, B.E., Olson, E.N., Colbran, R.J., Anderson, M.E. (2006). Death, cardiac dysfunction, and arrhythmias are increased by calmodulin kinase II in calcineurin cardiomyopathy. Circulation, 114, 1352–1359.

134. Chung, M.K., Pogwizd, S.M., Miller, D.P., Cain, M.E. (1997). Three-dimensional mapping of the initiation of nonsustained ventricular tachycardia in the human heart. Circulation, 95, 2517–2527.

135. Pogwizd, S.M., Chung, M.K., Cain, M.E. (1997). Termination of ventricular tachycardia in the human heart. Insights from three-dimensional mapping of nonsustained and sustained ventricular tachycardias. Circulation, 95, 2528–2540.

136. January, C.T., Riddle, J.M. (1989). Early afterdepolarizations: Mechanism of induction and block. A role for L-type Ca^{2+} current. Circulation Research, 64, 977–990.

137. January, C.T., Riddle, J.M., Salata, J.J. (1988). A model for early afterdepolarizations: Induction with the Ca^{2+} channel agonist Bay K 8644. Circulation Research, 62, 563–571.

138. Priori, S.G., Corr, P.B. (1990). Mechanisms underlying early and delayed afterdepolarizations induced by catecholamines. American Journal Physiology, 258, H1796–H1805.

139. Marban, E., Robinson, S.W., Wier, W.G.1987). Mechanisms of arrhythmogenic delayed and early afterdepolarizations in ferret ventricular muscle. Journal of Clinical Investigation, 78, 1185–1192.

140. Carlsson, L., Drews, L., Duker, G. (1996). Rhythm anomalies related to delayed repolarization in vivo: influence of sarcolemmal Ca^{++} entry and intracellular Ca^{++} overload. Journal of Pharmacological and Experimental Therapeutics, 279, 231–239.

141. Wu, Y., Kimbrough, J.T., Colbran, R.J., Anderson, M.E. (2004). Calmodulin kinase is functionally targeted to the action potential plateau for regulation of L-type Ca^{2+} current in rabbit cardiomyocytes. Journal of Physiology, 554, 145–155.

142. Mazur, A., Roden, D.M., Anderson, M.E. (1999). Systemic administration of calmodulin antagonist W-7 or protein kinase A inhibitor H-8 prevents Torsade de Pointes in rabbits. Circulation, 100, 2437–2442.

143. Gbadebo, T.D., Trimble, R.W., Khoo, M.S.C., Temple, J., Roden, D.M., Anderson, M.E. (2002). Calmodulin inhibitor W-7 unmasks a novel electrocardiographic parameter that predicts initiation of Torsade de Pointes. Circulation, 105, 770–774.

144. Pogwizd, S.M., Schlotthauer, K., Li, L., Yuan, W., Bers, D.M. (2002). Arrhythmogenesis and contractile dysfunction in heart failure: Roles of sodium-calcium exchange, inward rectifier potassium current, and residual beta-adrenergic responsiveness. Circulation Research, 88, 1159–1167.

145. Wu, Y., Roden, D.M., Anderson, M.E. (1999). Calmodulin kinase inhibition prevents development of the arrhythmogenic transient inward current. Circulation Research, 84, 906–912.

146. De Ferrari, G.M., Viola, M.C., D'Amato, E., Antolini, R., Forti, S. (1995). Distinct patterns of calcium transients during early and delayed afterdepolarizations induced by isoproterenol in ventricular myocytes. Circulation, 91, 2510–2515.

147. Pogwizd, S.M., McKenzie, J.P., Cain, M.E. (1998). Mechanisms underlying spontaneous and induced ventricular arrhythmias in patients with idiopathic dilated cardiomyopathy. Circulation, 98, 2404–2414.

148. Hund, T.J., Decker, K.F., Kanter, E., Mohler, P.J., Boyden, P.A., Schuessler, R.B., Yamada, K.A., Rudy, Y. (2008). Role of activated CaMKII in abnormal calcium homeostasis and I_{Na} remodeling after myocardial infarction: insights from mathematical modeling. Journal of Molecular and Cellular Cardiology, 45, 420–428.

CHAPTER 13

Selective Targeting of Ventricular Potassium Channels for Arrhythmia Suppression: Feasible or Risible?

HUGH CLEMENTS-JEWERY and MICHAEL CURTIS

13.1 INTRODUCTION

Ventricular fibrillation (VF) is an accepted cause of sudden cardiac death (SCD) [1, 2], but it has proven proved to be an elusive target for drug therapy. VF is believed to consist of reentrant excitation of myocardium facilitated by slow conduction velocity; some evidence suggests that VF may also originate through the occurrence of stable rotors [3]. The result is a chaotic appearance on the electrocardiogram (ECG), in which individual cycles cannot be distinguished from each other and vary in cycle length and amplitude on a cycle-to-cycle basis. The loss of coordinated electrical activity results in a loss of contractile activity, and the consequent loss of cardiac output can soon cause death if it is not terminated.

Although VF represents a disturbance of normal electrical activation and conduction, the cause of VF may have complex underlying biochemical and syncitial mechanisms [4]. Therapeutic strategies to prevent VF have targeted the abnormal electrophysiological processes—that is, the activation of ion channels—that produce the disordered electrical activity. The goal has been to find drugs that suppress aberrant ventricular action potentials but do not suppress action potentials generated and conducted in the normal manner.

The drugs that have been developed and tested clinically for prevention of VF are classified according to the Vaughan-Williams system. Class I drugs, which are subclassified into classes IA, 1B, and 1C, target voltage-gated Na^+ channels in the myocardium, His-Purkinje system, and AV node. Class II drugs are β-adrenergic receptor antagonists, class III drugs are agents that prolong action potential duration, and class IV drugs block voltage-gated L-type Ca^{2+} channels. Of these classes of

Novel Therapeutic Targets for Antiarrhythmic Drugs, Edited by George Edward Billman
Copyright © 2010 John Wiley & Sons, Inc.

drugs, only β-adrenergic receptor antagonists have shown any benefit with respect to improvement in mortality from SCD [5], and even then a direct effect on VF is hard to prove, because of the lack of correlation between accumulation of catecholamines in ischemic tissue and the severity of ischemic arrhythmias [6–8]. There are no examples of effective and safe drugs for VF prevention from the other Vaughan-Williams classes. For instance, we now know that class IV drugs prevent VF in animal models of acute coronary ligation, but the drug doses required to achieve a therapeutic effect are profoundly vascular selective, precluding their use clinically based on inevitable hypotension [9]. Class I agents have failed catastrophically in humans despite once being considered to have the most therapeutic potential. Two class I agents, flecainide and encainide, paradoxically increased mortality, with proarrhythmia the inferred mechanism [10]. With the benefit of hindsight, we now know that the drugs tested had poor selectivity for ischemic versus nonischemic tissue, which likely had the effect of slowing conduction in nonischemic tissue, thus promoting reentry [11]. The goal of achieving a class I agent that may suppress VF effectively and safely remains a possibility, in theory, if the drug has high selectivity for ischemic tissue [11]. However, the drug industry and the regulatory bodies are wary of such an approach given the disaster of the CAST trial [10], and as a consequence, the only drug to be developed with this selectivity, vernakalant [12], has been approved only for supraventricular arrhythmias. Thus, the outlook for an effective and safe class I antiarrhythmic agent seems bleak.

What of class III drugs? By widening the action potential, class III drugs in theory suppress reentrant activity by prolongation of the effective refractory period that increases the duration of Na^+ channel inactivation (see Figure 13.1). However, this class of drugs has been plagued by a somewhat paradoxical proarrhythmic effect—an

Action potential widening extends inactivation of I_{Na}

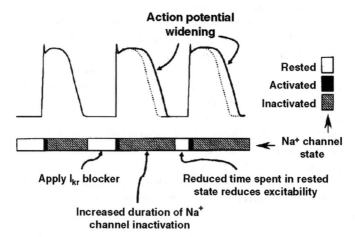

Figure 13.1. K^+ channel blockers inhibit reentry indirectly. Repolarization delay (an I_{Kr} blocker is shown here) prolongs the duration of Na^+ channel inactivation. Thus, class III agents are in effect indirectly acting class I agents.

increase in susceptibility to torsades de pointes, a syndrome characterized by an arrhythmia whose morphology on the ECG seems similar to VF [13]. This likely explains the adverse effect of d-sotalol on mortality in the clinic [14]. In fact, prolongation of action potential duration (or QT interval) by any drug, cardiac or not, is now more or less sufficient to kill its clinical development or severely limit its application.

How can this paradox be resolved? Some evidence indicates that not all class III drugs have torsadogenic potential at clinically relevant concentrations [15]. This suggests that QT or action potential duration (APD) prolongation *per se* is not necessarily torsadogenic, and it has led to the notion that arrhythmia suppression may be achieved safely by class III agents. Studies by Hondeghem [15, 16] have proposed that the effects of class III agents other than APD prolongation promote proarrhythmia, namely triangulation of the action potential (the time difference between the APD_{30} and the APD_{90}), instability (beat to beat variation in action potential duration), reverse use dependence (enhanced drug binding and effects on repolarization at low heart rates versus high heart rates), and dispersion of repolarization. Of these variables, the instability of APD has been proposed to be the most accurate predictor of proarrhythmia, whereas reverse use dependence, which presumably arises from a high affinity for the resting closed state of an ion channel, may be the "motor" of instability, in that in theory it can produce alternation of action potential duration [17].

With regard to triangulation of the action potential, the notion that changes in action potential shape may be somewhat more important than changes in action potential duration *per se* is intriguing. Some evidence for the importance of action potential triangulation exists when the effects of erythromycin and almokalant are compared; both agents prolong APD at therapeutic concentrations, but almokalant causes triangulation, whereas erythmoycin does not [18]. This tendency for action potential triangulation was correlated with the tendency to be proarrhythmic [18]. Hondeghem proposed that whether a drug produces triangulation of the action potential may be related to the phase of the action potential that is predominantly affected; erythromycin seems to affect predominantly the plateau region of the action potential, whereas almokalant affects the main repolarization phase, thereby inducing triangulation [18]. To consider the mechanisms by which these effects may be produced requires a thorough consideration of the form of the action potential and the ionic currents that underlie it.

The ventricular action potential has four phases: Phase 0 consists of the rapid upstroke of the action potential that is mediated by the opening of voltage-gated Na^+ channels ($Na_v1.5$) [19]. Following the peak of the action potential, a brief early repolarization phase (phase 1) produces a notch in the action potential waveform. This phase is produced by inactivation of I_{Na} and activation of the transient outward current, which actually consists of two separate currents, I_{to1} and I_{to2} [20]. I_{to1} itself consists of fast and slow components that are K^+ currents [21]. In contrast, I_{to2} is thought to be a Ca^{2+}-activated Cl^- current that occurs as a result of Ca^{2+} release from the sarcoplasmic reticulum inside the ventricular myocyte [22, 23]. Influx of Ca^{2+} via reverse-mode Na^+/Ca^{2+} exchange also contributes to repolarization during phase 1 [20]. The plateau of the action potential is termed phase 2; during this phase, the membrane potential does not change rapidly, reflecting the near balance between depolarizing currents and repolarizing currents during this time. Depolarizing currents during this phase are the L-type Ca^{2+} current and residual (late) Na^+ current that occur as a result of slowed inactivation of the Na^+ channels [24]. Three different repolarizing "delayed rectifier" K^+ currents balance these depolarizing currents during the plateau—I_{Kur}, I_{Kr}, and I_{Ks}. Of these, I_{Kur} is activated rapidly by depolarization, and the time course of changes in its magnitude roughly follows the shape of the action potential [20]. However, this current is less prominent in ventricular than atrial tissue. Compared to I_{Kur}, development of I_{Kr} is slower and that of I_{Ks} even more so; the increase in the magnitude of these currents cause the end of the action potential plateau. Subtle changes in the balance of these currents can profoundly affect the duration of the plateau region. For example, in the canine, midmyocardial cells typically have longer action potentials than epicardial or endocardial cells, and this is associated with reduced I_{Ks} expression in these cells [25].

The predominant phase of repolarization, phase 3, is produced mainly by I_{Kr} and I_{Ks}; initially, I_{Kr} actually increases as repolarization progresses, greatly accelerating repolarization [20]. During the final 30% of repolarization, I_{Kr} magnitude decreases, but another K^+ current, I_{K1}, is activated and contributes to the return to the resting membrane potential [26]. Phase 4 consists of the diastolic period between completion of repolarization and the onset of the next action potential upstroke. The negative membrane potential is maintained during this phase by a significant I_{K1} current that reduces tissue impedance and opposes the influence of any depolarizing currents [20]. Thus, I_{K1} activation helps to suppress aberrant action potential initiation from small depolarizing currents during diastole.

These descriptions of the ionic currents that underlie the action potential enable us to understand how different class III agents may cause changes in action potential shape to accompany action potential prolongation. Thus, if a drug prolongs phase 3 of the action potential, then the action potential is likely to become triangulated; in contrast, if a drug predominantly prolongs phase 2 of the action potential, then the action potential may be widened without substantial triangulation. As a result, agents that prolong the action potential by affecting phase 2 rather than phase 3 may be the safest antiarrhythmic drugs [18].

This hypothesis suggests that one might be able to design the ideal antiarrhythmic drug that is effective and safe (i.e., not proarrhythmic) based on what is known about drug properties that tend to be proarrhythmic. This requires consideration of the identity of and selectivity for the desired drug target. Based on the hypothesis that the ideal strategy involves APD prolongation without triangulation produced by selective prolongation of the action potential plateau, it would in theory seem that drugs that prolong the activation of the L-type Ca^{2+} current would increase the magnitude or duration of "late" I_{Na} or slow the activation of the "delayed rectifier" K^+ currents would be ideal antiarrhythmic drugs. However, there is some evidence that ATX-II, which is a drug that increases "late" I_{Na}, is proarrhythmic [27], and increasing the duration of the L-type Ca^{2+} current, e.g., by BayK8644, may trigger early afterdepolarizations [28]. Thus, better targets may be the "delayed rectifier" currents.

However, because these currents contribute substantially to phase 3 repolarization, the ideal drug would only slow "delayed rectifier" activation and then dissociate quickly to allow rapid phase 3 repolarization. In addition to this property, to minimize proarrhythmic potential, the ideal antiarrhythmic class III drug would not display reverse use dependence or cause instability of action potential duration, assuming that the triangulation, reverse use dependence, instability, and dispersion model of Hondeghem (TRIaD; [16]) is valid.

In the following section, we review the evidence concerning the antiarrhythmic and proarrhythmic effects of blockade of different K$^+$ currents present in ventricular myocardium in the context of ischemic heart disease, with the intention of providing evidence for or against the assertion that the action potential can be widened safely.

13.2   EFFECTS OF K$^+$ CHANNEL BLOCKADE ON APD AND ARRHYTHMOGENESIS

13.2.1   I$_{Kur}$ Blockade

Several different studies have identified compounds with apparent selectivity for Kv1.5, which is the channel believed to produce the I$_{Kur}$ current. These include diphenyl phosphine oxide compounds [29, 30] and an isoquinolinone (ISQ-1) [31]. The diphenyl phosphine oxide compounds seem to block the open state of the Kv1.5 channel preferentially. In rats, this causes an increase in atrial and ventricular refractoriness, presumably because of an increase in the action potential duration, but only an increase in atrial refractoriness is observed in African green monkeys, which is consistent with the differential myocardial expression of Kv1.5 in these two species [31]. Even though these drugs seem not to have been tested for efficacy against ventricular arrhythmias triggered by acute ischemia, as a consequence of a predominantly atrial effect in primates and lack of functional ventricular I$_{Kur}$ in humans, these drugs are being developed for the treatment of atrial fibrillation rather than VF [29]. Thus, their application for the treatment of ventricular arrhythmias is limited.

13.2.2   I$_{Kr}$ Blockade

I$_{Kr}$ is a target for methanesulfonanalide drugs (almokalant, dofetilide, d-sotalol, and E-4031), which seem to block the open state of the hERG channel preferentially and have low affinity for the closed and inactivated states [32]. Many other cardiac and noncardiac drugs also block I$_{Kr}$ as an ancillary mechanism [26]. In certain animal models of regional myocardial ischemia, selective I$_{Kr}$ block by dofetilide, E-4031, and d-sotalol has been reported to be antiarrhythmic [33–35]. However, we now know that d-sotalol increased mortality when tested clinically [14], and thus the safety of these drugs is a chief concern. With regard to the TRIaD model of proarrhythmia, d-sotalol has been recently shown to cause action potential triangulation along with prolongation of action potential duration and demonstrated reverse-use dependence in the isolated rabbit heart [36]. This would be expected from an open-state channel blocker. The possibility that an I_{Kr} blocker with selectivity for the inactivated state of the hERG channel might be safer seems not to have been explored. This may be interesting to test given that I_{Kr} has a relatively small magnitude during the action potential plateau because of rapid inactivation that follows channel activation after depolarization [37]; recovery from inactivation as repolarization proceeds accounts for the increase in I_{Kr} magnitude and rapid repolarization during phase 3 of the action potential. As a consequence, a drug that prolongs recovery from inactivation may prolong the action potential duration by predominantly affecting the duration of the plateau rather than the rate of phase 3 repolarization, thus preventing action potential triangulation. In addition, an inactivated state blocker would in theory not show any reverse use dependence, and it may thus minimize instability in action potential duration. Therefore, it may not be the case that I_{Kr} blockade is proarrhythmic in all cases.

13.2.3 I_{Ks} Blockade

I_{Ks} is selectively blocked by chromanol compounds, such as 293B and HMR-1556, in addition to other compounds such as thiopentone and propofol [26]. Block of I_{Ks} causes modest QT prolongation in dogs and rabbits *in vivo* [38]. However, because I_{Ks} magnitude is increased at high heart rates based on slow deactivation of the current that causes channels to accumulate in the "open" state, an I_{Ks} blocker would likely cause greater APD prolongation at high heart rates. Selective block of I_{Ks} has been reported to be effective against ischemic ventricular arrhythmias in the dog [39]. Because I_{Ks} is present during phase 2 and phase 3 of the action potential, the effect of I_{Ks} block on triangulation is not immediately obvious. One study that examined the safety of I_{Ks} blockade showed that I_{Ks} block alone did not induce triangulation nor show reverse use dependence, but it could potentiate the triangulation and proar-rhythmia observed with I_{Kr} block [36]. Therefore, there may be safety concerns of I_{Ks} block if there is lack of selectivity over I_{Kr} or it is combined with I_{Kr} block. In addition, congenital loss of I_{Ks} produces long QT syndromes 1 and 5 [40]. Finally, in a canine wedge preparation treated with isoproterenol, 30 µM chromanol 293B was found to increase the dispersion of repolarization and initiate torsades de pointes [41]. This observation reflects in part the intrinsic transmural variation in I_{Ks} magnitude and the differential activation of I_{Ks} in epicardium and endocardium versus midmyocardium by isoproterenol that was apparently not blocked by chromanol 293B. These studies therefore suggest that selective I_{Ks} block may not be a safe antiarrhythmic strategy. Nonetheless, confirmation of proarrhythmic effects in models of ischemic arrhyth-mogenesis *in vivo* is needed.

13.2.4 I_{K1} Blockade

There is some evidence in animal models of ischemic arrhythmogenesis that selective I_{K1} blockade is antiarrhythmic. For example, RP58866 reduced ischemic arrhythmias in isolated rat, rabbit, and marmoset hearts, and this antiarrhythmic effect was associated with QT widening [42]. These effects were attributed to block of I_{K1}

given that block of I_{Kr} could be ruled out by the fact that effects were observed in the rat heart, which is devoid of functional I_{Kr} (other studies have since revealed that RP58866 blocks I_{to}, I_{Kr}, and I_{Ks} in the micromolar range, [26]). Because I_{K1} is known to contribute to the final 30% of ventricular action potential repolarization, the QT widening effect is not surprising. However, because such a drug would only affect terminal repolarization, one would expect significant triangulation of the action potential, and this may be proarrhythmic. However, the block of I_{K1} by RP58866 did not seem to show reverse use dependence [42], and therefore it may not produce much instability in action potential duration. Certainly, the potential of I_{K1} blockade has not resulted in the development of new antiarrhythmic drugs, and safety concerns are probably the main reason. The RP58866 data notwithstanding, other theoretical concerns also may prevent the widespread development of I_{K1} blocking drugs. For example, observations in a nonischemic rabbit heart failure model suggest that reduced I_{K1} magnitude may be a mechanism for increased arrhythmia susceptibility in heart failure [43]. This is because normally I_{K1} buffers the resting membrane potential and prevents the triggering of aberrant action potentials by small depolarizing currents occurring in diastole; the loss of I_{K1} thus allows the possibility that delayed after depolarizations could trigger arrhythmias. Additional concerns make prediction of the overall effect of I_{K1} block on arrhythmias difficult. For instance, loss of I_{K1} would likely cause depolarization of the resting membrane potential that in ischemia may compound the depolarization caused by extracellular K$^+$ accumulation [44], resulting in inactivation of voltage-gated Na$^+$ channels that shortens the duration of the "critical window" for development of VF [11]. On the other hand, depolarization of nonischemic tissue by I_{K1} block may slow electrical conduction in this tissue and promote development of VF in ischemia. On the basis of these concerns, the therapeutic potential for I_{K1} blockers seems somewhat small.

13.2.5 I_{to} Blockade

I_{to} blockade can be produced by a range of drugs including ambasilide, clofilium, flecainide, propafenone, quinidine, and tedisamil [26]. Quinidine and propafenone are known to block the open state and accelerate the inactivation of the channel underlying I_{to1} [45]. Blockers of I_{to1} seem to prolong APD in ischemic ventricular muscle [46], but the overall effect on APD of I_{to} block can be complex because APD is determined by several other processes. For example, by slowing the rate of phase 1 repolarization, the magnitude of the L-type Ca^{2+} current may be increased and result in activation of Ca^{2+}-dependent repolarizing currents that shorten the action potential. Indeed, I_{to} current magnitude was found to have minimal influence on APD in one study [47].

I_{to} has been proposed to play some role in ischemic arrhythmogenesis. For example, the heterogeneous transmural distribution of I_{to1} in the ventricular myocardium has been suggested to increase the dispersion of repolarization in ischemia that may increase the potential for arrhythmogenesis [48]. Thus, I_{to} blockade may be antiarrhythmic. The main evidence concerning the effect of I_{to} blockade on ischemic arrhythmogenesis has been provided by studies using tedisamil. In isolated rat hearts that exhibit a large I_{to} current, tedisamil did not reduce the incidence of ischemic VF but interestingly reduced the duration of sustained VF; this effect was associated with QT prolongation prior to VF and to reduction of cycle frequency during VF [49]. However, there is limited information concerning the effect of I_{to} blockade on ischemic arrhythmias in other species, making it difficult to assess its proarrhythmic or antiarrhythmic potential. One study in transgenic mice revealed that I_{to} "knock down" prolonged APD but did not induce spontaneous arrhythmias, which suggests that I_{to} blockade may be safe from a proarrhythmic perspective [50]. Indeed, because I_{to} contributes directly only to early repolarization, it may not be that I_{to} blockade induces much action potential triangulation, although again this may be complicated by any indirect effects on L-type Ca^{2+} currents and delayed rectifier K^+ currents that contribute to phases 2 and 3 of the action potential, respectively. However, on the basis of the tedisamil data, it seems that I_{to} blockade may not be an effective antiarrhythmic strategy, regardless of its safety.

13.2.6 I_{KATP} Blockade

Ventricular myocardium exhibits an ATP-dependent K^+ current, I_{KATP}, which is activated during ischemia when ATP levels are diminished [51]. It was thought at one stage that I_{KATP} was responsible for the extracellular K^+ accumulation observed in ischemia that causes depolarization of the ischemic myocardium and potentially induces arrhythmias by the flow of injury current [52]. However, this was subsequently disproven [53]. In addition, activation of this current may explain the action potential shortening observed in many models of ischemia [54]; action potential shortening may also promote arrhythmogenesis by reducing tissue refractoriness. Thus, the blockade of I_{KATP} would seem to have antiarrhythmic promise if the above is true [55]. The data concerning the effects of I_{KATP} blockade, however, show a large degree of inconsistency. In the dog, guinea pig, and rat, glibenclamide has been reported to reduce arrhythmia severity [56–59]. However, these studies differ on whether glibenclamide is antifibrillatory or defibrillatory. Another study showed a proarrhythmic effect of glibenclamide [60]. Some of the agents used to block sarcolemmal I_{KATP}, e.g., 5-hydroxydecanoate, may also block the mitochondrial K_{ATP} channel that has been proposed to play a role in ischemic preconditioning [61], and thus an interpretation of the data is difficult because of lack of selectivity of effect. Finally, as described earlier, I_{KATP} blockers do not seem to reduce extracellular K^+ accumulation during ischemia [53].

I_{KATP} blockers have been reported to increase ventricular refractoriness in ischemia [62], but no studies have examined whether these drugs cause triangulation or instability in action potential duration. From a more global perspective on drug safety, because K_{ATP} channels are necessary for insulin secretion in the β-cells of the pancreas, the potential for systemic I_{KATP} blockers is limited given that these drugs are liable to cause hypoglycemia. This indicates the need for cardioselective drugs, such as HMR 1883 [62]. Thus, given the inconsistent data on their effectiveness as an antiarrhythmic agent together with a lack of data concerning drug safety, the potential for I_{KATP} blockade as an effective and safe antiarrhythmic strategy remains unclear.

13.3 CONCLUSIONS/FUTURE DIRECTIONS

Ventricular K^+ channels have the potential to represent useful targets for suppression of ventricular arrhythmias. To achieve benefit, repolarization delay sufficient to suppress reentry must be achieved without this leading to adverse effects. Repolarization delay may by itself provoke arrhythmias via adverse effects on TRIaD. It is not yet clear whether more selective targeting of a specific K^+ channel (e.g., I_{Kr}) or targeting of channels in a particular way (by state selectivity) or in a particular region (normal versus diseased tissue), or a combination of these approaches represents the best way forward. We recommend taking selective drugs into simple preclinical ventricular arrhythmia models early in drug discovery, and, in parallel conducting careful testing of proarrhythmic liability.

REFERENCES

1. Zipes, D.P., Wellens, H.J. (1998). Sudden cardiac death. Circulation, 98, 2334–2351.

2. Adgey, A.A., Devlin, J.E., Webb, S.W., Mulholland, H.C. (1982). Initiation of ventricular fibrillation outside hospital in patients with acute ischaemic heart disease. British Heart Journal, 47, 55–61.

3. Jalife, J. (2000). Ventricular fibrillation: Mechanisms of initiation and maintenance. Annual Review of Physiology, 62, 25–50.

4. Clements-Jewery, H., Curtis, M.J. (2003). Biochemical mediators of ventricular arrhythmias in ischaemic heart disease. In Cardiac Drug Development Guide, Pugsley, M.K., ed. Humana Press, Tottowa, NJ, pp. 203–226.

5. Antman, E.M., Lau, J., Kupelnick, B., Mosteller, F., Chalmers, T.C. (1992). A comparison of results of meta-analyses of randomized control trials and recommendations of clinical experts. Treatments for myocardial infarction. JAMA, 268, 240–248.

6. Cinca, J., Bardaji, A., Salas-Caudevilla, A. (1989). Ventricular arrhythmias and local electrograms after chronic regional denervation of the ischemic area in the pig heart. Journal of the American College of Cardiology, 14, 225–232.

7. Curtis, M.J., Botting, J.H., Hearse, D.J., Walker, M.J.A. (1989). The sympathetic nervous system, catecholamines and ischaemia-induced arrhythmias: Dependence upon serum potassium concentration. In Adrenergic System and Ventricular Arrhythmias in Myocardial Infarction, Brachmann, J., Schömig, A., eds. Springer-Verlag, Berlin, Germany, pp. 206–219.

8. Lameris, T.W., de Zeeuw, S., Alberts, G., Boomsma, F., Duncker, D.J., Verdouw, P.D., Veld, A.J., van Den Meiracker, A.H. (2000). Time course and mechanism of myocardial catecholamine release during transient ischemia in vivo. Circulation, 101, 2645–2650.

9. Farkas, A., Qureshi, A., Curtis, M.J. (1999). Inadequate ischaemia-selectivity limits the antiarrhythmic efficacy of mibefradil during regional ischaemia and reperfusion in the rat isolated perfused heart. British Journal of Pharmacology, 128, 41–50.

10. Echt, D.S., Liebson, P.R., Mitchell, L.B., Peters, R.W., Obias-Manno, D., Barker, A.H., Arensberg, D., Baker, A., Friedman, L., Greene, H.L., et al. (1991). Mortality and morbidity in patients receiving encainide, flecainide, or placebo. The Cardiac Arrhythmia Suppression Trial. New England Journal of Medicine, 324, 781–788.

11. Hondeghem, L.M. (1987). Antiarrhythmic agents: Modulated receptor applications. Circulation, 75, 514–520.

12. Roy, D., Pratt, C.M., Torp-Pedersen, C., Wyse, D.G., Toft, E., Juul-Moller, S., Nielsen, T., Rasmussen, S.L., Stiell, I.G., Coutu, B., et al. for the Atrial Arrhythmia Conversion Trial, I. (2008). Vernakalant hydrochloride for rapid conversion of atrial fibrillation: A phase 3, randomized, placebo-controlled trial. Circulation, 117, 1518–1525.

13. Curtis, M.J. (1991). Torsades de pointes: Arrhythmia, syndrome, or chimera? A perspective in the light of the Lambeth Conventions. Cardiovascular Drugs And Therapy, 5, 191–200.

14. Waldo, A.L., Camm, A.J., deRuyter, H., Friedman, P.L., MacNeil, D.J., Pauls, J.F., Pitt, B., Pratt, C.M., Schwartz, P.J., Veltri, E.P. (1996). Effect of d-sotalol on mortality in patients with left ventricular dysfunction after recent and remote myocardial infarction. The SWORD Investigators. Survival With Oral d-Sotalol. Lancet, 348, 7–12.

15. Hondeghem, L.M., Carlsson, L., Duker, G. (2001). Instability and triangulation of the action potential predict serious proarrhythmia, but action potential duration prolongation is antiarrhythmic. Circulation, 103, 2004–2013.

16. Hondeghem, L.M. (2007). Relative contributions of TRIaD and QT to proarrhythmia. Journal of Cardiovascular Electrophysiology, 18, 655–657.

17. Valentin, J.P., Hoffmann, P., De Clerck, F., Hammond, T.G., Hondeghem, L. (2004). Review of the predictive value of the Langendorff heart model (Screenit system) in assessing the proarrhythmic potential of drugs. Journal of Pharmacological and Toxicological Methods, 49, 171–181.

18. Hondeghem, L.M., Dujardin, K., De Clerck, F. (2001). Phase 2 prolongation, in the absence of instability and triangulation, antagonizes class III proarrhythmia. Cardiovascular Research, 50, 345–353.

19. Fozzard, H.A., Hanck, D.A. (1996). Structure and function of voltage-dependent sodium channels: comparison of brain II and cardiac isoforms. Physiology Review, 76, 887–926.

20. Bers, D.M. (2003). Excitation-Contraction Coupling and Cardiac Contractile Force 2nd ed) Kluwer Academic Publishers, Dordrecht, The Netherlands, pp. 78–94.

21. Nerbonne, J.M. (2000). Molecular basis of functional voltage-gated $K+$ channel diversity in the mammalian myocardium. Journal of Physiology, 525, 285–298.

22. Zygmunt, A.C. (1994). Intracellular calcium activates a chloride current in canine ventricular myocytes. American Journal of Physiology, 267, H1984–1995.

23. Kawano, S., Hirayama, Y., Hiraoka, M. (1995). Activation mechanism of $Ca(2+)$-sensitive transient outward current in rabbit ventricular myocytes. Journal of Physiology, 486, 593–604.

24. Maltsev, V.A., Sabbah, H.N., Higgins, R.S.D., Silverman, N., Lesch, M., Undrovinas, A.I. (1998). Novel, ultraslow inactivating sodium current in human ventricular cardiomyocytes. Circulation, 98, 2545–2552.

25. Liu, D.W., Antzelevitch, C. (1995). Characteristics of the delayed rectifier current (IKr and IKs) in canine ventricular epicardial, midmyocardial, and endocardial myocytes. A weaker IKs contributes to the longer action potential of the M cell. Circulation Research, 76, 351–365.

26. Tamargo, J., Caballero, R., Gomez, R., Valenzuela, C., Delpon, E. (2004). Pharmacology of cardiac potassium channels. Cardiovascular Research, 62, 9–33.

27. Michael, G., Dempster, J., Kane, K.A., Coker, S.J. (2007). Potentiation of E-4031-induced torsade de pointes by HMR1556 or ATX-II is not predicted by action potential short-term variability or triangulation. British Journal of Pharmacology, 152, 1215–1227.

28. January, C.T., Riddle, J.M., Salata, J.J. (1988). A model for early afterdepolarizations: Induction with the Ca2 + channel agonist Bay K 8644. Circulation Research, 62, 563–571.

29. Lagrutta, A., Wang, J., Fermini, B., Salata, J.J. (2006). Novel, potent inhibitors of human Kv1.5 K+ channels and ultrarapidly activating delayed rectifier potassium current. Journal of Pharmacology and Experimental Therapeutics, 317, 1054–1063.

30. Stump, G.L., Wallace, A.A., Regan, C.P., Lynch, J.J. Jr. (2005). In vivo antiarrhythmic and cardiac electrophysiologic effects of a novel diphenylphosphine oxide iKur blocker (2-Isopropyl-5-methylcyclohexyl) diphenylphosphine oxide. Journal of Pharmacological and Experimental Therapeutics, 315, 1362–1367.

31. Regan, C.P., Stump, G.L., Wallace, A.A., Anderson, K.D., McIntyre, C.J., Liverton, N.J., Lynch, J.J. Jr. (2007). In vivo cardiac electrophysiologic and antiarrhythmic effects of an isoquinoline IKur blocker, ISQ-1, in rat, dog, and nonhuman primate. Journal of Cardiovascular Pharmacology, 49, 236–245.

32. Mitcheson, J.S., Chen, J., Lin, M., Culberson, C., Sanguinetti, M.C. (2000). A structural basis for drug-induced long QT syndrome. Proceedings of the National Academy of Sciences USA, 97, 12329–12333.

33. Gout, B., Nichols, A.J., Feuerstein, G.Z., Bril, A. (1995). Antifibrillatory effects of BRL-32872 in anesthetized Yucatan minipigs with regional myocardial ischemia. Journal of Cardiovascular Pharmacology, 26, 636–644.

34. Lynch, J.J. Jr., Heaney, L.A., Wallace, A.A., Gehret, J.R., Selnick, H.G., Stein, R.B. (1990). Suppression of lethal ischemic ventricular arrhythmias by the class III agent E4031 in a canine model of previous myocardial infarction. Journal of Cardiovascular Pharmacology, 15, 764–775.

35. Thale, J., Haverkamp, W., Hindricks, G., Gulker, H. (1987). Comparative investigations on the antiarrhythmic and electrophysiologic effects of class I-IV antiarrhythmic agents following acute coronary artery occlusion. European Heart Journal, 8, 91–98.

36. Guerard, N.C., Traebert, M., Suter, W., Dumotier, B.M. (2008). Selective block of IKs plays a significant role in MAP triangulation induced by IKr block in isolated rabbit heart. Journal of Pharmacological and Toxicological Methods, 58, 32–40.

37. Tseng, G.N. (2001). I(Kr): The hERG channel. Journal of Molecular and Cellular Cardiology, 33, 835–849.

38. Lengyel, C., Varro, A., Tabori, K., Papp, J.G., Baczko, I. (2007). Combined pharmacological block of I(Kr) and I(Ks) increases short-term QT interval variability and provokes torsades de pointes. British Journal of Pharmacology, 151, 941–951.

39. Lynch, J.J. Jr., Houle, M.S., Stump, G.L., Wallace, A.A., Gilberto, D.B., Jahansouz, H., Smith, G.R., Tebben, A.J., Liverton, N.J., Selnick, H.G., Claremon, D.A., Billman, G.E. (1999). Antiarrhythmic efficacy of selective blockade of the cardiac slowly activating delayed rectifier current, IKs, in canine models of malignant ischemic ventricular arrhythmia. Circulation, 100, 1917–1922.

40. Splawski, I., Shen, J., Timothy, K.W., Lehmann, M.H., Priori, S., Robinson, J.L., Moss, A.J., Schwartz, P.J., Towbin, J.A., Vincent, G.M., Keating, M.T. (2000). Spectrum of mutations in Long-QT syndrome genes: KVLQT1, HERG, SCN5A, KCNE1, and KCNE2. Circulation, 102, 1178–1185.

41. Shimizu, W., Antzelevitch, C. (1998). Cellular basis for the ECG features of the LQT1 form of the long-QT syndrome: Effects of beta-adrenergic agonists and antagonists and sodium channel blockers on transmural dispersion of repolarization and torsade de pointes. Circulation, 98, 2314–2322.

42. Rees, S.A., Curtis, M.J. (1993). Specific IK1 blockade: A new antiarrhythmic mechanism? Effect of RP58866 on ventricular arrhythmias in rat, rabbit, and primate. Circulation, 87, 1979–1989.

43. Pogwizd, S.M., Schlotthauer, K., Li, L., Yuan, W., Bers, D.M. (2001). Arrhythmogenesis and contractile dysfunction in heart failure: Roles of sodium-calcium exchange, inward rectifier potassium current, and residual beta-adrenergic responsiveness. Circulation Research, 88, 1159–1167.

44. Hill, J.L., Gettes, L.S. (1980). Effect of acute coronary artery occlusion on local myocardial extracellular K$^+$ activity in swine. Circulation, 61, 768–778.

45. Wang, Z., Fermini, B., Nattel, S. (1995). Effects of flecainide, quinidine, and 4-aminopyridine on transient outward and ultrarapid delayed rectifier currents in human atrial myocytes. Journal of Pharmacological and Experimental Therapeutics, 272, 184–196.

46. Mubagwa, K., Flameng, W., Carmeliet, E. (1994). Resting and action potentials of nonischemic and chronically ischemic human ventricular muscle. Journal of Cardiovascular Electrophysiology, 5, 659–671.

47. Sun, X., Wang, H.-S. (2005). Role of the transient outward current (Ito) in shaping canine ventricular action potential—a dynamic clamp study. Journal of Physiology, 564, 411–419.

48. Lukas, A., Antzelevitch, C. (1993). Differences in the electrophysiological response of canine ventricular epicardium and endocardium to ischemia. Role of the transient outward current. Circulation, 88, 2903–2915.

49. Tsuchihashi, K., Curtis, M.J. (1991). Influence of tedisamil on the initiation and maintenance of ventricular fibrillation: Chemical defibrillation by Ito blockade? Journal of Cardiovascular Pharmacology, 18, 445–456.

50. Brunner, M., Guo, W., Mitchell, G.F., Buckett, P.D., Nerbonne, J.M., Koren, G. (2001). Characterization of mice with a combined suppression of Ito and IK, slow. American Journal of Physiology Heart Circulation Physiology, 281, H1201–1209.

51. Noma, A. (1983). ATP-regulated K+ channels in cardiac muscle. Nature, 305, 147–148.

52. Kleber, A.G., Riegger, C.B., Janse, M.J. (1987). Extracellular K+ and H+ shifts in early ischemia: Mechanisms and relation to changes in impulse propagation. Journal of Molecular and Cellular Cardiology, 19, 35–44.

53. Vanheel, B., Hemptinne, A.d. (1992). Influence of KATP channel modulation on net potassium efflux from ischaemic mammalian cardiac tissue. Cardiovascular Research, 26, 1030–1039.

54. Janse, M.J., Kleber, A.G. (1981). Electrophysiological changes and ventricular arrhythmias in the early phase of regional myocardial ischemia. Circulation Research, 49, 1069–1081.

55. Billman, G.E. (2008). The cardiac sarcolemmal ATP-sensitive potassium channel as a novel target for anti-arrhythmic therapy. Pharmacology & Therapeutics, 120, 54–70.

56. Billman, G.E., Avendano, C.E., Halliwill, J.R., Burroughs, J.M. (1993). The effects of the ATP-dependent potassium channel antagonist, glyburide, on coronary blood flow and susceptibility to ventricular fibrillation in unanesthetized dogs. Journal of Cardiovascular Pharmacology, 21, 197–204.

57. Gwilt, M., Henderson, C.G., Orme, J., Rourke, J.D. (1992). Effects of drugs on ventricular fibrillation and ischaemic K + loss in a model of ischaemia in perfused guinea-pig hearts in vitro. European Journal of Pharmacology, 220, 231–236.

58. D'Alonzo, A.J., Darbenzio, R.B., Hess, T.A., Sewter, J.C., Sleph, P.G., Grover, G.J. (1994). Effect of potassium on the action of the KATP modulators cromakalim, pinacidil, or glibenclamide on arrhythmias in isolated perfused rat heart subjected to regional ischaemia. Cardiovascular Research, 28, 881–887.

59. Rees, S.A., Curtis, M.J. (1995). Pharmacological analysis in rat of the role of the ATP-sensitive potassium channel as a potential target for antifibrillatory intervention in acute myocardial ischaemia. Journal of Cardiovascular Pharmacology, 26, 280–288.

60. Winter, S.A., Williams, K.I., Woodward, B. (1993). Detrimental effect of glibenclamide during ischemia and reperfusion in the isolated rat heart. British Journal of Pharmacology, 109, 42P.

61. Garlid, K.D., Paucek, P., Yarov-Yarovoy, V., Murray, H.N., Darbenzio, R.B., D'Alonzo, A.J., Lodge, N.J., Smith, M.A., Grover, G.J. (1997). Cardioprotective effect of diazoxide and its interaction with mitochondrial ATP-sensitive K + channels: Possible mechanism of cardioprotection. Circulation Research, 81, 1072–1082.

62. Billman, G.E., Englert, H.C., Scholkens, B.A. (1998). HMR 1883, a novel cardioselective inhibitor of the ATP-sensitive potassium channel. Part II: Effects on susceptibility to ventricular fibrillation induced by myocardial ischemia in conscious dogs. Journal of Pharmacology and Experimental Therapeutics, 286, 1465–1473.

CHAPTER 14

Cardiac Sarcolemmal ATP-sensitive Potassium Channel Antagonists: A Class of Drugs that May Selectively Target the Ischemic Myocardium

GEORGE E. BILLMAN

14.1 INTRODUCTION

To develop agents that will reduce cardiac mortality, one must first identify those factors that trigger the malignant arrhythmias responsible for these deaths. Ventricular tachyarrhythmias are known to be responsible for most sudden cardiac deaths [1–3]; yet only a minority of these patients had a known history of heart disease prior to the collapse. Postmortem examinations revealed that up to 90% of all sudden death patients were subsequently shown to have underlying coronary artery disease [4]. Furthermore, scar tissue from a previous infarction was found in one third of the victims of sudden death [5], and it was estimated that myocardial ischemia was responsible for up to 80% of the deaths in these patients [6]. Thus, it is likely that myocardial ischemia plays a crucial role in the induction of the lethal arrhythmias in these patients. If this hypothesis is correct, then it is crucial to identify the factor or factors that render the ischemic myocardium vulnerable to arrhythmia formation. Once identified, it should then be possible to develop therapeutic interventions that correct these ischemically induced changes in cardiac electrical stability and, thereby, prevent sudden death. The most effective antiarrhythmic agents would be those that target the ischemic myocardium with little or no action on the normal (i.e., nonischemic) cardiac tissue. As a consequence of this selectivity, one would expect that these drugs should also have a low propensity for proarrhythmic events and other off-target actions.

Novel Therapeutic Targets for Antiarrhythmic Drugs, Edited by George Edward Billman

It is well established that myocardial ischemia provokes abnormalities in the biochemical homeostasis of individual cardiac cells. These intracellular changes culminate in the disruption of cellular electrophysiologic properties, and as a result, life-threatening alterations in cardiac rhythm, such as ventricular fibrillation, frequently occur. Several different chemical substances have been proposed as possible causative factors in the genesis of ventricular fibrillation during myocardial ischemia, including catecholamines, amphiphilic products of lipid metabolism, various peptides, cytosolic calcium accumulation, and increases in extracellular potassium [7–9]. An accumulating body of evidence suggests that the activation of specific potassium channels, the adenosine triphosphate (ATP)-sensitive potassium channels, leads to potassium efflux from the ischemic cells thereby inducing the electrophysiologic changes that are ultimately responsible for the formation of lethal cardiac arrhythmias [10–12]. As such, drugs that selectively inhibit these channels should prove to be particularly effective in the prevention of sudden cardiac death. Therefore, this chapter will first discuss the relationship between ischemically induced alterations in extracellular potassium and arrhythmia formation and then evaluate the antiarrhythmic potential of ATP-sensitive potassium channel antagonists, drugs that may act selectively on the ischemic myocardium.

14.2 EFFECTS OF MYOCARDIAL ISCHEMIA ON EXTRACELLULAR POTASSIUM

Myocardial ischemia provokes both rapid increases in extracellular potassium and reductions in action potential duration. Harris and co-workers [13, 14] were the first to show that extracellular potassium rises dramatically after coronary artery ligation, which correlates with the onset of ventricular arrhythmias. They [13, 14] and others [15] further demonstrated that intracoronary injections of potassium chloride provoked electrocardiographic (ECG) changes and triggered ventricular arrhythmias similar to those induced by myocardial ischemia. They proposed that changes in extracellular potassium represented a major factor in the development of malignant arrhythmias during ischemia. Subsequent studies that used ion selective electrodes to measure potassium activity directly have confirmed these earlier observations [16–18]. Extracellular potassium increased within the first 15 s and reached a plateau within 5 to 10 min after the interruption of coronary perfusion [16–19]. Furthermore, regional differences or heterogeneities of potassium accumulation were recorded, accompanied by corresponding differences in ventricular electrical activity [16, 17, 19, 20]. This extracellular potassium accumulation resulted primarily from increases in potassium efflux rather than from decreased potassium influx caused by inhibition of the Na^+/K^+-ATPase [21–23].

A growing body of evidence demonstrates that the ischemically induced potassium accumulation and the corresponding reductions in action potential duration result primarily from the opening of ATP-sensitive potassium channels [24]. Using the patch clamp technique, Trube and Hescheler [25] were the first to record single ATP-sensitive potassium channel activity. Noma [26] and Trube and Hescheler [25] demonstrated that reductions in cellular ATP induced by cyanide exposure evoked an outward potassium current. The regulation of this channel has proven to be complex and beyond the scope of the present review. A detailed presentation of the biophysical regulation of this channel has been recently reviewed [27, 28]. To simplify, this channel is inhibited by cellular ATP but activated (opened) by adenosine diphosphate (ADP) [29–32]. Thus, as ATP levels fall and ADP levels increase during myocardial ischemia, the ATP-sensitive potassium channel opens and potassium leaves the cell. As such, the activation of an ATP-sensitive potassium channel might be responsible for the reductions in action potential duration induced by hypoxia. Indeed, several studies have implicated the activation of this current in the changes in cardiac action potential and extracellular potassium accumulation during myocardial ischemia [33–43]. The ATP-sensitive potassium channel inhibitor, glibenclamide, for example, has been shown either to attenuate or to abolish reductions in action potential duration in hypoxic myocytes [34, 35], isolated cardiac tissue [38–40, 42, 43], and regionally or globally ischemic hearts [33, 37, 44]. This sulfonylurea drug also reduced extracellular potassium accumulation induced by ischemia [30, 40–42]. Conflicting results have been obtained with ATP-sensitive potassium channel agonists. The ATP-sensitive potassium channel agonists (pinacidil, cromakalim) exacerbated ischemically induced reductions in action potential duration, as well as promoted extracellular potassium accumulation [33–35, 37–40, 44–47]. In contrast, there are a few reports in which ATP-sensitive potassium channel openers failed to alter extracellular potassium accumulation during ischemia [40, 43, 48]. Furthermore, Saito and co-workers [49] demonstrated that, although reductions in action potential duration induced by myocardial ischemia were significantly attenuated in ATP-sensitive potassium channel knockout mice, ischemia provoked similar increases in extracellular potassium in the knockout and wild-type mice. These data suggest that the activation of an ATP-sensitive potassium channel plays a significant role in the electrophysiological consequences of ischemia but is not solely responsible for the extracellular potassium that accompanies disruptions in myocardial perfusion. Other factors including sodium-activated potassium channels, the delayed rectifier potassium channel, potassium chloride ion cotransport, and lactate transport could contribute to extracellular potassium accumulation during ischemia [50–53].

It must also be emphasized that the ATP-sensitive potassium channel is activated only at low ATP concentrations with half maximum suppression of channel opening at $20\text{--}100\,\mu M$ [25–27, 54, 55]; yet intracellular concentrations are normally much higher (5–10 mM). Furthermore, cytosolic ATP levels remain in the millimolar range for the first 10 min of hypoxia, well after potassium accumulation begins [23, 56]. Therefore, the role that this channel plays in the response to myocardial ischemia can be questioned [24]. Several studies provide an explanation for this apparent paradox. Cardiac tissue contains a very high density of ATP-sensitive potassium channels. As a consequence, only a small increase in the open state probability ($<1\%$ of maximum) was required to shorten action potential duration during ischemia [27, 57–59]. Indeed, Faivre and Findlay [57] found, in guinea pig myocytes, that the opening of only 30 channels (less than 1% of the population) provoked a 50% reduction in action potential duration. They concluded that "physiologically relevant activity of the K_{ATP}

channel in cardiac membrane is confined to a very small percentage of the possible cell K_{ATP} current, and thus, intracellular ATP would not have to fall very far before the opening of K_{ATP} channels would influence cardiac excitability" [57]. In a similar manner, Deutsch et al. [60] correlated potassium current during hypoxia in an intact rabbit papillary muscle. They showed that during hypoxia, a significant shortening of action potential duration (blocked by glibenclamide) occurred when tissue ATP levels fell by approximately 25%. They also concluded that only modest changes in cellular ATP were required to induce major changes in cardiac electrical properties.

The activation of the ATP-sensitive potassium channel may also contribute significantly to the ST segment changes associated with myocardial ischemia. In anesthetized open chest dogs [61], the intracoronary injection of the ATP-sensitive potassium channel opener, pinacidil, elicited elevations in the ST segment very similar to those induced by myocardial ischemia. Abnormal electrocardiographic

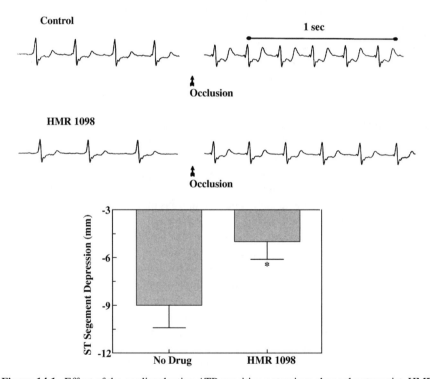

Figure 14.1. Effect of the cardioselective ATP-sensitive potassium channel antagonist, HMR 1098 on ischemic ECG changes. Representative recordings of the same animal before and on subsequent day alter HMR 1098 (3.0 mg/kg, i.v.). The bottom panel is composite data (n = 20) on the ST-depression induced by the myocardial ischemia (2 min left circumflex coronary artery occlusion conscious dogs). *P < 0.01 no drug versus HMR 1098.

(T-wave) changes suggestive of alterations of repolarization have also been reported in up to 30% of patients taking pinacidil as an antihypertensive medication [62]. Conversely, glibenclamide attenuated the ST segment elevations induced by the occlusion of the left anterior descending coronary artery [63]. Similar results were obtained in conscious dogs. Billman et al. [64] demonstrated that either glibenclamide or the cardioselective ATP-sensitive potassium channel antagonist HMR 1098 attenuated ischemically induced ST segment changes (Figure 14.1). They further reported that these drugs prevented ischemically induced increases in the descending portion of the T wave (an index of the dispersion of repolarization, [65, 66]) (Figure 14.2). In a similar manner, myocardial ischemia failed to alter the ECG of mice in which the Kir 6.2 gene (the gene responsible for the pore-forming subunit of the cardiac ATP-sensitive potassium channel, [67]) had been removed [68]. The large changes in the ECG that were induced by ligation of the left coronary artery in the wild-type control mice could be suppressed by prior treatment with the cardioselective ATP-sensitive potassium channel antagonist HMR 1098 [68]. It therefore seems likely that the activation of the ATP-sensitive potassium channel contributes significantly to alterations in cardiac electrical stability induced by myocardial ischemia, which leads to the formation of malignant arrhythmias.

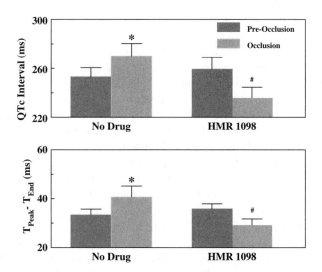

Figure 14.2. Effect of the cardioselective ATP-sensitive potassium channel antagonist, HMR 1098 on ischemically induced changes in indices of repolarization in conscious dogs ($n = 20$). Coronary occlusion (2 min left circumflex coronary artery occlusion) elicited significant increases in both QT interval corrected for hear rate (QT_C) and the descending portion of the T wave (Tpeak–Tend). Note that this increase was completed attenuated by the prior treatment with HMR 1098. *$P < 0.01$ preocclusion versus occlusion; #$P < 0.01$ No drug versus HMR 1098.

14.3   EFFECT OF EXTRACELLULAR POTASSIUM ON VENTRICULAR RHYTHM

Cardiac arrhythmias can result from either abnormal impulse generation or abnormal impulse conduction [69, see also Chapter 4]. The extracellular accumulation of potassium induced by myocardial ischemia can provoke these perturbations in cardiac electrical activity. Elevations in extracellular potassium promote the depolarization of the tissue surrounding the ischemic regions, as noted above. The flow of this injury current (electrotonic current flow between ischemic and normal cells) has been implicated as a potential cause for the initiation of premature ventricular beats. Under normal conditions, ventricular cells do not display a spontaneous rhythm. However, an automatic rhythm can be produced when the cells are partially depolarized [69, see also Chapter 4]. Coronel et al. [20, 70], in fact, demonstrated an increased excitability of normal tissue near the border of the ischemia, a region of the heart in which extracellular potassium concentrations were also increased.

Changes in action potential duration induced by alterations in potassium efflux can also provoke abnormalities of impulse conduction. As noted, increased potassium efflux from ischemic tissue triggers a reduction in action potential duration. A major factor contributing to ventricular fibrillation, particularly during myocardial ischemia, is a dispersion or heterogeneity of the refractory period that is related to regional differences in action potential duration [69, see also Chapter 4]. This allows for the fragmentation of impulse conduction during ensuing beats. As noted, the activation of the ATP-sensitive potassium channel produced large reductions in action potential duration [33–40, 42–44], which are inhibited by glibenclamide [33–35, 37–39, 44] but exacerbated by ATP-sensitive potassium channel agonists [40, 45, 71–73]. A differential ATP sensitivity of the ATP-dependent potassium channel has also been reported between endocardial and epicardial cells during ischemia such that smaller reductions in ATP were necessary to activate potassium channels located in epicardial tissue [74]. As a result, a heterogeneity in extracellular potassium and refractory period, as well as a gradient in action potential duration, was recorded between the epicardial and the endocardial tissue [74–76]. Nonuniformities in the refractory period could set the stage for the formation of irregular reentrant pathways and ventricular arrhythmias. In a similar manner, the ATP-sensitive potassium channel antagonist glibenclamide was shown to attenuate ischemically induced reductions in the refractory period [64, 77]. In contrast, activation of the ATP-sensitive potassium current with pinacidil elicited a marked dispersion of repolarization and refractory period between the epicardium and the endocardium, leading to the development of extrasystoles [78]. These effects could be abolished by glibenclamide [78]. Coromilas et al. [79] further demonstrated that the pinacidil restored excitability in the tissue adjacent to the ischemic region (i.e., the epicardial border zone). This reactivation of formerly inexcitable tissue led to the formation of reentrant circuits and the induction of ventricular tachycardia. Thus, the activation of the ATP-sensitive potassium channel could contribute significantly to the induction of malignant arrhythmias by changing impulse generation (depolarization induced changes in automaticity), conduction (refractory period dispersion), or a combination of both.

14.4   EFFECT OF ATP-SENSITIVE POTASSIUM CHANNEL ANTAGONISTS ON VENTRICULAR ARRHYTHMIAS

As noted, it is now generally accepted that the activation of the ATP-sensitive potassium channel during myocardial ischemia provokes a potassium efflux and reductions in action potential duration that lead to dispersion of repolarization. Since heterogeneity of repolarization plays a crucial role in the induction of ventricular fibrillation, drugs that prevent ATP-sensitive potassium channel activation should be particularly effective in the suppression of malignant arrhythmias induced by ischemia

14.4.1   Nonselective ATP-Sensitive Potassium Channel Antagonist

The sulfonylurea drug glibenclamide prevented hypoxia-induced reductions in action potential duration in single cells, isolated hearts, and intact animals [33, 34, 37–40, 42–44, 80–84]. Furthermore, glibenclaimide reduced the regional differences in action potential duration induced by hypoxia [74] and attenuated the ischemically induced changes in the ST segment in intact anesthetized or unanesthetized animals [63, 64]. Therefore, one would predict that glibenclamide should also prevent arrhythmias that develop as a consequence of these ischemically induced changes in cardiac electrical properties.

   Glibenclamide prevented arrhythmias induced by ischemia in a variety of experimental models (Table 14.1). For example, this drug abolished ventricular arrhythmias

Table 14.1.   Effect of Nonselective ATP-sensitive Potassium Channel Antagonist on Ischemic Cardiac Arrhythmias—Preclinical Studies

Model	Result	Reference
Rabbit heart	↓ VF	Pogatsa et al. [85]
Rat heart	↓ VF	Wolleben et al. [86]
Rat heart	↓ VF	Kantor et al. [37]
Dog and rabbit heart	No Effect	Smallwood et al. [44]
Guinea pig heart	↓ VF Duration	Gwilt et al. [87]
Anesthetized rat	↓ VF	Zhang et al. [88]
Rat heart	↓ VF Duration	Bril et al. [89]
Guinea pig tissue	↓ Re-entrant PVCs	Pasnani and Ferrier [90]
Conscious dog	↓ VF	Billman et al. [64, 91]
Rat heart	↓ VF	Tosaki et al. [92]
Rat heart	No Effect	Rees and Curtis [93]
Conscious rat	↓ VF	Lepran et al. [94]
Anesthetized rat	↓ VF	Baczko et al. [95]
Anesthetized rabbit	↓ VF	Barrett and Walker [96]
Anesthetized rat	↓ VF	El Reyani et al. [97]
Rabbit reart	↓ VF	Dhein et al. [81]
Conscious sheep	↑ reperfusion arrhythmias	del Valle et al. [98]
Anesthetized rat	↓ VF	Vajda et al. [99]

VF = Ventricular Fibrillation, PVCs = Premature Ventricular Contractions (activations).

induced by ischemia in isolated hearts [37, 81, 85–87, 92] or terminated ventricular fibrillation [87, 89] induced by myocardial ischemia in isolated hearts. Furthermore, both glibenclamide and glimepride reduced blood glucose and decreased the incidence of irreversible ventricular fibrillation induced by reperfusion (after a 6-min coronary occlusion) in anestheized rats [81, 88, 97, 99]. Glibenclamide also reduced the incidence of life-threatening arrhythmias induced by coronary artery ligation in the conscious rat [94] and anesthetized rabbit [96], as well as improved survival in anethetized rats during ischemia and reperfusion [95]. This drug also inhibited arrhythmias associated with the intracellular calcium overload induced by ouabain [88, 100]. Billman et al. [64, 91] further demonstrated that glibenclamide prevented ventricular fibrillation induced by the combination of acute ischemia during submaximal exercise in animals previously shown to be susceptible to sudden death (Figure 14.3). In contrast, glibenclamide failed to prevent ventricular tachyarrhythmias associated with reperfusion in anesthetized dogs (Billman, unpublished observation) and increased these reperfusion arrhtyhmias in conscious sheep [98]. It should also be noted that in conscious dogs glibenclamide significantly reduced both the exercise and reactive hyperemia induced increases in coronary blood flow, as well as depressed ventricular function (large reductions in left ventricular dP/dt maximum) [64, 91] (Figure 14.4). In the isolated working rabbit heart, glibenclamide provoked an immediate decrease in coronary blood flow reducing forward flow to zero [73]. Thus, glibenclamide both impairs ventricular contraction (negative inotropy) and exerts potent vasoconstrictor effects caused by the inhibiton of ATP-sensitive potassium channels located on the coronary vascular smooth muscle.

A few clinical studies illustrate the antiarrhythmic potential of ATP-sensitive potassium channels (Table 14.2). Cacciapuoti et al. [101] found that glibenclamide significantly reduced the frequency and severity of ventricular arrhythmias recorded during transient ischemia in non-insulin-dependent diabetic patients with coronary artery disease. This drug, however, did not affect nonischemic arrhythmias nor did it change the number or the length of the ischemic episodes. Glibenclamide significantly reduced the incidence of ventricular fibrillation in non-insulin-dependent diabetic patients with acute myocardial infarction [102]. The effects of sulfonylurea drugs on the incidence of ventricular arrhtyhmias (24-hr Holter monitoring) has also been evaluated in nondiabetic and diabetic patients with decompensated congestive heart failure [105]. These authors found that diabetic patients receiving sulfonylurea agents (glbenclamide or glipizide) exhibited a significantly lower incidence of both repetitive ventricular beats and runs of nonsustained ventricular tachycardia as compared with either nondiabetic patients or diabetic patients who did not receive sulfonlyurea drugs. Sulonyurea drugs attenuated the ST segment elevation during acute myocardial infarction in diabetic pateints [106].

It is important to emphasize that glibenclamide is not selective for cardiac tissue. As noted, this drug can profoundly reduce coronary blood flow via actions on vascular smooth muscle and can promote insulin release, thereby provoking hypoglycemia [64, 91]. These noncardiac actions would limit the antiarrhythmic potential of glibenclamide in the clinic. Cardioselective compounds should have fewer side

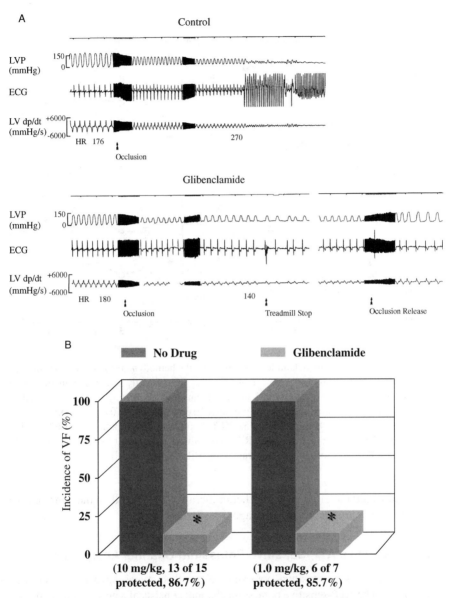

Figure 14.3. Effect of glibenclamide on susceptibility to ventricular fibrillation in a conscious canine model of sudden cardiac death. Panel A. Representative recordings before and after pretreatment with the ATP-sensitive potassium channel antagonist glibenclamide (10 mg/kg, i.v.) in the same dog. Note that glibenclamide abolished ventricular fibrillation induced by the combination of acute myocardial ischemia and exercise in dogs with healed myocardial infarctions. However, this drug provoked large reductions in left ventricular dP/dt and heart rate (HR). LVP = left ventricular pressure. Panel B. Composite data. Glibenclamide at either a high dose (10 mg/kg, i.v) or a low dose (1.0 mg/kg, i.v) significantly reduced the incidence of ventricular fibrillation protecting 13 of 15 and 6 of 7 dogs, respectively. $*P < 0.01$ glibenclamide versus no drug. (panel A, reprinted with permission, Billman et al. [91])

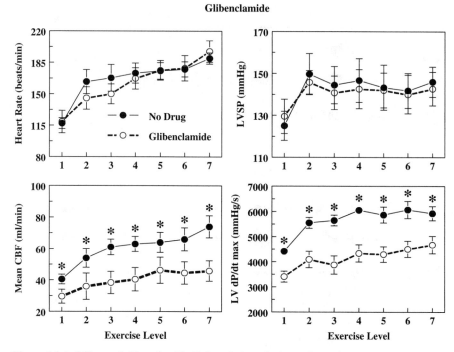

Figure 14.4. Effects of glibenclamide (1.0 mg/kg) on the hemodynamic response to submaximal exercise in conscious dogs. Note that this drug significantly reduced both the mean coronary blood flow (CBF) and left ventricular dP/dt (an index of inotropy) increases elicited by exercise. LVSP = left ventricular systolic pressure, Exercise levels: 1, 0%grade/0 kph; 2, 0%/4.8 kph; 3, 0%/6.4 kph; 4, 4%/6.4 kph; 5, 8%/6.4 kph; 6, 12%/6.4 kph; 7, 16%/6.4 kph.* $P < 0.01$ no drug versus glibenclamide. (Reprinted with permission of the American Society for Pharmacology and Experimental Therapeutics, Billman et al. [64])

effects and would therefore provide a better therapeutic option than the nonselective ATP-sensitive potassium channel antagonist glibenclamide.

14.4.2   Selective ATP-Sensitive Potassium Channel Antagonist

Several different ATP-sensitive potassium channel subtypes have been identified (Table 14.3). The ATP-sensitive potassium channel consists of a pore-forming subunit coupled to a sulfonylurea receptor [27, 113, 118–122]. The functional channel forms as a hetero-octomer composed of a tetramer of the pore and four sulfonyl receptor subunits. At present, two different pore-forming subunits have been identified, both of which produce an inward rectifier potassium current (Kir 6.1 and Kir 6.2) [68, 107]. Three different sulfonylurea receptor subtypes have been isolated: SUR1 (on pancreatic islet cells), SUR2A (on cardiac tissue), and SUR2B (on vascular smooth muscle) [119, 121, 123, 124]. Thus, six different potassium channel pore and sulfonylurea receptor combinations are possible (Table 14.3). Suzuki et al. [67] and

Table 14.2. Effect of Nonselective ATP-sensitive Potassium Channel Antagonists on Cardiac Arrhythmias – Clinical Studies

Patient Population	Result	Reference
Non-insulin-dependent diabetics treated with glibenclamide (n = 19)	Significant reduction in the frequency of PVCs and nonsustained VT	Cacciapuoti et al. [101]
Non-insulin-dependent diabetics (n = 232, 106 treated with glibenclamide, 126 with other hypoglycemic drugs) and nondiabetic patients all with acute myocardial infarction	Incidence of VF or sustained VT reduced in the glibenclamide treated patients. Cardiovascular mortality highest in non-glibenclamide treated diabetic patients	Lomuscio et al. [102] Lomuscio and Fiorentini [103]
Retrospective analysis of acute myocardial infarction patients (n = 5,715,745 diabetic patients)	VF rates similar in non-diabetic (11.0%) and diabetic patients taking glibenclamide (11.8%) but much higher in diabetic patients taking gliclazide (18%) or insulin (22.8%)	Davis et al. [104]
Diabetic patients with decompensated heart failure (n = 207)	Significant reduction in incidence of repetitive ventricular beats and nonsustained VT in patients treated with either glibenclamide or glipizide	Aronson et al. [105]

VF = Ventricular Fibrillation, VT = Ventricular Tachycardia, PVCs = Premature Ventricular Contractions (activations).

Manning-Fox et al. [120] recently demonstrated that Kir 6.2 and Kir 6.1 were required for cardiac and vascular smooth muscle ATP-sensitive potassium channel activity, respectively. They concluded that Kir 6.2/SUR2A most likely forms the cardiac cell membrane ATP-sensitive potassium channel, whereas Kir 6.1/SUR2B is located on vascular smooth muscle. In a similar manner, Lui et al. [107] reported that the actitivy to mitochondrial ATP-sensitive potassium channels was most closely mimicked by the Kir 6.1/SUR1 subtype, an conclusion that has not yet been confirmed [108]. A present, neither a specific action nor a traget tissue has been definitely identified for Kir6.1/SUR2A. However, overexpression of this channel is proarrhythmic and promotes premature death in transgenic mice [117]. Thus, cardiac sarcolemmal ATP-sensitive potassium channel hyperactivity decreases the electrical stability of the heart.

Given this apparent tissue specificity and the limited number of possible channel-receptor pairings, it should be possible to develop compounds that selectively inhibit (or activate) a particular ATP-sensitive potassium channel subtype. In particular, a drug that selectively blocks the Kir 6.2/SUR2A subtype should prevent ischemically

Table 14.3. Possible ATP-sensitive Potassium Channel Subtypes: Combinations of the Pore-Forming Units (Kir 6.1 or Kir 6.2) and the Sulphonylurea Receptors (SUR1, SUR2A, and SUR2B)

Channel	Tissue	Effect of Activation	Effect of Inhibition	Reference
Kir6.1/SUR1	Mitochondria?	Ischemic preconditioning	Prevents ischemic preconditioning	Liu et al. [107] Foster et al. [108]
Kir6.1/SUR2B	Vascular smooth muscle & coronary endothelial cells	Vasodilation & increase blood flow	Prevent vasodilation, promote vasoconstriction	Suzuki et al. [67] Schnitzler et al. [109]
Kir6.2/SUR1	Pancreatic β-cells	Hyperpolarization, Decreased insulin secretion	Insulin secretion, hypoglycemia	Aguilar-Bryan et al. [110] Koster et al., [111]
Kir6.2/SUR1	Neurons	Reduce excitability or neurotransmitter release	Increase excitability or neurotransmitter release	Liss and Roeper [112]
Kir6.2/SUR2A	Cardiac muscle	Decrease action potential duration	Prevent decrease in action potential duration	Inagaki et al. [113]
Kir6.2/SUR2A	Skeletal muscle	Prevent glucose uptake—fatigue	Glucose uptake	Chutkow et al. [114] Gong et al. [115]
Kir6.2/SUR2B	Nonvascular smooth muscle	Muscle relaxation (e.g., urinary bladder tone)	Prevent muscle relaxation	Gopalakrishnan et al. [116]

Note that neither specific actions nor a target tissue for Kir6.1/SUR2A have yet been identified. However, overexpression of this channel is proarrhythmic [117].

induced changes in cardiac electrical properties (e.g., reductions in action potential duration) and thereby prevent arrhythmias without the untoward side effects noted for the nonselective ATP-sensitive channel antagonist glibenclamide.

14.4.2.1 HMR 1883, a Cardioselective ATP-Potassium Channel Antagonist.

The sulfonylthiourea drug (1-[5-[2-5-chloro-o-ansamide)ethyl]2-methoxyphenyl]sulfonyl]-3-methylthiourea) HMR 1883 and its sodium salt HMR 1098 were recently developed to block the cardiac ATP-sensitive potassium channel [125]. HMR 1883 inhibited the sarcolemmal cardiac ATP-sensitive potassium channel activated by the channel opener rilmakalim at a much lower concentration (guinea pig myocytes $IC_{50} = 0.6–2.2\,\mu M$) than was required to promote insulin release (9–50-fold higher concentration was required to block rat pancreatic insulinoma, RIN m5F, cells) [126]. In a similar manner, HMR 1098 reversed the action potential shortening induced by rilmakalim in human cardiomycytes ($IC_{50} = 0.42 \pm 0.008\,\mu M$) and proved to be more potent in acidic condtions ($IC_{50} = 0.24 \pm 0.009\,\mu M$) as would occur during myocardial ischemia [126] Indeed, this drug attenuated hypoxia-induced shortening of cardiac action potential in rat and guinea pig tissue [127]. In contrast to glibenclamide, HMR 1883 did not alter hypoxia-induced increases in coronary blood flow in Langendorff perfused guinea pig hearts [127, 128]. HMR 1098 also inhibited Rb + efflux through Kir 6.2/SUR2A channels expressed in HEK293 cells (IC_{50} 181 nM), demonstrating that this system may be used to screen for compounds with a high affinity for the cardiac sarcolemmal channel [128]. Significantly, HMR 1883 did not alter flavoprotein autofluorescence, an index of mitochondrial redox state [129]. In contrast, 5-hydroxydecanoic acid, a selective blocker of mitochondrial channels, completely inhibited the flavoprotein fluorescence [130, 131]. In agreement with these *in vitro* findings, HMR 1883 did not prevent the cardioprotective effects induced by ischemic preconditioning in either rat [132] or rabbit [131, 133–135]. Accumulating evidence suggests that the activation of mitochondrial ATP-sensitive potassium channels plays a crucial role in the mechanical protection that results from ischemic preconditioning [136–138]. As noted, Liu et al. [107] demonstrated the mitochondrial ATP-sensitive potassium channel closely resembles the Kir 6.1/SUR1 subtype. Thus, HMR 1883 can inhibit cardiac membrane ATP-sensitive potassium channels with miminal effects on mitochondrial channels.

HMR 1883 also prevented ischemically induced changes in the ST segment in anesthetized mice [68], anesthetized swine [139], or conscious dogs (Figure 14.1) [140]. A similar response was also noted for glibenclamide but not for 5-hydroxydecanoic acid [141]. In the conscious dogs with healed myocardial infarctions, both HMR 1883 and glibenclamide prevented ischemically induced reductions in the effective refractory period [64]. Furthermore, HMR 1883 significantly reduced monophasic action potential shortening induced by coronary artery occlusion in anesthetized pigs [142] and prevented an ischemically induced dispersion of ventricular repolarization in isolated Langendorff perfused rabbit hearts [143].

As would be predicted based on these electrophysiological actions, HMR 1883/ 1098 prevented ischemically induced arrhtyhmias in most, but not all [144], animal models (Table 14.4). For example, HMR 1883 reduced cardiac mortality in

Table 14.4. Effect of Cardioselective ATP-sensitive Potassium Channel Antagonists on Ischemic Cardiac Arrhythmias

Model	Result	Reference
Anesthetized pig	HMR 1883, ↓ VF	Bohn et al. [145]
Conscious dog	HMR 1883, ↓ VF	Billman et al. [64]
Anesthetized pig	HMR 1883, ↓ VF	Wirth et al. [139]
Anesthetized rat	HMR 1883, ↓ VF	Wirth et al. [146]
Anesthetized dog	HMR 1098, ↓ Arrhythmias Induced by Programmed Electrical Stimulation dogs with Healed Myocardial Infarctions	Zhu et al. [147]
Rabbit heart	HMR 1098 ↓ VF by Programmed Electrical Stimulation	Behrens et al. [143]
Rabbit heart	HMR 1098, ↓ VF induced by pinacidil	Fischbach et al. [148]
Conscious dog	HMR 1402, ↓ VF	Billman et al. [149]
Rat heart	HMR 1098, No Effect	Gok et al. [144]
Anesthetized rat	HMR 1098 ↓ VF	Vajda et al. [92]

VF = Ventricular Fibrillation.

anesthetized pigs [139, 145] and prevented ventricular fibrillation induced by myocardial ischemia and reperfusion in rats [146]. HMR 1098 also significantly reduced arrhythmias induced by programmed electrical stimulation in dogs with healed myocardial infarctions without altering blood glucose levels [147]. In a similar manner, both glibenclamide and HMR 1883 (Figure 14.5 & 14.6) [64], but not 5-hydoxydecanoic acid (Figure 14.6 & 14.7) [141], significantly reduced the incidence of ventricular fibrillation induced by myocardial ischemia in conscious dogs with healed anterior wall myocardial infarctions. HMR 1098, but not 5-hydoxydecanoic acid, also prevented ventricular fibrillation induced by the ATP-sensitive potassium channel agonist pinacidil in isolated rabbit hearts subjected to hypoxic perfusion [148]. These data strongly suggest that the selective opening of sarcolemmal ATP-sensitive potassium channels during ischemia provokes ventricular fibrillation, whereas activation of the mitochodrial channels does not. Since, as noted, ischemic preconditioning may result, at least in part, from the activation of mitochondrial channels, it may be possible to develop drugs that selectively activate these channels. However, nonspecific ATP-sensitive potassium channel agonists should be avoided because of the enhanced risk for malignant arrhythmias that would result from the activation of the sarcolemmal channels.

In contrast to glibenclamide, HMR 1883 did not alter plasma insulin or blood glucose levels in these animals (Figure 14.8) [64, 91]. Furthermore, glibenclamide but not HMR 1883 significantly reduced an exercise-induced increase in mean cornary blood flow and provoked large reductions in left ventricular dP/dt maximum (both at rest and during exercise, Figure 14.9) [64, 91]. Thus, HMR 1883 seems to act selectively on the cardiac cell membrane ATP-sensitive potassium channel and thereby prevents ischemically induced arrhythmias with minimal effects on either pancreatic or smooth muscle channels.

Control

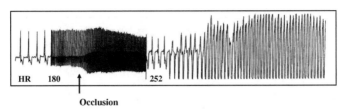

HMR 1098

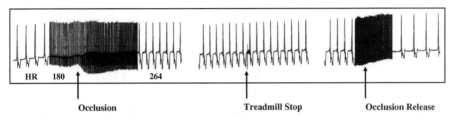

Figure 14.5. Effect of the cardioselective ATP-sensitive potassium channel antagonist, HMR 1098, on susceptibility to ventricular fibrillation in a conscious canine model of sudden cardiac death. Representative recordings from the same dog are displayed before and after pretreatment with the ATP-sensitive potassium channel antagonist HMR 1098 (3.0 mg/kg, i.v.). HMR 1098 abolished ventricular fibrillation induced by the combination of acute myocardial ischemia and exercise in dogs with healed myocardial infarctions, protecting 16 of 20 dogs tested. (Reprinted with permission of the American Society for Pharmacology and Experimental Therapeutics, Billman et al. [64])

14.4.2.2 HMR 1402, a Cardioselective ATP-Sensitive Potassium Antagonist.

As noted, at least six different K_{ATP} channels are possible and further that the Kir 6.2/SUR2A combination is restricted to cardiac muscle [67, 120]. Thus, substances that preferentially inhibit this channel should display selectivity for cardiac tissue. Recently, a second cardioselective ATP-sensitive potassium channel antagonist, HMR 1402, 1-[[5-[2(5-chloro-o-anisamido)ethyl]-β-methoxyethoxyphe-nyl]sulfonyl]-3-methylthioura, has been developed [121]. This compound is structurally similar to HMR 1883/1098. As was noted for HMR 1883/1098, HMR 1402 had no significant effects on action potential duration (APD_{90}), the resting potential, the amplitude of the phase 1 of the action potential, or on the upstroke velocity [149]. These data suggest that HMR 1402 did not affect potassium channels (i.e., I_{K1}, I_K, and I_{Ks}) or the sodium channel at rest. This conclusion that was directly confirmed by patch clamp experiments performed in either rat or guinea pig ventricular myocytes [149]. In contrast, HMR 1402 potently blocked the rilmaka-lim-activated K_{ATP} channels in both guinea pig papillary muscles and rat ventricular myocytes [149]. At an external pH of 6.0, this inhibition was approximately 6.1 times more potent than that reported for HMR 1883 (IC_{50} for HMR 1402: 98 nM, 123, vs. IC_{50} for HMR 1883: 0.6 μM, [127]). Similarly, hypoxia consistently elicited a marked reduction in APD_{90} that was potently antagonized by HMR 1402 [128, 149]. This

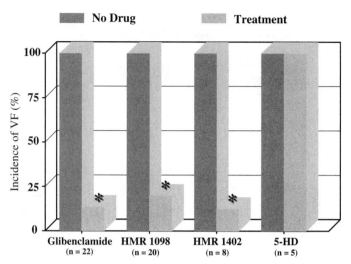

Figure 14.6. The effect of ATP-sensitive potassium channel antagonists on the susceptibility to ventricular fibrillation in a canine model of sudden cardiac death. Ventricular fibrillation was induced by a combination of acute myocardial ischemia during submaximal exercise in dogs with healed myocardial infarctions. The nonselective antagonist glibenclamide (1.0 or 10 mg/kg, i.v.) protected 19 of 22; the cardioselective antagonists, HMR 1098 (3.0 mg/kg), and HMR 1402 (3.0 mg/kg, i.v.) protected 16 of 20 and 7 of 8 dogs, respectively. In contrast, the mitochondrial selective antagonist 5-hydroxydecanoic acid (5-HD) failed to protect any animal tested (0 of 5). $*P < 0.01$ no drug versus the corresponding drug treatment.

inhibition of the hypoxia-induced shortening of the action potential duration was more potent for HMR 1402 than has been previously reported for HMR 1883 [127]. For example, 0.5 µM of HMR 1883 had no significant effect [127], whereas 0.3 µM of HMR 1402 produced a significant inhibition of reductions in APD_{90} induced by hypoxia [149]. Thus, one may conclude that HMR 1402 is more potent in blocking rilmakalim-activated and hypoxia-activated K_{ATP} channels than HMR 1883.

In contrast, HMR 1402 exhibited slightly more potent inhibition of vascular smooth and pancreatic β-cells than had been previously reported for HMR 1883/1098. For example, HMR 1402, in contrast to HMR 1883/1098, reduced hypoxia-induced increases in coronary flow at low concentrations [127, 149]. However, the same dose of glibenclamide (10 µM) provoked much larger reductions in coronary flow under normoxic conditions as well as hypoxic conditions [127]. As such, in isolated guinea pig hearts, HMR 1402 was more potent in inhibiting hypoxia-induced vasodilation than HMR 1883 but was still much less potent than glibenclamide. In a similar manner, HMR 1402 only partially inhibited the effect of diazoxide on the pancreatic β cell membrane potential ($IC_{50} = 3.9$ µM, [149]). This inhibition was somewhat more potent than that of HMR 1883 (IC_{50} approximately 20 µM) [120, 127] but considerably less than that of glibenclamide ($IC_{50} = 9.3$ nM) [127]. HMR 1402, like HMR 1883/1098, did not alter either plasma insulin or blood glucose levels in conscious dogs [149]. This was in marked contrast to the pronounced hypoglycemia and the

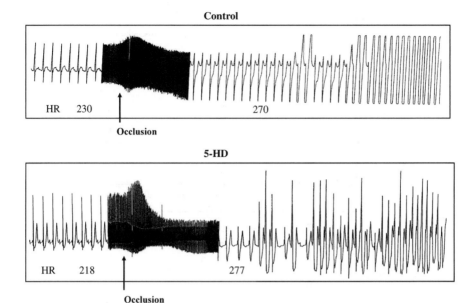

Figure 14.7. Effect of the mitochondrial selective ATP-sensitive potassium channel antagonist, 5-hydroxydecanoic acid (5-HD), on susceptibility to ventricular fibrillation in a conscious canine model of sudden cardiac death. Representative recordings from the same dog are displayed before and after pretreatment with 5-HD (30 mg/kg, i.v.). The 5-HD treatment failed to prevent ventricular fibrillation induced by the combination of acute myocardial ischemia and exercise in any animal test (0 of 5 dogs).

increase in plasma insulin provoked by glibenclamide [64, 149]. These *in vitro* and *in vivo* data strongly suggest that HMR 1402 acts preferentially on cardiac K_{ATP} channels but with slightly less selectively than HMR 1883/1098.

As would one might predict, HMR 1402 was found to reduce the incidence of ventricular fibrillation induced by myocardial ischemia, protecting seven of eight animals tested (Figure 14.6 & 14.10) [149]. This protection was very similar to that noted for both HMR 1883 and glibenclamide (Figure 14.6) [64, 91]. However, it is important to emphasize that, in contrast to the actions of either HMR 1402 or HMR 1883 (Figure 14.9), glibenclamide significantly reduced both exercise (Figure 14.4) and reactive hyperemia-induced increases in coronary blood flow, as well as depressed ventricular function (large reductions in left ventricular dP/dt maximum) in animals [64, 91]. Therefore, nonselective K_{ATP} channel antagonist may protect against ischemic arrhythmias but not without potentially significant adverse side effects.

14.4.3   Proarrhythmic Effects of ATP-sensitive Potassium Channel Agonists

In contrast to ATP-sensitive potassium channel antagonists, channel agonists induced arrhythmias during ischemia in both isolated hearts and intact animals [86, 150, 151].

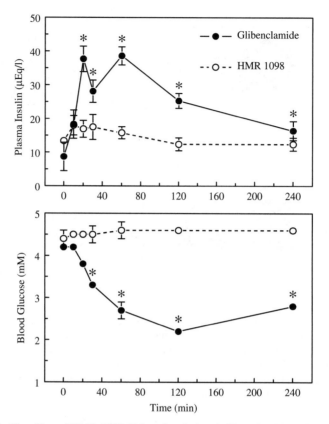

Figure 14.8. The effect of HMR 1098 (3.0 mg/kg, i.v.) and glibenclamide (1.0 mg/kg, i.v.) on plasma insulin concentration and blood glucose levels in conscious dogs. Note that glibenclamide but not HMR 1098 elicited significant changes in both blood glucose and plasma insulin levels. (Reprinted with permission of the American Society for Pharmacology and Experimental Therapeutics, Billman et al. [64])

The ATP-sensitive potassium channel agonist pinacidil facilitated ventricular fibrillation during myocardial ischemia in isolated rat [86], guinea pig [151], or rabbit [150] hearts with reduced potassium levels. Di Diego and Antzelevitch [78] found that the activation of the ATP-sensitive potassium channel with pinacidil caused marked heterogeneities of the refractory period, which provoked extrasystoles. These extrasystoles were blocked by glibenclamide in strips of isolated canine myocardium. They concluded that this dispersion of repolarization and refractory period formed a substrate for reentry. Indeed, the ATP-sensitive potassium channel opener cromakalim reduced effective refractory period and increased vulnerability for reentrant arrhythmias [72]. Furthermore, this drug also increased interventricular dispersion of refractory period and induced ventricular fibrillation in 5 of 12 isolated rabbit hearts under normoxic conditions [73]. However, neither cromakalim nor tedisamil altered the incidence of ventricular fibrillation induced by regional ischemia in isolated rat

HMR 1098

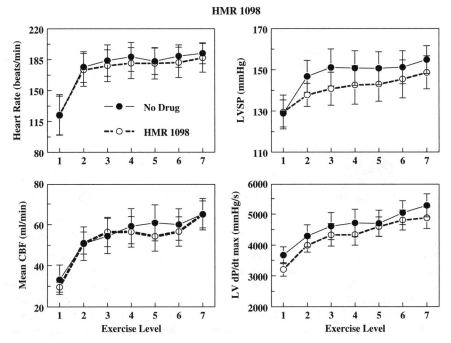

Figure 14.9. Effects of HMR 1098 (3.0 mg/kg) on the hemodynamic response to submaximal exercise in conscious dogs. Note that this drug did not significantly alter any hemodynamic parameter. Coronary blood flow = CBF, LVSP = left ventricular systolic pressure. Exercise levels: 1, 0%grade/0 kph; 2, 0%/4.8 kph; 3, 0%/6.4 kph; 4, 4%/6.4 kph; 5, 8%/6.4 kph; 6, 12%/6.4 kph; 7, 16%/6.4 kph. (Reprinted with permission of the American Society for Pharmacology and Experimental Therapeutics, Billman et al. [64])

hearts [153], whereas nicorandil produced only a modest proarrhythmic response; ventricular fibrillation was induced in two of nine hearts during reperfusion [154]. Chi et al. [152] further demonstrated that pinacidil increased the frequency of ventricular fibrillation during myocardial ischemia in unanesthetized dogs. This drug had no effect on arrhythmias induced by electrical stimulation in normally perfused tissue [152]. Coromilas et al. [79] also demonstrated that the pinacidil restored excitability in the tissue adjacent to the ischemic region (i.e., the epicardial border zone). This reactivation of formerly inexcitable tissue led to the formation of reentrant circuits and the induction of ventricular tachycardia.

Although proarrhythmic events have not been associated with ATP-sensitive potassium channel agonists in the clinical setting [156, 157], these drugs can alter ECG parameters that have been linked to arrhythmia formation. Indeed, abnormal T-wave changes suggestive of alteration in cardiac repolarization were reported in 30% of the hypertensive patients taking pinacidil [62]. In the presence of ischemia, these cardiac electrophysiological actions of nonselective ATP-sensitive potassium channel agonists could become more pronounced, increasing the propensity for life-threatening arrhythmias. However, nicorandil reduced the number of episodes of

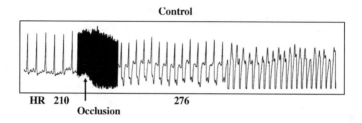

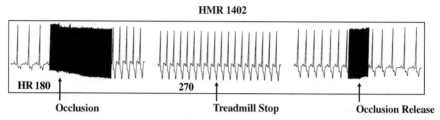

Figure 14.10. Effect of the cardioselective ATP-sensitive potassium channel antagonist, HMR 1402, on susceptibility to ventricular fibrillation in a conscious canine model of sudden cardiac death. Representative recordings from the same dog are displayed before and after pretreatment with the ATP-sensitive potassium channel antagonist HMR 1402 (3.0 mg/kg, i.v.). HMR 1402 abolished ventricular fibrillation induced by the combination of acute myocardial ischemia and exercise in dogs with healed myocardial infarctions, protecting seven of eight dogs tested. (Reprinted with permission of the American Society for Pharmacology and Experimental Therapeutics, Billman et al. [149])

nonsustained ventricular tachycardia in patients with unstable angina [157]. This drug also reduced the episodes of transient ischemia. Thus, it is likely that the antiarrhythmic effects of this drug probably resulted secondarily from reductions in ischemia rather than a direct action on the ventricular myocardium. Remme and Wilde [158] concluded that since clinical studies of ATP-sensitive potassium channel agonists have not reported any major adverse effects on cardiac rhythm, the proarrhythmic potential of these agents may be "overestimated."

In contrast to these nonselective agonists, mitochondrial selective agonists may lack proarrhythmic effects. For example, the novel mitochondrial agonist, BMS-191095 [159], reduced myocardial infarction size and preserved mechanical function during ischemia/reperfusion without adversely affecting cardiac electrophysiological parameters or the induction of arrhythmias [160].

When considered together, these reports indicate that the activation of sarcolemmal ATP-sensitive potassium channels promote arrhythmias, particularly in the setting of acute myocardial ischemia. In contrast, the selective activation of mitochondrial ATP-sensitive potassium channels contribute to ischemic preconditioning and, thereby, reduce the mechanical dysfunction induced by ischemia without affecting cardiac electrical stability. Therefore, the "ideal" modulator of ATP-sensitive potassium channels would both inhibit sarcolemmal channels and increase the activation (open) of mitochondrial channels in cardiac tissue. Recently, bepridil, an arrhythmic drug that modulates intracellular calcium, has been shown to both inhibit sarcolemmal ATP-sensitive potassium channels and to activate mitochondrial ATP-sensitive potassium channels [161]. As such, this compound may serve as model for future antiarrhythmic drug development.

14.5 SUMMARY

The activation of cardiac cell membrane ATP-sensitive potassium channels during myocardial ischemia promotes potassium efflux, reductions in action potential duration, and heterogeneities in repolarization, thereby creating a substrate for reentrant arrhythmias. Drugs that block this channel should be particularly effective antiarrhythmic agents. Indeed, it is interesting to note that many currently available antiarrhythmic drugs, including verapamil, mibefradil, quinidine, lidocaine, and amiodarone, have also been reported to inhibit ATP-sensitive potassium channels at therapeutic concentrations [162–165]. Of particular note, amiodarone selectively inhibited sarcolemmal ATP-sensitive potassium channels without affecting mito-chondrial channels [166]. Therefore, the inhibition of the ATP-sensitive potassium channel may be required for antiarrhythmic actions during myocardial ischemia. HMR 1883 (or its sodium salt HMR 1098) or HMR 1402 selectively blocks cardiac sarcolemmal ATP-sensitive potassium channels. As such, these drugs attenuate ischemically induced changes in cardiac electrical properties, thereby preventing malignant arrhythmias without the untoward effects of other drugs. Since, as noted, the ATP-sensitive potassium channel only becomes active as ATP levels fall, these drugs have the added advantage that they would have effects *only* on ischemic tissue with little or no effect noted on normal tissue. Thus, selective antagonists of the cardiac cell surface ATP-sensitive potassium channel may represent the first truly ischemia selective antiarrhythmic medications and should be free of the proarrhyth-mic actions that have plagued many of the currently available antiarrhythmic drugs.

REFERENCES

1. Bayes de Luna, A., Coumel, P., LeClercq, J.F. (1989). Ambulatory sudden cardiac death: Mechanisms of production of fatal arrhythmia on the basis of data from 157 cases. American Heart Journal, 117, 151–159.
2. Hinkle, L.E.J., Thaler, H.T. (1982). Clinical classification of cardiac deaths. Circulation, 65, 457–464.
3. Greene, H.L. (1990). Sudden arrhythmic cardiac death: Mechanisms, resuscitation and classification: The Seattle perspective. American Journal of Cardiology, 65, 4B–12B.
4. Abildstrom, S.Z., Kobler, L., Torp-Pedersen, C. (1999). Epidemiology of arrhythmic and sudden death in the chronic phase of ischemic heart disease. Cardiac Electrophysiology Reviews, 3, 177–179.
5. Zipes, D.P., Wellens, H.J. (1998). Sudden cardiac death. Circulation, 98, 2334–2351.
6. Rubart, M., Zipes, D.P. (2005). Mechanism of sudden cardiac death. Journal of Clinical Investigation, 115, 2305–2315.

7. Opie, L.H., Nathan, D., Lubbe, W.F. (1979). Biochemical aspects of arrhythmogenesis. American Journal of Cardioliogy, 43, 131–148.

8. Curtis, M.J., Pugsley, M.K., Walker, M.J.A. (1993). Endogenous chemical mediators of ventricular arrythmias in ischaemic heart disease. Cardiovascular Research, 27, 703–719.

9. Billman, G.E. (1991). The antiarrhythmic and antifibrillatory effects of calcium antagonists. Journal of Cardiovascular Pharmacology, 18(Suppl 10), S107–S117.

10. Billman, G.E. (1994). The role of the ATP-sensitive K^+ channel in K^+ accumulation and cardiac arrhythmias during myocardial ischemia. Cardiovascular Research, 28, 762–769.

11. Wilde, A.A.M. (1993). Role of ATP-sensitive K^+ channel current in ischemic arrhythmias. Cardiovascular Drugs and Therapy, 7, 521–526.

12. Wilde, A.M.M., Aksnes, G. (1995). Myocardial potassium loss and cell depolarization in ischaemia and hypoxia. Cardiovascular Research, 29, 1–15.

13. Harris, A.S. (1966). Potassium and experimental coronary occlusion. American Heart Journal, 71, 797–802.

14. Harris, A.S., Bisteni, A., Russell, R.A., Brigham, J.C., Firestone, J.E. (1954). Excitatory factors in ventricular tachycardia resulting from myocardial ischemia: potassium a major excitant. Science, 119, 200–203.

15. Curtis, M.J. (1991). The rabbit dual coronary perfusion model: A new method for assessing pathological relevance of individual products of the ischaemeic milieu: role of potassium in arrhythmogenesis. Cardiovascular Research, 25, 1010–1022.

16. Coronel, R., Fiolet, J.W., Wilms-Schopman, F.J., Schaapherder, A.F., Johnson, T.A., Gettes, L.S., Janse, M.J. (1988). Distribution of extracellular potassium and its relation to electrophysiologic changes during acute myocardial ischemia in the isolated perfused porcine heart. Circulation, 77, 1125–1138.

17. Hill, J.L., Gettes, L.S. (1980). Effect of acute coronary artery occlusion on local myocardial extracellular K^+ activity in swine. Circulation, 61, 768–778.

18. Kleber, A.G. (1984). Extracellular potassium accumulation in acute myocardial ischemia. Journal of Molecular and Cellular Cardiology, 16, 389–394.

19. Johnson, T.A., Engle, C.L., Boyd, L.M., Koch, G.G., Gwinn, M., Gettes, L.S. (1991). Magnitude and time course of extracellular potassium inhomogeneities during acute ischemia in pigs. Effect of verapamil. Circulation, 83, 622–634.

20. Coronel, R., Wilms-Schopman, F.J., Opthof, T., van Capelle, F.J., Janse, M.J. (1991). Injury current and gradients of diastolic stimulation threshold, TQ potential, and extracellular potassium concentration during acute regional ischemia in the isolated perfused pig heart. Circulation Research, 68, 1241–1249.

21. Kleber, A.G. (1983). Resting membrane potential, extracellular potassium activity, and intracellular sodium activity during acute global ischemia in isolated perfused guinea pig hearts. Circulation Research, 52, 442–450.

22. Rau, E.E., Shine, K.I., Langer, G.A. (1977). Potassium exchange and mechanical performance in anoxic mammalian myocardium. American Journal of Physiology—Heart and Circulatory Physiology, 232, H85–H94.

23. Shine, K.I., Douglas, A.M., Ricchiuti, N. (1977). ^{42}K exchange during myocardial ischemia. American Journal of Physiology—Heart and Circulatory Physiology, 232, H564–H570.

24. Wilde, A.M.M. (1998). ATP and the role of I_{KATP} during acute myocardial ischaemia: Controversies revive. Cardiovascular Research, 35, 181–183.

25. Trube, G., Hescheler, J. (1984). Inward-rectifying channels in isolated patches of the heart cell membrane: ATP-dependence and comparison with cell-attached patches. Pflugers Archiv—European Journal of Physiology, 401, 178–184.

26. Noma, A. (1983). ATP-regulated K^+ channels in cardiac muscle. Nature, 305, 147–148.

27. Nichols, C.G. (2006). K_{ATP} channels as molecular sensors of cellular metabolism. Nature, 440, 470–476.

28. Flagg, T.P., Nichols, C.G. (2005). Sarcolemmal K_{ATP} channels: What do we really know? Journal of Molecular and Cellular Cardiology, 39, 61–70.

29. Nichols, C.G., Shyng, S.L., Nestorowicz, A., Glaser, B., Celment, J.P., IV, Gonzalez, G., Aguilar-Bryan, L., Permutt, M.A., Bryan, J. (1996). Adenosine diphosphate as intracellular regulator of insulin section. Science, 272, 1785–1787.

30. Gribble, F.M., Tucker, S.J., Ashcroft, F.M. (1997). The essential role of Walker A motifs of SUR1 in K-ATP channel activation by MgADP and diazoxide. EMBO Journal, 16, 1145–1152.

31. Dunne, M.J., Petersen, O.H. (1986). Intracellular ADP activates K^+ channels that are inhibited by ATP in an insulin secreting cell line. FEBS Letters, 208, 59–62.

32. Kakei, M., Kelly, R.P., Ashcroft, S.J., Ashcroft, F.M. (1986). The ATP-sensitivity of K^+ channels in rat pancreatic β-cells is modulated by ADP. FEBS Letters, 208, 63–66.

33. Bekheit, S.S., Restivo, M., Boutjdir, M., Henkin, R., Gooyandeh, K., Assadi, M., Khatib, S., Gough, W.B., El-Sherif, N. (1990). Effects of glyburide on ischemia-induced changes in extracellular potassium and local myocardial activation: A potential new approach to the management of ischemia-induced malignant ventricular arrhythmias. American Heart Journal, 119, 1025–1033.

34. Benndorf, K., Friedrich, M., Hirche, H. (1991). Anoxia opens ATP regulated K channels in isolated heart cells of the guinea pig. Pflugers Archiv—European Journal of Physiology, 419, 108–110.

35. Fosset, M., De Weille, J.R., Green, R.D., Schmid-Antomarchi, H., Lazdunski, M. (1988). Antidiabetic sulfonylureas control action potential properties in heart cells via high affinity receptors that are linked to ATP- dependent K^+ channels. Journal of Biological Chemistry, 263, 7933–7936.

36. Hicks, M.N., Cobbe, S.M. (1991). Effect of glibenclamide on extracellular potassium accumulation and the electrophysiological changes during myocardial ischaemia in the arterially perfused interventricular septum of rabbit. Cardiovascular Research, 25, 407–413.

37. Kantor, P.F., Coetzee, W.A., Carmeliet, E.E., Dennis, S.C., Opie, L.H. (1990). Reduction of ischemic K^+ loss and arrhythmias in rat hearts: Effect of glibenclamide, a sulfonylurea. Circulation Research, 66, 478–485.

38. Nakaya, H., Takeda, Y., Tohse, N., Kanno, M. (1991). Effects of ATP-sensitive K^+ channel blockers on the action potential shortening in hypoxic and ischaemic myocardium. British Journal of Pharmacology, 103, 1019–1026.

39. Ruiz-Petrich, E., Leblanc, N., deLorenzi, F., Allard, Y., Schanne, O.F. (1992). Effects of K^+ channel blockers on the action potential of hypoxic rabbit myocardium. British Journal of Pharmacology, 106, 924–930.

40. Vanheel, B., De Hemptinne, A. (1992). Influence of KATP channel modulation on net potassium efflux from ischaemic mammalian cardiac tissue. Cardiovascular Research, 26, 1030–1039.

41. Venkatesh, N., Lamp, S.T., Weiss, J.N. (1991). Sulfonylureas, ATP-sensitive K^+ channels, and cellular K^+ loss during hypoxia, ischemia, and metabolic inhibition in mammalian ventricle. Circulation Research, 69, 623–637.

42. Weiss, J.N., Venkatesh, N., Lamp, S.T. (1992). ATP-sensitive K^+ channels and cellular K^+ loss in hypoxic and ischaemic mammalian ventricle. Journal of Physiology (London), 447, 649–673.

43. Wilde, A.A., Escande, D., Schumacher, C.A., Thuringer, D., Mestre, M., Fiolet, J.W., Janse, M.J. (1990). Potassium accumulation in the globally ischemic mammalian heart. A role for the ATP-sensitive potassium channel. Circulation Research, 67, 835–843.

44. Smallwood, J.K., Ertel, P.J., Steinberg, M.I. (1990). Modification by glibenclamide of the electrophysiological consequences of myocardial ischaemia in dogs and rabbits. Naunyn Schmiedebergs Archives of Pharmacology, 342, 214–220.

45. Edwards, G., Weston, A.H. (1993). The pharmacology of ATP-sensitive potassium channels. Annual Review of Pharmacology and Toxicology, 33, 597–637.

46. Mitani, A., Kinoshita, K., Fukamachi, K., Sakamoto, M., Kurisu, K., Tsuruhara, Y., Fukumura, F., Nakashima, A., Tokunaga, K. (1991). Effects of glibenclamide and nicorandil on cardiac function during ischemia and reperfusion in isolated perfused rat hearts. American Journal of Physiology—Heart and Circulatory Physiology, 261, H1864–H1871.

47. Venkatesh, N., Stuart, J.S., Lamp, S.T., Alexander, L.D., Weiss, J.N. (1992). Activation of ATP-sensitive K^+ channels by cromakalim: Effects on cellular K^+ loss and cardiac function in ischemic and reperfused mammalian ventricle. Circulation Research, 71, 1324–1333.

48. Kanda, A., Watanabe, I., Williams, M.L., Engle, C.L., Li, S., Koch, G.G., Gettes, L.S. (1997). Unanticipated lessening of the rise in extracellular potassium during ischemia by pinacidil. Circulation, 95, 1937–1944.

49. Saito, T., Sato, T., Takashi, M., Seino, S., Nakaya, H. (2005). Role of ATP-sesntive K^+ cahnnels in electrophysiological altetions during myocardial ischemia: a study using Kir6.2-null mice. American Journal of Physiology—Heart and Circulatory Physiology, 288, H352–H357.

50. Mitani, A., Shattock, M.J. (1992). Role of Na-activated K channel, Na-K-Cl cotransport, Na-K pump and $[K]_e$ changes during ischemia in the rat heart. American Journal of Physiology—Heart and Circulatory Physiology, 263, H333–H340.

51. Shieh, R.C., Goldhaber, J.I., Stuart, J.S., Weiss, J.N. (1994). Lactate transport in mammalian ventricle: General properties and relation to K^+ efflux. Circulation Research, 74, 829–838.

52. Yan, G.X., Yamada, K.A., Kleber, A.G., McHowat, J., Corr, P.B. (1993). Dissociation between cellular $K +$ loss, reduction in repolarization time, and tissue ATP levels during myocardial hypoxia and ischemia. Circulation Research, 72, 560–570.

53. Wang, J., Wang, H., Han, H., Zhang, Y., Yang, B., Nattel, S., Wang, Z. (2001). Phospholipid metabolite 1-palmitoyl-lysophosphatidylcholine enhances human ether-a-go-go-related gene (HERG) K^+ channel function. Circulation, 104, 2645–2648.

54. Findlay, I. (1988). ATP4- and ATP.Mg inhibit the ATP-sensitive $K +$ channel of rat ventricular myocytes. Pflugers Archiv—European Journal of Physiology, 412, 37–41.

55. Nichols, C.G., Lederer, W.J. (1990). The regulation of ATP-sensitive K^+ channel activity in intact and permeabilized rat ventricular myocytes. Journal of Physiology (London), 423, 91–110.

56. Rovetto, M.J., Whitmer, J.T., Neely, J.R. (1973). Comparison of the effects of anoxia and whole heart ischemia on carbohydrate utilization in isolated working rat hearts. Circulation Research, 32, 699–711.

57. Faivre, J.F., Findlay, I. (1990). Action potential duration and activation of ATP-sensitive potassium current in isolated guinea-pig ventricular myocytes. Biochimica Biophysica Acta, 1029, 167–172.

58. Nichols, C.G., Lederer, W.J. (1991). Adenosine triphosphate-sensitive potassium channels in the cardiovascular system. American Journal of Physiology—Heart and Circulatory Physiology, 261, H1675–H1686.

59. Nichols, C.G., Ripoll, C., Lederer, W.J. (1991). ATP-sensitive potassium channel modulation of the guinea pig ventricular action potential and contraction. Circulation Research, 68, 280–287.

60. Deutsch, N., Klitzner, T.S., Lamp, S.T., Weiss, J.N. (1991). Activation of cardiac ATP-sensitive K^+ current during hypoxia: Correlation with tissue ATP levels. American Journal of Physiology—Heart and Circulatory Physiology, 261, H671–H676.

61. Kubota, I., Yamaki, M., Shibata, T., Ikeno, E., Hosoya, Y., Tomoike, H. (1993). Role of ATP-sensitive K^+ channel on ECG ST segment elevation during a bout of myocardial ischemia. A study on epicardial mapping in dogs. Circulation, 88, 1845–1851.

62. Goldberg, M.R. (1988). Clinical pharmacology of pinacidil, a prototype for drugs that affect potassium channels. Journal of Cardiovascular Pharmacology, 12(Suppl 2), S41–S47.

63. Kondo, T., Kubota, I., Tachibana, H., Yamaki, M., Tomoike, H. (1996). Glibenclamide attenuates peaked T wave in early phase of myocardial ischemia. Cardiovascular Research, 31, 683–687.

64. Billman, G.E., Englert, H.C., Schoelkens, B.A. (1998). HMR 1883, a novel cardioselective inhibitor of the ATP- sensitive potassium channel;Part II: Effects on susceptibility to ventricular fibrillation induced by myocardial ischemia in conscious dogs. Journal of Pharmacology and Experimental Therapeutics, 286, 1465–1473.

65. Yan, G.X., Antzelevitch, C. (1998). Cellular basis for the normal T wave and the electrocardiographic manifestations of the long-QT syndrome. Circulation, 98, 1928–1936.

66. Opthof, T., Coronel, R., Wilms-Schopman, F.J.G., Plotnikov, A.N., Shlapakova, I.N., Danilo, P., Jr., Rosen, M.R., Janse, M.J. (2007). Dispersion of repolarization in canine ventricle and electrocardiographic T wave: T_{p-e} interval does not reflect transmural dispersion. Heart Rhythm, 4, 341–348.

67. Suzuki, M., Li, R.A., Miki, T., Uemura, H., Sakamoto, N., Ohmoto-Sekine, Y., Tamagawa, M., Ogura, T., Seino, S., Marban, E., Nakaya, H. (2001). Functional roles of cardiac and vascular ATP-sensitive potassium channels clarified by Kir6.2-knockout mice. Circulation Research, 88, 570–577.

68. Li, R.A., Leppo, M., Miki, T., Seino, S., Marban, E. (2000). Molecular basis of electrocardiographic ST-segment elevation. Circulation Research, 87, 837–839.

69. Wit, A.L., Janse, M.J. (1989). Electrophysiological mechanisms of ventricular arrhythmias resulting from myocardial ischemia and infarction. Physiological Reviews, 69, 1049–1169.

70. Coronel, R., Wilms-Schopman, F.J., Dekker, L.R., Janse, M.J. (1995). Heterogenties in [K +]o and TQ potential and the inducinbillity of ventricular fibrillation during acute regional ischemia in the isolated perfused porcine heart. Circulation, 92, 120–129.

71. Krause, E., Englert, H., Gögelein, H. (1995). Adenosine triphosphate-dependent K^+ currents activated by metabolic inhibition in rat ventricular myocytes differ from those elicited by the channel opener rilmakalim. Pflugers Archiv—European Journal of Physiology, 429, 625–635.

72. Uchida, T., Yashima, M., Gotoh, M., Qu, Z., Garfinkel, A., Weiss, J.N., Fishbein, M.C., Mandel, W.J., Chen, P.S., Karagueuzian, H.S. (1999). Mechanism of acceleration of functional reentry in the ventricle: Effects of ATP-sensitive potassium channel opener. Circulation, 99, 704–712.

73. Wolk, R., Cobbe, S.M., Kane, K.A., Hicks, M.N. (1999). Relevance of inter- and intraventricular electrical dispersion to arrhythmogenesis in normal and ischaemic rabbit myocardium: A study with cromakalim, 5-hydroxydecanoate and glibenclamide. Journal of Cardiovascular Pharmacology, 33, 323–334.

74. Furukawa, T., Kimura, S., Furukawa, N., Bassett, A.L., Myerburg, R.J. (1992). Potassium rectifier currents differ in myocytes of endocardial and epicardial origin. Circulation Research, 70, 91–103.

75. Gilmour, R.F. Jr, Zipes, D.P. (1980). Different electrophysiological responses of canine endocardium and epicardium to combined hyperkalemia, hypoxia, and acidosis. Circulation Research, 46, 814–825.

76. Kimura, S., Bassett, A.L., Kohya, T., Kozlovskis, P.L., Myerburg, R.J. (1986). Simultaneous recording of action potentials from endocardium and epicardium during ischemia in the isolated cat ventricle: Relation of temporal electrophysiologic heterogeneities to arrhythmias. Circulation, 74, 401–409.

77. Tweedie, D., Henderson, C., Kane, K. (1993). Glibenclamide, but not class III drugs, prevents ischaemic shortening of the refractory period in guinea-pig hearts. European Journal of Pharmacology, 240, 251–257.

78. Di Diego, J.M., Antzelevitch, C. (1993). Pinacidil-induced electrical heterogeneity and extrasystolic activity in canine ventricular tissues. Does activation of ATP- regulated potassium current promote phase 2 reentry? Circulation, 88, 1177–1189.

79. Coromilas, J., Costeas, C., Deruyter, B., Dillon, S.M., Peters, N.S., Wit, A.L. (2002). Effects of pinacidil on electrophysiological properties of epicardial border zone of healing canine infarcts: Possible effects of K_{ATP} channel activation. Circulation, 105, 2309–2317.

80. Bellemin-Baurreau, J., Poizot, A., Hicks, P.E., Rochette, L., Armstrong, J.M. (1994). Effects of ATP-dependent K^+ channel modulators on an ischemia-reperfusion rabbit isolated heart model with programmed electrical stimulation. European Journal of Pharmacology, 256, 115–124.

81. Dhein, S., Pejman, P., Krusemann, K. (2000). Effects of the $I_{K.ATP}$ blockers glibenclamide and HMR1883 on cardiac electrophysiology during ischemia and reperfusion. European Journal of Pharmacology, 398, 273–284.

82. Hamada, K., Yamazaki, J., Nagao, T. (1998). Shortening of monophasic action potential duration during hyperkalemia and myocardial ischemia in anesthetized dogs. Japanese Journal of Pharmacology, 76, 149–154.

83. Koumi, S.I., Martin, R.L., Sato, R. (1997). Alterations in ATP-sensitive potassium channel sensitivity to ATP in failing human hearts. American Journal of Physiology—Heart and Circulatory Physiology, 272, H1656–H1665.

84. MacKenzie, I., Saville, V.L., Waterfall, J.F. (1993). Differential class III and glibenclamide effects on action potential duration in guinea-pig papillary muscle during normoxia and hypoxia/ischaemia. British Journal of Pharmacology, 110, 531–538.

85. Pogatsa, G., Koltai, M.Z., Balkanyi, I., Devai, I., Kiss, V., Koszeghy, A. (1988). The effect of various hypoglycaemic sulphonylureas on the cardiotoxicity of glycosides and arrhythmogenic activity due to myocardial ischaemia. Acta Physiologica Hungarica, 71, 243–250.

86. Wolleben, C.D., Sanguinetti, M.C., Siegl, P.K. (1989). Influence of ATP-sensitive potassium channel modulators on ischemia-induced fibrillation in isolated rat hearts. Journal of Molecular and Cellular Cardiology, 21, 783–788.

87. Gwilt, M., Henderson, C.G., Orme, J., Rourke, J.D. (1992). Effects of drugs on ventricular fibrillation and ischaemic K^+ loss in a model of ischaemia in perfused guinea-pig hearts in vitro. European Journal of Pharmacology, 220, 231–236.

88. Zhang, H.L., Li, Y.S., Fu, S.X., Yang, X.P. (1991). Effects of glibenclamide and tolbutamine on ischemia-induced and ouabain-induced arrhythmias and membrane potentials of ventricular myocardium from rat and guinea-pig. Acta Pharmcologica Sinica, 12, 398–402.

89. Bril, A., Laville, M.-P., Gout, B. (1992). Effects of glibenclamide on ventricular arrhythmias and cardiac function in ischaemia and reperfusion in isolated rat heart. Cardiovascular Research, 26, 1069–1076.

90. Pasnani, J.S., Ferrier, G.R. (1992). Differential effects of glyburide on premature beats and ventricular tachycardia in an isolated tissue model of ischemia and reperfusion. Journal of Pharmacology and Experimental Therapeutics, 262, 1076–1084.

91. Billman, G.E., Avendano, C.E., Halliwill, J.R., Burroughs, J.M. (1993). The effects of the ATP-dependent potassium channel antagonist glyburide on coronary blood flow and susceptibility to ventricular fibrillation. Journal of Cardiovascular Pharmacology, 21, 197–204.

92. Tosaki, A., Engelman, D.T., Engelman, R.M., Das, D.K. (1995). Diabetes and ATP-sensitive potassium channel openers and blockers in isolated ischemic/reperfused hearts. Journal of Pharmacology and Experimental Therapeutics, 27, 1115–1123.

93. Rees, S.A., Curtis, M.J. (1995). Pharmacological analysis in rat of the role of the ATP-sensitive potassium channels as a potential target fro antifibrillatory intervention in acute myocardial-ischemia. Journal of Cardiovascular Pharmacology, 26, 280–288.

94. Lepran, I., Baczko, I., Varro, A., Papp, J.G. (1996). ATP-sensitive potassium channel modulators: Both pinacidil and glibenclamide produce antiarrhythmic activity during acute myocardial infarction in conscious rats. Journal of Pharmacology and Experimental Therapeutics, 277, 1215–1220.

95. Baczko, I., Lepran, I., Papp, J.G. (1997). KATP channel modulators increase survival rate during coronary occlusion-reperfusion in anaesthetized rats. European Journal of Pharmacology, 324, 77–83.

96. Barrett, T.D., Walker, M.J. (1998). Glibenclamide does not prevent action potential shortening induced by ischemia in anesthetized rabbits but reduces ischemia-induced arrhythmias. Journal of Molecular and Cellular Cardiology, 30, 999–1008.

97. El Reyani, N.E., Bozdogan, O., Baczko, I., Lepran, I., Papp, J.G. (1999). Comparison of the efficacy of glibenclamide and glimepiride in reperfusion-induced arrhythmias in rats. European Journal of Pharmacology, 365, 187–192.

98. del Valle, H.F., Lascano, E.C., Negroni, J.A., Crottogini, A.J. (2001). Glibenclamide effects reperfusion-induced malignant arrhythmias and left ventricular mechanical recovery from stunning in conscious sheep. Cardiovascular Research, 50, 474–485.

99. Vajda, S., Baczko, I., Lepran, I. (2007). Selective cardiac plasma-membrane K_{ATP} channel inhibition is defibrillatory and improves survival during acute myocardial ischemia and reperfusion. European Journal of Pharmacology, 577, 115–123.

100. Yazar, A., Polat, G., Levant, A., Kaygusuz, A., Camdeviren, H., Buyukafsar, K. (2002). Effects of glibenclamide, metaformin and insulin on the incidence and latency of death by ouabain-induced arrhythmias. Pharmaceutical Research, 45, 183–187.

101. Cacciapuoti, F., Spiezia, R., Bianchi, M., Lama, D., D'Avino, M., Varricchio, M. (1991). Effectiveness of glibenclamide on myocardial ischemic ventricular arrhythmias in non-insulin dependent diabetes mellitus. American Journal of Cardiology, 67, 843–847.

102. Lomuscio, A., Vergani, D., Marano, L., Castagnone, M., Fiorentini, C. (1994). Effects of glibenclamide on ventricular fibrillation in non-insulin- dependent diabetics with acute myocardial infarction. Coronary Artery Disease, 5, 767–771.

103. Lomuscio, A., Fiorentini, C. (1996). Influence of oral antidiabetic treatment on electrocardiac alterations induced by myocardial infarction. Diabetes Research and Clinical Practice, 31(Suppl), S21–S26.

104. Davis, T.M., Parsons, R.W., Broadhurst, R.J., Hobbs, M.S., Jamrozik, K. (1998). Arrhythmias and mortality after myocardial infarction in diabetic patients. Relationship to diabetes treatment. Diabetes Care, 21, 637–640.

105. Aronson, D., Mittleman, M.A., Burger, A.J. (2003). Effects of sulfonylurea agents and adenosine triphosphate dependent potassium channel antagonists on ventricular arrhythmias in patients with decompensated heart failure. PACE—Pacing and Clinical Electrophysiology, 26, 1254–1261.

106. Huizar, J.F., Gonzalez, L.A., alderman, J., Smith, H.S. (2003). Sulfonylureas attenuate electrocardiographic ST-segment elevations during acute myocardial infarction in diabetics. Journal of the American College of Cardiology, 42, 1017–1021.

107. Liu, Y., Ren, G., O'Rourke, B., Marban, E., Seharaseyon, J. (2001). Pharmacological comparison of native mitochondrial K_{ATP} channels with molecularly defined surface K_{ATP} channels. Molecular Pharmacology, 59, 225–230.

108. Foster, D.B., Rucker, J.J., Marban, E. (2008). Is Kir6.1 a subunit of mitoK_{ATP}? Biochemical and Biophysical Research Communications, 266, 649–656.

109. Schnitzler, M.M.Y., Derst, C., Daut, J., Preisig-Muller, R. (2000). ATP-sensitive potassium channels in capillaries isolated from guinea-pig heart. Journal of Physiology (London), 525, 307–317.

110. Aguilar-Bryan, L., Nichols, C.G., Wechsler, S.W., Clement, J.P., Boyd, A.E., Gonzales, G., Herrera-Sosa, H., Nguy, K., Bryan, J., Nelson, D. (1995). Cloning of the beta cell high affinity sulfonylurea receptor: a regulator of insulin secretion. Science, 268, 423–426.

111. Koster, J.C., Permutt, M.A., Nichols, C.G. (2005). Diabetes and insulin secretion the ATP-sensitive K^+ channel (K_{ATP}) connection. Diabetes, 54, 3065–3072.

112. Liss, B., Roeper, J. (2001). Molecular physiology of neuronal K-ATP channels. Molecular Membrane Biology, 18, 117–127.

113. Inagaki, N., Gonoi, T., Clement, J.P., Namba, N., Inazawa, J., Gonzalez, G., Aguilar-Bryan, L., Seino, S., Bryan, J. (1995). Reconstitution of I_{KATP}: an inward rectifier subunit plus the sulfonylurea receptor. Science, 270, 1166–1170.

114. Chutkow, W.A., Samuel, V., Hansen, P.A., Pu, J., Valdivia, C.R., Makielshi, J.C., Burant, C.F. (2001). Disruption of Sur2-containg K_{ATP} channels enhances insulin-stimulated

glucose uptake in skeletal muscle. Proceeding of the National Academy of Sciences (USA), 98, 11760–11764.

115. Gong, B., Miki, T., Seino, S., Renaud, J.M. (2000). A K_{ATP} channel deficiency affects resting tension, not contractile force, during fatigue in skeletal muscle. American Journal of Physiology—Cellular Physiology, 279, C1351–1358.

116. Gopalakrishnan, M., Whiteaker, K.L., Molinari, E.J., Davis-Taber, R., Scott, V.E.s., Shieh, C.C., Buckner, S.A., Milicic, I., Cain, J.C., Postl, S., Sullivan, J.P., Brioni, J.D. (1999). Characterization of the ATP-Sensitive potassium channels (K-ATP) expressed in guinea pig bladder smooth muscle cells. Journal of Pharmacology and Experimental Therapeutics, 289, 551–558.

117. Flagg, T.P., Patton, B., Masia, R., Mansfield, C., Lopatin, A.N., Yamada, K.A., Nichols, C. G. (2007). Arrhythmia susceptibility and premature death in transgenic mice over-expressing both SUR1 and Kir6.2[ΔN30,K185Q] in the heart. American Journal of Physiology—Heart Circulatory Physiology, 293, H836–H845.

118. Gögelein, H. (2001). Inhibition of cardiac ATP-dependent potassium channels by sulfonylurea drugs. Current Opinion of Investigational Drugs, 2, 71–80.

119. Gögelein, H., Hartung, J., Englert, H.C. (1999). Molecular basis, pharmacology and physiological role of cardiac K_{ATP} channels. Cellular Physiology and Biochemistry, 9, 227–241.

120. Manning-Fox, J.E.M., Kanji, H.D., French, R.J., Light, P.E. (2002). Cardioselectivity of the sulphonylurea HMR 1098: studies on native and recombinant cardiac and pancreatic K-ATP channels. British Journal of Pharmacology, 135, 480–488.

121. Englert, H.C., Heitsch, H., Gerlach, U., Knieps, S. (2003). Blockers of the ATP-sensitive potassium channel SURA/Kir6.2: A new approach to prevent sudden cardiac death. Current Medicinal Chemistry, 1, 253–271.

122. Gribble, F.M., Reimann, F. (2003). Sulphonylurea action revisited: The post-cloning era. Diabetologia, 46, 875–891.

123. Gribble, F.M., Tucker, S.J., Seino, S., Ashcroft, F.M. (1998). Tissue specificity of sulfonylureas: studies on cloned cardiac and beta- cell K_{ATP} channels. Diabetes, 47, 1412–1418.

124. Reimann, F., Proks, P., Ashcroft, F.M. (2001). Effects of mitiglinide (S 21403) on Kir6.2/ SUR1, Kir6.2/SUR2A and Kir6.2/SUR2B types of ATP-sensitive potassium channel. British Journal of Pharmacology, 132, 1542–1548.

125. Englert, H.C., Gerlach, U., Goegelein, H., Hartung, J., Heitsch, H., Mania, D., Scheidler, S. (2001). Cardioselective K(ATP) channel blockers derived from a new series of m- anisamidoethylbenzenesulfonylthioureas. Journal of Medicinal Chemistry, 44, 1085–1098.

126. Kaab, S., Zwermann, L., Barth, A., Hinterseer, M., Englert, H.C., Gögelein, H.R., Nabauer, M. (2003). Selective block of sarcolemmal IKATP in human cardiomyocytes using HMR 1098. Cardiovascular Drugs and Therapy, 17, 435–441.

127. Gögelein, H., Hartung, J., Englert, H.C., Scholkens, B.A. (1998). HMR 1883, a novel cardioselective inhibitor of the ATP-sensitive potassium channel. Part I: Effects on cardiomyocytes, coronary flow and pancreatic beta-cells. Journal of Pharmacology and Experimental Therapeutics, 286, 1453–1464.

128. Weyermann, A., Vollert, H., Busch, A.E., Bleich, M., Gögelein, H. (2004). Inhibitors of ATP-sensitive potassium channels in guinea pig isolated ischemic hearts. Naunyn Schmiedebergs Archives of Pharmacology, 369, 374–381.

129. Sato, T. (1999). Signaling in late preconditioning: involvement of mitochondrial K_{ATP} channels. Circulation Research, 85, 1113–1114.

130. Liu, Y., Sato, T., O'Rourke, B., Marban, E. (1998). Mitochondrial ATP-dependent potassium channels: Novel effectors of cardioprotection? Circulation, 97, 2463–2469.

131. Sato, T., Marban, E. (2000). The role of mitochondrial K_{ATP} channels in cardioprotection. Basic Research in Cardiology, 95, 285–289.

132. Fryer, R.M., Eells, J.T., Hsu, A.K., Henry, M.M., Gross, G.J. (2000). Ischemic preconditioning in rats: role of mitochondrial K_{ATP} channel in preservation of mitochondrial function. American Journal of Physiology—Heart and Circulatory Physiology, 278, H305–H312.

133. Jung, O., Englert, H.C., Jung, W., Gögelein, H., Scholkens, B.A., Busch, A.E., Linz, W. (2000). The K_{ATP} channel blocker HMR 1883 does not abolish the benefit of ischemic preconditioning on myocardial infarct mass in anesthetized rabbits. Naunyn Schmiedebergs Archives of Pharmacology, 361, 445–451.

134. Sato, T., Sasaki, N., Seharaseyon, J., O'Rourke, B., Marban, E. (2000). Selective pharmacological agents implicate mitochondrial but not sarcolemmal K_{ATP} channels in ischemic cardioprotection. Circulation, 101, 2418–2423.

135. Das, B., Sarkar, S. (2005). Is the sarcolemmal or mitochondrial K_{ATP} channel activation important in the antiarrhythmic and cardioprotective effects during acute ischemia/ reperfusion in the intact anesthetized rabbit model? Life Science, 77, 1226–1248.

136. Gross, G.J., Fryer, R.M. (1999). Sarcolemmal versus mitochondrial ATP-sensitive K^+ channels and myocardial preconditioning. Circulation Research, 84, 973–979.

137. O'Rourke, B. (2000). Myocardial K_{ATP} channels in preconditioning. Circulation Research, 87, 845–855.

138. Grover, G.J., Garlid, K.D. (2000). ATP-sensitive potassium channels: A review of their cardioprotective pharmacology. Journal of Molecular and Cellular Cardiology, 32, 677–695.

139. Wirth, K.J., Rosenstein, B., Uhde, J., Englert, H.C., Busch, A.E., Scholkens, B.A. (1999). ATP-sensitive potassium channel blocker HMR 1883 reduces mortality and ischemia-associated electrocardiographic changes in pigs with coronary occlusion. Journal of Pharmacology and Experimental Therapeutics, 291, 474–481.

140. Billman, G.E., Houle, M.S., Englert, H.C., Goegelein, H. (1999). Ischemically-induced changes in the T-wave and susceptibility to sudden death: Evidence that activation of the ATP-sensitive potassium channel may contribute to ventricular fibrillation. Circulation, 100(Suppl I), I–52.

141. Billman, G.E., Englert, H.C., Goegelein, H., Busch, A. (2001). Selective sarcolemmal, but not selective mitochondrial, ATP-sensitive potassium channel antagonists prevent ventricular fibrillation induced by ischaemia. European Heart Journal, 22(abstract suppl), 246.

142. Wirth, K.J., Uhde, J., Rosenstein, B., Englert, H.C., Gögelein, H., Schölkens, B.A., Busch, A.E. (2000). K_{ATP} channel blocker HMR 1883 reduces monophasic action potential shortening during coronary ischemia in anesthetised pigs. Naunyn Schmiedebergs Archives of Pharmacology, 361, 155–160.

143. Behrens, S., Zabel, M., Janssen, A., Barbierato, M., Schultheiss, H.P. (2001). Influence of a new ATP-sensitive potassium-channel antagonist (HMR 1098) on ventricular fibrillation inducibility during myocardial ischemia. European Heart Journal, 22(abstract suppl), 546.

144. Gok, S., Vural, K., Sekuri, C., Onur, R., Tezcan, A., Izanli, A. (2006). Effects of the blockade of cardiac sarcolemmal ATP-sensitive potassium channels on arrhythmias and coronary flow in ischemia-reperfusion model in isolated rat hearts. Vascular Pharmacology, 44, 197–205.

145. Bohn, H., Englert, H.C., Schoelkens, B.A. (1998). The K_{ATP} channel blocker HMR 1883 attenuates the effects of ischemia on MAP duration and improves survival during LAD occlusion in anaesthetized pig. British Journal of Pharmacology, 124, 23P.

146. Wirth, K.J., Klaus, E., Englert, H.G., Schölkens, B.A., Linz, W. (1999). HMR 1883, a cardioselective K(ATP) channel blocker, inhibits ischaemia- and reperfusion-induced ventricular fibrillation in rats. Naunyn Schmiedebergs Archives of Pharmacology, 360, 295–300.

147. Zhu, B.M., Miyamoto, S., Nagawa, Y., Wajima, T., Hashimoto, K. (2003). Effect of sarcolemmal K-ATP blocker HMR 1098 on arrhythmias induced by programmed electrical stimulation in canine old myocardial infarction model: Comparison with glibenclamide. Journal of Pharmacological Sciences, 93, 106–113.

148. Fischbach, P.S., White, A., Barrett, T.D., Lucchesi, B.R. (2004). Risk of ventricular proarrhythmia with the selective opening of the myocardial sarcolemmal versus mitochondrial ATP-gated potassium channel. Journal of Pharmacology and Experimental Therapeutics, 309, 554–559.

149. Billman, G.E., Houle, M.S., Englert, H.C., Gögelein, H. (2004). Effects of a novel cardioselective ATP-sensitive potassium channel antagonist 1-[[5-[2(5-chloro-o-anisamido)ethyl]-β-methoxyethoxyphenyl]sulfonyl]-3-methylthioura, sodium salt (HMR 1402), on susceptibility to ventricular fibrillation induced by myocardial ischemia: in vitro and in vivo studies. Journal of Pharmacology and Experimental Therapeutics, 309, 182–192.

150. Chi, L., Black, S.C., Kuo, P.I., Fagbemi, S.O., Lucchesi, B.R. (1993). Actions of pinacidil at a reduced potassium concentration - a direct cardiac effect possibly involving the ATP-sensitive potassium channel. Journal of Cardiovascular Pharmacology, 21, 179–190.

151. D'Alonzo, A.J., Zhu, J.L., Darbenzio, R.B., Dorso, C.R., Grover, G.J. (1998). Proarrhythmic effects of pinacidil are partially meditated through enhancement of catecholamine release inisloated perfused guinea-pig hearts. Journal of Molecular and Cellular Cardiology, 30, 415–423.

152. Chi, L., Uprichard, A.C.G., Lucchesi, B.R. (1990). Profibrillatory actions of pinacidil in a conscious canine model of sudden coronary death. Journal of Cardiovascular Pharmacology, 15, 452–464.

153. Rees, S.A., Tsuchihashi, K., Hearse, D.J., Curtis, M.J. (1993). Combined administration of an Ik(ATP) activator and Ito blocker increases coronary blood flow independently of effects on heart rate, QT interval, and ischaemia-induced ventricular fibrillation in rats. Journal of Cardiovascular Pharmacology, 22, 343–349.

154. Kempsford, R.D., Hawgood, B.J. (1989). Assessment of the antiarrhythmic activity of nicorandil during myocardial ischemia and reperfusion. European Journal of Pharmacology, 163, 61–68.

155. Friedel, H.A., Brogden, R.N. (1990). Pinacidil—a review of its pharmacodynamic and pharmacokinetic properties and therapeutic potential in the treatment of hypertension. Drugs, 39, 929–967.

156. Krumenacker, M., Roland, E. (1992). Clinical profile of nicorandil—an overview of its hemodynamic properties and therapeutic efficacy. Journal of Cardiovascular Pharmacology, 20(Suppl 3), S93–S102.

157. Patel, D.J., Purcell, H.J., Fox, K.M. (1999). Cardioprotection by opening of the K_{ATP} channel in unstable angina. European Heart Journal, 20, 51–57.

158. Remme, C.A., Wilde, A.M.M. (2000). K_{ATP} channel opener, myocardial ischemia and arrhythmias—should the electrophysiologist worry? Cardiovascular Drugs and Therapy, 14, 17–22.

159. Grover, G.J., D'Alonzo, A.J., Garlid, K.D., Bajgar, R., Lodge, N.J., Sleph, P.G., Darbenzio, R.B., Hess, T.A., Smith, M.A., Paucke, P., Atwal, K.S. (2001). Pharmacologic characterization of BMS-191095, a mitochondrial K_{ATP} opener with no peripheral vasodilator or cardiac action potential shortening activity. Journal of Pharmacology and Experimental Therapeutics, 297, 1184–1192.

160. Grover, G.J., D'Alonzo, A.J., Darbenzio, R.B., Parhaqm, C.S., Hess, T.A., Bathala, M.S. (2002). In vivo characterization of the mitochondrial selective K_{ATP} opener (3R)-trans-4-((4-chlorophenyl)-N-(1H-imidazol-2-ylmethyl)dimethyl-2H-1-benzopyran-6-carbonitril monohydrochloride (BMS-191095): Cardioprotective, hemodynamic, and electrophysiological effects. Journal of Pharmacology and Experimental Therapeutics, 303, 132–140.

161. Sato, T., Costa, A.D.T., Saito, T., Ogura, T., Ishida, H., Garlid, K.D., Nakaya, H. (2006). Bepridil, an antiarrhythmic drug, opens mitochondrial K_{ATP} channels, blocks sarcolemmal K_{ATP} channels, and confers cardioprotection. Journal of Pharmacology and Experimental Therapeutics, 316, 182–188.

162. Colatsky, T.J., Follmer, C.H., Starmer, C.F. (1990). Channel specificity in antiarrhythmic drug action. Mechanism of potassium channel block and its role in suppressing and aggravating cardiac arrhythmias. Circulation, 82, 2235–2242.

163. Haworth, R.A., Goknur, A.B., Berkoff, H.A. (1989). Inhibition of ATP-sensitive potassium channels of adult rat heart cells by antiarrhythmic drugs. Circulation Research, 65, 1157–1160.

164. Holmes, D.S., Sun, Z.Q., Porter, L.M., Bernstein, N.E., Chinitz, L.A., Artman, M., Coetzee, W.A. (2000). Amiodarone inhibits cardiac ATP-sensitive potassium channels. Journal of Cardiovascular Electrophysiology, 11, 1152–1158.

165. Olschewski, A., Brau, M.E., Olschewski, H., Hempelmann, G., Vogel, W. (1996). ATP-dependent potassium channel in rat cardiomyocytes is blocked by lidocaine. Possible impact on the antiarrhythmic action of lidocaine. Circulation, 93, 656–659.

166. Sato, T., Takizawa, T., Saito, T., Kobayashi, S., Hara Nakaya, H. (2003). Amiodarone inhibits sarcolemmal but not mitchondrial K-ATP channels in guinea pig ventricular cells. Journal of Pharmacology and Experimental Therapeutics, 307, 955–960.

CHAPTER 15

Mitochondrial Origin of Ischemia-Reperfusion Arrhythmias

BRIAN O'ROURKE

15.1 INTRODUCTION

Having the advantage of more than a century of research into the complex mechanisms involved in the synchronization of electrical and contractile function in the heart, we now move toward an understanding of myocardial function spanning from the gene, to the cell, to the whole organ and beyond. It is now almost possible to predict, with some degree of accuracy, the influence of an ion channel gene mutation or an untoward pharmaceutical compound side effect on the vulnerability to arrhythmias using high-throughput screening methods, advanced computational models, and high-resolution diagnostic mapping techniques. Despite this wealth of basic knowledge, approximately 700,000 people die of heart disease in the United States each year (29% of all deaths) and 63% of these deaths are attributable to sudden cardiac death [1].

Although prevention of progressive cardiovascular disease is the ultimate solution to this problem, the increasing average age of the population, the lack of an effective preventive medicine strategy, or the lack of the public's motivation to change their lifestyle has led to yearly increases in the incidence of cardiac deaths. Because of several cases involving drug recalls, liability issues, and financial losses originating from unexpected side effects of pharmaceutical agents on ion channels [2] or mitochondria [3], as well as the remaining uncertainties associated with predicting the effect of a compound on the electrical stability of the heart, an alarming trend away from drug development for cardiac arrhythmias is underway, leaving clinicians with a relatively limited armamentarium for dealing with acute cardiac arrest.

Part of the solution to this problem is to continue to strive for a complete understanding of the cellular and organ level events leading from a coronary occlusion to catastrophic cardiac arrhythmias. In this vein, many factors are known to change

Novel Therapeutic Targets for Antiarrhythmic Drugs, Edited by George Edward Billman
Copyright © 2010 John Wiley & Sons, Inc.

during the acute, prolonged, and chronic phases of ischemia and reperfusion. What is lacking is a comprehensive understanding of how each of these changes impinge on the integrated function of the myocyte and the myocardial syncytium, which involves complex nonlinear control systems for regulating energy production, Ca^{2+} cycling, contraction, cell-cell coupling, and signal propagation in the heart.

Descriptive mechanistic studies of the origin of ischemia-related arrhythmias based on tissue level recordings and the macroscopic properties of the excitable medium are abundant in the literature and are remarkable for their elegance and insight (for an excellent compendium see ref. 4). At a subcellular level, however, less is known about the sequence of events leading up to the important changes in the myocardial substrate that set the stage for arrhythmias. Our approach to studying this problem, based on observations of single cardiomyocyte behavior, has been to view the organ level dysfunction as a cascade of failures that scale from the collapse of the ability of individual mitochondria to maintain energy production, to the failure of the mitochondrial network, to the failure of the electrical and Ca^{2+} cycling systems of the myocyte, and ultimately, to the emergence of unsynchronized and uncoordinated behavior of the tissue as a consequence of the underlying functional heterogeneity of the connected cells. Hopefully, this new way of thinking about the origin of arrhythmias, which, of course, requires further validation and elaboration in future studies, will lead to novel therapeutics targets and alternative approaches that might permit an acute cardiac patient to break out of the emergent pathological state by attacking the triggers or sustaining factors at the root of the cascade.

15.2   MECHANISMS OF ARRHYTHMIAS

Although the intent of this chapter is to focus on one particular subcellular mechanism as a possible contributor to (primarily) post-ischemic arrhythmias, it is worth reviewing some of the generally accepted mechanisms of arrhythmogenesis in the context of ischemia-reperfusion. These include alterations in conduction, refractory period, abnormal automaticity, ectopic triggering of excitation, and the development of reentrant circuits.

15.2.1   Automaticity

Automaticity refers to activity of spontaneous pacemakers located in the sinoatrial (SA) node, atrioventricular (AV) node, and the ventricle (bundle of His and Purkinje fibers). Under normal conditions, the intrinsic rate of electrical activation of the heart is determined by the fastest pacemaker in the SA node. Through the mechanism of overdrive suppression [5], subsidiary pacemakers are silenced, but they may potentially emerge under pathological conditions (or during intense vagal nerve stimulation) that lead to AV nodal block. During ischemia or reperfusion, abnormal automaticity may originate consequent to depolarization of the resting membrane potential either within or outside of (i.e., ectopic sources) the normal pacemaker locations, for example, near the border of the ischemic and nonischemic zones [6].

Enhanced sympathetic stimulation also increases the firing rate of subsidiary pacemakers [7], which could be a factor during ischemia-reperfusion. Several studies have examined whether the intrinsic idioventricular rate is altered after reperfusion and have found no increase [8–10], although others have observed an increase [11, 12]. Hence, any modification of normal automaticity could, theoretically, contribute to reperfusion arrhythmias. One explanation for variability in the reported results could be related to the duration of the ischemia before reperfusion. Notably, the most commonly observed change in automaticity upon reperfusion is after thrombolytic treatment (i.e. typically after a long ischemia), where the idioventricular rate is increased to 70–95 bpm [11, 13–15]. However, the general consensus is that rapid ectopic rhythms associated with ischemia or reperfusion are more strongly correlated with either triggered activity near the ischemic border [16–18] or by reentrant circuits [19, 20].

15.2.2 Triggered Arrhythmias

Triggered arrhythmias are defined as those occurring after the onset of a normal excitation, i.e., early- or delayed-afterdepolarizations. Early afterdepolarizations (EADs), which often trigger runs of spontaneous action potentials (APs), are prominent under conditions of drug-induced AP prolongation or genetic mutations of ion channels (long QT syndrome). The mechanism of EAD generation is thought to involve the reactivation of Ca^{2+} channels when the plateau potential hovers too long at a vulnerable membrane potential (usually between $-40\,mV$ and $0\,mV$), allowing the L-type Ca^{2+} channels to recover from inactivation [21]. Delayed afterdepolarizations (DADs), on the other hand, represent triggered APs that originate from spontaneous depolarization of the resting membrane potential to the firing threshold after a normal AP. DADs are prominent under conditions of $Na^+{}_i$ overload such as during digitalis treatment [22], and the mechanism involves a spontaneous release of Ca^{2+} from the sarcoplasmic reticulum and the associated activation of the sarcolemmal Na^+/Ca^{2+} exchange current [23]. DADs tend to be favored when the SR Ca^{2+} load is high (e.g., during catecholamine stimulation) when the probability of a spontaneous Ca^{2+} release is increased (for example, with genetic mutations of the ryanodine receptor linked to catecholamine-induced polymorphic ventricular tachycardia (CPVT) [24, 25], or in some models of heart failure when the Na^+/Ca^{2+} exchanger is increased and the inward rectifier K^+ current density is decreased [26, 27]. There is evidence that arrhythmias occurring on recovery from ischemia may be associated with the formation of EADs or DADs [28, 29]. However, other evidence suggests that EADs are present during I/R but are not correlated with ventricular fibrillation (VF) induction [30]. Depending on the specific ischemia-reperfusion protocol (e.g., global ischemia versus regional, low flow versus total), it is safe to say that both reentrant and non-reentrant mechanisms can contribute to potentially lethal arrhythmias [31].

15.2.2.1 *Reentrant Arrhythmias.* Reentry involves waves of excitation that circle around to encounter myocardium that has recovered from refractoriness so as to permit reexcitation in a manner that does not follow the normal conduction pathway.

Reentry is favored by slowed conduction, unidirectional block, and an increase in the dispersion of refractoriness in the tissue, factors that can change dramatically during ischemia-reperfusion. Some important considerations that contribute to the suscepti- bility of the myocardial substrate for reentry include the architecture of the heart, including the fiber orientation, the overall mass of the heart, and the transitions between wide and narrow conduction pathways (that promote current source-sink mismatches), as well as the functional alterations that may play a role in diseased hearts, such as regional changes in K^+_o, gap junctional uncoupling, altered AP restitution, and abnormal dispersion of AP repolarization. Both anatomical and functional factors contribute to ischemia-related arrhythmias and must be considered together to understand arrhythmogenesis comprehensively.

15.2.2.2 Conduction. Conduction changes during ischemia have been reported by many investigators (for review see, refs. 4 and 32) and consist of a transient elevation of conduction velocity during the first few minutes of ischemia, followed by conduction slowing (in the longitudinal direction, with respect to fiber orientation, from the normal 50 cm/s to ~33 cm/s in the ischemic zone and in the transverse direction from 21 to 13 cm/s [33]). Several factors are thought to contribute to conduction slowing, including resting membrane potential depolarization related to extracellular K^+ accumulation, metabolic acidification, and decreased gap junctional channel conductance, which reduces cell-cell electrical coupling.

Over the first 10 min of ischemia, resting membrane potential depolarizes by approximately 10 mV while K^+_o rises monotonically from 4 mM to between 10 and 20 mM [34]. Several factors may contribute to the K^+_o increase, including partial inhibition of the Na^+/K^+ ATPase caused by a decrease in ΔG_{ATP} 55 to 46 kJ/mol (<4 min), an osmotically induced decrease of the volume of the extracellular space, and an increase in cellular K^+ loss. K^+ efflux might occur as a result of K^+ transport coupled to anaerobic lactate accumulation (i.e., anion loss) or from the activation of sarcolemmal K_{ATP} channels [35], although both mechanisms have been chal- lenged [36, 37]. Other factors including metabolic acidification [32] and Na^+_i loading [36] have also been linked to ischemia-induced K^+_o accumulation. Metabolic acidification occurs rapidly at the onset of ischemia because of an increase in tissue PCO_2, and the changes in external (pH_o decreases from 7.4 to 6.5) and internal pH (pH_i decreases from 7.0 to 6.5) can influence a large number of sarcolemmal ion channels, as well as gap junctional channels. Lysophospholipids and acylcarnitines begin to accumulate within minutes of the onset of ischemia and may alter ion channel activities to trigger arrhythmias [38, 39]. Na^+_i rises rapidly (3–5-fold over 15 min) and may contribute to K^+ loss [36] and later Ca^{2+} overload [40–42]. Also within the first 10 min of ischemia, significant shortening of the AP occurs, its amplitude is diminished, and the upstroke velocity slows—effects that contribute to diminished tissue conduction velocity. These changes in the AP can be blunted by inhibiting K_{ATP} channels or by compounds that prevent mitochondrial depolarization (discussed below) [43].

Additional changes occur during the 2nd 10 min of ischemia, including a further decrease in conduction velocity [44], gap junctional uncoupling, catecolamine release (at $\sim$15–20 min), an increase in Ca^{2+}_i (2–3 fold), a second phase of ATP_i decrease, and an increase in Mg^{2+} (>3-fold).

15.2.2.3 Refractory Period. For reentry to be initiated, the path length of the circuit must exceed the wavelength of the propagating wave or else the wave will be terminated. The wavelength is a function of the product of the conduction velocity (CV) and the effective refractory period (ERP). Thus, either a decrease in CV or decrease in ERP may establish a short enough wavelength for the formation of a reentrant circuit. The refractory period is only partly determined by the AP duration during ischemia, and it has been observed that the ERP can lengthen even during the period when the AP is shortening [45], a phenomenon that has been referred to as post-repolarization refractoriness [46, 47]. The mechanism underlying this effect is not well understood, although it has been correlated with a slowed recovery from inactivation of Na^+ and Ca^{2+} currents [33], perhaps related to partial depolarization of the resting membrane potential. Although post-repolarization refractoriness can partially counteract decreased ERP during ischemia, many studies have demonstrated that ERP is abbreviated along with the AP after coronary occlusion [48–50].

CV slowing and abbreviation of ERP during ischemia can enhance susceptibility to reentry but, by themselves, may not be sufficient to trigger it. Mechanistic models of reentry generally require that unidirectional block occur in part of the conduction pathway, in order for the distal part of the loop to remain excitable when the wavefront returns. One way in which functional unidirectional block can occur is if the ERP is significantly different in two arms of a conduction pathway, for example, if the action potential duration differs (creating an effective block in one direction at fast stimulus rates if the AP is long, but not in the region of short AP and ERP). In the ventricular myocardium, the critical difference between the shortest and longest ERP required to support ventricular tachycardia in response to a premature stimulus in normal tissue is in the range of 95–145 ms [51–54]. During ischemia-reperfusion, such an increase in the regional heterogeneity of ERP, also known as "dispersion of refractoriness," has been linked to the onset of reentrant arrhythmias and depends on the duration of the ischemia, with a significant increase in the fibrillation incidence with reperfusion after 20–30 min of ischemia, correlated with a large increase in AP heterogeneity [55]. Thus, for reentrant arrhythmias to originate after ischemia-reperfusion, the likely requirements include slowed CV, shortened ERP with dispersion of refractoriness, and transient unidirectional block perhaps resulting from a triggered premature stimulus.

15.3   ISCHEMIA-REPERFUSION ARRHYTHMIAS

The arrhythmias associated with acute ischemia may differ depending on the model used (for example, low-flow ischemia, regional, global ischemia), but they have generally been classified into two types. Early, or type 1a, arrhythmias occur between 2 and 10 min after coronary occlusion, with a peak at approximately 5 min [4, 56, 57] and late type. Type 1a arrhythmias occur when there is delayed activation in the subepicardial ischemic region, and they are often associated with electrical alternans. There is evidence that reentry may be involved [58, 59]. Phase 1a arrhythmias are usually followed by a short arrhythmia-free period followed by a second increase occurring between 15 and 45 min (type 1b). Type 1b arrhythmias occur when epicardial conduction has normalized somewhat and may vary depending on species (cf. page 236 of ref. 4). The mechanisms underlying both types of arrhythmias are still not completely understood.

Reperfusion arrhythmias can occur after as little as 3 min of ischemia [60] but are greatly increased in incidence when the ischemia is prolonged for 20–30 min [55]. Extension of the ischemia period beyond 30 min tends to decrease the occurrence of arrhythmias [61], probably as the extent of reperfusion injury increases, which limits the mass of viable (and electrically active) myocardium. Two phases of reperfusion arrhythmias have been noted in the dog after 30 min of ischemia [57], the first being almost immediate induction of ventricular fibrillation. If this does not occur, then a second period of arrhythmias, consisting of ventricular premature depolarizations and ventricular tachycardia, is observed at 2–7 min of reperfusion.

15.4   MITOCHONDRIAL CRITICALITY: THE ROOT OF ISCHEMIA-REPERFUSION ARRHYTHMIAS

As discussed, a plethora of changes in ion gradients, channel activities, and metabolic factors are present during ischemia and when oxidative phosphorylation and electron flow are restored on reperfusion. Unraveling the complex network of interactions that lead up to electrical and contractile dysfunction after a long ischemia is challenging; yet most of the key alterations can be plausibly linked to the failure of the mitochondria to maintain the energy state and limit the accumulation of protons, Na^+, Ca^{2+}, and reactive oxygen species (ROS). Several successful protective strategies have focused on mitigating one or more of these factors (e.g., inhibition of the sarcolemmal Na^+/H^+ or Na^+/Ca^{2+} exchangers, inhibition of L-type Ca^{2+} channels, and antioxidant treatment); however, a detailed understanding of why the mitochondrial network of the myocyte fails could indicate new strategies to head off the problem at its root cause. Our work over the years has gradually led us to view arrhythmias associated with metabolic stress as the result of a chain of events spanning from failure of mitochondria to cellular and organ level spatiotemporal dysfunction.

The spatial organization of cardiac myocyte reflects a tripartite relationship between the sites of excitation and Ca^{2+} release (the dyads), the main sites of energy consumption (the myofilaments), and the sites of ATP production (mitochondria). Mitochondria form a regular three-dimensional lattice, packed between the myofilaments and surrounding the t-tubules. Both feedforward and feedback signaling takes place between these three compartments. An increase in work initiates a rapid mitochondrial response as ATP is hydrolyzed by the myosin ATPase, whereas an increase in the Ca^{2+} transient amplitude facilitates mitochondrial Ca^{2+} uptake to stimulate oxidative phosphorylation. Mitochondria are also a major source of ROS in the cell, which can alter the activity of ion channels, Ca^{2+} handling proteins, and contractile proteins. Moreover, the generation of metabolic intermediates (e.g., NADH, isocitrate, etc.) provides the reducing equivalents required to maintain the negative redox potential of the antioxidant pathways (such as the thioredoxin and GSH pools), driven by the $NADPH/NADP^+$ redox potential. Thus, mitochondrial redox regulation will have an impact on neighboring structures like the SR Ca^{2+} release channel.

Because of the central role played by the mitochondria in coordinating the integrative function of the cell, any deficiency of mitochondrial function is amplified. When metabolism becomes severely compromised by ischemia, reperfusion, or other forms of metabolic stress (e.g., oxidative stress, and substrate deprivation), the vulnerability of the mitochondrial network is revealed and cell injury or death is the outcome (for review, see refs. 62 and 63). Prior to the irreversible cell injury, however, the collapse of mitochondrial inner membrane potential ($\Delta\Psi_m$) mediates changes in energy sensitive channels, because uncoupled mitochondria begin to consume ATP via reversal of the mitochondrial ATP synthase. In particular, sarcolemmal K_{ATP} channels are activated and cellular electrical excitability is strongly affected [64–66].

More than a decade ago, we observed that metabolic stress (substrate deprivation) in isolated guinea pig myocytes precipitated spontaneous, self-organized oscillations in NADH, K_{ATP} current, and Ca^{2+} transient amplitude [67]. We hypothesized that such spatiotemporal changes in electrical excitability, if present in the whole heart, might underlie reentrant arrhythmias associated with ischemia and reperfusion. Consequently, we sought to elucidate the mechanisms responsible for triggering this emergent network property [68], and subsequent studies have led us to a mechanism involving ROS-dependent mitochondrial oscillator [69, 70].

The concept of mitochondrial ROS-induced ROS release, first described by the group of Sollott and coworkers [71], was conceived to explain how laser excitation of mitochondria leads to rapid $\Delta\Psi_m$ depolarization (an effect observed by several laboratories [72–74]), which involves the activation of an energy dissipating ion channel (presumably the permeability transition pore) in the inner membrane. The process is autocatalytic; that is, a small amount of triggering ROS causes a larger leak of ROS to be produced by the electron transport chain. Having observed, in some cases, highly synchronized mitochondrial depolarization/repolarization cycles within and between myocytes subjected to metabolic stress, and in other cases, rather localized clusters of mitochondria behaving independently [68], we employed a variation of the laser method to ask the question of what would be the effect of local laser excitation of a few mitochondria on the mitochondrial network as a whole. In other words, does a small amount of oxidative stress propagate to the many thousands of mitochondria within a heart cell? Using two-photon microscopy, we were able to scan a small focal volume of a cell (approximately 8 μm square and 1 μm thick) loaded with the $\Delta\Psi_m$ sensor TMRE and the ROS sensor CM-DCF to effect a local depolarization and ROS burst in the flashed region. This procedure has no immediate effect on mitochondria outside of the scanned region, but after several minutes of delay, triggers coordinated $\Delta\Psi_m$, NADH and ROS oscillations throughout the cell. The oscillations had a period of approximately one every 90–100 s, consisting of a rapid depolarization phase, a short period of stable low potential, and then a slow recovery of $\Delta\Psi_m$ before the cycle begins again [69]. Furthermore, prior to the first global $\Delta\Psi_m$ depolarization, gradual spreading of the oxidative stress to mitochondria across the length and width of the cell was noted, and we observed the first fast depolarization corresponded to the time when $\sim$56% of the mitochondrial network had oxidative stress above a certain threshold level (indicated by the intensity of the ROS sensor CM-DCF). This number fit the theoretical framework of a percolation matrix near its critical threshold (the point at which the probability of a given mitochondrion belonging to a spanning cluster from one end of the cell to the other rises rapidly) [75]. This indicated that the mitochondrial network behaves in a manner similar to many other nonlinear excitable systems [76], and that close to the critical percolation threshold, the mitochondrial network can collapse in a highly coordinated manner. We referred to this state as the point of "mitochondrial criticality." The concept that biological systems can operate at the edge of dynamic instability to achieve physiological control has been put forward by several investigators [76–78]. This adaptation may have evolved to favor a quick and flexible response to environmental change. However, there are dire consequences for the function of the myocardial syncytium when the network is pushed too far. The emergent macroscopic patterns of $\Delta\Psi_m$ depolarization depend on the spatial arrangement and on the proximity of the mitochondria to each other; that is, the lattice-like organization and neighbor-neighbor interaction of mitochondria in the heart cell are important determinants of the spatiotemporal response.

Other experimental studies examining the mechanism of $\Delta\Psi_m$ oscillation revealed that ROS production from complex III of the electron transport chain triggers the opening of a mitochondrial ion channel that can be inhibited by ligands of the mitochondrial (peripheral) benzodiazepine receptor (mBzR) [69], which are known to block an inner membrane anion channel (IMAC) [79, 80]. Since small molecular weight markers were retained by the mitochondria and there was no sensitivity of the oscillator to Ca^{2+} or cyclosporin A [69], the PTP was ruled out as the mediator of ROS-induced ROS release in our experiments. Oscillations with a similar period could also be reproduced in a single mitochondrion computational model that incorporated ROS production by the electron transport chain, a ROS-activated IMAC, and ROS scavenging [70]. The model is able to simulate a relaxation-type oscillator: ROS produced by the electron transport chain accumulate to a threshold level and then trigger the opening of IMAC in a positive feedback loop. Termination of the cycle occurs when ROS at the activator site of the channel decrease as a result of both membrane depolarization (decreasing the electrochemical driving force for superoxide efflux from the mitochondrial matrix) and ROS scavenging by the antioxidant enzymes.

15.5 K_{ATP} ACTIVATION AND ARRHYTHMIAS

K_{ATP} channels are rapidly activated by cytoplasmic ATP removal or metabolic inhibition and mediate a weakly inwardly rectifying background K^+ current

[64, 65]. The increased K^+ conductance tends to lock the resting membrane potential close to the equilibrium potential for K^+ (E_K) and after 10 min of ischemia resting membrane potential is equal to E_K [81]. K_{ATP} activation can occur even though total cellular ATP has not been fully depleted because the open probability is increased when cofactors like ADP, pH, and Mg^{2+} increase. K_{ATP} current activates rapidly when mitochondria uncouple because the drop in $\Delta\Psi_m$ caused by an increased proton leak causes the ATP synthase to run in reverse, thus consuming cytoplasmic ATP and decreasing the phosphorylation potential. Tight coupling between the mitochondrial energy state and the sarcolemmal K_{ATP} current is facilitated by the high-energy phosphoryl transfer reactions of the cytoplasm [82].

K_{ATP} current activation accounts for most of the AP shortening during ischemia, as evidenced by the ability of K_{ATP} channel inhibitors (e.g., glibenclamide) to prevent the decrease in AP duration occurring over the first 10 min of ischemia [43]. After 10–15 min of global ischemia, cellular electrical excitability diminishes and eventually ceases (by about 20 min), roughly paralleling the time course of increased tissue resistance [44]. Glibenclamide treatment does not prevent the latter failure of AP generation. Concomitant with the AP shortening, there is a monotonic decrease in the AP amplitude and upstroke velocity during the first 10 min of ischemia [43]. This is also partially prevented by glibenclamide treatment, suggesting that K_{ATP} channels may be responsible for both the AP shortening and the depolarization of resting membrane potential, most likely because of their contribution to extracellular K^+ accumulation.

The effect of K_{ATP} channel inhibition on ischemia-reperfusion injury and arrhythmogenesis is variable and very species dependent. For example, in mice treated with the KATP channel blocker HMR1098, ischemia causes a much more rapid contracture of the isolated perfused heart (within 5 min of the onset of ischemia) compared with untreated hearts [83]. In this species, APs are already very short and the heart rate is extremely high (~600 bpm), which could potentially explain why K_{ATP} channel activation during ischemia is essential to prevent a tetanus-like depolarization of the membrane potential under metabolic stress. In contrast, in larger animals with slower heart rates and longer AP plateau potentials (e.g., guinea pig, dogs, and humans), glibenclamide treatment does not accelerate ischemic contracture, although it does prevent the protective effects of ischemic or chemical preconditioning [84]. In fact, K_{ATP} channel inhibition has been shown to prevent VF after acute myocardial infarction in non-insulin-dependent diabetic patients [85]. Furthermore, in a model of VF induced by the combination of acute myocardial ischemia and exercise in dogs with healed myocardial infarctions, K_{ATP} channel inhibition effectively prevented arrhythmias [86–89]. Notably, the antiarrhythmic effect was observed with compounds (HMR1883 and congeners) that were designed to selectively inhibit the heart sarcolemmal K_{ATP} channel (i.e., Kir6.2-SUR2A isoforms combination) without affecting pancreatic insulin release. It is also not very likely that the antiarrhythmic effect of the HMR compound was due to inhibition of mitochondrial K_{ATP} channels, since we, and others, have previously shown that this compound does not block the cardioprotective effect of diazoxide [90].

The arrhythmogenic effect of K_{ATP} channel activation during ischemia-reperfusion could be attributable to an increased dispersion of repolarization and shortening of the effective refractory period of the myocardium, especially if the activation of K_{ATP} currents occurs heterogeneously in the heart. In this light, it is important to understand that mitochondrial $\Delta\Psi_m$ depolarization is tightly coupled to K_{ATP} channel activation and AP duration changes in cardiac cells undergoing mitochondrial oscillations [43, 69]. Hence, the spatiotemporal behavior of the mitochondrial energy state of myocytes in the syncytium could govern the susceptibility of the whole organ to arrhythmias.

15.6 METABOLIC SINKS AND REPERFUSION ARRHYTHMIAS

The data discussed above led us to hypothesize that if individual myocytes, or clusters of myocytes, in intact hearts subjected to ischemia-reperfusion undergo $\Delta\Psi_m$ oscillations, or simply display a heterogeneous regional $\Delta\Psi_m$ distribution, the associated increases in local K_{ATP} current density could create regional current sinks, which we called "metabolic sinks," that could either block the wave from propagating (metabolic sink/block) or dramatically shorten the wavelength in those regions. Theoretically, this dispersion of repolarization could provide a substrate for reentry. In particular, the finding that ROS-induced ROS release occurs in normally oxygenated myocytes when there is electron flow in the respiratory chain, we speculated that the mechanism might be important upon reperfusion after ischemia, since the criteria for mitochondrial criticality would be fulfilled, that is, increased oxidative stress, depletion of the antioxidant pool, and restoration of substrate oxidation. Subsequent studies then focused on establishing the link between mitochondrial depolarization and post-ischemic arrhythmias using an isolated perfused heart, global ischemia model. Global ischemia was employed to eliminate the complicating issue of ischemic border zone behavior, where there is an interface between normal and ischemic tissue, where other mechanisms for triggered arrhythmias may be present (see discussion above).

Optical mapping of Langendorff-perfused guinea pig hearts subjected to 30 min of ischemia followed by reperfusion revealed that tachyarrhythmias and VF occurs in >90% of the hearts upon reperfusion [43]. In hearts treated with the mBzR ligand/ IMAC inhibitor, 4′chlorodiazepam (4′Cl-DZP), AP shortening during ischemia was significantly blunted, and unlike controls, electrical activation continued to be present more than 20 min into the ischemic phase. The reduction of the AP amplitude and the decreased overshoot velocity were also partially prevented by 4′Cl-DZP treatment. These data indicated that mitochondrial depolarization is the primary factor driving K_{ATP} channel activation in early ischemia and contributes to the failure of excitation late in the ischemic phase (20–30 min). Most remarkably, ventricular tachyarrhythmias on reperfusion were almost completely eliminated by 4′Cl-DZP, even when it was applied only upon reperfusion. More recently, the protective effect of 4′Cl-DZP on both electrical and contractile post-ischemic function was also demonstrated in a rabbit heart model [91]. The antiarrhythmic effect was not evident in hearts treated with CsA, again arguing against the PTP as the earliest target involved in ROS-induced ROS release in hearts exposed to ischemia-reperfusion (although we do not deny that the permeability transition pore opens later in the reperfusion phase and may contribute to cell death and increased infarct size).

The argument that metabolic sinks exist in the intact heart is strengthened by imaging studies demonstrating that individual myocytes, or groups of myocytes, lose $\Delta\Psi_m$ both during ischemia and, even more so, upon reperfusion [92, 93]. The loss of $\Delta\Psi_m$ in individual myocytes is correlated with high levels of ROS in the same cells and is decreased when the hearts are treated with 4'Cl-DZP [93].

15.7 ANTIOXIDANT DEPLETION

The synchronized collapse of $\Delta\Psi_m$ can be induced, not only by an increase in mitochondrial ROS production, but also by depletion of the intracellular antioxidant pool. For example, we have previously reported that depletion of the GSH pool with diamide can trigger $\Delta\Psi_m$ oscillations that were similar to those induced by laser flash [94]. To analyze the specific cytoplasmic GSH/GSSG ratio that triggers the initial reversible $\Delta\Psi_m$ loss, we studied partially permeabilized cardiomyocytes that were exposed to various GSH:GSSG combinations. We found that a decrease in the ratio from 300:1 to approximately 150:1 could depolarize the mitochondrial network in a 4'Cl-DZP sensitive manner. A further decrease in the GSH:GSSG ratio to 50:1 provoked the opening of the PTP, suggesting that ROS-induced ROS release involves a hierarchy of energy dissipating ion channels that have different sensitivities to the mitochondrial redox state.

Extending these observations to the whole heart level, we demonstrated that diamide treatment of normoxic isolated perfused hearts also induces heterogeneous ROS production and mitochondrial network depolarization [93]. Furthermore, ventricular fibrillation could also be induced by diamide treatment [95]. Taken together, the findings support the idea that mitochondrial criticality initiates a cascade of failures that scales to produce organ level electrical and contractile dysfunction.

15.8 MITOCHONDRIA AS THERAPEUTIC TARGETS

Understanding the mechanisms involved in the interaction among the mitochondrial network, the Ca^{2+} handling subsystem, sarcolemmal membrane electrical excitability, and the contractile element holds out the promise of being able to intervene at the very onset of the catastrophic scaling phenomenon. Preservation of mitochondrial function has an advantage over other protective strategies since mitochondria will impact every other component of the cell. Defects in mitochondrial ATP production, redox status, and ROS generation stand upstream from most of the changes occurring during ischemia and reperfusion—thus, attacking only a single downstream target such as the K_{ATP} channel, Na^+/H^+ exchanger, Na^+/Ca^{2+} exchanger, or voltage-gated Na^+ channel would be expected to be only partially effective in preventing arrhythmias, contractile dysfunction, and infarction.

The development of effective therapeutic strategies targeting the mitochondria is currently hampered by a lack of solid molecular information about the identity of many of the major players behind mitochondrial network failure. For example, none of the proteins involved in mitochondrial Ca^{2+} homeostasis have been unequivocally resolved. Effective pharmacological tools point us toward targets like the mBzR, IMAC, or the PTP, but the actual structures causing the observed changes in $\Delta\Psi_m$ are the subject of extensive debate. The field is therefore ripe for discovery as new proteomic and genomic tools are applied. Meanwhile, an integrative multiscale approach, involving both experimental and computational models of the cardiac cell and the myocardial syncytium is essential for understanding how failure at the level of the organelle can scale to produce an arrhythmia in the whole organ.

REFERENCES

1. CDC. Available at http://www.cdc.gov/mmwr/preview/mmwrhtml/mm5106a3.htm.

2. Egan, W., Zlokarnik, G., Grootenhuis, D. (2004). In silico prediction of drug safety: Despite progress there is abundant room for improvement. Drug Discovery Today, 1, 381–387.

3. Dykens, J.A., Will, Y. (2007). The significance of mitochondrial toxicity testing in drug development. Drug Discovery Today, 12, 777–785.

4. Wit, A.L., Janse, M.J. The Ventricular Arrhythmias of Ischemia and Infarction: Electrophysiological Mechanisms. Futura, Mount Kisco, NY, 1993.

5. Vassalle, M. (1970). Electrogenic suppression of automaticity in sheep and dog purkinje fibers. Circulation Research, 27, 361–377.

6. Hauer, R.N., de Bakker, J.M., de Wilde, A.A., Straks, W., Vermeulen, J.T., Janse, M.J. (1991). Ventricular tachycardia after in vivo DC shock ablation in dogs. Electrophysiologic and histologic correlation. Circulation, 84, 267–278.

7. Hume, J., Katzung, B.G. (1980). Physiological role of endogenous amines in the modulation of ventricular automaticity in the guinea-pig. Journal of Physiology, 309, 275–286.

8. Levites, R., Banka, V.S., Helfant, R.H. (1975). Electrophysiologic effects of coronary occlusion and reperfusion. Observations of dispersion of refractoriness and ventricular automaticity. Circulation, 52, 760–765.

9. Ramanathan, K.B., Bodenheimer, M.M., Banka, V.S., Helfant, R.H. (1977). Electrophysiologic effects of partial coronary occlusion and reperfusion. American Journal of Cardiology, 40, 50–54.

10. Murdock, D.K., Loeb, J.M., Euler, D.E., Randall, W.C. (1980). Electrophysiology of coronary reperfusion. A mechanism for reperfusion arrhythmias. Circulation, 61, 175–182.

11. Goldberg, S., Greenspon, A.J., Urban, P.L., Muza, B., Berger, B., Walinsky, P., Maroko, P.R. (1983). Reperfusion arrhythmia: A marker of restoration of antegrade flow during intracoronary thrombolysis for acute myocardial infarction. American Heart Journal, 105, 26–32.

12. Penkoske, P.A., Sobel, B.E., Corr, P.B. (1978). Disparate electrophysiological alterations accompanying dysrhythmia due to coronary occlusion and reperfusion in the cat. Circulation, 58, 1023–1035.

13. Sclarovsky, S., Strasberg, B., Agmon, J. (1978). Multiform accelerated idioventricular rhythm in acute myocardial infarction. Journal of Electrocardiology, 11, 197–200.

14. Sclarovsky, S., Strasberg, B., Martonovich, G., Agmon, J. (1978). Ventricular rhythms with intermediate rates in acute myocardial infarction. Chest, 74, 180–182.

15. Rentrop, P., Blanke, H., Karsch, K.R., Kaiser, H., Kostering, H., Leitz, K. (1981). Selective intracoronary thrombolysis in acute myocardial infarction and unstable angina pectoris. Circulation, 63, 307–317.

16. Janse, M.J., van Capelle, F.J., Electrotonic interactions across an inexcitable region as a cause of ectopic activity in acute regional myocardial ischemia. A study in intact porcine and canine hearts and computer models. Circulation Research, 50, (1982). 527–537.

17. Ideker, R.E., Klein, G.J., Harrison, L., Smith, W.M., Kasell, J., Reimer, K.A., Wallace, A. G., Gallagher, J.J. (1981). The transition to ventricular fibrillation induced by reperfusion after acute ischemia in the dog: A period of organized epicardial activation. Circulation, 63, 1371–1379.

18. Pogwizd, S.M., Corr, P.B. (1987). Electrophysiologic mechanisms underlying arrhythmias due to reperfusion of ischemic myocardium. Circulation, 76, 404–426.

19. Wu, J., Zipes, D.P. (2001). Transmural reentry during acute global ischemia and reperfusion in canine ventricular muscle. American Journal of Physiology Heart and Circulatory Physiology, 280, H2717–2725.

20. Yan, G.X., Joshi, A., Guo, D., Hlaing, T., Martin, J., Xu, X., Kowey, P.R. (2004). Phase 2 reentry as a trigger to initiate ventricular fibrillation during early acute myocardial ischemia. Circulation, 110, 1036–1041.

21. Zeng, J., Rudy, Y. (1995). Early afterdepolarizations in cardiac myocytes: Mechanism and rate dependence. Biophysical Journal, 68, 949–964.

22. Lederer, W.J., Tsien, R.W. (1976). Transient inward current underlying arrhythmogenic effects of cardiotonic steroids in Purkinje fibres. Journal of Physiology, 263, 73–100.

23. Berlin, J.R., Cannell, M.B., Lederer, W.J. (1989). Cellular origins of the transient inward current in cardiac myocytes. Role of fluctuations and waves of elevated intracellular calcium. Circulation Research, 65, 115–126.

24. Priori, S.G., Napolitano, C., Memmi, M., Colombi, B., Drago, F., Gasparini, M., DeSimone, L., Coltorti, F., Bloise, R., Keegan, R., Cruz Filho, F.E., Vignati, G., Benatar, A., DeLogu, A. (2002). Clinical and molecular characterization of patients with catecholaminergic polymorphic ventricular tachycardia. Circulation, 106, 69–74.

25. Marks, A.R, Priori, S., Memmi, M., Kontula, K., Laitinen, P.J. (2002). Involvement of the cardiac ryanodine receptor/calcium release channel in catecholaminergic polymorphic ventricular tachycardia. Journal of Cell Physiology, 190, 1–6.

26. Pogwizd, S.M., Schlotthauer, K., Li, L., Yuan, W., Bers, D.M. (2001). Arrhythmogenesis and contractile dysfunction in heart failure: Roles of sodium-calcium exchange, inward rectifier potassium current, and residual beta-adrenergic responsiveness. Circulation Research, 88, 1159–1167.

27. Pogwizd, S.M., Qi, M., Yuan, W., Samarel, A.M., Bers, D.M., Upregulation of Na($+$)/Ca ($2+$) exchanger expression and function in an arrhythmogenic rabbit model of heart failure. Circulation Research, 85, (1999). 1009–1019.

28. Rozanski, G.J., Witt, R.C. (1991). Early afterdepolarizations and triggered activity in rabbit cardiac Purkinje fibers recovering from ischemic-like conditions. Role of acidosis. Circulation, 83, 1352–1360.

29. Pogwizd, S.M., Corr, B. (1992). The contribution of nonreentrant mechanisms to malignant ventricular arrhythmias. Basic Research in Cardiology, 87Suppl, 2, 115–129.

30. Vera, Z., Pride, H.P., Zipes, D.P. (1995). Reperfusion arrhythmias: Role of early afterdepolarizations studied by monophasic action potential recordings in the intact canine heart during autonomically denervated and stimulated states. Journal of Cardiovascular Electrophysiology, 6, 532–543.

31. Pogwizd, S.M., Corr, P.B. (1986). Mechanisms of arrhythmogenesis during myocardial ischemia and reperfusion: A perspective of our current understanding. Journal of Molecular and Cellular Cardiology, 18 Suppl 4, 43–47.

32. Kleber, A.G., Fleischhauer, J., Cascio, W.E., Ischemia-induced propagation failure in the heart. In Jalife, J., Zipes, D.P., eds. , Cardiac electrophysiology: From cell to bedside. W. B. Saunders, Philadelphia, P.A., 1995.

33. Kleber, A.G., Janse, M.J., Wilms-Schopmann, F.J., Wilde, A.A., Coronel, R. (1986). Changes in conduction velocity during acute ischemia in ventricular myocardium of the isolated porcine heart. Circulation, 73, 189–198.

34. Cascio, W.E., Yan, G.X., Kleber, A.G. (1990). Passive electrical properties, mechanical activity, and extracellular potassium in arterially perfused and ischemic rabbit ventricular muscle. Effects of calcium entry blockade or hypocalcemia. Circulation Research, 66, 1461–1473.

35. Wilde, A.A., Escande, D., Schumacher, C.A., Thuringer, D., Mestre, M., Fiolet, J.W., Janse M.J. (1990). Potassium accumulation in the globally ischemic mammalian heart. A role for the ATP-sensitive potassium channel. Circulation Research, 67, 835–843.

36. Shivkumar, K., Deutsch, N.A., Lamp, S.T., Khuu, K., Goldhaber, J.I., Weiss, J.N. (1997). Mechanism of hypoxic K loss in rabbit ventricle. Journal of Clinical Investigation, 100, 1782–1788.

37. Weiss, J.N., Shieh, R.C. (1994). Potassium loss during myocardial ischaemia and hypoxia: Does lactate efflux play a role? Cardiovascular Research, 28, 1125–1132.

38. DaTorre, S.D., Creer, M.H., Pogwizd, S.M., Corr, P.B. (1991). Amphipathic lipid metabolites and their relation to arrhythmogenesis in the ischemic heart. Journal of Molecular and Cellular Cardiology, 23 Suppl 1, 11–22.

39. Pogwizd, S.M., Onufer, J.R., Kramer, J.B., Sobel, B.E., Corr, P.B. (1986). Induction of delayed afterdepolarizations and triggered activity in canine Purkinje fibers by lysophosphoglycerides. Circulation Research, 59, 416–426.

40. Pierce, G.N., Meng, H. (1992). The role of sodium-proton exchange in ischemic/reperfusion injury in the heart. Na(+)-H + exchange and ischemic heart disease. American Journal of Cardiovascular Pathology, 4, 91–102.

41. Ravens, U., Himmel, H.M. (1999). Drugs preventing Na + and Ca2 + overload. Pharmacological Research, 39, 167–174.

42. Ver Donck, L., Borgers, M., Verdonck, F. (1993). Inhibition of sodium and calcium overload pathology in the myocardium: A new cytoprotective principle. Cardiovascular Research, 27, 349–357.

43. Akar, F.G., Aon, M.A., Tomaselli, G.F., O'Rourke, B. (2005). The mitochondrial origin of postischemic arrhythmias. Journal of Clinical Investigation, 115, 3527–3535.

44. Kleber, A.G., Riegger, C.B., Janse, M.J. (1987). Electrical uncoupling and increase of extracellular resistance after induction of ischemia in isolated, arterially perfused rabbit papillary muscle. Circulation Research, 61, 271–279.

45. Downar, E., Janse, M.J., Durrer, D. (1977). The effect of acute coronary artery occlusion on subepicardial transmembrane potentials in the intact porcine heart. Circulation, 56, 217–224.

46. el-Sherif, N., Scherlag, B.J., Lazarra, R., Samet, P. (1974). Pathophysiology of tachycardia- and bradycardia-dependent block in the canine proximal His-Purkinje system after acute myocardial ischemia. American Journal of Cardiology, 33, 529–540.

47. Lazzara, R., El-Sherif, N., Scherlag, B.J. (1975). Disorders of cellular electrophysiology produced by ischemia of the canine His bundle. Circulation Research, 36, 444–454.

48. Brooks, C.M., Gilbert, J.L., Greenspan, M.E., Lange, G., Mazzella, H.M. (1960). Excitability and electrical response of ischemic heart muscle. American Journal of Physiology, 198, 1143–1147.

49. Han, J., Moe, G.K. (1964). Nonuniform recovery of excitability in ventricular muscle. Circulation Research, 14, 44–60.

50. Russell, D.C., Oliver, M.F. (1978). Ventricular refractoriness during acute myocardial ischaemia and its relationship to ventricular fibrillation. Cardiovascular Research, 12, 221–227.

51. Wallace, A.G., Mignone, R.J. (1966). Physiologic evidence concerning the re-entry hypothesis for ectopic beats. American Heart Journal, 72, 60–70.

52. Kuo, C.S., Amlie, J.P., Munakata, K., Reddy, C.P., Surawicz, B. (1983). Dispersion of monophasic action potential durations and activation times during atrial pacing, ventricular pacing, and ventricular premature stimulation in canine ventricles. Cardiovascular Research, 17, 152–161.

53. Kuo, C.S., Munakata, K., Reddy, C.P., Surawicz, B. (1983). Characteristics and possible mechanism of ventricular arrhythmia dependent on the dispersion of action potential durations. Circulation, 67, 1356–1367.

54. Kuo, C.S., Reddy, C.P., Munakata, K., Surawicz, B. (1985). Mechanism of ventricular arrhythmias caused by increased dispersion of repolarization. European Heart Journal, 6 Suppl D, 63–70.

55. Corr, P.B., Witkowski, F.X. (1983). Potential electrophysiologic mechanisms responsible for dysrhythmias associated with reperfusion of ischemic myocardium. Circulation, 68, 16–24.

56. Janse, M.J., Wit, A.L. (1989). Electrophysiological mechanisms of ventricular arrhythmias resulting from myocardial ischemia and infarction. Physiological Reviews, 69, 1049–1169.

57. Kaplinsky, E., Ogawa, S., Balke, C.W., Dreifus, L.S. (1979). Two periods of early ventricular arrhythmia in the canine acute myocardial infarction model. Circulation, 60, 397–403.

58. Janse, M.J., van Capelle, F.J., Morsink, H., Kleber, A.G., Wilms-Schopman, F., Cardinal, R., d'Alnoncourt, C.N., Durrer, D. (1980). Flow of "injury" current and patterns of excitation during early ventricular arrhythmias in acute regional myocardial ischemia in isolated porcine and canine hearts. Evidence for two different arrhythmogenic mechanisms. Circulation Research, 47, 151–165.

59. Pogwizd, S.M., Corr, P.B. (1987). Reentrant and nonreentrant mechanisms contribute to arrhythmogenesis during early myocardial Ischemia: results using three-dimensional mapping. Circulation Research, 61, 352–371.

60. Corbalan, R., Verrier, R.L., Lown, B. (1976). Differing mechanisms for ventricular vulnerability during coronary artery occlusion and release. American Heart Journal, 92, 223–230.

61. Manning, A.S., Hearse, D.J. (1984). Reperfusion-induced arrhythmias: Mechanisms and prevention. Journal of Molecular and Cellular Cardiology, 16, 497–518.

62. Duchen, M.R. (1999). Contributions of mitochondria to animal physiology: From homeostatic sensor to calcium signalling and cell death. Journal of Physiology, 516, 1–17.

63. Crompton, M. (1999). The mitochondrial permeability transition pore and its role in cell death. Biochemical Journal, 341, 233–249.

64. Noma, A. (1983). ATP-regulated K+ channels in cardiac muscle. Nature, 305, 147–148.

65. Lederer, W.J., Nichols, C.G., Smith, G.L. (1989). The mechanism of early contractile failure of isolated rat ventricular myocytes subjected to complete metabolic inhibition. Journal of Physiology, 413, 329–349.

66. Venkatesh, N., Lamp, S.T., Weiss, J.N. (1991). Sulfonylureas, ATP-sensitive K+ channels, and cellular K+ loss during hypoxia, ischemia, and metabolic inhibition in mammalian ventricle. Circulation Research, 69, 623–637.

67. O'Rourke, B., Ramza, B.M., Marban, E. (1994). Oscillations of membrane current and excitability driven by metabolic oscillations in heart cells. Science, 265, 962–966.

68. Romashko, D.N., Marban, E., O'Rourke, B. (1998). Subcellular metabolic transients and mitochondrial redox waves in heart cells. Proceedings of the National Academy of Science USA, 95, 1618–1623.

69. Aon, M.A., Cortassa, S., Marban, E., O'Rourke, B. (2003). Synchronized whole-cell oscillations in mitochondrial metabolism triggered by a local release of reactive oxygen species in cardiac myocytes. Journal of Biological Chemistry, 278, 44735–44744.

70. Cortassa, S., Aon, M.A., Winslow, R.L., O'Rourke, B. (2004). A mitochondrial oscillator dependent on reactive oxygen species. Biophysical Journal, 87, 2060–2073.

71. Zorov, D.B., Filburn, C.R., Klotz, L.O., Zweier, J.L., Sollott, S.J. (2000). Reactive oxygen species (ROS)-induced ROS release: A new phenomenon accompanying induction of the mitochondrial permeability transition in cardiac myocytes. Journal of Experimental Medicine, 192, 1001–1014.

72. Siemens, A., Walter, R., Liaw, L.H., Berns, M.W. (1982). Laser-stimulated fluorescence of submicrometer regions within single mitochondria of rhodamine-treated myocardial cells in culture. Proceedings of the National Academy of Science USA, 79, 466–470.

73. Loew, L.M., Tuft, R.A., Carrington, W., Fay, F.S. (1993). Imaging in five dimensions: Time-dependent membrane potentials in individual mitochondria. Biophysical Journal, 65, 2396–2407.

74. Huser, J., Rechenmacher, C.E., Blatter, L.A. (1998). Imaging the permeability pore transition in single mitochondria. Biophysical Journal, 74, 2129–2137.

75. Aon, M.A., Cortassa, S., O'Rourke, B. (2004). Percolation and criticality in a mitochondrial network. Proceedings of the National Academy of Sciences USA, 101, 4447–4452.

76. Bak, P. How Nature Works: The Science of Self-Organized Criticality. Copernicus, New York, 1996.

77. Kauffman, S.A. Origins of Order: Self-Organization and Selection in Evolution. Oxford University Press, New York, 1993.

78. Sornette, D. Critical Phenomena in Natural Sciences. Chaos, Fractals, Self Organization and Disorder: Concepts and Tools. Springer, Berlin, Germany, 2000.

79. Beavis, A.D. (1989). On the inhibition of the mitochondrial inner membrane anion uniporter by cationic amphiphiles and other drugs. Journal of Biological Chemistry, 264, 1508–1515.

80. Beavis, A.D. (1992). Properties of the inner membrane anion channel in intact mitochondria. Journal of Bioenergetics and Biomembranes, 24, 77–90.

81. Kleber, A.G. (1983). Resting membrane potential, extracellular potassium activity, and intracellular sodium activity during acute global ischemia in isolated perfused guinea pig hearts. Circulation Research, 52, 442–450.

82. Sasaki, N., Sato, T., Marban, E., O'Rourke, B. (2001). ATP consumption by uncoupled mitochondria activates sarcolemmal K(ATP) channels in cardiac myocytes. American Journal of Physiology Heart Circulation Physiology, 280, H1882–1888.

83. Suzuki, M., Saito, T., Sato, T., Tamagawa, M., Miki, T., Seino, S., Nakaya, H. (2003). Cardioprotective effect of diazoxide is mediated by activation of sarcolemmal but not mitochondrial ATP-sensitive potassium channels in mice. Circulation, 107, 682–685.

84. O'Rourke, B. (2004). Evidence for mitochondrial K+ channels and their role in cardioprotection. Circulation Research, 94, 420–432.

85. Lomuscio, A., Vergani, D., Marano, L., Castagnone, M., Fiorentini, C. (1994). Effects of glibenclamide on ventricular fibrillation in non-insulin-dependent diabetics with acute myocardial infarction. Coronary Artery Disease, 5, 767–771.

86. Billman, G.E. (2008). The cardiac sarcolemmal ATP-sensitive potassium channel as a novel target for anti-arrhythmic therapy. Pharmacology and Therapeutics, 120, 54–70.

87. Billman, G.E., Houle, M.S., Englert, H.C., Gogelein, H. (2004). Effects of a novel cardioselective ATP-sensitive potassium channel antagonist, 1-[[5-[2-(5-chloro-o-anisamido)ethyl]-beta-methoxyethoxyphenyl]sulfonyl]-3 -methylthiourea, sodium salt (HMR 1402), on susceptibility to ventricular fibrillation induced by myocardial ischemia: in vitro and in vivo studies. Journal of Pharmacology and Experimental Therapies, 309, 182–192.

88. Billman, G.E., Englert, H.C., Scholkens, B.A. (1998). HMR 1883, a novel cardioselective inhibitor of the ATP-sensitive potassium channel. Part II: Effects on susceptibility to ventricular fibrillation induced by myocardial ischemia in conscious dogs. Journal of Pharmacology and Experimental Therapy, 286, 1465–1473.

89. Billman, G.E., Avendano, C.E., Halliwill, J.R., Burroughs, J.M. (1993). The effects of the ATP-dependent potassium channel antagonist, glyburide, on coronary blood flow and susceptibility to ventricular fibrillation in unanesthetized dogs. Journal of Cardiovascular Pharmacology, 21, 197–204.

90. Sato, T., Sasaki, N., Seharaseyon, J., O'Rourke, B., Marban, E. (2000). Selective pharmacological agents implicate mitochondrial but not sarcolemmal K(ATP) channels in ischemic cardioprotection. Circulation, 101, 2418–2423.

91. Brown, D.A., Aon, M.A., Akar, F.G., Liu, T., Sorarrain, N., O'Rourke, B. (2008). Effects of 4′-chlorodiazepam on cellular excitation-contraction coupling and ischaemia-reperfusion injury in rabbit heart. Cardiovascular Research, 79, 141–149.

92. Matsumoto-Ida, M., Akao, M., Takeda, T., Kato, M., Kita, T. (2006). Real-time 2-photon imaging of mitochondrial function in perfused rat hearts subjected to ischemia/reperfusion. Circulation, 114, 1497–1503.

93. Slodzinski, M.K., Aon, M.A., O'Rourke, B. (2004). Intracellular and intercellular mitochondrial membrane potential oscillations in the Langendorff perfused heart. Biophysical Journal, 86, 461a.

94. Aon, M.A., Cortassa, S., Maack, C., O'Rourke, B. (2007). Sequential opening of mitochondrial ion channels as a function of glutathione redox thiol status. Journal of Biological Chemistry, 282, 21889–21900.

95. Brown, D., Aon, M., Akar, F., O'Rourke, B. (2008). A ligand to the mitochondrial benzodiazepine receptor prevents ventricular arrhythmias and LV dysfunction after ischemia or glutathione depletion. FASEB Journal, 22, 747.747

Cardiac Gap Junctions: A New Target for New Antiarrhythmic Drugs: Gap Junction Modulators

ANJA HAGEN and STEFAN DHEIN

16.1 INTRODUCTION

The successful propagation of a cardiac action potential is a prerequisite for a normal rhythm. Propagation depends on several factors, including the availability of sodium channels for the fast depolarization of the fibers and the conduction along a single cell [1], the existence of intercellular communication channels (gap junctions), by which the action potential can spread from cell to cell [2], as well as by structural factors such as fibrotic strands that—as nonexcitable tissue—can impede propagation. Moreover, the heart is typically a nonuniform anisotropic tissue, which means that the longitudinal and transverse electrical resistance is different (transverse resistance ≫ longitudinal) and that this changes from area to area [3, 4]. The anisotropic nature is related to the elongated shape of the cells and to the predominant localization of gap junction channels at the cell poles. This structure and a certain degree of anisotropy seem to be necessary to allow conduction with a preferential direction. The situation becomes more complex if differences in the action potential duration exist (dispersion; see below), which elicit voltage differences between two areas and may lead to current flowing between them.

Although antiarrhythmic therapy for decades was a domain of drug therapy, today electrophysiological methods, such as catheter-based ablation therapy, pacemaker implantation, and implantable cardioverter defibrillator (ICD) implantation, have increasing impact. This is the consequence of a plethora of past studies that demonstrated the risk of the common antiarrhythmic drugs. Thus, class I antiarrhythmics exert marked proarrhythmic effects if given in the presence of a structural heart disease, in

Novel Therapeutic Targets for Antiarrhythmic Drugs, Edited by George Edward Billman
Copyright © 2010 John Wiley & Sons, Inc.

particular if given after myocardial infarction [5–7]. These proarrhythmic effects include life-threatening ventricular fibrillation, ventricular tachycardia, and ventricular extrasystoles. Besides this, many drugs can cause bradycardia, atrioventricular (AV)-block and asystoles, as well as supraventricular arrhythmias.

The mechanism responsible for the proarrhythmic activity of class I antiarrhythmic drugs that leads to ventricular fibrillation and tachycardia is complex: Class I antiarrhythmic drugs are sodium channel blockers and, thus, reduce I_{Na}. However, I_{Na} availability is the main factor responsible for the longitudinal conduction velocity [1]. The slowing of conduction is a prerequisite for reentrant arrhythmia [8, 9], because it allows that the activation wavefront can propagate around an obstacle and reach its own repolarization front later in time. At normal conduction velocities, reentry is less probable, because a possible reentrant pathway at high velocity needs to be long to allow sustained reentry, because at shorter pathways the activation wavefront at normal conduction velocity would encounter refractory areas (areas that are still depolarized). At slow conduction velocities, the wavefront may reach the same area after the end of refractoriness [3, 4, 8–12]. Thus, after I_{an} blockade, smaller reentry circuits will either be made possible or favored. The reentrant circuit is assumed to be stable if the reentry path length L equals the wavelength Λ, i.e., the product of local refractory period (RP) and local conduction velocity (CV) (stable reentrant conditions: L = RP * CV).

Another factor contributing to reentrant arrhythmia is heterogeneity in the action potential duration, which is the so-called action potential dispersion. If differences in action potential duration, e.g., by ischemia-induced opening of I_{KATP} channels, occur at a certain location, this will result in a voltage difference, which will be equalized by a current flowing via gap junction channels between the cell with the longer and that with the shorter action potential. In the case of reduced gap junction conductance, this current will be minimized, so that the differences in action potential duration will be maintained. Thus, gap junction blockade can unmask differences in action potential duration [13]. If conduction is slowed by I_{Na} blockade, then the time period during which activated and nonactivated cells (or cells with different action potential durations) are neighbored will be prolonged. If this occurs together with reduced gap junction coupling, it will enhance dispersion as was shown by computer simulation [14]. Experimentally, it was also shown that sodium channel blockade enhances dispersion in nonuniform anisotropic tissue [15]. The resulting compensatory currents may be large enough to depolarize adjacent cells and, thereby, promote arrhythmia. This effect can be expected to be enhanced if myocardial scars or infarcted areas are present, because these represent nonuniformities [3, 4]. The increase in collagen deposition with increasing age may also contribute to this effect [3, 4]. However, it should be kept in mind that sodium channel blocking agents possess use-dependent blocking kinetics and that recovery of excitability is not equivalent to action potential repolarization. Currently, it might be speculated that similar phenomena (i.e., increased dispersion of action potential duration under reduced sodium conductance in nonuniform anisotropic tissue) may at least partially contribute to the well-known proarrhythmic risk of class I antiarrhythmic drugs during the postinfarction period.

At that point, it could be theoretically assumed that gap junction opening should reduce dispersion by enhancing the compensatory currents. However, this enhancement might—if reaching a certain level over a certain period—be large enough to elicit activation. However, because of enhanced coupling, the current (source) is distributed to a larger area (sink), so that it probably does no longer reach the threshold needed for activation (see also below and the section: "Short overview about cardiac gap junctions").

Regarding other antiarrhythmic drugs, class II antiarrhythmics also exhibit proarrhythmic activity mainly leading to AV block, arrest, or bradycardia. The molecular basis of their use in ventricular arrhythmia is not well understood, yet, regarding the therapeutic concentration range. However, recent findings show that the β-adrenergic receptor regulates the expression of the cardiac ventricular gap junction protein connexin (Cx43), [16], which might open a new perspective on the effects of β-adrenergic receptors blockers as well. Class III antiarrhythmics can also exhibit proarrhythmia in the form of polymorphic ventricular tachycardia, torsades de pointes. Class IV antiarrhythmics, which are effective against certain supraventricular tachycardic arrhythmia, can cause AV block, arrest, or bradycardia.

Taken together, all classic ion-channel-blocking antiarrhythmics exert important side effects and possess a considerable proarrhythmic risk. Thus, there is an urgent need for new developments in that field and for the quest for new targets. From the above considerations, the intercellular communication could be a candidate for a new antiarrhythmic target. Once this was recognized, the development of antiarrhythmic peptides started several years ago.

16.2   THE DEVELOPMENT OF GAP JUNCTION MODULATORS AND AAPs

In 1993, we became aware of the effects of intercellular coupling on the homogeneity of activation spreading and on action potential dispersion. At that time, by chance, we found an old article from 1980, where a natural antiarrhythmic peptide (H-Gly-Pro-Hyp-Gly-Ala-Gly), a hexapeptide isolated from bovine atrium, was described that enhanced the synchronization of spontaneously beating embryonic chick heart cell aggregates [17]. The promising first experiments of this group were not pursued after others reported that AAPnat had no effect on action potential parameters of Purkinje fibers [18]. The effects of this peptide on conductive parameters had not been investigated at that time.

First, we started to synthesize this natural antiarrhythmic peptide using classic Merrifield synthesis. We tested the product in cultures of spontaneously beating embryonic chick heart cell aggregates and, indeed, observed enhanced synchronisation between the clusters about 10 minutes after addition of the peptide. After this proof of concept had been established, we performed systematic research: We synthesized the natural antiarrhythmic peptide, AAPnat, and several derivatives. Then, we tested these in isolated rabbit hearts, perfused according to the Langendorff technique, and investigated the spread of activation and the homogeneity of repolarization by 256 channel epicardial potential mapping. The effects were weak, but consistently produced a reduction in local dispersion with EC_{50} values around 10^{-9} mol/L [19–21], as assessed by the standard deviation of the activation-recovery intervals at 256 electrodes and by an increase in homogeneity (defined as the percentage of electrodes exhibiting an ARI which is ±5 ms around the mean ARI). (A selection of peptides, which are still under investigation is shown in Figure 16.1) These derivatives did not affect on any other cardiovascular parameter (Table 16.1). The peptides exhibited similar effects and seemingly the effect could be observed with 1–10 nM. For several reasons (pharmacological and chemical), the antiarrhythmic peptide AAP10 (H-Gly-Ala-Gly-Hyp-Pro-Tyr-$CONH_2$) was selected as the lead compound for all investigations.

The finding that only dispersion was affected by the AAPs was similar to our computer simulations findings where the increase in dispersion resulted as a consequence of increased coupling resistance [14]. Thus, the above findings suggested that the effect of these peptides could be related to intercellular coupling.

To test this hypothesis, papillary muscle experiments were performed as follows: Isolated, Tyrode solution superfused guinea pig papillary muscles were electrically stimulated at their basis (1 Hz, double threshold), and the propagated action potential was measured at the tip of the papillary muscle via a sharp KCl-filled glass

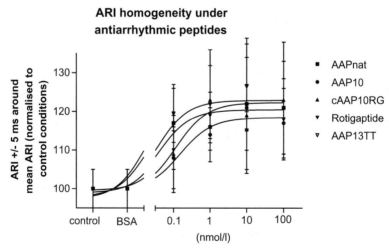

Figure 16.1. Concentration-response curves for the enhancement in homogeneity of activation recovery intervals (ARIs) by various antiarrhythmic peptides in isolated rabbit hearts under standard conditions. ARI homogeneity was defined as the percentage of 256 electrodes exhibiting an ARI, which did not deviate more than 5 ms from the mean ARI, normalized to the control level of homogeneity (100%). Under control conditions, $49 \pm 4\%$ of all ARI were ± 5 ms around the mean ARI. (AAPnat: H_2N-Gly-Pro-4Hyp-Gly-Ala-Gly-COOH; AAP10: H_2N-Gly-Ala-Gly-4Hyp-Pro-Tyr-$CONH_2$; cAAP10RG: Cyclo(C−CF_3(OH)-Gly-Ala-Gly-4Hyp-Pro-Tyr); rotigaptide: H_2N-Gly-D-Ala-Gly-D-4Hyp-D-Pro-D-Tyr-Ac; AAP13TT: H2N-Gly-Ala-Gly-4Hyp-Pro-I-Tyr-$CONH_2$).

Table 16.1. Effects of Vehicle (Vehicle Treated Time Control Series), AAP10, and Rotigaptide (ZP123) (0, 10, or 100 nM) on Cardiovascular Parameters Obtained from Isolated Rabbit Hearts, Exposed to AAPs. Abbreviations: LVP = Left Ventricular Pressure, CF = Coronary Flow, TAT = Total Activation Time, ARI = Activation-Recovery Interval, PQ = AV-Conduction Time. (Means ± SEM, $n = 5$ For Each Series)

Vehicle			AAP10			Rotigaptide			Parameter
T1	T2	T3	0	10	100	0	10	100 nM	
110 ± 1	87 ± 3	83 ± 4	99 ± 6	82 ± 4	81 ± 4	103 ± 6	81 ± 6	74 ± 4	LVP [mm Hg]
35 ± 2	28 ± 2	26 ± 2	49 ± 3	44 ± 3	41 ± 2	48 ± 2	40 ± 2	38 ± 2	CF [mL/min]
7.2 ± 0.4	7.3 ± 0.4	7.5 ± 0.4	7.3 ± 0.5	7.3 ± 1	7.7 ± 0.9	6.9 ± 0.5	7 ± 0.5	6.7 ± 0.5	TAT [ms]
126 ± 5	133 ± 3	137 ± 4	147 ± 7	145 ± 9	148 ± 9	157 ± 12	165 ± 14	174 ± 16	ARI [ms]
63 ± 2	62 ± 1	63 ± 2	55 ± 3	56 ± 2	56 ± 2	52 ± 3	55 ± 3	56 ± 4	PQ [ms]

microelectrode (10–20 MΩ) connected to an amplifier for intracellular potential recordings. The upstroke velocity and the time delay between stimulus and propagated action potential as stimulus-response interval (SRI) were measured. Using 1 μM AAP10 in the superfusion solution, the stimulus-response interval was shortened from 4.8 ± 0.16 ms to 4.3 ± 0.13 ms ($P < 0.05$), although there was no effect on action potential duration (165 ± 5 ms vs 164 ± 6 ms), resting membrane potential (-84 ± 1 vs -84 ± 3 mV) or overshoot potential (29 ± 2 vs 30 ± 4 mV). Furthermore, the maximum upstroke velocity (dU/dt_{max}) was not changed by AAP10 (181 ± 10 vs 190 ± 12 V/s) [22]. A lower concentration of AAP10 (10 nM) had no significant effect under control conditions, although even this low concentration showed a tendency for shortened SRI and enhanced dU/dt_{max}. However, this lower dose was effective under hypoxic conditions [23] (see below under "Site- and condition-specific effects of AAPs"). Similarly, the AAP10 derivative rotigaptide did not exhibit any effect on transmembrane ion channels or action potential [24], whereas the natural antiarrhythmic peptide AAPnat did not affect the action potential [18]. The fact that, in papillary muscle experiments, the stimulus response interval was shortened with unchanged action potential duration, unaffected maximum upstroke velocity and unchanged resting membrane potential, when taken together with the finding of reduced dispersion (mapping studies) support the hypothesis that AAP10 affects intercellular coupling and conduction.

16.3 MOLECULAR MECHANISMS OF ACTION OF AAPs

To test the above hypothesis, dual whole-cell voltage clamp experiments were performed on isolated ventricular guinea pig cardiomyocytes. Each cell of a pair of two cardiomyocytes, superfused at 37 °C with Tyrode's solution (composition: [mM]: NaCl 135, KCl 4, CaCl$_2$ 2, MgCl$_2$ 1, NaH$_2$PO$_4$ 0.33, HEPES 10, glucose 10, pH 7.4), was patched with a 3 MΩ glass microelectrode filled with intracellular solution (composition: [mM]: CsCl 125, NaCl 8, CaCl$_2$ 1, EGTA 10, Na$_2$-ATP 2, Mg-ATP 3, Na$_2$-GTP 0.1, HEPES 10, pH 7.2, with CsOH), and clamped to a holding potential of -40 mV to inactivate I$_{Na}$. Thereafter, one cell was in 10 mV steps clamped to potentials ranging from -90 to $+10$ mV for 200 ms, thereby establishing transjunctional voltage gradients from -50 to $+50$ mV.

According to the formulas for current in cell 1 (I_1) and in cell 2 (I_2),

$$I_1 = (V_1/R_{m1}) + [V_1 - V_2/R_j]$$
$$I_2 = (V_2/R_{m2}) + [V_2 - V_1/R_j]$$

with V$_1$ and V$_2$ being the voltage relative to the holding potential and R_{m1} and R_{m2} the membrane resistance in cell 1 and 2, respectively, the current I$_2$ is

$$I_2 = V_1/R_j$$

if V_2 is kept at the holding potential so that I_2 is a direct measure of the gap junction current.

These experiments revealed that 10–50 nM AAP10 increased the gap junction conductance (gj) [23]. Thus, the application of 10 nM AAP10 resulted in a rise in gap junction conductance from 88.4 nS to 112.5 nS within 5 min. It was observed in this study and others [22, 23, 25] that under normal conditions, the gap junction conductance slowly decreases with time (-2.5 ± 2 nS/min). A common explanation for this rundown is a possible dephosphorylation of the gap junction proteins (connexins) [26–28], which could result from either an inhibition of protein kinases, from the activation of phosphatases [28] or from a loss of adenosine triphosphate (ATP) [29]. The latter can usually be avoided by addition of ATP to the pipette solution (as commonly used and as used in our studies), in concentrations corresponding the physiological intracellular level of 3–7.5 mM. Addition of 10–50 nM AAP10, however, reversed this gj rundown in guinea pig cardiomyocytes and in HeLa-cells transfected with connexin 43 [25]. Because this was also seen in HeLa cells, that are much smaller than cardiomyocytes, an artefact related to space clamp problems can be ruled out. An original example of the effect of AAP10 on cardiac gap junction current is displayed in Figure 16.2.

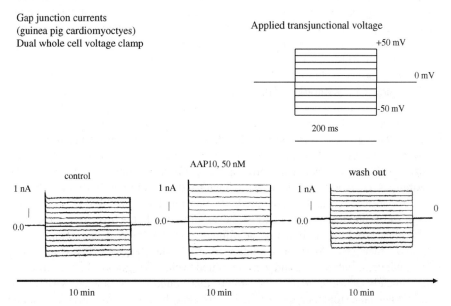

Figure 16.2. Gap junction currents from pairs of guinea pig cardiomyocytes during control conditions (with 0.05% bovine serum albumin), after 10 min application of 50-nM AAP10 and after 10 min washout. Using a dual whole-cell voltage clamp, transjunctional voltages ranging from -50 mV to $+50$ mV (steps: 10 mV; duration: 200 ms; holding potential: -40 mV) were applied. Cardiomyocytes were kept at 37 °C, superfused with Tyrode solution (1 mL/min) (Na^+ 161.02, K^+ 5.36, Ca^{++} 1.8, Mg^{++} 1.05, Cl^- 147.86, HCO_3^- 23.8, PO_4^{2-} 0.42 and glucose 11.1 mmol/L, equilibrated with 95% O_2 and 5% CO_2, supplemented with 1-mM $BaCl_2$) and patched with glassed capillaries of 2–3 MΩ, filled with intracellular solution [(mM): CsCl 125, NaCl 8, $CaCl_2$ 1, EGTA 10, Na_2ATP 2, MgATP 3, Na_2GTP 0.1, HEPES 10, pH 7.2 with CsOH].

Because protein kinase C (PKC) is often involved in the regulation of gap junction conductance [30–32], it was tempting to hypothesize that PKC may be involved in the action of AAP10. Therefore, the effect of PKC inhibition was investigated, first using bisindolylmaleimide I, an inhibitor of classic PKC, which completely antagonized the effect of AAP10. Furthermore, it became evident from radioactive ^{32}P-experiments that AAP10 led to the phosphorylation of Cx43, which also was completely inhibited by bisindolylmaleimide I [25]. These experiments, thus, showed that AAP10 acts via PKC on the phosphorylation of Cx43. More experiments revealed that AAP10 activates PKCα [25]. Because PKC normally is activated via G-protein–coupled receptors, we tested whether GDP-βS, a G-protein inhibitor, can antagonize the AAP10 effects on Cx43 phosphorylation. This G-protein inhibitor did, in fact, block the effects of AAP10; data suggest that G-proteins mediate the actions of AAP10. It could be shown that Ser-368 on the C-terminus of Cx43 is one of the targets that is phosphorylated by AAP10 [33] and rotigaptide (H2N-Gly-D-Ala-Gly-D-4Hyp-D-Pro-D-Tyr-Ac), which was formerly named ZP123 [34]. Moreover, AAP10 stimulated PKC activity [35]. Because PKC normally is activated by G-protein–mediated mechanisms, the transduction of the AAP effect by PKCα implied the existence of a G-protein coupled receptor that can bind AAP10. Therefore, radioligand binding studies were performed using ^{14}C-AAP10. In isolated plasma membranes from rabbit hearts, we found a saturable binding of ^{14}C-AAP10 with a K_D of 0.88 nM and a B_{max} of 2.2 pmol/mg (=receptor density), using AAPnat as the heterologous competitor. Similar findings were obtained when AAPnat was used as a competitor. Displacement binding studies, i.e., saturation of the membranes with $5*10^{-5}$ mol/L 14C-AAP10 and displacing the resulting bound agonist by increasing concentrations of AAP10 (10^{-10} to 10^{-4} mol/L in 10 steps), revealed a biphasic displacement unmasking a high ($K_{D.high}$ 19 nmol/L) and a low affinity binding site ($K_{D.low}$ 23 μmol/L) [25]. Because this result demonstrated the existence of a membrane-binding protein for AAPs, we then tried to identify or isolate this protein. Using affinity chromatography, membrane preparations of rabbit ventricles were incubated on columns with immobilized AAP10, washed out, and fractionated. By this procedure, a 200-kDa membrane protein was found that was retained on the column [25]. In the inverse experiment, a chemical crosslinking study using the bifunctional crosslinker disuccinimidylsuberate, and either ^{14}C-AAP10 or in another trial FITC-labeled AAP10 was incubated with rabbit ventricular tissue and then submitted to chromatography. In both cases, an approximately 200-kDa membrane protein that bound to the labeled AAP10 was found. When taken together, these experiments show the existence of an AAP-binding membrane protein that might serve as the AAP receptor [25]. Unfortunately, it was not possible to isolate enough receptor material for a reliable sequence analysis.

The finding that the gap junction conductance was slowly, but steadily, increasing after application of and under the influence of AAP10 (onset of effect about 10 min) or other AAPs allowed us to make the hypothesis that the mechanism downstream of PKCα activation and Cx43 phosphorylation might involve the transfer of connexins from the sarcoplasmic reticulum (SR) or Golgi apparatus to the plasma membrane or their insertion into the membrane. The typical way gap junction channels are built is as follows: First the connexin subunits are synthesized in the rough SR then transferred to the trans-Golgi network, where they are oligomerized to hexameric hemichannels, followed by transfer to the plasma membrane where they are inserted, allowing contact to another hemichannel provided by the neighboring cell, so that both hemichannels can form a complete (dodecameric) gap junction channel (for review see ref. 36). This protein trafficking from the Golgi to the plasma membrane can be inhibited with monensine. In support of the hypothesis, we found that monensine completely suppressed the effect of AAP10 on gap junction conductance and that PKCα-induced Cx43 phosphorylation could result in enhanced transfer of Cx43 to the membrane and/or enhanced formation of functional channels [37]. The mechanism of action of AAPs is depicted in Figure 16.3.

A new aspect has been identified with the observation of enhanced synthesis of Cx43 under the subchronic influence (12–24 h) of AAP10 [38, 39]. The acute effects observed within 10–30 min probably are caused not by enhanced synthesis but by the above mentioned mechanisms. However, these findings suggest that AAPs open the possibility for a second cell–cell communication-enhancing effect of AAPs beyond their acute action.

Taken together, AAP10 was the first drug shown to exert an antiarrhythmic action by enhancing gap junction conductance, and thereby decreasing action potential dispersion. This was the first drug to support the new principle of gap junction modulation. In between, it was also shown by others that AAP10 prevents from Cx43-dephosphorylation [40, 41] and decreases incidence of ventricular fibrillation [42]. Moreover, others also described a binding site for iodinated AAP10 ($[^{125}I]$-di-I-AAP10) with a KD of 0.1 nM and a density of 15 fmol/mg protein [43]. AAP10 was also found to be effective in delaying the onset of ouabain-induced AV-block in mice [44]. The AAP10-derivative rotigaptide (formerly named ZP123) yielded similar results; the key results were protections against ischemia-induced ventricular fibrillation [45, 46], reduced action potential dispersion [35, 44], and discordant action potential alternans [47], increased PKC activity [35], the prevention of Cx43-dephosphorylation that lead to enhanced Ser368 phosphorylation [34], inhibition of acidosis-induced conduction slowing [48], improved atrial conduction [49, 50], enhanced resting gap junction current [46, 51], enhanced intercellular communication [52], and increased Cx43 expression [53]. The latter finding may be still a matter of debate since Clarke et al. [52] did not find this increase.

16.4   ANTIARRHYTHMIC EFFECTS OF AAPs

The next question to be answered was: Are antiarrhythmic peptides antiarrhythmic? Because impairment and slowing of conduction is an important cause for arrhythmia, in particular for reentrant tachycardia, but also may play a role in AV-block, it was tempting to speculate that drugs that improve cardiac gap junction coupling may exert antiarrhythmic effects. Antiarrhythmic peptides have been evaluated in various arrhythmia models long before the mechanism of action was known. Thus, improvement of synchronization of cell clusters was initially described for many derivatives of AAPnat (see Table 16.2). The most intriguing

440

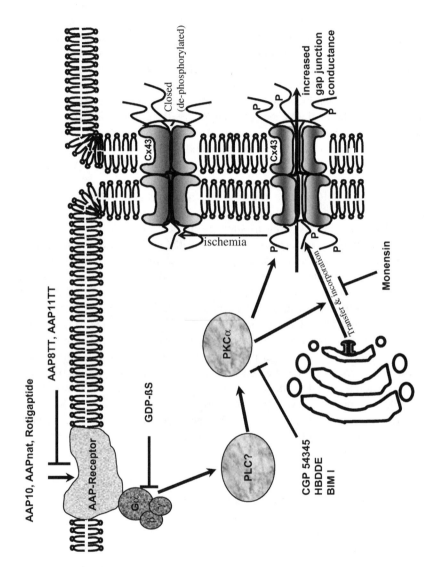

Figure 16.3. Schematic drawing of the molecular mechanism of action of AAP10.

Table 16.2. Survey of the Antiarrhythmic Peptides: − = **Inactive;** (+) = **Weak Activity;** + = **Active;** + + = **Activity > AAPnat**

Peptide	Activity	Concentration	Model	Reference
AAPnat: H₂N-Gly-Pro-4Hyp-Gly-Ala-Gly-COOH	+	0.1 μg/ml	Cell clusters, 0.5 mM K +	[17]
	+	10 mg/kg	Mice, CaCl$_2$	[60]
	+	0.1–100 nM	Rabbit heart, dispersion	[21]
H₂N-Gly-Pro-4Hyp-COOH	(+)	500 μg/mL	Cell clusters, 0.5 mM K +	[61]
H₂N-Gly-Pro-COOH	−	500 μg/mL	Cell clusters, 0.5 mM K +	[17]
H₂N-Gly-Pro-Leu-COOH	−	500 μg/mL	Cell clusters, 0.5 mM K +	[17]
H₂N-Gly-Pro-4Hyp-Gly-COOH	−	500 μg/mL	Cell clusters, 0.5 mM K +	[61]
H₂N-Gly-Pro-Leu-Gly-Pro-COOH	−	500 μg/mL	Cell clusters, 0.5 mM K +	[17]
H₂N-4Hyp-Gly-COOH	−	500 μg/mL	Cell clusters, 0.5 mM K +	[61]
H₂N-Gly-Ala-Gly-COOH	−	500 μg/mL	Cell clusters, 0.5 mM K +	[61]
H₂N-Gly-Gly-Gly-COOH	−	500 μg/mL	Cell clusters, 0.5 mM K +	[61]
(H₂N-Pro-Pro-Gly-COOH)₅	−	500 μg/mL	Cell clusters, 0.5 mM K +	[61]
H₂N-Pro-4Hyp-Gly-Ala-Gly-COOH	+	10 mg/kg	Mice, CaCl$_2$	[60]
H₂N-Pro-4Hyp-COOH	(+)	10 mg/kg	Mice, CaCl$_2$	[60]
H₂N-Pro-4Hyp-Gly-COOH	−	10 mg/kg	Mice, CaCl$_2$	[60]
H₂N-Pro-4Hyp-Gly-Ala-COOH	−	10 mg/kg	Mice, CaCl$_2$	[60]
N-3-(4-Hydroxyphenyl)propionyl-Pro-4Hyp-Gly-Ala-Gly-COOH	+ +	10 mg/kg	Mice, CaCl$_2$	[60]
N-3-Phenylpropionyl-Pro-4Hyp-Gly-Ala-Gly-COOH	+	10 mg/kg	Mice, CaCl$_2$	[60]
N-3-Phenylpropyl-Pro-4Hyp-Gly-Ala-Gly-COOH	−	10 mg/kg	Mice, CaCl$_2$	[60]
N-3-(4-Hydroxyphenyl)propionyl-Pro-4Hyp-Gly-Ala-COOH	−	10 mg/kg	Mice, CaCl$_2$	[60]
N-3-(4-Hydroxyphenyl)propionyl-Pro-4Hyp-Gly-COOH	(+)	10 mg/kg	Mice, CaCl$_2$	[60]
N-3-(4-Hydroxyphenyl)propionyl-				

(continued)

Table 16.2 (*Continued*)

Peptide	Activity	Concentration	Model	Reference
Pro-Pro-Gly-Ala-Gly-COOH	+ +	10 mg/kg	Mice, $CaCl_2$	[62]
AAP10: H₂N-Gly-Ala-Gly-4Hyp-Pro-Tyr-CONH₂	+ +	$1-5 \times 10^{-8}$ mol/L	VF, Ischemia, rabbit heart	[21, 33]
	+ +	$1-5 \times 10^{-8}$ mol/L	Rabbit heart, dispersion	[19, 33]
	+ +	80n mol/L	Ischemia, rabbit heart	[42]
	+ +	10^{-8} mol/L	Guinea pig, papillary muscle	[63]
	+ +	10^{-8} mol/L	**cardiomyocytes, GJ-coupling**	[22, 25]
	+ +	500 nmol/L	Suppress. of TdP, rabbit	[40]
		30 mg/kg	*In vivo*, rat, aconitine	[55]
		0.1 mg/kg/min	*In vivo*, pig, ischemia	[55]
Pro-4Hyp-Gly-Ala-COOH	–	10^{-10} mol/L	Ischemia, rabbit heart	[64]
N-3-(4-Hydroxyphenyl)propionyl-				
H₂N-Gly-Ala-Gly-4Hyp-Pro-Tyr-COOH	(+)	10^{-8} mol/L	Rabbit heart, dispersion	[21]
H₂N-Ala-Gly-4Hyp-Pro-Tyr-CONH₂	–	10^{-8} mol/L	Rabbit heart, dispersion	[21]
H₂N-Gly-Ser-Gly-4Hyp-Pro-Tyr-CONH₂	–	10^{-7} mol/L	Rabbit heart, dispersion	[21]
H₂N-Gly-Ala-Gly-4Hyp-His-Tyr-CONH₂	+	10^{-10} mol/L	Rabbit heart, dispersion	[21]
H₂N-Gly-Ala-Gly-4Hyp-Ile-Tyr-CONH₂	–	10^{-7} mol/L	Rabbit heart, dispersion	[21]
H₂N-Gly-Ala-Gly-4Hyp-Pro-Phe-CONH₂	(+)	10^{-7} mol/L	Rabbit heart, dispersion	[21]
H₂N-Ala-Ala-Gly-4Hyp-Pro-Tyr-CONH₂	(+)	10^{-7} mol/L	Rabbit heart, dispersion	[21]

H_2N-Gly-Ala-Gly-Pro-Pro-Tyr-$CONH_2$	–	10^{-7} mol/L	Rabbit heart, dispersion	[21]
H_2N-Arg-Ala-Gly-4Hyp-Pro-Tyr-$CONH_2$	(+)	10^{-7} mol/L	Rabbit heart, dispersion	[21]
H_2N-Val-Ala-Gly-4Hyp-Pro-Tyr-$CONH_2$	(+)	10^{-7} mol/L	Rabbit heart, dispersion	[21]
H_2N-Gly-Ala-Gly-4Hyp-Pro-I-Tyr-$CONH_2$	+ +	10^{-8} mol/L	Rabbit heart, dispersion	[21]
H_2N-Gly-Ala-Gly-4Hyp-Pro-F-Tyr-$CONH_2$	–	10^{-8} mol/L	Rabbit heart, dispersion	[21]
Cyclo($C\_CF_3(OH)$-Gly-Ala-Gly-4Hyp-Pro-Tyr)	+ +	10^{-8} mol/L	Rabbit heart, dispersion	[20, 21]
H_2N-Gly-Sar-Pro-Gly-Ala-Gly-COOH	–	10 mg/kg	Rat, aconitine	[65]
H_2N-Gly-Pro-Sar-Gly-Ala-Gly-COOH	+	10 mg/kg	Rat, aconitine	[65]
H_2N-Gly-Sar-Sar-Gly-Ala-Gly-COOH	+	10 mg/kg	Rat, aconitine	[65]
ZP123/Rotigaptide:				
H_2N-Gly-D-Ala-Gly-D-4Hyp-D-Pro-D-Tyr-Ac	+ +	10^{-7} mol/L	Rabbit heart, dispersion	[35, 44]
	+ +	1 μg/kg/h	Dog, VT, ischemia	[45, 46]
	+ +	10 nmol/L	Cardiomyocytes, **Gap junction coupling**	[46]
	+ +	100 nmol/L	Metabolic stress, Enhanced atrial conduction	[24]

question, however, was, are antiarrhythmic peptides effective against atrial fibrillation (AF), ventricular fibrillation (VF), or reentrant arrhythmia? Only a few of these peptides have been investigated with regard to efficacy against AF or VF: AAP10, rotigaptide, and Pro-4Hyp-Gly-Ala-COOH, the latter being ineffective (Table 16.2).

16.4.1 Ventricular Fibrillation and Ventricular Tachycardia

Only AAP10 and rotigaptide presently have been shown to act against VF: AAP10 prevents late ischemic (type IB; i.e., after 20 min of local ischemia) VF as shown in isolated rabbit hearts with a left coronary ligation (local ischemia) [21]. Similarly, AAP10 was effective in the suppression of VF in rabbits with healed myocardial infarction [42], which is an important observation in a remodeled tissue. In these rabbits, the effects of AAP10 were evaluated three months after a myocardial infarction. Typically, class I antiarrhythmic drugs cannot be given after myocardial infarction has healed. Rotigaptide has been shown to prevent spontaneous ventricular arrhythmias (ventricular extrasystoles and ventricular tachycardia) during myocardial ischemia/reperfusion in dogs [45, 46]. However, 1–4 h after occlusion (fresh myocardial infarction), rotigaptide failed to reduce focal arrhythmia, triggered activity, or DADs, as investigated by programmed stimulation in dogs [54].

In a series of studies performed on 18 male pigs (German landrace, 16–25 kg), the left anterior descending coronary artery (LAD) was occluded for 90 minutes. For 15 min prior to LAD occlusion, the pigs received a bolus of 10 mg/kg AAP10 followed by an infusion at a rate of 0.1 mg/kg/min (or in the control series they received the vehicle). The incidence of late ischemic (type IB) ventricular fibrillation was monitored; 70% (7/10) of the untreated pigs developed type IB VF, whereas in AAP10 treated animals, only 37.5% (3/8) exhibited type IB VF [55]. AAP10 (bolus: 30 mg/kg) also proved to be effective in the prevention of VF-induced aconitine intoxication. Using anaesthetized rats, we found that $45 \pm 2 \mu g/kg$ aconitine were needed for induction of VF in vehicle-treated animals, whereas a significantly lower amount was required after AAP10 ($38 \pm 1 \mu g/kg$, $P < 0.05$, aconitine infusion rate: $3 \mu g/kg/min$) [55]. Aconitine intoxication leads to VF via opening of fast I_{Na} channels that results not only in an enhanced automaticity but also in gap junctional uncoupling via increased intracellular Na^+.

16.4.2 Atrial Fibrillation

Regarding atrial fibrillation, one could assume that improving gap junction communication may be effective. However, the situation in humans is rather complex, and often fibrosis accompanies the process of atrial fibrillation (chronic AF). The fibrotic depositions are mostly found along the lateral border of the cell, thereby separating cells from each other. In these cases, there are probably only few functional gap junctions, and it might be questionable whether a drug-enhancing gap junction conductance can overcome the increased cell-to-cell resistance caused by collagen fibers. In addition, in the atrium cells are probably mostly coupled by Cx40, with fewer cells coupled either by Cx43 or by Cx45 (the latter might be related to cardiomyocyte-fibroblast contacts). In agreeement with these considerations, rotigaptide (ZP123) does not affect resting conduction in isolated rat atrial tissue. However, this drug prevented atrial conduction slowing during metabolic stress [24]. Similarly, AAP10 did not affect AF in rats [56].

Comparing AF induced in dogs by atrial tachypacing, AF induced by congestive heart failure, and AF induced by atrial ischemia, Shiroshita-Takeshita et al. [49] found that an antifibrillatory effect for rotigaptide was only observed in the atrial ischemia AF model. Although rotigaptide slightly improved conduction in the other models, it did not affect duration of AF. Similarly, Haugan et al. [50] found, using a rabbit model of chronic volume overload-induced atrial dilation, that rotigaptide slightly improved conduction velocity, but it did not decrease susceptibility to the induction of AF. In chronic mitral regurgitation in dogs, however, Guerra et al. [57] reported that 50 nM rotigaptide shortened the duration of AF.

Thus, it would seen that it is necessary to discriminate between types of atrial fibrillation when deciding whether a gap junction modulator would be effective. The structural uncoupling because fibrosis (most forms of chronic AF) would probably not respond to a functional improvement of intercellular communication, whereas forms of AF with a functional uncoupling (e.g., because of ischemia, metabolic stress, or ATP loss) would will probably be more sensitive to antiarrhythmic peptide treatment. Moreover, it is important to recall that all previous investigations examined the effect of AAPs on Cx43, but the effects of these agents on Cx40 and Cx45 remain to be determined. Because in atrial tissue (human), coupling is maintained mostly by Cx40, and only in part by Cx43, an AAP that was more selective for Cx40 could be more effective in the treatment of atrial arrhythmias. Currently, no such compound has been developed. However, in rat atria, in contrast to other species, the cell-to-cell coupling is provided by Cx43 [58]. This observation might explain better the effects of rotigaptide that have been reported for rat models of AF.

16.4.3 Others

In addition, both AAP10 and rotigaptide were effective in delaying the onset of ouabain-induced AV-block in mice [44]. This is interesting insofar as ouabain can lead to gap junctional uncoupling probably by increases in intracellular Na^+ and Ca^{2+} [59].

Moreover, various antiarrhythmic peptides, starting with AAPnat, have been proven to be efficacious against tachycardic arrhythmias induced by injection of $CaCl_2$ (500 µg/mL) in mice (see Table 16.2). Furthermore, several antiarrhythmic peptides, such as AAP10, its derivatives, AAPnat, and rotigaptide, have been shown to reduce local dispersion of activation-recovery interval (as a measure of dispersion of action potential duration and is often used as a surrogate parameter for possible antifibrillatory effects) (Table 16.2).

16.5 SITE- AND CONDITION-SPECIFIC EFFECTS OF AAPs; EFFECTS IN ISCHEMIA OR SIMULATED ISCHEMIA

We had the impression from the stages of our research that the AAP10 effect on gap junction conductance might be enhanced in situations of partial uncoupling. The first hint that this is true came from the experiments using a glucose-free hypoxic superfusion medium in guinea pig papillary muscles. During the normoxic phase, a low concentration of AAP10 (10 nM) had no effect on the SRI (delay between electric stimulus at the muscles basis and the propagated action potential at the muscles tip) [23], whereas a high concentration (1000 nM) led to SRI shortening [22]. Simulated ischemia (glucose-free, hypoxia) resulted in significant SRI prolongation, which indicates conduction slowing that could be completely inhibited by 10 nM AAP10 [23].

Similarly, the effects of AAP10 were tested on guinea pig papillary muscle previously uncoupled by sodium propionate [63]. Under control conditions, 10 nM of AAP10 did not shorten the SRI. However, after uncoupling with sodium propionate, 10 nM AAP10 significantly accelerated conduction and antagonized SRI prolongation. Similar results were obtained using a model of acidosis-induced uncoupling. Eloff et al. [48] showed that rotigaptide (ZP123) prevented acidosis-induced conduction slowing but had no effect on conduction under control conditions. Furthermore, the positive effect of rotigaptide on atrial conduction was only detectable in atria undergoing metabolic stress [24] or ischemia-induced atrial fibrillation [49].

Because of these findings, the site-specific effects of AAP10 were recently investigated in a model of 30-min local ischemia (LAD occlusion, isolated rabbit heart) [33]. In isolated rabbit hearts, a 30 min LAD occlusion was performed with or without AAP10 treatment (50 nM). Ischemia leads to dephosphorylation of Cx43 in the ischemic area but not in the nonischemic area. The ischemia-induced Cx43 dephosphorylation (including Ser368; but obviously other sites were also involved) was significantly antagonized by AAP10, whereas AAP10 did not affect phoshporylation in the nonischemic area. Interestingly, ischemia led to a loss of Cx43 from the cell poles and lateral sides in the ischemic area and border zone. AAP10 completely prevented the ischemia-induced decrease in polar Cx43 presence. Moreover, AAP10 (but not vehicle) reduced dispersion in the ischemic area. Within the border zone of the ischemic area, wave propagation velocity was significantly slowed (from 0.7 m/s to 0.4 m/s); this action was significantly antagonized by AAP10 (0.6 m/s). Thus, this chapter clearly shows that AAP10 at 50 nM exerts effects in the ischemic area and its border zone, but it does not affect parameters in the nonischemic area. This means that AAP10 acts in an ischemia-specific manner such that its action is confined to the site of ischemia. This selectivity would provide a great advantage in comparison with other common antiarrhythmic drugs (class IA, IB, IC), that affect ionic membrane channels and—more or less uniformly— lead to slowed conduction in all ischemic and nonischemic areas, thereby imposing a lower or higher proarrhythmic risk.

16.6 CHEMISTRY OF AAPs

Antiarrhythmic peptides are classic peptides with peptide bonds (R-COO-NH-R) of 4–7 amino acids, most of them containing one or two proline or 4-hydroxyproline residues and a Gly-Ala-Gly sequence. According to our structure-activity data [21], the proline residues are necessary to induce a semicyclic structure. The classic secondary structures of peptide chains are the α-helix and the β-sheet. Because in proline residues, the N-atom is part of the ring structure, the inclusion of proline into the peptide would induce a kinking of the α-helix.

According to the published structure-activity data [21], the horseshoe-like semicyclic structure of a certain diameter is essential for the activity. The effects of AAP10 could be mimicked with cAAP10RG, a cyclic peptide, where the N- and C-terminus were bridged by a C-CF$_3$-group, whereas in contrast, spontaneous cyclization (induction of a peptide bond between the N- and C-terminus) led to a smaller ring and an inactive compound. Enlargement of the ring by introduction of a disulfide bond for cyclization also leads to an inactive compound. The deduced proposed semicyclic structure of AAP10 could be verified using 2-dimensional nuclear magnetic resonance techniques, such as correlated spectroscopy (COSY), rotating frame Overhauser enhancement spectroscopy (ROESY), and total correlated spectroscopy (TOCSY). These techniques allowed definition of neighbored H-atoms and C-atoms as well as long-range coupling. Thus, nuclear Overhauser effects (NOE) could be detected between the protons of δPro and αOHPro, as well as between NH-Tyr and α-Ala. Other interactions derived from TOCSY data were among αCH$_2$-Gly', βCH$_2$-Pro, and γCH$_2$-Pro resonances, as well as among δCH$_2$-Pro, γCHOH-Pro, and βCH-OHPro. Furthermore, interaction occurred between NH-Ala and αCH-OHPro [20]. From these data, it was possible to construct the dimensional (three-dimensional) horseshoe-like semicyclic structure of AAP10 (Figure 16.4)

The idea of a semicyclic peptide, which is a structure that was also found for AAPnat, led to the construction of a hypothetical receptor pouch (computerized) and to the finding that the assumed functional groups could be brought into the fitting positions by rotation of AAPnat, AAP10, or cAAP10RG within the pouch [21]. These ideas lead to the assumption that it should be possible to replace all or some of the l-amino acids by d-amino acids, if one simultaneously inverts the sequence, so that the functional groups are at the same location with regard to the hypothetical receptor pouch. This was the idea that finally led to the design of ZP123 by the Zealand chemists; this peptide is now called rotigaptide.

16.7 SHORT OVERVIEW ABOUT CARDIAC GAP JUNCTIONS

One important difference between an accumulation of cells and an organized tissue is that cells in (most) tissues communicate with each other. Cell-adhesion molecules form surface receptors, release mediators, and allow direct cell-to-cell communication to occur. The direct cell-to-cell communication often is realized via intercellular gap

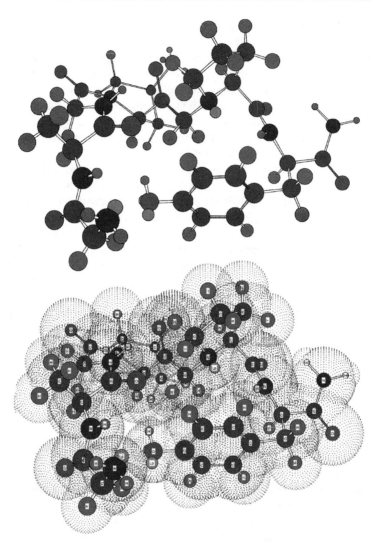

Figure 16.4. Spatial horseshoe-like semicyclic structure of AAP10 as revealed by ROESY, COSY, and computer simulation using MM2- and molecular dynamics simulation. See color insert.

junction channels that connect the cytoplasma of the neighboring cells with each other through the channel pore, which electrically acts similar to an Ohmic resistor. In the cardiovascular system, gap junction channels provide the basis for intercellular communication. They form low-resistance pathways connecting cells and allowing the transfer of current, thereby enabling action potential spreading and the exchange of small molecules (molecules < 1000 Da or with an ionic radius < 0.8–1.0 nm; there is a slightly higher conductivity for cations over anions) between neighboring cells. It was shown by Weingart and Maurer [59] that an action potential can only be transferred from cell to cell via functional gap junctions and that ephaptic or electrical field coupling is unlikely to occur under normal conditions. Gap junction channels (approx. length: 100–150 Å, approx. pore width: 12.5 Å, bridging the 20 Å gap between the cells) are composed from proteins, the so-called connexins. Each neighboring cell provides a hexameric hemichannel, a connexon, that consists of six connexins, and two connexons to form the complete gap junction channel. Currently, the Cx comprise a gene family of 20 members in mouse and 21 in human [66] (see also [67]) (hCx23, hCx25, hCx26, hCx30.2, hCx30, hCx31.9, hCx30.3, hCx31, hCx31.1, hCx32, hCx36, hCx37, hCx40.1, hCx40, hCx43, hCx45, hCx46, hCx47, hCx50, hCx59, and hCx62; h = human, and the number gives the approximate molecular weight in kDa). The various connexin isoforms differ with regard to their molecular weight because of different lengths of their C-terminals. A connexin is a protein with four transmembrane spanning domains, two extracellular and 1 intracellular loop, and N- and C-terminals at the intracellular side [68]. Connexins are synthetized in the rough endoplasmic reticulum, and they are folded and inserted into vesicles for transfer to the Golgi apparatus, where they are oligomerized to hexameric hemichannels. Thereafter, they are transported along microtubular structures to the plasma membrane and dock to another hemichannel of the neighboring cell, thereby forming a complete gap junction channel [69–71]. This process includes interaction with the cytoskeletal apparatus, in particular with zonula occludens protein 1 (ZO-1; for review see ref. 72). Connexins are degraded with short half-lives (see below) via either the lysosomal or (predominantly) the proteasomal pathway.

In contrast to transmembrane ionic channels, gap junction channels (see Figure 16.5) do not exhibit only one conductance state but can switch between various substates, which seem (at least in some cases, but see below) to depend on the

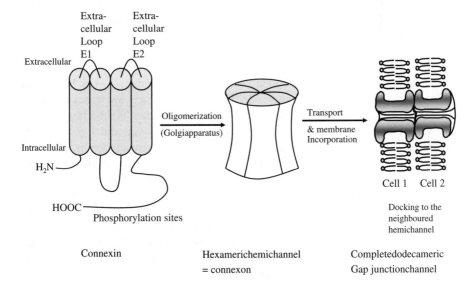

Figure 16.5. Structure of a gap junction channel.

phosphorylation state of the connexins. It should be mentioned that the role of the substates in regulation of the channel conductance is a matter of discussion, because the regulation is related to the portion a certain substate represents (for details see ref. 73).

Intercellular coupling can be regulated by either the number of channels, the mean open time, the mean closed time, or the single-channel conductance. The number of channels is either controlled by the rate of synthesis of connexins, their transport from the sarcoplasmic reticulum to the trans-Golgi network [69] and their integration and assembly in the membrane [74], or by their degradation [75]. The half-life time (1–5 h) of these channels is rather short [76, 77] (Cx43: about 90 min; Cx45 about 2.9 h [78]). Function and lifetime of connexins including connexin trafficking, assembly, disassembly, degradation, and control of gating are controlled—at least partially—by phosphorylation and dephosphorylation [79]. For a review of the pharmacological and physiological modulation of gap junction channels, please see ref. 80; for a review regarding the role of gap junctions in arrhythmia, see refs. 81–83.

The role of gap junctions in the biophysics of cardiac electrical networking, anisotropy, defined as the ratio $V_{longitudinal}/V_{transverse}$, and nonuniformity are important features of the tissue. Propagation of the action potential is determined by the following three factors: (1) sodium channel availability [1], (2) tissue architecture including cell size and shape and interstitial collagen depositions [84], and (3) gap junctions [85]. Typically, action potential propagation is faster along the longitudinal axis of the fibers (propagation velocity along the fiber axis mainly depends on the sodium channel availability [1]) than in transverse direction because of higher intercellular resistance perpendicular to the fiber axis. On the microscopic basis, propagation is discontinuous; the heterogeneous and anisotropic distribution of the cellular connections influence action potential upstroke and the safety factor of propagation [86]. The difference between the two forms of anisotropy, i.e., uniform versus nonuniform, is important for the understanding of arrhythmia. Thus, the action potential upstroke velocity and amplitude are greater during transverse propagation, which is accompanied by a faster foot potential. This finding led to the hypothesis that longitudinal propagation is—although faster—more vulnerable to block because of its lower upstroke velocity and amplitude. The upstroke velocity increases as a result of reduced coupling [87], because current cannot pass to the neighboring cells.

Concerning the role of coupling on transverse and longitudinal propagation, Delmar et al. [87] investigated longitudinal and transverse propagation in thin layers of sheep cardiac muscle before and after superfusion with the gap junction uncoupler heptanol. They found that transverse propagation is more sensitive to electrical uncoupling, which indicates a lower safety factor under these circumstances. With regard to the findings of Spach et al. [86], these authors suggested that uncoupling can have opposite directional effects to those observed when sodium conductance is reduced. One might speculate that the smaller number of gap junctions at the side-to-side border as compared with the intercalated disks might form the basis for a higher sensitivity of transverse propagation to uncoupling. However, some arguments against a role of gap junctions in uncoupling are as follows:

1. Jongsma and Wilders [88] found that a 90% decrease in the number of gap junctions was necessary to reduce conduction velocity by only 25%. It should be noted that this observations refers to normoxic standard conditions.

2. Heterozygous Cx43 knock out mice exhibited only a small effect on conduction, with about 25% reduction [89–91].

3. In simulated ischemia in cell pairs, gap junction coupling remained large enough to equilibrate action potential duration between the coupled cells until inexcitability occurred [92].

However, evidence suggests a role of gap junctions in uncoupling. It has been reported that the number of hearts exhibiting pacing-induced ventricular tachycardia in Cx43 +/+ or in Cx43 +/- mice was clearly higher in Cx43 +/- mice than in Cx43 +/+ population [90]. This finding suggests a role of gap junctions in arrhythmogenesis. This conclusion is supported by the numerous studies that demonstrated an antiarrhythmic effect of peptides like AAP10, AAPnat, or rotigaptide, all of which enhance gap junction conductance (see Table 16.2).

The safety of propagation has been described by the use of the safety factor (SF), which is defined as the quotient of charge produced by a given membrane patch during activation divided by the charge consumed during the activation process. As long as SF is larger than 1.0, conduction will be possible; as SF drops below 1.0, conduction will fail [93, 94]. Reduction of I_{Na} conductance from 100% to 10% leads to decreased conduction velocity and finally failure, as conduction velocity approaches 17 cm/s from initially 54 cm/s, whereas concomitantly SF is reduced from 1.6 to 1.0, and dU/dt_{max} decreases from about 240 to 25 V/s [94]. In the same model, a progressive decrease in intercellular coupling from 3 to 0.008 µS also led to a drop in conduction velocity, but not until the value reached 0.01 µS, SF and dU/dt_{max} increased under these conditions. Finally, below 0.009 µS, SF and dU/dt_{max} started to decrease and conduction failure occurred. The increase in dU/dt_{max} and SF can be explained by a diminished current loss to nondepolarized cells. Thus, if gap junction uncoupling occurs in concert with reduced I_{Na} conductance, as during acute ischemia, the closure of gap junctions would limit current shunting downstream and enhance availability of inward current for local depolarization. In that way, gap junction uncoupling may—partially—compensate for reduced SF (because of reduced I_{Na} availability) preserving slow but still effective conduction. Under these ischemic conditions, even smaller changes in gap junction conductance may affect the biophysics of propagation, whereas under normal conditions gap junction conductance probably exerts a lower effect on conduction velocity. It is necessary to mention the finding by Rohr et al. [95], which indicates that the balance between current source and sink (= area to which current is flowing from the activated site) is important for successful conduction. In this regard, enhanced gap junction coupling may even cause conduction failure if the current source is small and the sink is large, or vice versa—reduced gap junction coupling may limit current loss, thus keeping SF > 1.0 and providing effective conduction. However, this should not be simply generalized because the local conditions, architecture, and the resulting current source/sink ratios have to be taken into account. Thus, opening of gap junctions may act antiarrhythmically in those cases, in which arrhythmia is caused by functional uncoupling, although it may lead to conduction failure in certain other situations.

16.8   GAP JUNCTION MODULATION AS A NEW ANTIARRHYTHMIC PRINCIPLE

First suggested by Dhein and Tudyka [96], the enhancement of gap junction communication has proven in between to be a possible new antiarrhythmic principle. The development started with AAP10 as the first drug, for which the acute enhancement of cardiac gap junction conductance was described as the mechanism for its antiarrhythmic effect [19, 22, 23]. In between the suggestion and the testing of the first drug, other investigators also proposed the modulation of gap junctions as a new therapeutic approach for managing arrhythmias [97, 98].

A long standing debate, has discussed whether an improvement in gap junction conductance might enlarge infarct zones, because the closing of gap junctions during ischemia by ATP loss, increases in intracellular Na^+, H^+, and Ca^{2+}, and by the accumulation of acylcarnitines it may prevent from further loss of ATP. However, it was shown that the antiarrhythmic peptides AAP10 [33] or rotigaptide [45, 99] did not enlarge the infarct zone. The most intriguing question at present probably is: Which types of arrhythmia might be best treated by gap junction openers? The findings presented above suggest that antiarrhythmic peptides act by preventing from dephosphorylation of Cx43 and by phopshorylation of Cx43. Whether other connexin isoforms are targeted is currently not known. Functionally, this net phosphorylation would produce an increased gap junction current. However, a prerequisite for this action is the existence of a close contact with neighboring cells, so that gap junction channels can be formed or existing channels can be opened or kept open. The findings described in the preceding sections suggest that, in particular, the effect of AAPs is enhanced in situations with reduced cell-to-cell coupling, such as ischemia or metabolic stress. AAP10 seems to exhibit some preference for action in ischemic area [33]. Thus, arrhythmias that are related to reduced coupling caused by a functional uncoupling involving ischemia or metabolic stress, probably involving dephosphorylation of connexin43, seem to be amenable to treatment with AAPs. The most relevant arrhythmia of this type probably is type IB (late ischemic) ventricular fibrillation. According to the data cited above, AAP treatment offers prophylaxis against VF, because these studies all have used AAPs as a pretreatment (i.e., before the onset of ischemia). It is not clear whether ongoing VF also can be targeted with AAPs or whether these agents would be useful only as preventative treatments.

However, if VF has occurred in the clinical situation, then defibrillation is the only treatment of choice that is available today. Unfortunately, this treatment frequently fails, and it has been suggested that this might be related to the defibrillation threshold. Interestingly, it has been shown that rotigaptide decreases the defibrillation threshold by about 30% in rabbits with prolonged VF [100]. Thereby, rotigaptide improved the ability to defibrillate these hearts even after prolonged VF.

From these considerations, one could conclude that the mechanism of action of AAPs probably does not allow for improved conduction if cells are structurally uncoupled, e.g., by fibrotic strands. This is of particular importance considering a possible use in atrial fibrillation (AF), since in this arrhythmia typically the atrium is remodelled and (chronic) AF is associated with extensive fibrosis in humans [101]. Most investigations discussed above did not find an effect of AAPs on AF or AF duration in various models. In contrast, a therapeutic effect was found in atria undergoing metabolic stress [24] or in ischemia-induced atrial fibrillation [49]. In addition, a positive effect was also observed in a 6-week canine mitral regurgitation model [57]; this time period might be too short to induce the degree of fibrosis as observed in humans in chronic AF.

Taken together, AAPs offer a new perspective for the prophylaxis of ventricular tachycardia, especially in ischemia/reperfusion or acute myocardial infarction. In addition, certain types of AF, in particular AF associated with atrial ischemia, may also be positively treated by AAPs. In particular, the possibility of a prophylaxis against ventricular fibrillation with a new kind of drugs, which does not affect transmembrane currents but does affect intercellular communication, is an interesting new step in antiarrhythmic drug therapy.

REFERENCES

1. Buchanan, J.W., Saito, T., Gettes, L.S. (1985). The effect of antiarrhythmic drugs, stimulation frequency and potassium induced resting membrane potential changes on conduction velocity and dV/dtmax in guinea pig myocardium. Circulation Research, 56, 696–703.
2. Weingart, R., Maurer, P. (1988). Action potential transfer in cell pairs isolated from adult rat and guinea pig ventricles. Circulation Research, 63, 72–80.
3. Spach, M.S., Dolber, P.C., Anderson, A.W. (1989). Multiple regional differences in cellular properties that regulate repolarization and contraction in the right atrium of adult and newborn dogs. Circulation Research, 65, 1594–1611.
4. Spach, M.S., Dolber, P.C., Heidlage, J.F. (1989). Interaction of inhomogeneities of repolarization with anisotropic propagation in dog atria. A mechanism for both preventing and initiating reentry. Circulation Research, 65, 1612–1631.
5. Echt, D.S., Liebson, P.R., Mitchell, L.B., et al. (1991). Mortality and morbidity in patients receiving encainide, flecainide or placebo. The cardiac arrhythmia suppression trial. New England Journal of Medicine, 324, 781–788.
6. Roden, D.M., Andersen, M.E. (2006). Proarrhythmia. Handbook of Experimental Pharmacology, 171, 73–97.
7. Morganroth, J. (1992). Proarrhythmic effects of antiarrhythmic drugs: evolving concepts. American Heart Journal, 123, 1137–1139.
8. Spach, M.S., Josephson, M.E. (1994). Initiating reentry: The role of non-uniform anisotropy in small circuits. Journal of Cardiovascular Electrophysiology, 5, 182–209.
9. Wit, A.L., Rosen, M.R. (1983). Pathophysiologic mechanisms of cardiac arrhythmias. American Heart Journal, 106, 798–811.

10. Janse, M.J., Wit, A.L. (1989). Electrophysiological mechanisms of ventricular arrhythmias resulting from myocardial ischemia and infarction. Physiological Reveiws, 69, 1049–1169.

11. Janse, M.J., van Capelle, F.J.L. (1982). Electrotonic interactions across an inexcitable region as a cause of ectopic activity in acute regional myocardial ischemia. Circulation Research, 50, 527–537.

12. Janse, M.J., van Capelle, F.J.L., Morsink, H., Kléber, A.G., Wilms-Schopman, F., Cardinal, R., Naumann d'Alnoncourt, C., Durrer, D. (1980). Flow of "injury current" and patterns of excitation during early ventricular arrhythmias in acute myocardial ischemia in isolated porcine and canine hearts. Circulation Research, 47, 151–165.

13. Lesh, M.D., Pring, M., Spear, J.F. (1989). Cellular uncoupling can unmask dispersion of action potential duration in ventricular myocardium. Circulation Research, 65, 1426–1440.

14. Müller, A., Dhein, S. (1993). Sodium channel blockade enhances dispersion of the cardiac action potential duration. A computer simulation study. Basic Research Cardiology, 88, 11–15.

15. Dhein, S., Müller, A., Gerwin, R., Klaus, W. (1993). Comparative study on the proarrhythmic effects of some antiarrhythmic agents. Circulation, 87, 617–630.

16. Salameh, A., Frenzel, C., Boldt, A., Rassler, B., Glawe, I., Schulte, J., Muhlberg, K., Zimmer, H.G., Pfeiffer, D., Dhein, S. (2006). Subchronic alpha- and beta-adrenergic regulation of cardiac gap junction protein expression. FASEB Journal, 20, 365–7.

17. Aonuma, S., Kohama, Y., Akai, K., Komiyama, Y., Nakajima, S., Wakabayashi, M., et al. (1980). Studies on heart. XIX. Isolation of an atrial peptide that improves the rhythmicity of cultured myocardial cell clusters. Chemical and Pharmaceutical Bulletin, 28, 3332–33329.

18. Argentieri, T., Cantor, E., Wiggins, J.R. (1989). Antiarrhythmic peptide has no direct cardiac actions. Experientia, 45, 737–738.

19. Dhein, S., Manicone, N., Müller, A., Gerwin, R., Ziskoven, U., Irankhahi, A., Minke, C., Klaus, W. (1994). A new synthetic antiarrhythmic peptide reduces dispersion of epicardial activation recovery interval and enhances cellular communication. Antiarrhythmic properties in regional ischemia. Naunyn Schmiedeberg's Archive of Pharmacology, 350, 174–184.

20. Grover, R., Dhein, S. (1998). Spatial structure determination of antiarrhythmic peptide using nuclear magnetic resonance spectroscopy. Peptides, 19, 1725–1729.

21. Grover, R., Dhein, S. (2001). Structure-activity relationships of novel peptides related to the antiarrhythmic peptide AAP10 which reduce the dispersion of epicardial action potential duration. Peptides, 22, 1011–1021.

22. Müller, A., Gottwald, M., Tudyka, T., Linke, W., Klaus, W., Dhein, S. (1997a). Increase in gap junction conductance by an antiarrhythmic peptide. European Journal of Pharmacology, 327, 65–72.

23. Müller, A., Schaefer, T., Linke, W., Tudyka, T., Gottwald, M., Klaus, W., Dhein, S. (1997b). Actions of the antiarrhythmic peptide AAP10 on cellular coupling. Naunyn Schmiedeberg's Archive of Pharmacology, 356, 76–82.

24. Haugan, K., Olsen, K.B., Hartvig, L., Petersen, J.S., Holstein-Rathlou, N.H., Hennan, J. K., Nielsen, M.S. (2005). The antiarrhythmic peptide analog ZP123 prevents atrial conduction slowing during metabolic stress. Journal of Cardiovascular Electrophysiology, 16, 537–45.

25. Weng, S., Lauven, M., Schaefer, T., Polontchouk, L., Grover, R., Dhein, S. (2002). Pharmacological modification of gap junction coupling by an antiarrhythmic peptide via protein kinase C activation. FASEB Journal, 16, 1114–1116.

26. Verrecchia, F., Hervé, J.C. (1997). Reversible blockade of gap junctional communication by 8-butanedione monoxime in rat cardiac myocytes. American Journal of Physiology, 272, C875–C885.

27. Verrecchia, F., Duthe, F., Duval, S., Duchatelle, I., Sarrouilhe, D., Hervé, J.C. (1999). ATP counteracts the rundown of gap junctional channels of rat ventricular myocytes by promoting protein phosphorylation. Journal of Physiology (London), 516, 447–459.

28. Moreno, A.P., Saéz, J.C., Fishman, G.I., Spray, D.C. (1994). Human connexin43 gap junction channels: Regulation of unitary conductances by phosphorylation. Circulation Research, 74, 1050–1057.

29. Sugiura, H., Toyama, J., Tsuboi, N., Kamiya, K., Kodama, I. (1990). ATP directly affects junctional conductance between paired ventricular myocytes isolated from guinea pig heart. Circulation Research, 66, 1095–1102.

30. Kwak, B.R., Van Veen, T.A.B., Analbers, L.J.S., Jongsma, H.J. (1995). TPA increases conductance but decreases permeability in neonatal rat cardiomyocyte gap junction channels. Experimental Cellular Research, 220, 456–463.

31. Kwak, B.R., Jongsma, H.J. (1996). Regulation of cardiac gap junction channel permeability and conductance by several phosphorylating conditions. Molecular and Cellular Biochemistry, 157, 93–99.

32. Doble, B.W., Ping, P., Kardami, E. (2000). The ε subtype of protein kinase C is required for cardiomyocyte connexin-43 phosphorylation. Circulation Research, 86, 293–301.

33. Jozwiak, J., Dhein, S. (2008). Local effects and mechanisms of antiarrhythmic peptide AAP10 in acute regional myocardial ischemia: electrophysiological and molecular findings. Naunyn Schmiedebergs Archive Pharmacology, 2008 Jun 24. [Epub ahead of print].

34. Axelsen, L.N., Stahlhut, M., Mohammed, S., Larsen, B.D., Nielsen, M.S., Holstein-Rathlou, N.H., Andersen, S., Jensen, O.N., Hennan, J.K., Kjølbye, A.L. (2006). Identification of ischemia-regulated phosphorylation sites in connexin43: A possible target for the antiarrhythmic peptide analogue rotigaptide (ZP123). Journal of Molecular Cellular Cardiology, 40, 790–8.

35. Dhein, S., Larsen, B.D., Petersen, J.S., Mohr, F.W. (2003). Effects of the new antiarrhythmic peptide ZP123 on epicardial activation and repolarization pattern. Cell Communication and Adhesion, 10, 371–378.

36. Salameh, A. (2006). Life cycle of connexins: Regulation of connexin synthesis and degradation. Advanced Cardiology, 42, 57–70.

37. Dhein, S., Schaefer, T., Polonchouk, L., Weng, S. (2001). Involvement of protein kinase C (PKC) in the effect of antiarrhythmic peptide (AAP) on cardiac gap junctions. British Journal of Pharmacolgy, 133, 26P.

38. Neef, M., Frenzel, C., Mühlberg, K., Dhein, S., Pfeiffer, D., Salameh, A. (2004). Growth factors and antiarrhythmic peptide AAP10 regulate connexin43 expression. European Journal of Physiology, 447, S131.

39. Martin, P., Petersen, J.S., Easton, J. (2007). The antiarrhythmic peptide AAP10 enhances Cx43 and Cx40 expression and functionality by a protein kinase C dependent mechanism. Proceedings of the International Gap Junction Conference, Elsinore, UT, 2007, abstract book. p. 92.

40. Quan, X.Q., Bai, R., Liu, N., Chen, B.D., Zhang, C.T. (2007). Increasing gap junction coupling reduces transmural dispersion of repolarization and prevents torsade de pointes in rabbit LQT3 model. Journal of Cardiovascular Electrophysiology, 8, 1184–1189.

41. Wang, R., Zhang, C., Ruan, Y., Liu, N., Wang, L. (2007). Changes in phosphorylation of connexin43 in rats during acute myocardial hypoxia and effects of antiarrhythmic peptide on the phosphorylation. Journal of Huazhong University of Science Technology and Medical Science, 27, 241–244.

42. Ren, Y., Zhang, C.T., Wu, J., Ruan, Y.F., Pu, J., He, L., Wu, W., Chen, B.D., Wang, W.G., Wang, L. (2006). The effects of antiarrhythmic peptide AAP10 on ventricular arrhythmias in rabbits with healed myocardial infarction. Zhonghua Xin Xue Guan Bing Za Zhi, 34, 825–828.

43. Jørgensen, N.R., Teilmann, S.C., Henriksen, Z., Meier, E., Hansen, S.S., Jensen, J.E., Sørensen, O.H., Petersen, J.S. (2005). The antiarrhythmic peptide analog rotigaptide (ZP123) stimulates gap junction intercellular communication in human osteoblasts and prevents decrease in femoral trabecular bone strength in ovariectomized rats. Endocrinology, 146, 4745–4754.

44. Kjølbye, A.L., Knudsen, C.B., Jepsen, T., Larsen, B.D., Petersen, J.S. (2003). Pharmacological characterization of the new stable antiarrhythmic peptide analog Ac-D-Tyr-D-Pro-D-Hyp-Gly-D-Ala-Gly-NH2 (ZP123): In vivo and in vitro studies. Journal of Pharmacology and Experimental Therapy, 306, 1191–1199.

45. Hennan, J.K., Swillo, R.E., Morgan, G.A., Keith, J.C. Jr., Schaub, R.G., Smith, R.P., Feldman, H.S., Haugan, K., Kantrowitz, J., Wang, P.J., Abu-Qare, A., Butera, J., Larsen, B.D., Crandall, D.L. (2006). Rotigaptide (ZP123) prevents spontaneous ventricular arrhythmias and reduces infarct size during myocardial ischemia/reperfusion injury in open-chest dogs. Journal of Pharmacological and Experimental Therapy, 317, 236–243.

46. Xing, D., Kjølbye, A.L., Nielsen, M.S., Petersen, J.S., Harlow, K.W., Holstein-Rathlou, N.H., Martins, J.B. (2003). ZP123 increases gap junctional conductance and prevents reentrant ventricular tachycardia during myocardial ischemia in open chest dogs. Journal of Cardiovascular Electrophysiology, 14, 510–520.

47. Kjølbye, A.L., Dikshteyn, M., Eloff, B.C., Deschênes, I., Rosenbaum, D.S. (2008). Maintenance of intercellular coupling by the antiarrhythmic peptide rotigaptide suppresses arrhythmogenic discordant alternans. American Journal of Physiology Heart Circulation Physiology, 294, H41–9.

48. Eloff, B.C., Gilat, E., Wan, X., Rosenbaum, D.S. (2003). Pharmacological modulation of cardiac gap junctions to enhance cardiac conduction: Evidence supporting a novel target for antiarrhythmic therapy. Circulation, 108, 3157–3163.

49. Shiroshita-Takeshita, A., Sakabe, M., Haugan, K., Hennan, J.K., Nattel, S. (2007). Model-dependent effects of the gap junction conduction-enhancing antiarrhythmic peptide rotigaptide (ZP123) on experimental atrial fibrillation in dogs. Circulation, 115, 310–318.

50. Haugan, K., Miyamoto, T., Takeishi, Y., Kubota, I., Nakayama, J., Shimojo, H., Hirose, M. (2006). Rotigaptide (ZP123) improves atrial conduction slowing in chronic volume overload-induced dilated atria. Basic and Clinical Pharmacology and Toxicology, 99, 71–79.

51. Lin, X., Zemlin, C., Hennan, J.K., Petersen, J.S., Veenstra, R.D. (2008). Enhancement of ventricular gap-junction coupling by rotigaptide. Cardiovascular Research, 79, 416–26.

52. Clarke, T.C., Thomas, D., Petersen, J.S., Evans, W.H., Martin, P.E. (2006). The antiarrhythmic peptide rotigaptide (ZP123) increases gap junction intercellular communication in cardiac myocytes and HeLa cells expressing connexin 43. British Journal of Pharmacology, 147, 486–495.

53. Stahlhut, M., Petersen, J.S., Hennan, J.K., Ramirez, M.T. (2006). The antiarrhythmic peptide rotigaptide (ZP123) increases connexin 43 protein expression in neonatal rat ventricular cardiomyocytes. Cell Communication and Adhesion, 13, 21–27.

54. Xing, D., Kjølbye, A.L., Petersen, J.S., Martins, J.B. (2005). Pharmacological stimulation of cardiac gap junction coupling does not affect ischemia-induced focal ventricular tachycardia or triggered activity in dogs. American Journal of Physiology Heart Circulation Physiology, 288, H511–H516.

55. Gottwald, M. (1998). Verbesserung der zellulären Kopplung auf der Ebene der gap junction Kanäle alsm neuer antiarrhythmischer Therapieansatz bei Herzrhythmusstörungen. Thesis, University of Cologne, Germany.

56. Haugan, K., Lam, H.R., Knudsen, C.B., Petersen, J.S. (2004). Atrial fibrillation in rats induced by rapid transesophageal atrial pacing during brief episodes of asphyxia: a new in vivo model. Journal of Cardiovascular Pharmacology, 44, 125–135.

57. Guerra, J.M., Everett, T.H. 4th, Lee, K.W., Wilson, E., Olgin, J.E. (2006). Effects of the gap junction modifier rotigaptide (ZP123) on atrial conduction and vulnerability to atrial fibrillation. Circulation 114, 110–118.

58. Gros, D., Jary-Guichard, T., ten Velde, I., et al. (1994). Restricted distribution of connexin40, a gap junctional protein, in mammalian heart. Circulation Research, 74, 839–851.

59. Weingart, R., Maurer, P. (1987). Cell-to-cell coupling studied in isolated ventricular cell pairs. Experientia, 43, 1091–1094.

60. Kohama, Y., Okimoto, N., Mimura, T., Fukaya, C., Watanabe, M., Yokoyama, K. (1987). A new antiarrhythmic peptide, N-3-(4-hydroxyphenyl) propionyl-Pro-Hyp-Gly-Ala-Gly. Chemical Pharmacology Bulletin, 35, 3928–3930.

61. Aonuma, S., Kohama, Y., Makino, T., Fujisawa, Y. (1982). Studies on heart. XXI. Amino acid sequence of antiarrhythmic peptide (AAP) isolated from atria. Journal of Pharmaceuticals, 5, 40–48.

62. Kohama, Y., Kuwahara, S., Yamamoto, K., Aonuma, S. (1988). Effect of N-3-(4-hydroxyphenyl)propionyl-Pro-Pro-Gly-Ala-Gly on calcium-induced arrhythmias. Chemical Pharmacology Bulletin, 36, 4597–4599.

63. Dhein, S., Gottwald, M., Schaefer, T., Müller, A., Tudyka, T., Krüsemann, K., Grover, R. (1998). Effects of an antiarrhythmic peptide on intercellular coupling via gap junctions, In: Werner, R.ed., Gap Junctions. Proceedings of International Gap Junction Conference. IOS Press, Amsterdam, The Netherlands, 1998, pp. 163–167.

64. Kjolbye, A.L., Kanters, J.K., Holstein-Rathlou, N.H., Pertersen, J.S. (2000). The antiarrhythmic peptide HPP-5 reduces APD90 dispersion and prevents ventricular fibrillation in isolated perfused rabbit hearts. FASEB Journal, 14, A698.

65. Kundu, B., Rizvi, S.Y., Mathur, K.B. et al. (1990). Antiarrhythmic activity of a novel analogue of AAP. Collective Czech Chemical Communications, 55, 575–580.

66. Söhl, G., Willecke, K. (2004). Gap junctions and the connexion protein family. Cardiovascular Research, 62, 228–232.

67. Cruciani, V., Mikalsen, S.O. (2007). Evolutionary selection pressure and family relationships among connexin genes. Biologic Chemistry, 388, 253–264.

68. Kumar, N.M., Gilula, N.B. (1996). The gap junction communication channel. Cell, 84, 381–388.

69. Musil, L.S., Goodenough, D.A. (1993). Multisubunit assembly of an integral plasma membrane channel protein, gap junction connexin43, occurs after exit from the ER. Cell, 74, 1065–1077.

70. Musil, L.S., Goodenough, D.A. (1995). Biochemical analysis of connexon assembly. In Kanno, Y., Kataoka, K., Shiba, Y., Shibata, Y., Shimazu, T.eds., Intercellular Communication Through Gap Junctions. Progress in Cell Research Vol. 4. Elsevier Science, Amsterdam, The Netherlands, 1995, pp. 327–330.

71. Falk, M.M. (2000). Connexin-specific distribution within gap junctions revealed in living cells. Journal of Cellular Science, 113, 4109–4120.

72. Giepmans, B.N.G. (2004). Gap junctions and connexion interacting proteins. Cardiovascular Research, 62, 233–245.

73. Christ, G.J., Brink, P.R. (1999). Analysis of the presence and physiological relevance of subconducting states of connxin43-derived gap junction channels in cultured human corporal vascular smooth muscle cells. Circulation Research, 85, 797–803.

74. Lauf, U., Giepmans, B.N., Lopez, P., Braconnot, S., Chen, S.C., Falk, M.M. (2002). Dynamic trafficking and delivery of connexons to the plasma membrane and accretion to gap junctions in living cells. Proceedings of the National Academy of Sciences USA, 99, 10446–10451.

75. Brink, P.R. (1998). Gap junctions in vascular smooth muscle. Acta Physiology Scandanavia, 164, 349–356.

76. Fallon, R.F., Goodenough, D.A. (1981). Five hour half-life of mouse liver gap junction protein. Journal of Cellular Biology, 127, 343–355.

77. Laird, D.W. (1996). The life cycle of a connexin: Gap junction formation removal and degradation. Journal of Bioenergetics and Biomembranes, 28, 311–317.

78. Darrow, B.J., Laing, J.G., Lampe, P.D., Saffitz, J.E., Beyer, E.C. (1995). Expression of multiple connexins in cultured neonatal rat ventricular myocytes. Circulation Research, 76, 381–387.

79. Lampe, P.D., Lau, A.F. (2000). Regualtion of gap junctions by phosphorylation of connexins. Archives of Biochemistry and Biophysics, 384, 205–215.

80. Salameh, A., Dhein, S. (2005). Pharmacology of gap junctions. New pharmacological targets for treatment of arrhythmia, seizure and cancer? Biochimica and Biophysica Acta, 1719, 36–58.

81. Dhein, S. (1998). Cardiac Gap Junctions. Physiology, Regulation, Pathophysiology and Pharmacology, S. Karger Verlag, Basel, Switzerland, 1998.

82. Dhein, S. (2006). Role of connexins in atrial fibrillation. Advanced Cardiology, 42, 161–174.

83. Dhein, S. (2006). Cardiac ischemia and uncoupling: Gap junctions in ischemia and infarction. Advanced Cardiology, 42, 198–212.

84. Kawara, T., Derksen, R., de Groot, J.R., Coronel, R., Tasseron, S., Linnenbank, A.C., Hauer, R.N., Kirkels, H., Janse, M.J., de Bakker, J.M. (2001). Activation delay after

premature stimulation in chronically diseased human myocardium relates to the architecture of interstitial fibrosis. Circulation, 104, 3069–3075.

85. Spach, M.S., Heidlage, J.F., Dolber, P.C., Barr, R.C. (2000). Electrophysiological effects of remodeling cardiac gap junctions and cell size: Experimental and model studies of normal cardiac growth. Circulation Research, 86, 302–311.

86. Spach, M.S., Dolber, P.C. (1990). Discontinuous anisotropic propagation. In: Rosen, M. R., Janse, M.J., Wit, A.L., eds., Cardiac Electrophysiology: A Textbook. Futura Publishing Company Inc, Mount Kisco, New York. 1990, pp. 517–534.

87. Delmar M., Michaels, D.C., Johnson, T., Jalife, J. (1987). Effects of increasing intercellular resistance on transverse and longitudinal propagation in sheep epicardial muscle. Circulation Research, 60, 780–785.

88. Jongsma, H.J., Wilders, R. (2000). Gap junctions in cardiovascular disease. Circulation Research, 86, 1193–1197.

89. Morley, G.E., Vaidya, D., Samie, F.H., Lo, C., Delmar, M., Jalife, J. (1999). Characterization of conduction in the ventricles of normal and heterozygous Cx43 knockout mice using optical mapping. Journal of Cardiovascular Electrophysiology, 10, 1361–1375.

90. Lerner, D.L., Yamada, K.A., Schuessler, R.B., Saffitz, J.E. (2000). Accelerated onset and increased incidence of ventricular arrhythmias induced by ischemia in Cx43-deficient mice. Circulation, 101, 547–552.

91. Thomas, S.P., Kucera, J.P., Bircher-Lehmann, L., Rudy, Y., Saffitz, J.E., Kleber, A.G. (2003). Impulse propagation in synthetic strands of neonatal cardiac myocytes with genetically reduced levels of connexin43. Circulation Research, 92, 1209–1216.

92. De Groot, J.R., Schumacher, C.A., Verkerk, A.O., Baartscheer, A., Fiolet, J.W.T., Coronel, R. (2003). Intrinsic heterogeneity in repolarization is increased in isolated failing rabbit cardiomyocytes during simulated ischemia. Cardiovascular Research, 59, 705–714.

93. Shaw, R.M., Rudy, Y. (1997). Electrophysiologic effects of acute myocardial ischemia. A mechanistic investigation of action potential conduction and conduction failure. Circulation Research, 80, 124–138.

94. Shaw, R.M., Rudy, Y. (1997). Ionic mechanisms of propagation in cardiac tissue: roles of the sodium and L-type calcium currents during reduced excitability and decreased gap-junction coupling. Circulation Research, 81, 727–741.

95. Rohr, S., Kucera, J.P., Fast, V.G., Kleber, A.G. (1997). Paradoxical improvement of impulse conduction in cardiac tissue by partial cellular uncoupling. Science, 275, 841–844.

96. Dhein, S., Tudyka, T. (1995). The therapeutic potential of antiarrhythmic peptides. Cellular coupling as a new antiarrhythmic target. Drugs, 49, 851–855.

97. Naccarelli, G.V., Wolbrette, D.L., Samii, S., Banchs, J.E., Penny-Peterson, E., Gonzalez, M.D. (2007). New antiarrhythmic treatment of atrial fibrillation. Expert Review of Cardiovascular Therapy, 5, 707–714.

98. Wit, A.L., Duffy, H.S. (2008). Drug development for treatment of cardiac arrhythmias: targeting the gap junctions. American Journal of Physiology Heart Circulation Physiology, 294, H16–H18.

99. Haugan, K., Marcussen, N., Kjølbye, A.L., Nielsen, M.S., Hennan, J.K., Petersen, J.S. (2006). Treatment with the gap junction modifier rotigaptide (ZP123) reduces infarct size in rats with chronic myocardial infarction. Journal of Cardiovascular Pharmacology, 47, 236–242.

100. Zhong, J.Q., Laurent, G., So, P.P., Hu, X., Hennan, J.K., Dorian, P. (2007). Effects of rotigaptide, a gap junction modifier, on defibrillation energy and resuscitation from cardiac arrest in rabbits. Journal of Cardiovascular and Pharmacological Therapy, 12, 69–77.

101. Boldt, A., Wetzel, U., Lauschke, J., Weigl, J., Gummert, J., Hindricks, G., Kottkamp, H., Dhein, S. (2004). Fibrosis in left atrial tissue of patients with atrial fibrillation with and without underlying mitral valve disease. Heart, 90, 400–405.

CHAPTER 17

Novel Pharmacological Targets for the Management of Atrial Fibrillation

ALEXANDER BURASHNIKOV and CHARLES ANTZELEVITCH

17.1 INTRODUCTION

Atrial fibrillation (AF) is a growing clinical problem associated with increased morbidity and mortality. Despite significant progress in nonpharmacological AF treatments (largely because of the use of catheter ablation techniques), pharmacological agents remain first-line therapy for rhythm control management of AF [1]. Antiarrhythmic drugs are also used in postablation periods for a better success rate [2].

Clinically available anti-AF agents, which primarily target ionic channels, are generally only moderately effective and are associated with a risk of inducing ventricular arrhythmias and/or organ toxicity. Agents that inhibit the early sodium current (I_{Na}, such as flecainide and propafenone) and the rapidly activating delayed rectified potassium current (I_{Kr}, such as dofetilide) have proven to be effective in terminating paroxysmal episodes of AF, but these agents are far less effective in dealing with persistent AF. I_{Na} blockers are known to cause serious ventricular arrhythmias in patients with structural heart diseases, which account for more than 70% of the AF population. I_{Kr} blockers can induce acquired long QT syndrome (LQTS) and torsades de pointes (TdP) arrhythmias [1]. Amiodarone, which is a mixed ion channel blocker, is widely used for the long-term maintenance of sinus rhythm [3]. The use of amiodarone is rarely associated with ventricular proarrhythmia, and this agent can be safely used in patients with structural heart disease. A major disadvantage of long-term use of amiodarone is the risk of multiple organ toxicity. Consequently, safer and more effective anti-AF agents are needed.

Recent pharmacological approaches for the management of AF include the development of agents that target (a) atrial-specific ion channels, (b) structural substrates that predispose to AF, (c) gap junctions, and (d) intracellular calcium

Novel Therapeutic Targets for Antiarrhythmic Drugs, Edited by George Edward Billman
Copyright © 2010 John Wiley & Sons, Inc.

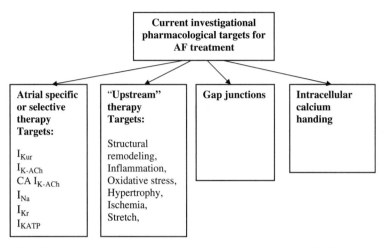

Figure 17.1. Current investigational targets for rhythm control of atrial fibrillation. Modified from Burashnikov and Antzelevitch [4] with permission.

homeostasis (Figure 17.1). This chapter describes our current understanding of these new pharmacological approaches for the rhythm control of AF.

17.2 NOVEL ION CHANNEL TARGETS FOR ATRIAL FIBRILLATION TREATMENT

The search for new ion channel targets for the treatment of AF has largely been focused on the delineation of atrial-specific agents. This strategy was conceived in the early 1990s with the intention of avoiding the adverse effects of traditional anti-AF agents [5]. Atrial-specific targets for AF treatment are those that are present exclusively or almost exclusively in the atria and include the ultrarapid delayed rectified potassium current (I_{Kur}), the conventional acetylcholine-regulated inward rectifying potassium current (I_{K-ACh}), and the constitutively active I_{K-ACh} (i.e., which does not require acetylcholine or muscarinic receptors for activation) [6, 7].

A recent development is the elucidation of atrial-selective sodium channel blockers, which effectively suppress AF without significantly influencing ventricular electrophysiology [8]. Atrial-selective ionic channel targets are those that are present in both chambers of the heart, but inhibition of these targets produces greater effects in atria than in ventricles. Included among atrial selective/predominant targets are early I_{Na} and I_{Kr} [8–10]. These AF targets are not newly discovered channels but rather are novel in the context of their potential use for atrial-selective AF strategies.

17.2.1 The Ultrarapid Delayed Rectifier Potassium Current (I_{Kur})

The atrial-specific current, I_{Kur} (carried by Kv1.5 channels encoded by KCNA5) was first described by Wang et al. in 1993 [5]. I_{Kur} is among the most investigated ion channel and is widely considered to be the most promising among atrial-specific or selective targets [7, 11] for the treatment of AF. This consideration stems largely from the fact that agents capable of blocking I_{Kur} selectively (such as AVE0118, AVE1231, S9947, S20951, ISQ-1, TAEA, DPO-1, vernakalant, AZD7009, NIP141, NIP-142, and acacetin) selectively prolong atrial effective refractory period (ERP) and thus can suppress AF [12–22]. At concentrations that effectively control AF, these agents also potently block other currents (e.g., I_{Na} is inhibited by vernakalant and AZD7009 and I_{to}/I_{KACh} are inhibited by AVE0118) [12, 23, 24]. Even though I_{Kur} block may contribute to the antiarrhythmic efficacy of these agents, recent studies suggest that "pure" I_{Kur} block may not suffice to suppress AF effectively and that inhibition of additional currents may be required (e.g., I_{Na}, I_{to}, I_{K-ACh}, and/or I_{Kr}) [10, 25]. At concentrations that specifically inhibit I_{Kur} ($\leq 50\,\mu M$), 4-amiopyridine (4-AP) neither terminates sustained AF nor prevents its initiation in an acetylcholine-mediated AF model [25]. 4-AP is capable of AF suppression only at concentrations that strongly block I_{to}. It has been reported that I_{Kur} density is reduced at rapid activation rates [26, 27] and that density of I_{Kur} can be reduced in cells isolated from chronic AF atria [28]. These data indicate that the relative contribution of I_{Kur} to atrial repolarization during AF may not be crucial and that blockade of this current alone may not be sufficient for effective AF suppression.

There is an apparent inconsistency between prolongation of the ERP [12–20] and abbreviation of action potential duration (APD_{90}) induced by I_{Kur} blockers in "healthy" atria (Figure 17.2) [25, 29, 30]. The prolongation of ERP without lengthening of APD_{90} is caused by the development of postrepolarization refractoriness (PRR), which is generally secondary to inhibition of I_{Na}, rather than I_{Kur}. Because I_{Na} blockers can selectively prolong atrial ERP [8], the atrial selectivity of at least some I_{Kur} blockers (such as AZD7009 and vernakalant) can be explained by a concomitant inhibition of I_{Na}. AZD7009 has been shown to display characteristics of an atrial-selective sodium channel blocker, slowing conduction and increasing diastolic threshold of excitation in atria, but not in the canine ventricle *in vivo* [17].

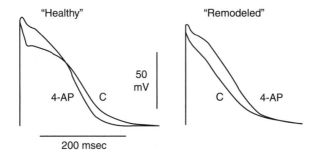

Figure 17.2. Block of I_{Kur} with 4-AP ($50\,\mu M$) abbreviates APD_{90} in "healthy" (plateau-shaped action potential), but prolongs it in "acutely remodeled" (triangular-shaped action potential) canine coronary-perfused atrial preparations (pectinate muscles). Low flow ischemia was used to generate the "acutely remodeled" atria. Modified from Burashnikov et al. [25, 29] with permission.

ISQ1 and TAEA also slow conduction velocity in atria *in vivo* [31], indicating that they block I_{Na}.

Recent clinical and experimental data suggest that reduction of I_{Kur} may actually predispose to the development of AF [25, 32]. Loss-of-function mutations in *KCNA5*, which is the gene that encodes the $K_v1.5$ channels responsible for I_{Kur}, was found to be associated with AF, suggesting that a reduction in I_{Kur} may predispose to the development of AF [31]. A test of this hypothesis was recently performed in the coronary-perfused canine right atrial model using low concentrations of 4-AP to block I_{Kur} selectively [25]. 4-AP (25–50 uM) greatly abbreviated APD in the canine right atrium, permitting the induction of, AF., thus providing evidence in support of the hypothesis that reduction of I_{Kur} is proarrhythmic in healthy canine right atrial preparations. Abbreviation of, APD, whether from 4-AP or other agents [25, 29, 30], is well known to be associated with an increase in AF vulnerability [33]. It is noteworthy that in remodeled atria (typically displaying a triangular-shaped AP morphology), a reduction of I_{Kur} prolongs APD (Figure 17.2) and does not promote AF [25, 30].

17.2.2 The Acetylcholine-Regulated Inward Rectifying Potassium Current ($I_{K\text{-}ACh}$) and the Constitutively Active (CA) $I_{K\text{-}ACh}$

$I_{K\text{-}ACh}$ is carried the through channels constituted by Kir3.1/Kir3.4 alpha subunits, and under normal conditions, it is activated by the parasympathetic neurotransmitter acetylcholine through the muscarinic (M2) receptors. Another form of $I_{K\text{-}ACh}$, the so-called constitutively active $I_{K\text{-}ACh}$ (CA $I_{K\text{-}ACh}$), does not require cholinergic agonist stimulation or acetylcholine receptors for activation [6, 34–36]. This current is only marginally present in healthy nonfibrillating human or canine atria and is significantly increased in atria of chronic AF patients and canine tachycardia-remodeled atria [6, 35–37]. The CA $I_{K\text{-}ACh}$ is thought to contribute importantly to abbreviation of atrial APD and AF maintenance in remodeled atria [6, 36, 37]. The CA $I_{K\text{-}ACh}$ has been suggested recently to be an atrial-specific as well as pathology-specific target for AF treatment [36, 38]. Indeed, CA $I_{K\text{-}ACh}$ could be a valuable target for safe AF treatment, if it can be inhibited independently of conventional $I_{K\text{-}ACh}$ channels present in many organs other than the heart (e.g., in the central nervous system). However, no selective CA $I_{K\text{-}ACh}$ blocker is available currently. Clinical studies indicate that a vagal component may contribute to the initiation of some paroxysmal AF in the clinic [39, 40], suggesting that block of I_{KACh} may exert an antiarrhythmic action in such cases [7]. In experimental AF models, block of $I_{K\text{-}ACh}$ currents (presumably both the conventional I_{KACh} and the CA I_{KACh}) with tertiapin prolongs atrial APD and suppresses AF [37, 41]. An atrial-specific M_2 receptor antagonist, cisatracurium, prevents vagally mediated APD abbreviation and AF in dogs [42].

17.2.3 The Early Sodium Current (I_{Na})

It has recently been shown that some I_{Na} blockers (e.g., ranolazine and chronic amiodarone) can produce atrial-selective depression of sodium channel-dependent parameters and effectively suppress AF in canine coronary-perfused atrial preparations [8, 43]. Based on these findings, we have recently suggested atrial-selective sodium channel block as a novel strategy for the management of AF [8]. The mechanisms underlying the atrial-selective effects of I_{Na} blockers are gradually coming into focus [9]. These factors include a more negative steady-state inactivation relationship, a more positive resting membrane potential (RMP), and a more gradual phase 3 of the action potential in atrial versus ventricular cells (Figure 17.3 and Figure 17.4) [4, 8, 9, 43]. The more negative half-inactivation voltage and more positive RMP importantly reduce the availability of sodium channels, translating to a smaller fraction of channels in the resting state in atria versus ventricles at RMP. Because recovery from sodium channel block occurs principally during the resting state of the channel, accumulation of sodium channel block is greater in atria versus ventricles at rapid rates of activation. At rapid rates, the slower phase 3 in atria versus ventricles results in the elimination of the diastolic interval in the former but not in the latter, which leads to greater accumulation of drug-induced sodium channel block in atria versus ventricles.

Available data suggest significant variability in the degree to which sodium channel blockers are atrial selective [4, 9, 43]. I_{Na} blockers possessing rapid versus slow unbinding kinetics tend to be atrial selective (e.g., ranolazine, chronic amiodarone, and lidocaine, but not propafenone) [8, 9, 43, 44]. The degree of atrial selectivity as well as the anti-AF potency of ranolazine or chronic amiodarone is much greater than those of lidocaine, principally because of the ability of ranolazine and chronic amiodarone to prolong atrial APD, secondary to their effect to inhibit I_{Kr}. The

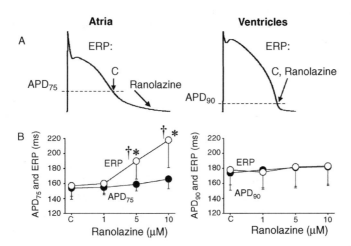

Figure 17.3. Ranolazine induces prolongation of the ERP and development of PRR in atria (PRR = the difference between ERP and APD_{75} in atria and between ERP and APD_{90} in ventricles; ERP corresponds to APD_{75} in atria and APD_{90} in ventricles). CL = 500 ms. C = control. The arrows in panel A illustrate the position on the action potential corresponding to the end of the ERP in atria and ventricles and the effect of ranolazine to shift the end of the ERP in atria but not in ventricles. *$P < 0.05$ vs. control. †$P < 0.05$ vs. APD_{75} values in atria and APD_{90} in ventricles; ($n = 5$–18). From Burashnikov et al. [8] with permission.

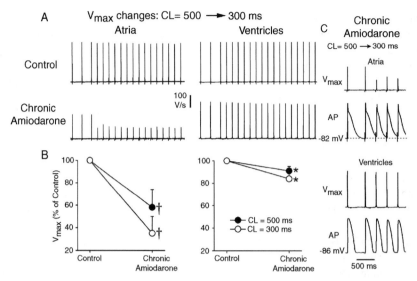

Figure 17.4. Chronic amiodarone produces a preferential rate-dependent depression of maximum rate of rise of the action potential upstroke (V_{max}) in atria versus ventricles. **A:** Atrial-selective rate-dependent depression of V_{max} following chronic amiodarone. CL = cycle length. **B**: Plot of normalized reduction in V_{max} ($n = 4$–14). "Atria" represent combined PM and CT data of canine right atrium. "Ventricles" represent combined epicardial and M cell data of canine left ventricle. $*P < 0.05$ vs. untreated control. $\dagger P < 0.001$ vs. control. **C:** Mechanism contributing to atrial selectivity of chronic amiodarone to depress V_{max} at rapid activation rates: Gradual phase 3 of the atrial action potential and prolongation of atrial APD lead to greater reduction or elimination of diastolic interval and a more positive takeoff potential at rapid rates. The dashed line indicates RMP in atria. From Burashnikov et al. [43] with permission.

prolongation of APD in atria greatly potentiates the I_{Na} inhibitory effects of these drugs because it leads to the reduction or elimination of the diastolic interval at rapid rates as well as a greater depolarization of takeoff potential. Lidocaine is less atrial selective because it abbreviates APD [8, 43].

AZD7009 produces atrial selective depression of sodium-channel-dependent parameters in *in vivo* dogs [17] and effectively suppresses clinical AF [22]. Whether vernakalant blocks I_{Na} in an atrial-selective manner has not been established, but the rapid unbinding of vernakalant from the sodium channels [23] is consistent with this notion. It is not clear whether I_{Na} or I_{Kur} block plays a greater role in the atrial selectivity and anti-AF actions of AZD7009 and vernakalant (see "I_{Kur} section" for more discussion on this topic).

The effectiveness of ranolazine to suppress AF in experimental models is consistent with the results of the recently reported MERLIN-TIMI 36 study, where ranolazine treatment was associated with reduced incidence of supraventricular arrhythmias and a 30% reduction in new onset AF in patients with non-ST segment elevation acute coronary syndrome [45].

17.2.4   Block I_{Kr} and Its Relation to Atrial Selectivity of I_{Na} Blockade

Recent studies have demonstrated that I_{Kr} block produces a much greater prolongation of APD and ERP in atria versus ventricles at normal activation rates (cycle length [CL] = 500 ms) [43]. These findings explain the results of many experimental and clinical studies) showing a preferential prolongation of ERP in atria versus ventricles by I_{Kr} blockers [46–52]. In the presence of bradycardia and long pauses, however, it is the ventricles, rather than the atria, that develop the greater APD prolongation and early afterdepolarization (EAD), which leads to the development of torsades de pointes arrhythmias [53, 54]. This effect of I_{Kr} block limits the widespread use of drugs with I_{Kr} blocking properties in the treatment of AF.

Whereas "pure" I_{Kr} block possess the highest probability of inducing bradycardia-dependent TdP, agents that also exert inhibition of opposing late I_{Na} and/or I_{Ca}, such as amiodarone and ranolazine, are rarely associated with TdP [55, 56]. Accordingly, a balanced combination of atrial-selective sodium and potassium-channel blockade may be the most effective approach to a safe and effective treatment for AF. It seems that the degree of atrial selectivity of I_{Na} blockers as well as their anti-AF efficacy are importantly related to the ability of I_{Na} blockers to produce concomitant atrial selective prolongation of APD because of the inhibition of I_{Kr} [8, 9, 43]. Atrial-selective APD prolongation greatly potentiates the actions of drug-induced inhibition of the sodium channel to depress I_{Na}-dependent parameters by reducing or eliminating the diastolic interval (during which the recovery from the sodium channel blockade typically occurs) at fast activation rates preferentially in the atria (Figure 17.4) [8, 43]. Thus, block of I_{Kr} exerts direct anti-AF influences by prolonging APD and also promotes sodium-channel inhibitory actions (see Figure 17.4). Pure I_{Na} blockers such as lidocaine are generally not effective in suppressing AF in the clinic, although at high concentration, beyond the therapeutic range, they can be demonstrated to be effective in experimental and theoretical studies [57, 58]). All clinically effective anti-AF I_{Na} blockers inhibit I_{Kr} as well (e.g., propafenone and flecainide) [1].

17.2.5   Other Potential Atrial-Selective Ion Channel Targets for the Treatment of AF

4-AP blocks I_{to} much more effectively in atrial versus ventricular myocytes, with an IC_{50} in atrial myocytes one third that in ventricular myocytes (471 ± 97 and 1486 ± 261 μM, respectively) [59, 60]. The predominant α-subunit of the I_{to} channel, Kv4.3, is expressed significantly more strongly in human atria versus ventricles [61]. I_{to} inhibition likely contributes to the atrial-specific and anti-AF effects of I_{Kur} blockers because all agents that block I_{Kur} also inhibit I_{to}. Propafenone also blocks the adenosine triphosphate (ATP)-sensitive potassium current (I_{KATP}) with a 4-fold higher affinity in atrial than ventricular rabbit myocytes [62]. Data indicate that $I_{K\text{-}ATP}$ may be involved in the generation of some forms of AF [28, 63]. In theory, atrial-selective block of I_{KATP} may be of benefit in the management of I_{KATP}-mediated forms of AF.

17.2.5.1   Atrial Selectivity in Remodeled Atria. It is important to recognize that the atrial selectivity of I_{Na} and I_{Kr} blockers has been demonstrated largely in "healthy" atria and ventricles [8, 46–48, 50, 64]. Changes associated with AF (electrical and structural remodeling) can significantly modify the pharmacologic response of atria to I_{Na} and I_{Kr} blockers [30, 65, 66], thereby modulating the atrial selectivity of these agents and their ability to suppress AF (as it well recognized with I_{Kur} blockers [30]). The triangulation of atrial action potential (typically observed in electrically remodeled atria) reduces the ability of I_{Kr} blockers to prolong atrial APD. In contrast, the ability of I_{Kur} blockers to prolong APD_{70-90} is augmented or even revealed in remodeled atria [25, 29, 30]. In a tachypacing-induced AF goat model, I_{Kur}/I_{to} block has been shown to restore the ability of I_{Kr} blockers to prolong atrial repolarization, greatly improving anti-AF efficacy, compared wtih I_{Kur}/I_{to} or I_{Kr} block alone [67].

The depolarization of RMP promotes and abbreviation of APD normally reduces the efficacy of sodium channel blockers [68]. Of note, the prolongation of APD/ERP or depression of I_{Na}-mediated parameters by pharmacological agents may not necessarily correlate with the ability of these agents to suppress clinical AF. For instance, sodium channel blockers essentially lose their ability to terminate effectively persistent AF [1] but not their efficacy to depress I_{Na} mediated parameters in remodeled atria [65, 69]. Whereas I_{Kr} blockers are the most effective in terminating persistent AF in the clinic [1], their ability to prolong APD/ERP is remarkably reduced in remodeled atria in the goat model [65]. The pharmacologic response of electrically remodeled atria is also likely to be influenced by the extent to which the atria undergo structural remodeling.

17.2.6   Influence of Atrial- Selective Agents on Ventricular Arrhythmias?

Like atrial arrhythmias, ventricular rhythm disturbances also commonly occur under pathophysiological conditions associated with ischemia, infarction, long QT syndrome, hypotrophy, and so on. These conditions can importantly modulate the efficacy of sodium and potassium channel blockers. This may explain why atrial-selective agents can exert significant electrophysiological and antiarrhythmic actions in "abnormal" ventricles. For instance, atrial selective I_{Kur}/I_{to} blocker AVE0118 effectively suppresses ventricular ischemic arrhythmias in dogs, presumably because of its I_{to} blockade [70]. Ranolazine also reduces the incidence of ventricular arrhythmias associated with acute coronary and long QT syndrome; this effect is attributed to the action of ranolazine to block late I_{Na} [45, 55, 71]. The ability of chromic amiodarone to prevent ventricular arrhythmias is also well recognized [56].

17.3   UPSTREAM THERAPY TARGETS FOR ATRIAL FIBRILLATION

It is becoming increasingly clear that the maintenance of persistent AF may be primarily determined by atrial structural remodeling and that effective anti-AF actions can be achieved by preventing or reversing the structural AF substrate and/or by affecting the factors that cause this structural AF substrate [72–74]. This anti-AF strategy is generally referred to as "upstream therapy." Structural remodeling is composed of several pathological changes (such as interstitial fibrosis, fibroblast proliferation, dilatation, hypertrophy, pathological collagen accumulation, and its abnormal distribution or redistribution) and can be mediated by several interrelated factors (such as stretch, oxidative stress, inflammation, and ischemia) [72–75]. Even though stretch and oxidative injury by themselves can induce arrhythmic-triggered activity, inflammation does not seem to cause arrhythmias directly. The pro-AF influence of atrial structural remodeling is thought to be largely mediated by conduction disturbances, which promotes reentrant arrhythmias.

Many factors and many signaling pathways exist, the activities of which have been associated with atrial structural remodeling. Among these factors are angiotensin II., transforming growth factor-$\beta 1$ (TGF-$\beta 1$), mitogen-activated protein kinase (MAPK), platelet-derived growth factor (PDGF), matrix metalloproteinases, peroxisome pro-liferator-activated receptor-λ (PPAR- λ), Janus kinase (JAK), Rac1, nicotinamide adenine dinucleotide phosphate (NADPH) oxidase, signal transducers and activators of transcription (STAT), calcineurin, and so on. [72, 74, 76–80]. Angiotensin II and its angiotensin II type 1 (AT1) receptors are critically involved in the initiation of most signaling cascades [72, 74]. Unfortunately, a cause-effect relationship of these factors with AF is poorly defined or unknown, so that many changes observed in the factors/signaling pathways could be mere consequences of AF [74].

The precise contribution of structural remodeling, inflammation, oxidative injury, ischemia, and stretch (and numerous mediating factors/signaling pathways) in the development of AF remains poorly understood and is likely to vary significantly among different AF pathologies [74, 75, 81]. Experimental and clinical evidence indicate that angiotensin-converting enzyme (ACE) inhibitors, angiotensin receptors blockers (ARBs), statins, aldosterone antagonists, and omega-3 polyunsaturated fatty acids (PUFAs) may or may not be beneficial for AF treatments [72, 73, 82–85]. The anti-AF mechanisms of these interventions are not well established and are presumed to be largely caused by their antihypertensive, anti-inflammatory, and antioxidative stress actions, which reduce structural remodeling. To develop "upstream therapy" approaches successfully, it is vitally important to identify and understand the factors and signaling pathways involved in various AF pathologies. Interestingly, atria can develop structural remodeling to a greater degree or even independently of the ventricles [76, 78, 80, 86–89], pointing to the presence of potential atrial-selective targets for "upstream" AF therapy [90].

17.4 GAP JUNCTION AS TARGETS FOR AF THERAPY

It has long been appreciated that conduction disturbances may have a pivotal role in the generation of AF. Conduction abnormalities in the heart can occur because of 1) disturbances in the sodium and/or calcium channel activity, 2) gap junction abnor-malities (impairing cell-to-cell communications), and 3) structural changes in the myocardium. Although the gap junction has long been known for its important contribution to cardiac propagation, the gap junction was not considered to be a potential antiarrhythmic target until recently. Improving gap junction conductance using the gap junction modulator rotigaptide has been shown to exert an antiarrhythmic effect in ischemic ventricles [91, 92]. The feasibility of this antiarrhythmic approach was later demonstrated in a canine chronic mitral regurgitation AF model [93] and in the canine acute ischemia AF model [94]. Rotigaptide, however, did not affect the AF development in AF models associated with heart failure or atrial tachypacing [93, 94]. The improvement of gap junction conductance can not only improve impulse propagation, but also can reduce dispersion of repolarization [92], which is a principal proarrhythmic substrate [53].

It has been reported that some forms of AF are associated with a reduction *Cx40*, which is a principal connexin involved in the conduction of electrical excitation in atrial muscle [95]. Somatic mutations in the *Cx40* gene (GJA5) have recently been found in patients with idiopathic AF [96].

It is noteworthy that *Cx40* is commonly included in the list of potential atrial-specific targets for AF treatment because *Cx40* is found in atrial but not ventricular myocardium, with the exception of the conduction system in the ventricles [6, 97]. No specific *Cx40* modulators are available yet.

17.5 INTRACELLULAR CALCIUM HANDLING AND AF

A growing body of evidence suggests that abnormal intracellular calcium homeostasis, which is observed in experimental and clinical AF studies, may play a role in the generation of AF and that normalization of sarcoplasmic reticulum (SR) calcium release may be a potential therapeutic approach [54, 98–102]. Electrophysiological mechanisms responsible for atrial arrhythmias caused by abnormal intracellular calcium handling could be delayed afterdepolarization-(DAD) and EAD-induced triggered activity, secondary to spontaneous SR calcium release. Also, a specific form of, EAD, termed the late phase 3 EAD, is caused by augmented normal SR calcium release under conditions of abbreviated, APD, when the calcium transient extends beyond the end of final repolarization [54, 98]. Multielectrode and optical mapping studies have shown that some forms of AF can be initiated and/or maintained by SR calcium release-mediated triggered activity, which often originates from pulmonary vein (PV) muscle sleeves [103–106].

An increase in spontaneous SR Ca^{2+} release as well as a significant SR calcium leak have been observed in atrial myocytes isolated from AF patients and dogs with tachypacing-induced atrial remodeling [99, 100]. This SR calcium leak may be mediated by protein kinase A (PKA) hyperphosphorylation and calstabin2 (a ryanodine receptor inhibitory subunit, FKBP12.6) [100]. Calstabin2-deficient mice displaying an augmented SR calcium leak are prone to develop AF [102]. A pharmacological normalization of SR calcium release with JTV519 and tetracaine has been shown to exert antiarrhythmic actions in experimental models of AF [102, 107].

REFERENCES

1. Fuster, V., Ryden, L.E., Cannom, D.S., Crijns, H.J., Curtis, A.B., Ellenbogen, K.A., et al. (2006). ACC/AHA/ESC 2006 guidelines for the management of patients with atrial fibrillation—executive summary: A report of the American College of Cardiology/ American Heart Association Task Force on Practice Guidelines and the European Society of Cardiology Committee for Practice Guidelines (Writing Committee to Revise the 2001 Guidelines for the Management of Patients With Atrial Fibrillation). Journal of the American College of Cardiology, 48, 854–906.

2. Naccarelli, G.V., Gonzalez, M.D. (2008). Atrial fibrillation and the expanding role of catheter ablation: Do antiarrhythmic drugs have a future? Journal of Cardiovascular Pharmacology, 52, 203–209.

3. Zimetbaum, P. (2007). Amiodarone for atrial fibrillation. New England Journal of Medicine, 356, 935–941.

4. Burashnikov, A., Antzelevitch, C. (2009). New pharmacological strategies for the treatment of atrial fibrillation. Annals of Noninvasive Electrocardiology, 14, 290–300.

5. Wang, Z.G., Fermini, B., Nattel, S. (1993). Sustained depolarization-induced outward current in human atrial myocytes: Evidence for a novel delayed rectifier K^+ current similar to Kv1.5 cloned channel currents. Circulation Research, 73, 1061–1076.

6. Dobrev, D., Friedrich, A., Voigt, N., Jost, N., Wettwer, E., Christ, T., et al. (2005). The G protein-gated potassium current, $I_{K.,ACh}$ is constitutively active in patients with chronic atrial fibrillation. Circulation, 112, 3697–3706.

7. Nattel, S., Carlsson, L. (2006). Innovative approaches to anti-arrhythmic drug therapy. Nature Reviews Drug Discovery, 5, 1034–1049.

8. Burashnikov, A., Di Diego, J.M., Zygmunt, A.C., Belardinelli, L., Antzelevitch, C. (2007). Atrium-selective sodium channel block as a strategy for suppression of atrial fibrillation: Differences in sodium channel inactivation between atria and ventricles and the role of ranolazine. Circulation, 116, 1449–1457.

9. Burashnikov, A., Antzelevitch, C. (2008). Atrial-selective sodium channel blockers: Do they exist? Journal of Cardiovascular Pharmacology, 52, 121–128.

10. Burashnikov, A., Antzelevitch, C. (2008). How do atrial-selective drugs differ from antiarrhythmic drugs currently used in the treatment of atrial fibrillation? Journal of Atrial Fibrillation, 1, 98–107.

11. Ford, J.W., Milnes, J.T. (2008). New drugs targeting the cardiac ultra-rapid delayed-rectifier current (I_{Kur}): Rationale, pharmacology and evidence for potential therapeutic value. Journal of Cardiovascular Pharmacology, 52, 105–120.

12. Blaauw, Y., Gogelein, H., Tieleman, R.G., van, H.A., Schotten, U., Allessie, M.A. (2004). "Early" class III drugs for the treatment of atrial fibrillation: Efficacy and atrial selectivity of AVE0118 in remodeled atria of the goat. Circulation, 110, 1717–1724.

13. Knobloch, K., Brendel, J., Rosenstein, B., Bleich, M., Busch, A.E., Wirth, K.J. (2004). Atrial-selective antiarrhythmic actions of novel Ikur vs. Ikr, Iks, and IKAch class Ic drugs and beta blockers in pigs. Medical Science Monitor, 10, BR221–BR228.

14. Wirth, K.J., Brendel, J., Steinmeyer, K., Linz, D.K., Rutten, H., Gogelein, H. (2007). In vitro and *in vivo* effects of the atrial selective antiarrhythmic compound AVE1231. Journal of Cardiovascular Pharmacology, 49, 197–206.

15. Regan, C.P., Stump, G.L., Wallace, A.A., Anderson, K.D., McIntyre, C.J., Liverton, N.J., Lynch, J.J. Jr. (2007). In vivo cardiac electrophysiologic and antiarrhythmic effects of an isoquinoline IKur blocker, ISQ-1, in rat, dog, and nonhuman primate. Journal of Cardiovascular Pharmacology, 49, 236–245.

16. Dorian, P., Pinter, A., Mangat, I., Korley, V., Cvitkovic, S.S., Beatch, G.N. (2007). The effect of vernakalant (RSD1235), an investigational antiarrhythmic agent, on atrial electrophysiology in humans. Journal of Cardiovascular Pharmacology, 50, 35–40.

17. Goldstein, R.N., Khrestian, C., Carlsson, L., Waldo, A.L. (2004). Azd7009: A new antiarrhythmic drug with predominant effects on the atria effectively terminates and prevents reinduction of atrial fibrillation and flutter in the sterile pericarditis model. Journal of Cardiovascular Electrophysiology, 15, 1444–1450.

18. Seki, A., Hagiwara, N., Kasanuki, H. (2002). Effects of NIP-141 on K currents in human atrial myocytes. Journal of Cardiovascular Pharmacology, 39, 29–38.

19. Matsuda, T., Takeda, K., Ito, M., Yamagishi, R., Tamura, M., Nakamura, H., et al. (2005). Atria selective prolongation by NIP-142, an antiarrhythmic agent, of refractory period and action potential duration in guinea pig myocardium. Journal of Pharmacology Sciences, 98, 33–40.

20. Li, G.R., Wang, H.B., Qin, G.W., Jin, M.W., Tang, Q., Sun, H.Y., et al. (2008). Acacetin, a natural flavone, selectively inhibits human atrial repolarization potassium currents and prevents atrial fibrillation in dogs. Circulation, 117, 2449–2457.

21. Roy, D., Pratt, C.M., Torp-Pedersen, C., Wyse, D.G., Toft, E., Juul-Moller, S., et al. (2008). Vernakalant hydrochloride for rapid conversion of atrial fibrillation. A phase 3, randomized, placebo-controlled trial. Circulation, 117, 1518–1525.

22. Crijns, H.J., Van, G.I., Walfridsson, H., Kulakowski, P., Ronaszeki, A., Dedek, V., et al. (2006). Safe and effective conversion of persistent atrial fibrillation to sinus rhythm by intravenous AZD7009. Heart Rhythm, 3, 1321–1331.

23. Fedida, D. (2007). Vernakalant (RSD1235): A novel, atrial-selective antifibrillatory agent. Expert Opinon on Investigation Drugs, 16, 519–532.

24. Carlsson, L., Chartier, D., Nattel, S. (2006). Characterization of the in vivo and in vitro electrophysiological effects of the novel antiarrhythmic agent AZD7009 in atrial and ventricular tissue of the dog. Journal of Cardiovascular Pharmacology, 47, 123–132.

25. Burashnikov, A., Antzelevitch, C. (2008). Can inhibition of I_{Kur} promote atrial fibrillation? Heart Rhythm, 5, 1304–1309.

26. Feng, J., Xu, D., Wang, Z., Nattel, S. (1998). Ultrarapid delayed rectifier current inactivation in human atrial myocytes: properties and consequences. American Journal of Physiology, 275, H1717–H1725.

27. Ehrlich, J.R., Ocholla, H., Ziemek, D., Rutten, H., Hohnloser, S.H., Gogelein, H. (2008). Characterization of human cardiac $K_v1.5$ inhibition by the novel atrial-selective antiarrhythmic compound AVE1231. Journal of Cardiovascular Pharmacology, 51, 380–387.

28. Workman, A.J., Kane, K.A., Rankin, A.C. (2008). Cellular bases for human atrial fibrillation. Heart Rhythm, 5, S1–S6.

29. Burashnikov, A., Mannava, S., Antzelevitch, C. (2004). Transmembrane action potential heterogeneity in the canine isolated arterially-perfused atrium: Effect of I_{Kr} and I_{to}/I_{Kur} block. American Journal of Physiology, 286, H2393–H2400.

30. Wettwer, E., Hala, O., Christ, T., Heubach, J.F., Dobrev, D., Knaut, M., et al. (2004). Role of I_{Kur} in controlling action potential shape and contractility in the human atrium: influence of chronic atrial fibrillation. Circulation, 110, 2299–2306.

31. Regan, C.P., Kiss, L., Stump, G.L., McIntyre, C.J., Beshore, D.C., Liverton, N.J., et al. (2008). Atrial antifibrillatory effects of structurally distinct I_{Kur} blockers 3-[(dimethylamino)methyl]-6-methoxy-2-methyl-4-phenylisoquinolin-1(2H)-one and 2-phenyl-1,1-dipyridin-3-yl-2-pyrrolidin-1-yl-ethanol in dogs with underlying heart failure. Journal of Pharmacology and Experimental Therapies, 324, 322–330.

32. Olson, T.M., Alekseev, A.E., Liu, X.K., Park, S.J., Zingman, L.V., Bienengraeber, M., et al. (2006). Kv1.5 channelopathy due to KCNA5 loss-of-function mutation causes human atrial fibrillation. Human Molecular Genetics, 15, 2185–2191.

33. Nattel, S. (2002). New ideas about atrial fibrillation 50 years on. Nature, 415, 219–226.

34. Heidbuchel, H., Callewaert, G., Vereecke, J., Carmeliet, E. (1992). Membrane-bound nucleoside diphosphate kinase activity in atrial cells of frog, guinea pig, and human. Circulation Research, 71, 808–820.

35. Ehrlich, J.R., Cha, T.J., Zhang, L., Chartier, D., Villeneuve, L., Hebert, T.E., Nattel, S. (2004). Characterization of a hyperpolarization-activated time-dependent potassium current in canine cardiomyocytes from pulmonary vein myocardial sleeves and left atrium. Journal of Physiology, 557, 583–597.

36. Voigt, N., Friedrich, A., Bock, M., Wettwer, E., Christ, T., Knaut, M., et al. (2007). Differential phosphorylation-dependent regulation of constitutively active and muscarinic receptor-activated, $I_{K,ACh}$ channels in patients with chronic atrial fibrillation. Cardiovascular Research, 74, 426–437.

37. Cha, T.J., Ehrlich, J.R., Chartier, D., Qi, X.Y., Xiao, L., Nattel, S. (2006). Kir3-based inward rectifier potassium current: potential role in atrial tachycardia remodeling effects on atrial repolarization and arrhythmias. Circulation, 113, 1730–1737.

38. Ravens, U. (2008). Potassium channels in atrial fibrillation: Targets for atrial and pathology-specific therapy? Heart Rhythm, 5, 758–759.

39. Bettoni, M., Zimmermann, M. (2002). Autonomic tone variations before the onset of paroxysmal atrial fibrillation. Circulation, 105, 2753–2759.

40. Pappone, C., Santinelli, V., Manguso, F., Vicedomini, G., Gugliotta, F., Augello, G., et al. (2004). Pulmonary vein denervation enhances long-term benefit after circumferential ablation for paroxysmal atrial fibrillation. Circulation, 109, 327–334.

41. Hashimoto, N., Yamashita, T., Tsuruzoe, N. (2006). Tertiapin, a selective, $I_{K,ACh}$ blocker, terminates atrial fibrillation with selective atrial effective refractory period prolongation. Pharmacology Research, 54, 136–141.

42. Patterson, E., Scherlag, B.J., Zhou, J., Jackman, W.M., Lazzara, R., Coscia, D., Po, S. (2008). Antifibrillatory actions of cisatracurium: an atrial specific m receptor antagonist. Journal of Cardiovascular Electrophysiology, 19, 861–868.

43. Burashnikov, A., Di Diego, J.M., Sicouri, S., Ferreiro, M., Carlsson, L., Antzelevitch, C. (2008). Atrial-selective effects of chronic amiodarone in the management of atrial fibrillation. Heart Rhythm, 5, 1735–1742.

44. Burashnikov, A., Belardinelli, L., Antzelevitch, C. (2007). Ranolazine and propafenone both suppress atrial fibrillation but ranolazine unlike propafenone does it without prominent effects on ventricular myocardium. Heart Rhythm, 4, S163.

45. Scirica, B.M., Morrow, D.A., Hod, H., Murphy, S.A., Belardinelli, L., Hedgepeth, C.M., et al. (2007). Effect of ranolazine, an antianginal agent with novel electrophysiological properties, on the incidence of arrhythmias in patients with non ST-segment elevation acute coronary syndrome: Results from the Metabolic Efficiency With Ranolazine for Less Ischemia in Non ST-Elevation Acute Coronary Syndrome Thrombolysis in Myocardial Infarction 36 (MERLIN-TIMI 36) randomized controlled trial. Circulation, 116, 1647–1652.

46. Spinelli, W., Parsons, R.W., Colatsky, T.J. (1992). Effects of WAY-123,398, a new Class-III antiarrhythmic agent, on cardiac refractoriness and ventricular fibrillation threshold in anesthetized dogs—a comparison with UK-68798, e-4031, and DL- Sotalol. Journal of Cardiovascular Pharmacology, 20, 913–922.

47. Wiesfeld, A.C., De Langen, C.D., Crijns, H.J., Bel, K.J., Hillege, H.L., Wesseling, H., Lie, K.I. (1996). Rate-dependent effects of the class III antiarrhythmic drug almokalant on refractoriness in the pig. Journal of Cardiovascular Pharmacology, 27, 594–600.

48. Baskin, E.P., Lynch, J.J. Jr. (1998). Differential atrial versus ventricular activities of class III potassium channel blockers. Journal of Pharmacology and Experimental Therapeutics, 285, 135–142.

49. Stump, G.L., Wallace, A.A., Regan, C.P., Lynch, J.J. Jr. (2005). In vivo antiarrhythmic and cardiac electrophysiologic effects of a novel diphenylphosphine oxide IKur blocker (2-isopropyl-5-methylcyclohexyl) diphenylphosphine oxide. Journal of Pharmacology and Experimental Therapeutics, 315, 1362–1367.

50. Wang, J., Feng, J., Nattel, S. (1994). Class III antiarrhythmic drug action in experimental atrial fibrillation. Differences in reverse use dependence and effectiveness between d-sotalol and the new antiarrhythmic drug ambasilide. Circulation, 90, 2032–2040.

51. Echt, D.S., Berte, L.E., Clusin, W.T., Samuelson, R.G., Harrison, D.C., Mason, J.W. (1982). Prolongation of the human monophasic action potential by sotalol. American Journal of Cardiology, 50, 1082–1086.

52. Buchanan, L.V., LeMay, R.J., Walters, R.R., Hsu, C.Y., Brunden, M.N., Gibson, J.K. (1996). Antiarrhythmic and electrophysiologic effects of intravenous ibutilide and sotalol in the canine sterile pericarditis model. Journal of Cardiovascular Electrophysiology, 7, 113–119.

53. Antzelevitch, C., Shimizu, W., Yan, G.X., Sicouri, S., Weissenburger, J., Nesterenko, V.V., et al. (1999). The M cell: Its contribution to the ECG and to normal and abnormal electrical function of the heart. Journal of Cardiovascular Electrophysiology, 10, 1124–1152.

54. Burashnikov, A., Antzelevitch, C. (2006). Late-phase 3 EAD. A unique mechanism contributing to initiation of atrial fibrillation. PACE, 29, 290–295.

55. Antzelevitch, C., Belardinelli, L., Wu, L., Fraser, H., Zygmunt, A.C., Burashnikov, A., et al. (2004). Electrophysiologic properties and antiarrhythmic actions of a novel antianginal agent. Journal of Cardiovascular Pharmacology Therapeutics, 9, S65–S83.

56. Singh, B.N. (2006). Amiodarone: A multifaceted antiarrhythmic drug. Current Cardiology Reports, 8, 349–355.

57. Kneller, J., Kalifa, J., Zou, R., Zaitsev, A.V., Warren, M., Berenfeld, O., et al. (2005). Mechanisms of atrial fibrillation termination by pure sodium channel blockade in an ionically-realistic mathematical model. Circulation Research, 96, e35–e47.

58. Comtois, P., Sakabe, M., Vigmond, E.J., Munoz, M.A., Texier, A., Shiroshita-Takeshita, A., Nattel, S. (2008). Mechanisms of atrial fibrillation termination by rapidly unbinding

Na$^+$ channel blockers. Insights from mathematical models and experimental correlates. American Journal of Physiology Heart Circulation Physiology, 295, H1489–H1504.

59. Amos, G.J., Wettwer, E., Metzger, F., Li, Q., Himmel, H.M., Ravens, U. (1996). Differences between outward currents of human atrial and subepicardial ventricular myocytes. Journal of Physiology, 491, 31–50.

60. Nattel, S., Matthews, C., De Blasio, E., Han, W., Li, D., Yue, L. (2000). Dose-dependence of 4-aminopyridine plasma concentrations and electrophysiological effects in dogs: Potential relevance to ionic mechanisms in vivo. Circulation, 101, 1179–1184.

61. Gaborit, N., Le, B.S., Szuts, V., Varro, A., Escande, D., Nattel, S., Demolombe, S. (2007). Regional and tissue specific transcript signatures of ion channel genes in the non-diseased human heart. Journal of Physiology, 582, 675–693.

62. Christe, G., Tebbakh, H., Simurdova, M., Forrat, R., Simurda, J. (1999). Propafenone blocks ATP-sensitive K$^+$ channels in rabbit atrial and ventricular cardiomyocytes. European Journal of Pharmacology, 373, 223–232.

63. Olson, T.M., Alekseev, A.E., Moreau, C., Liu, X.K., Zingman, L.V., Miki, T., et al. (2007). K$_{ATP}$ channel mutation confers risk for vein of Marshall adrenergic atrial fibrillation. Nature Clinical Practice. Cardiovascular Medicine, 4, 110–116.

64. Burashnikov, A., Di Diego, J.M., Zygmunt, A.C., Belardinelli, L., Antzelevitch, C. (2008). Atrial-selective sodium channel block as a strategy for suppression of atrial fibrillation. Annals of NY Academy of Sciences, 1123, 105–112.

65. Duytschaever, M., Blaauw, Y., Allessie, M. (2005). Consequences of atrial electrical remodeling for the anti-arrhythmic action of class IC and class III drugs. Cardiovascular Research, 67, 69–76.

66. Linz, D.K., Afkham, F., Itter, G., Rutten, H., Wirth, K.J. (2007). Effect of atrial electrical remodeling on the efficacy of antiarrhythmic drugs: comparison of amiodarone with I_{Kr}- and I_{to}/I_{Kur}-blockade *in vivo* strial electrical remodeling and antiarrhythmic drugs. Journal of Cardiovascular Electrophysiology, 18, 1313–1320.

67. Blaauw, Y., Schotten, U., van, H.A., Neuberger, H.R., Allessie, M.A. (2007). Cardioversion of persistent atrial fibrillation by a combination of atrial specific and non-specific class III drugs in the goat. Cardiovascular Research, 75, 89–98.

68. Whalley, D.W., Wendt, D.J., Grant, A.O. (1995). Basic concepts in cellular cardiac electrophysiology: Part II: Block of ion channels by antiarrhythmic drugs. PACE, 18, 1686–1704.

69. Eijsbouts, S., Ausma, J., Blaauw, Y., Schotten, U., Duytschaever, M., Allessie, M.A. (2006). Serial cardioversion by class IC drugs during 4 months of persistent atrial fibrillation in the goat. Journal of Cardiovascular Electrophysiology, 17, 648–654.

70. Billman, G.E., Kukielka, M. (2008). Novel transient outward and ultra-rapid delayed rectifier current antagonist, AVE0118, protects against ventricular fibrillation induced by myocardial ischemia. Journal of Cardiovascular Pharmacology, 51, 352–358.

71. Antzelevitch, C. (2008). Ranolazine: A new antiarrhythmic agent for patients with non-ST-segment elevation acute coronary syndromes? Nature Clinical Practice Cardiovascular Medicine, 5, 248–249.

72. Goette, A., Bukowska, A., Lendeckel, U. (2007). Non-ion channel blockers as anti-arrhythmic drugs (reversal of structural remodeling). Current Opinion Pharmacology, 7, 219–224.

73. Savelieva, I., Camm, J. (2008). Statins and polyunsaturated fatty acids for treatment of atrial fibrillation. Nature Clinical Practice Cardiovascular Medicine, 5, 30–41.

74. Nattel, S., Burstein, B., Dobrev, D. (2008). Atrial remodeling and atrial fibrillation: Mechanisms and implications. Circulation: Arrhythmia and Electrophysiology, 1, 62–73.

75. Van Wagoner, D.R. (2008). Oxidative stress and inflammation in atrial fibrillation: Role in pathogenesis and potential as a therapeutic target. Journal of Cardiovascular Pharmacology, 52, 306–313.

76. Nakajima, H., Nakajima, H.O., Salcher, O., Dittie, A.S., Dembowsky, K., Jing, S., Field, L.J. (2000). Atrial but not ventricular fibrosis in mice expressing a mutant transforming growth factor-b_1 transgene in the heart. Circulation Research, 86, 571–579.

77. Dudley, S.C. Jr., Hoch, N.E., McCann, L.A., Honeycutt, C., Diamandopoulos, L., Fukai, T., et al. (2005). Atrial fibrillation increases production of superoxide by the left atrium and left atrial appendage: Role of the NADPH and xanthine oxidases. Circulation, 112, 1266–1273.

78. Burstein, B., Libby, E., Calderone, A., Nattel, S. (2008). Differential behaviors of atrial versus ventricular fibroblasts: A potential role for platelet-derived growth factor in atrial-ventricular remodeling differences. Circulation, 117, 1630–1641.

79. Shimano, M., Tsuji, Y., Inden, Y., Kitamura, K., Uchikawa, T., Harata, S., et al. (2008). Pioglitazone, a peroxisome proliferator-activated receptor-gamma activator, attenuates atrial fibrosis and atrial fibrillation promotion in rabbits with congestive heart failure. Heart Rhythm, 5, 451–459.

80. Tsai, C.T., Lai, L.P., Kuo, K.T., Hwang, J.J., Hsieh, C.S., Hsu, K.L., et al. (2008). Angiotensin II activates signal transducer and activators of transcription 3 via Rac1 in atrial myocytes and fibroblasts: Implication for the therapeutic effect of statin in atrial structural remodeling. Circulation, 117, 344–355.

81. Lin, C.S., Pan, C.H. (2008). Regulatory mechanisms of atrial fibrotic remodeling in atrial fibrillation. Cellular and Molecular Life Sciences, 65, 1489–1508.

82. Ducharme, A., Swedberg, K., Pfeffer, M.A., Cohen-Solal, A., Granger, C.B., Maggioni, A.P., et al. (2006). Prevention of atrial fibrillation in patients with symptomatic chronic heart failure by candesartan in the Candesartan in Heart failure: Assessment of reduction in mortality and morbidity (CHARM) program. American Heart Journal, 152, 86–92.

83. Salehian, O., Healey, J., Stambler, B., Alnemer, K., Almerri, K., Grover, J., et al. (2007). Impact of ramipril on the incidence of atrial fibrillation: Results of the Heart Outcomes Prevention Evaluation study. American Heart Journal, 154, 448–453.

84. Berkowitsch, A., Neumann, T., Kuniss, M., Zaltsberg, S., Pitschner, H.F. (2008). Effects of angiotensin converting enzyme inhibitors and angiotensin receptor blockers in patients with hypertension and atrial fibrillation after pulmonary vein isolation. Heart Rhythm, 5, S265.

85. Jang, J.K., Park, J.S., Kim, Y.H., Choi, J., Lim, H.E., Pak, H.N., et al. (2008). Effects of the therapy with statins, angiotensin-converting enzyme inhibitors, and angiotensin II receptor blocker on the outcome after catheter ablation of atrial fibrillation. Heart Rhythm, 5, S324.

86. Hanna, N., Cardin, S., Leung, T.K., Nattel, S. (2004). Differences in atrial versus ventricular remodeling in dogs with ventricular tachypacing-induced congestive heart failure. Cardiovascular Research, 63, 236–244.

87. Xiao, H.D., Fuchs, S., Campbell, D.J., Lewis, W., Dudley, S.C. Jr., Kasi, V.S., et al. (2004). Mice with cardiac-restricted angiotensin-converting enzyme (ACE) have atrial enlargement, cardiac arrhythmia, and sudden death. American Journal of Pathology, 165, 1019–1032.

88. Verheule, S., Sato, T., Everett, T., Engle, S.K., Otten, D., Rubart-von der, L.M., et al. (2004). Increased vulnerability to atrial fibrillation in transgenic mice with selective atrial fibrosis caused by overexpression of TGF-beta1. Circulation Research, 94, 1458–1465.

89. Adam, O., Frost, G., Custodis, F., Sussman, M.A., Schafers, H.J., Bohm, M., Laufs, U. (2007). Role of Rac1 GTPase activation in atrial fibrillation. Journal of the American College of Cardiology, 50, 359–367.

90. Burashnikov, A. (2008). Are there atrial selective/predominant targets for "upstream" atrial fibrillation therapy?. Heart Rhythm, 5, 1294–1295.

91. Xing, D., Kjolbye, A.L., Nielsen, M.S., Petersen, J.S., Harlow, K.W., Holstein-Rathlou, N.H., Martins, J.B. (2003). ZP123 increases gap junctional conductance and prevents reentrant ventricular tachycardia during myocardial ischemia in open chest dogs. Journal of Cardiovascular Electrophysiology, 14, 510–520.

92. Eloff, B.C., Gilat, E., Wan, X., Rosenbaum, D.S. (2003). Pharmacological modulation of cardiac gap junctions to enhance cardiac conduction: Evidence supporting a novel target for antiarrhythmic therapy. Circulation, 108, 3157–3163.

93. Guerra, J.M., Everett, T.H., Lee, K.W., Wilson, E., Olgin, J.E. (2006). Effects of the gap junction modifier rotigaptide (ZP123) on atrial conduction and vulnerability to atrial fibrillation. Circulation, 114, 110–118.

94. Shiroshita-Takeshita, A., Sakabe, M., Haugan, K., Hennan, J.K., Nattel, S. (2007). Model-dependent effects of the gap junction conduction-enhancing antiarrhythmic peptide rotigaptide (ZP123) on experimental atrial fibrillation in dogs. Circulation, 115, 310–318.

95. Gollob, M.H. (2008). Begetting atrial fibrillation: Connexins and arrhythmogenesis. Heart Rhythm, 5, 888–891.

96. Gollob, M.H., Jones, D.L., Krahn, A.D., Danis, L., Gong, X.Q., Shao, Q., et al. (2006). Somatic mutations in the connexin 40 gene (GJA5) in atrial fibrillation. New England Journal of Medicine, 354, 2677–2688.

97. Ehrlich, J.R., Biliczki, P., Hohnloser, S.H., Nattel, S. (2008). Atrial-selective approaches for the treatment of atrial fibrillation. Journal of the American College of Cardiology, 51, 787–792.

98. Burashnikov, A., Antzelevitch, C. (2003). Reinduction of atrial fibrillation immediately after termination of the arrhythmia is mediated by late phase 3 early afterdepolarization-induced triggered activity. Circulation, 107, 2355–2360.

99. Hove-Madsen, L., Llach, A., Bayes-Genis, A., Roura, S., Rodriguez, F.E., Aris, A., Cinca, J. (2004). Atrial fibrillation is associated with increased spontaneous calcium release from the sarcoplasmic reticulum in human atrial myocytes. Circulation, 110, 1358–1363.

100. Vest, J.A., Wehrens, X.H., Reiken, S.R., Lehnart, S.E., Dobrev, D., Chandra, P., et al. (2005). Defective cardiac ryanodine receptor regulation during atrial fibrillation. Circulation, 111, 2025–2032.

101. Dobrev, D., Nattel, S. (2008). Calcium handling abnormalities in atrial fibrillation as a target for innovative therapeutics. Journal of Cardiovascular Pharmacology, 52, 293–298.

102. Sood, S., Chelu, M.G., van Oort, R.J., Skapura, D., Santonastasi, M., Dobrev, D., Wehrens, X.H. (2008). Intracellular calcium leak due to FKBP12.6 deficiency in mice facilitates the inducibility of atrial fibrillation. Heart Rhythm, 5, 1047–1054.

103. Zhou, S., Chang, C.M., Wu, T.J., Miyauchi, Y., Okuyama, Y., Park, A.M., et al. (2002). Nonreentrant focal activations in pulmonary veins in canine model of sustained atrial fibrillation. American Journal of Physiology Heart Circulation Physiology, 283, H1244–H1252.

104. Fenelon, G., Shepard, R.K., Stambler, B.S. (2003). Focal origin of atrial tachycardia in dogs with rapid ventricular pacing-induced heart failure. Journal of Cardiovascular Electrophysiology, 14, 1093–1102.

105. Chou, C.C., Nihei, M., Zhou, S., Tan, A., Kawase, A., Macias, E.S., et al. (2005). Intracellular calcium dynamics and anisotropic reentry in isolated canine pulmonary veins and left atrium. Circulation, 111, 2889–2897.

106. Hirose, M., Laurita, K.R. (2007). Calcium-mediated triggered activity is an underlying cellular mechanism of ectopy originating from the pulmonary vein in dogs. American Journal of Physiology Heart Circulation Physiology, 292, H1861–H1867.

107. Kumagai, K., Nakashima, H., Gondo, N., Saku, K. (2003). Antiarrhythmic effects of JTV-519, a novel cardioprotective drug, on atrial fibrillation/flutter in a canine sterile pericarditis model. Journal of Cardiovascular Electrophysiology, 14, 880–884.

CHAPTER 18

I$_{Kur}$, Ultra-rapid Delayed Rectifier Potassium Current: A Therapeutic Target for Atrial Arrhythmias

ARUN SRIDHAR and CYNTHIA A. CARNES

18.1 INTRODUCTION

Cardiac repolarization occurs via a multitude of potassium (K^+) channels, which are voltage-gated or ligand gated [1]. Most notable among them are the voltage-gated potassium channels, which exhibit both time- and voltage-dependent activation. These voltage-gated K^+ channels open and close based on the voltage perceived by the cardiac myocytes during the action potential. In addition to opening at various phases of the action potential based on the voltage dependence, the uniqueness of a cardiac voltage-gated K^+ channel stems from channel activity that originates from secondary effects on other types of channels (e.g., sarcolemmal Ca^{2+} channels and the sarcoplasmic reticulum Ca^{2+} release channels) [2, 3]. Alterations in repolarizing K^+ currents may occur as primary ion channelopathies or as acquired defects caused by disease or drugs, which alter channel activity. This property can be exploited in certain disease pathologies, when blocking one of the K^+ channels contributing to early repolarization can have secondary effects on other ion channels that follow during the action potential. For example, the use of I$_{Kur}$ blockers could have electrophysiologic effects, as well as increasing contractility because of feedback on other ion channels [4]. The data supporting these concepts will be presented in the following sections.

This chapter focuses on one such ion channel contributing to repolarization of the cardiac action potential, the K$_v$1.5 channel, which encodes a distinct delayed rectifier current called the ultrarapid delayed rectifier current. Before understanding the pharmacology of the K$_v$1.5 channel and its blockers, the reader needs to understand the structure of voltage-gated K^+ channels, which are similar in their ion conducting

Novel Therapeutic Targets for Antiarrhythmic Drugs, Edited by George Edward Billman
Copyright © 2010 John Wiley & Sons, Inc.

properties to gain a deeper appreciation of the potential of voltage-gated K$^+$ channel blockers.

18.2   MOLECULAR BIOLOGY OF THE K$_V$1.5 CHANNELS:

Voltage-gated K$^+$ channels exist as tetramers in the cell membrane. Each monomer has six transmembrane helices as shown in the Figure 18.1. The helices (segments) are numbered S1 to S6 and are interconnected. One of the most widely studied voltage-gated K$^+$ channels is a member of the Shaker family, which is isolated from the shaker gene locus of drosophila. This channel is homologous to many mammalian and eukaryotic K$^+$ channels [5, 6]. (For more detailed information, refer to Chapter 2 in this volume). Each monomer of the channel possesses six membrane-spanning α-helices that are interconnected [6, 7]. Most voltage-gated K$^+$ channels have an amino (N-) and carboxy (C-) terminus, and both ends of the protein play specific roles in the opening and closing of the channel. The most distinct and preserved part of the voltage-gated K$^+$ channel are the residues located in the pore loop between helices S5 and S6 (Figure 18.1). These residues form a distinct signature sequence of amino acids (GYG), which serve to determine the selectivity of the K$^+$ channel, and are conserved among both prokaryotic and eukaryotic K$^+$ channels [7].

18.2.1   K$_V$1.5 Activation and Inactivation

Two distinct processes must be considered in ion channel physiology: activation and inactivation. Activation is the process of opening an ion channel pore, whereas

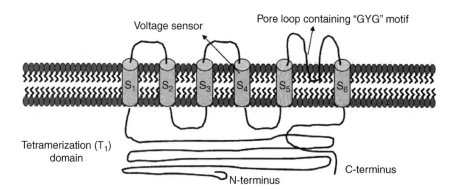

Figure 18.1. Topology of a voltage-gated K$^+$ channel showing the six transmembrane helices (numbered S1 through S6). Also shown is the amino acid sequence between S5 and S6 helices, which forms the pore loop. The GYG motif that resides in this loop is responsible for the selectivity of the channel. The N-terminus is usually ∼60 amino acids long, but in some ion channels, an additional tetramerization (T1) domain is present, which serves to interact with the N-terminus of the channels. The T1 domain may also act as a point of interaction between other accessory subunits that might interact with the transmembrane α subunit.

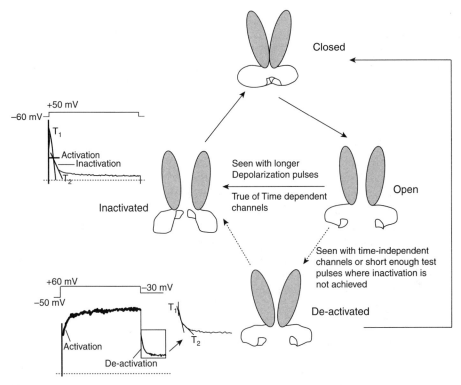

Figure 18.2. Representation of ion channel processes that govern ion flow. For the sake of simplicity, only two monomers are shown. (Most voltage gated K$^+$ channels exist as tetramers.) N-type inactivation via the ball and chain model is shown here. However, it must be kept in mind that other proposed mechanisms of inactivation and deactivation exist, which are beyond the scope of discussion for this chapter [4]. For more information, see ref. 4.

inactivation is the process by which the channel limits ion flux during prolonged stimulation. Inactivation can be confused with the closed state of the ion channel, which it is not. The inactivated state is a step in the ion channel cycle that lies between a fully open state and a closed state, and it serves as a pathway in the process of closing the ion channel pore (Figure 18.2). The molecular mechanisms involved in this process are briefly described below.

18.2.1.1 Activation. The process of activation was described by the work of Hodgkin and Huxley, and the exact mechanisms have been elucidated by the work from the laboratories of multiple eminent scientists, including Clay Armstrong, Bertil Hille, and Francisco Bezanilla [4, 8]. A voltage sensor is created by the presence of positively charged amino acid molecules (arginine and histidine) on the S4 helix of the channel. Because a tetramer forms the channel, four such voltage sensors act in synergy to open the channel pore [7]. This conformational change results from the twisting and upward and outward motion of the S$_4$ channel helix, which opens the channel by the mechanical pull of the S_4 on its other helical counterparts. This motion of the S_4 helices opens the channel and results in the activation properties of the channel, with the degree of the movement controlled by the degree of change in the membrane voltage registered by the S4 voltage sensors. *So, the higher the voltage change perceived by the S4 voltage, the greater the movement, degree of activation, and channel open times* [8]. This relationship is true of most voltage-gated K^+ channels that open more at positive potentials.

18.2.1.2 Inactivation. The first 20 amino acids of the N-terminus of the ion channel form a "ball" structure, whereas the remaining amino acids of the N-terminus form the "chain" structure. This forms the "ball and chain" of the N-terminus, which can block the channel pore on the cytoplasmic (intracellular) side and thereby block ion current flow through the channel [8]. This mechanism is referred to as N-type inactivation, which is so named because of the effect of the N-terminus of each monomer on inactivation. The other type of channel inactivation mechanism is called C-type inactivation. This involves the combined movement of S_5 and S_6 helices in concert with the C-terminus, which mechanically push into the lumen of the channel producing an electrostatic hindrance to ion current flow through the pore of the channel.

18.2.2 Where Does I_{Kur} Fit Into the Cardiac Action Potential?

Seminal studies about I_{Kur} from Nerbonne and colleagues [9, 10] demonstrated that when rat cardiac myocytes were voltage clamped to isolate K^+ currents (by using a combination of a holding potential of $-60\,mV$ to inactivate sodium channels, and an L-type calcium channel blocker), depolarization elicited an outward current that peaked early with a steady-state current component. The peak current rapidly inactivated, whereas the steady-state current showed little to no inactivation (Figure 18.3).

More studies showed that the peak current (later identified as I_{to}) was sensitive to millimolar concentrations of 4-aminopyridine (4-AP). The steady-state current was insensitive to 4-AP but highly sensitive to tetraethylammonium (TEA) chloride [11]. However, even in the presence of TEA, a TEA-insensitive steady-state current remained. This residual current was sensitive to micromolar concentrations of 4-AP [11]. Nerbonne's group, as well as other investigators, elucidated the molecular basis of the peak and steady-state currents. They identified that mouse and rat ventricles have a multitude of voltage-gated K^+ channel subunits, such as $K_v4.2$ and $K_v4.3$ (encoding I_{to}), as well as $K_v1.4$, $K_v1.5$, $K_v1.2$ and $K_v2.1$ (encoding sustained current), which result in the peak and sustained K^+ currents [1, 12–14]. Details of the transgenic studies that lead to elucidation of each current component are beyond the scope of this chapter, but certain transgenic studies with $K_v1.5$ knock out mice deserve special mention.

Transgenic studies have shed light on K_v1-encoded currents and their relation to the QT interval on the electrocardiogram (ECG). $K_v1.5$ knock out mice exhibit prolongation of action potential duration and QT interval on the ECG, suggesting that

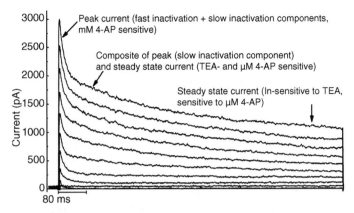

Figure 18.3. Potassium currents recorded from a mouse ventricular myocyte. The currents were elicited in response to 800-ms voltage steps from -50 mV to $+50$ mV, from a holding potential of -60 mV. The current trace elicited shows an early peak that is now regarded as I_{to} (fast, sensitive to mM 4-AP), a slowly inactivating component of I_{to}, and a steady-state current. The steady-state current has two components [9–12]. One component inactivates slowly and is sensitive to 30 mM TEA. The second steady-state component (observed toward the end of the 800-ms test pulse) is a µM 4-AP sensitive I_{Kur}.

the K$_v$1.5-encoded steady-state current plays an important role in the repolarization of murine ventricles [15, 16]. A similar plateau current was found in rat atria, confirming the presence of K$_v$1.5 as the putative subunit encoding I_{Kur} [17]. These studies confirmed the role of K$_v$1.5 as a major repolarizing current in the rat ventricle, but that finding raises the question about I_{Kur} in other species.

Yue and Marban [18] reported a plateau current in guinea pig ventricle, I_{Kp}. Through a combination of whole-cell and single-channel recording approaches, the authors found that the current was selective for K$^+$ ions and opened at voltages close to plateau potential (thus naming the current I_{Kp}) of the action potential. Recently, this current has been suggested to be similar to I_{Kur} (see a recent review on K$^+$ channels by Nerbonne and Kass) [1].

Notably, the gene encoding Kv1.5, KCNA5, has been found in the ventricles and atria of rabbits, canines, and humans [1]. Canines are considered a reliable surrogate model to study human cardiac electrophysiology. Canine atria and ventricles have abundant Kv1.5 expression, and a study by Fedida et al. [19] demonstrated that Kv1.5 encodes I_{Kur} in canine atrium. Another electrophysiological characterization of I_{Kur} in canine and human atria has suggested that canine and human atrial I_{Kur} is similar to rodent I_{Kur} (in atria and ventricle) in its sensitivity to micromolar concentrations of 4-AP [19, 20]. In addition, they clearly delineated the differences in I_{Kur} and I_{to}, based on their differences in sensitivity to 4-AP, with I_{Kur} blocked by micromolar 4-AP, whereas I_{to} block required millimolar concentrations.

As stated above, Kv1.5, which is the protein encoding I_{Kur}, is present in both canine and human atria and ventricles [1, 21]. Evidence for I_{Kur} in the human heart came from a report by Wettwer et al. [22] that showed human atrial I_{Kur} is composed of two components. The first current component corresponding to the early peak current in $K_v1.5$ expressing cells (found in heterologous cultured cells and in human atrial myocytes) was a fast inactivating component. The second current component had a slowly inactivating component (slower time constant) and corresponded to steady-state plateau current, suggesting that human atrial I_{Kur} mirrors Kv1.5 expressing cultured cells [22].

I_{Kur} in human cardiac myocytes has been described only in atrial myocytes, and the current is reportedly absent in ventricular myocytes. However, the expression of $K_v1.5$ is similar when comparing canine and human atrial and ventricular tissue [19, 21]. A study by Sridhar et al. [24] examined canine ventricular myocytes for the presence of a plateau current sensitive to micromolar 4-AP (similar to the concentration used by to inhibit atrial I_{Kur}, Figure 18.4), and they found an "I_{Kur}-like" current [24]. This current shares all the features attributed to I_{Kur}, including 1) an activation voltage range corresponding to plateau voltages 2) sensitivity to micromolar concentrations of 4-AP, and 3) increased density during isoproterenol stimulation. In addition, an envelope of tails test confirmed that the "I_{Kur}-like" current resulted from a single current component. More studies are required to establish definitively that $K_v1.5$ encodes a "I_{Kur}-like" current in the canine ventricle. This study suggests that a current similar or identical to canine atrial I_{Kur} exists in the canine ventricle. Human ventricular myocardium expresses $K_v1.5$ at a level similar to canine ventricular myocardium; the

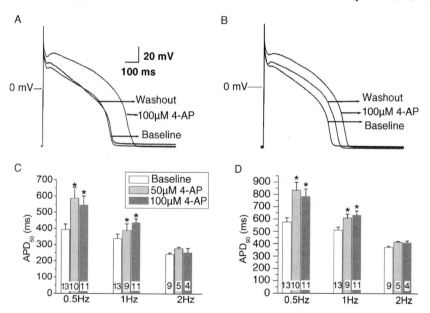

Figure 18.4. Evidence of micromolar 4-AP–induced prolongation of the canine ventricular action potential. Panels A and B show action potentials recorded at 0.5 and 1 Hz at baseline, after superfusion with 100-μM 4-AP and following washout of 4-AP. Panels C and D show the action potential duration at 50% (APD50) and 90% repolarization, respectively, expressed as a function of stimulation frequency. *$P < 0.05$ vs. baseline. Adapted by permission from Macmillan Publishers Ltd, British Journal of Pharmacology, copyright 2007 [24].

existence of human ventricular I$_{Kur}$ remains understudied, particularly in structurally normal hearts, at this time.

Notably, Feng et al. [25] documented an absence of I$_{Kur}$ in human ventricular myocytes by using antisense oligonucleotides (AsODNs) for the K$_v$1.5 protein. They showed that in human atrial myocytes, K$_v$1.5 AsODNs reduced the I$_{Kur}$ current (4-AP-sensitive current), whereas no effect was observed in the currents recorded with and without AsODNs in ventricular myocytes. This led the authors to conclude that in humans, I$_{Kur}$ exists only in the atria. Caveats that must be considered are that the myocytes in this study were from the right ventricle of explanted failing human hearts. Of note, the right ventricle has been documented to be more dependent on transient outward K$^+$ current than the left ventricle for repolarization [26]. Thus, the role of I$_{Kur}$ in repolarization of the left ventricle of patients with structurally normal hearts remains undefined.

18.2.3 Adrenergic Modulation of I$_{Kur}$

Isolated canine atrial myocytes show an increase in I$_{Kur}$ density after exposure to 1 μM isoproterenol [27]. In addition to the increase in the step current density, a significant increase occurred in the tail current density, without alteration of the reversal potential or the activation time constant. Superfusion with 8-bromo-cyclic adenosine 3'5'-monophosphate (cAMP) and forskolin have been reported to augment I$_{Kur}$ density significantly, whereas pretreatment with protein kinase A inhibiting (PKI) peptide prevents augmentation of I$_{Kur}$ by isoproterenol. These lines of evidence suggest that I$_{Kur}$ is modulated in canine atrial myocytes via the β-adrenergic receptor signaling pathway, specifically through protein kinase A and cAMP. Conversely, α-adrenergic stimulation with phenylephrine reduces I$_{Kur}$ density, and this effect is blocked by the α-adrenergic receptor antagonist prazosin. Thus, I$_{Kur}$ density can increase or decrease based on the type of adrenergic receptors that are activated in canine atrial myocytes.

18.3 I$_{KUR}$ AS A THERAPEUTIC TARGET

Based on the limited studies evaluating the presence of I$_{Kur}$ in the human ventricle (described above), I$_{Kur}$ has been suggested as an "atrial-selective" therapeutic target for the treatment of atrial arrhythmias (e.g., see a recent review by Page and Roden [28]). The advantage of atrial selectivity is the potential avoidance of ventricular proarrhythmia. Atrial fibrillation (AF) is the most common sustained cardiac arrhythmia and is a leading cause of stroke in the United States. Ion current remodeling during human AF has been described as reductions in I$_{Kur}$, I$_{to}$, and I$_{Ca-L}$. In agreement with the observed reduction in I$_{Kur}$ during AF, Kv1.5 protein is reduced in human AF tissue by ∼50% [29]. Similar reductions have also been observed in canine models of AF [30, 31] A recent report suggests that during chronic canine heart failure, there is a reduction in I$_{Kur}$, while Kv 1.5 is preserved [32]. Thus, atrial I$_{Kur}$ is reduced by atrial fibrillation, and possibly by heart failure.

Evidence that I_{Kur} blockade might be beneficial in AF came from studies by Wettwer et al. [33], who studied the electrophysiology of atrial trabeculae from AF patients in comparison with sinus rhythm patients. In this study, the blockade of I_{Kur} (with 5 µM 4-AP) resulted in a greater degree of augmentation of both action potential duration at 20% repolarization (APD_{20}) and plateau amplitude in the AF tissues relative to controls. This effect on the plateau and APD_{20} coincided with an increased force of contraction in AF trabeculae. In addition, this study evaluated an investigational mixed I_{Kur} blocker, AVE0118, and it reported that the effects of AVE0118 were similar to the effects of 4-AP. An *in vivo* study with AVE0118 was conducted by Blaauw et al. [34], using a goat model of AF to compare AVE0118 with ibutilide and dofetilide (I_{Kr} blockers). AVE0118 terminated AF in 68% of the treated animals, and the efficacy of AVE0118 was dose dependent [35].

Although studies with I_{Kur} blockers reveal effects on action potential duration in tissues from patients with AF, it raises a question regarding the mechanism of I_{Kur} blockade in atrial fibrillation. Specifically, because I_{Kur} (as stated above) is reduced in AF, how can pathologically reduced I_{Kur} be pharmacologically blocked and result in greater APD prolongation in AF than in control myocytes? This point has been addressed in a recent study of AVE0118 in human atrial myocytes [23]. The authors dissected three components of human atrial I_{Kur} by fitting the time constants of decay of the K^+ current trace: a fast inactivating current, a slow inactivating current, and a noninactivating current. Atrial myocytes from patients in sinus rhythm showed blockade of all three components with AVE0118, whereas in AF myocytes, only the peak and slowly inactivating components were blocked by AVE0118. Therefore, this finding suggests that in human AF, a noninactivating component of I_{Kur} is resistant to pharmacologic blockade. This observation explains the mechanisms for the greater effects of I_{Kur} blockers on atrial repolarization in AF patient samples compared with controls.

18.4 ORGANIC BLOCKERS OF I_{KUR}

The most widely studied investigational I_{Kur} blockers to date are reviewed here. Consideration is given to compounds with the most currently available data.

18.4.1 Mixed Channel Blockers

18.4.1.1 In-Vitro Effects. AVE0118 and AVE1231 are drugs currently in development for the treatment of AF [36–38]. AVE0118 inhibits $hK_v1.5$ ($IC_{50} \sim 1.1$–6.0 µM), and also blocks $hK_v4.3/KChIP2.2$ (molecular correlates of cardiac I_{to}) with an IC_{50} value of 3.4 ± 0.5 µM, and it also blocks I_{KACh} in pig atrial myocytes ($IC_{50} = 4.5$ µM) [34]. Notably, the concentration required for hERG (protein encoding I_{Kr}) blockade is ~ 10 µM [36]. In addition, AVE0118 also blocks the L-type calcium current, I_{Ks} and $I_{K(ATP)}$ at concentrations between 5–10 µM. Therefore, AVE0118 blocks many ion channels at concentrations of 1–4 µM, with I_{Kur}, I_{to}, and I_{KACh} expected to be affected at this concentration range. A small amount of hERG blockade is possible at this concentration range based on the relative IC_{50}s (IC_{50} for hERG block is 10 µM; while in comparison, the IC_{50} for Kv1.5 is 1.1–6.0 µM) [36].

A second mixed I_{Kur} blocker, AVE1231, blocks hKv1.5 and hKv4.3/KChIP2.2 with IC_{50} concentrations of 3.6 and 5.9 µM, respectively [37]. The IC_{50} for blockade of I_{KACh} is 8.4 µM, whereas L-type calcium current, I_{Ks}, and I_{KATP} are only minimally blocked (~8–12% at 10 µM AVE1231). I_{Kr} tail current was 25% and 50% blocked at 10 and 30 µM AVE1231, respectively, whereas atrial dV/dt and APD_{90} were unaffected by either 10 or 30 µM AVE1231. Thus, AVE1231 seems to be relatively more selective for I_{to} and I_{Kur}, with potential for only 10% block of I_{Kr} at the concentration where I_{Kur} is fully blocked [37, 38].

18.4.1.2   *Vernakalant (RSD1235).* RSD1235 is a mixed blocker of cardiac Na^+ and K^+ channels [39]. It blocks $K_v4.2$ ($IC_{50} = 38$ µM) and $K_v4.3$ ($IC_{50} = 30$ µM), whereas $K_v1.5$ is blocked with an IC_{50} value of 13 µM [39–41]. No block of cardiac inward rectifier current (I_{K1}) or L-type calcium current (I_{Ca}) was observed at concentrations blocking $K_v1.5$ channels (IC_{50} values were 1 mM and 220 µM, respectively). hERG channels exhibited an IC50 of ~21 µM. RSD1235 exhibits mild open-channel inhibition of Nav1.5 ($IC_{50} = 43$ µM at 1 Hz). Cells expressing $Na_v1.5$ and treated with RSD1235 showed a rapid recovery from current inactivation after a rate reduction (when the interpulse interval to 1 Hz from 10 Hz) [42]. In addition, the $Na_v1.5$ blocking potency of RSD1235 was use dependent, with an IC_{50} of 40 µM at 0.25 Hz and an IC_{50} of 9 µM at 20 Hz. The IC_{50} for hERG channel blockade is ~21 µM. In addition, RSD1235 also blocks late sodium current (0.5–30 µM) and has shown efficacy in the prevention of torsades de pointes [42]. These data suggest that RSD1235's efficacy results from the block of a multitude of K^+ channels, combined with the frequency- and voltage-dependent blockade of Na^+ channels.

18.4.2   Mixed Channel Blockers

18.4.2.1   *In-Vivo effects.* As noted, AVE0118 produced atrial-specific prolongation of the effective refractory period (ERP) and terminated AF (5/8 goats) in a goat model of atrial fibrillation, with no effect on ventricular repolarization as assessed by QT_c [34]. One caveat when considering the reported lack of effect on ventricular repolarization (QT_c) is that these animals had rapid ventricular response rates, which would physiologically shorten the QT interval. Notably, most I_{Kr} blockers exhibit reverse use dependence, i.e., they prolong ventricular repolarization more at slower than rapid ventricular rates [43], and rate dependence of AVE0118 block of I_{Kr} is currently unknown. Impaired atrial contractility is a significant contributor to the pathology of AF, and interestingly, AVE0118 restored atrial contractility in the goat model of AF (as might be predicted based on the increased phase 2 amplitude of the action potential) [33, 35].

Potential ventricular proarrhythmic effects of AVE0118 were investigated in a chronic canine atrioventricular (AV) block model (a model to evaluate the propensity for drug-induced torsades de pointes [TdP]) [44]. In this model, plasma concentrations of 12.7 µM AVE0118 did not significantly prolong QTc or cause TdP. Similarly, infusions of AVE1231 at 3 mg/kg intravenously (IV) had no effect on the QTc on the surface electrocardiogram. In another study in a goat model of tachypacing-induced atrial fibrillation, AVE1231 prolonged the atrial ERP at baseline, while AVE1231 showed more selective atrial ERP prolongation after 72 h of atrial tachypacing in goats with no change in ventricular ERP [37].

In a randomized, controlled trial of RSD1235 infusion in patients with recent onset AF (AF persisting for 3–72 h), infusion of 2 mg/kg followed by 3 mg/kg (if AF was observed) resulted in termination of AF in 61% of the patients compared with 5% of those treated with placebo [45]. The RSD1235 infusion group had 56% in sinus rhythm compared with 5% of the placebo group; median time to convert to sinus rhythm was significantly shorter in the RSD1235 group (14 vs 162 min in the drug and placebo groups, respectively). No serious adverse events were reported with only 2 patients of 56 who experienced ventricular premature beats.

In another multicenter randomized study [46], 356 patients were studied. Sixty-six percent (237) had AF lasting for 3 h to 7 days (short duration), whereas 119 (34%) had AF lasting for 8 to 45 days (long duration). Patients in each group were randomized to vernakalant (RSD1235—3 mg/kg for 10 min, followed by second infusion of 2 mg/kg) or placebo in a 2:1 ratio. In the short-term AF group, 51% of the patients reverted to sinus rhythm compared with 4% of the placebo group. Another interesting finding was that RSD1235 was most efficacious when infusion was given early (3–72 h) after AF onset (62% vs 4.9% in the placebo group). In the long-term AF patients, only 7% of the active treatment group converted to sinus rhythm. Changes in QRS duration and QTc were observed at end of the 10-min period only in the vernakalant group, and these were unchanged in controls ($P < 0.001$). However, within 90 min, the QTc values in the placebo and vernakalant groups was similar ($P = $ ns). These findings suggest that the interval immediately after drug infusion has an increased propensity for QTc prolongation (half life is 2–3 hrs), but so far no significant arrhythmic episodes are reported. No significant changes in hemodynamic parameters were observed after vernakalant infusion. These studies suggest that RSD1235's multiple ion channel blocking activities have promise in the treatment of AF in humans.

18.4.3 Selective Kv1.5 Blockers

Diphenyl phosphine oxide (DPO-1) is reportedly relatively selective for $hK_v1.5$ and human I_{Kur} ($IC_{50} \sim 30$ nM for both) [47, 48]. DPO-1 seems to be selective for I_{Kur} as the IC_{50}s for I_{to}, I_{K1}, I_{Kr}, and I_{Ks} are reported to be $\sim$20-fold higher in human atrial myocytes than for I_{Kur} [48]. DPO-1 also seems to be atrial selective when evaluated in human myocytes, as 1 μM blocked I_{Kur} and prolonged atrial action potentials (APD_{50} after DPO-1 was 120% longer, whereas APD90 was 25% longer after DPO-1) [49]. The authors reported a lack of ventricular action potential prolongation with DPO-1 in ventricular myocytes isolated from explanted failing hearts at the time of transplantation, although this was not quantified in the report.

In vivo electrophysiologic effects of DPO-1 were assessed in African green monkeys where atrial selective ERP prolongation was observed ($\sim$12% prolongation) [48]. In a canine atrial flutter model, DPO-1 terminated atrial flutter in 6/6 dogs with an intravenous dose of 5.5 ± 2 mg/kg, with no effect observed on ventricular effective refractory period [47]. Notably, these *in vivo* atrial flutter experiments were performed during pentobarbital anesthesia, which has been reported to prolong ventricular APD_{95}, confounding the interpretation of this result [50]. In addition, DPO-1 superfusion in canine ventricular myocytes prolonged both APD_{50} and APD_{90}, suggesting a potential I_{Kur} blockade effect in the canine ventricle [25]. In contrast to the finding in human ventricular myocytes from explanted failing hearts, DPO-1 prolonged APD_{50} and APD_{90} by ~20–25% in canine ventricular myocytes, suggesting that the selective I_{Kur} blocker also prolonged ventricular APs in the dog. This finding confirms our report [24] suggesting that an "I_{Kur}-like" current is present in the canine ventricle.

In addition to vernakalant, AVE0118, and DPO-1, multiple other investigational compounds are in development, which are described as being relatively specific for Kv1.5 [49].

At this time, the presence of human ventricular I_{Kur} in structurally normal hearts remains undefined. Notably (as above), Kv1.5 is expressed in human ventricle [21, 52]. More studies are required to assess fully the proarrhythmic potential of I_{Kur} blockade in both healthy and diseased hearts over a wide range of heart rates.

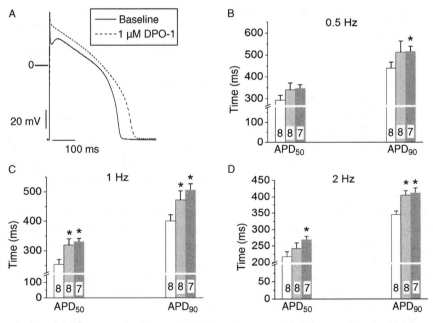

Figure 18.5. Effects of DPO-1 on canine ventricular myocyte action potential. Panel A shows canine ventricular action potentials recorded before and after DPO-1 superfusion. The average APD_{50} and APD_{90} values at 0.5, 1, and 2 Hz are shown in Panels B, C, and D, respectively. White bars represent baseline, gray and black represent data after 0.3- and 1-μM DPO-1. (*$P < 0.05$ vs. baseline). Adapted by permission from Macmillan Publishers Ltd, British Journal of Pharmacology, copyright 2007 [24].

18.5 CONCLUSIONS

I_{Kur} is an important component of repolarization in rodent, canine, and human atria, as well as in rodent, guinea pig, and canine ventricles. Multiple I_{Kur} blockers have been developed with varying degrees of selectivity for Kv1.5/I_{Kur} blockade. Interest in the development of these compounds has been driven by the potential atrial selectivity of this therapeutic approach. However, studies in patients with structurally normal hearts conducted at physiologic heart rates are needed to evaluate fully the safety of I_{Kur} blockers in humans.

REFERENCES

1. Nerbonne, J.M., Kass, R.S. (2005). Molecular physiology of cardiac repolarization. Physiological Reviews, 85, 1205–1253.

2. Sah, R., Ramirez, R.J., Oudit, G.Y., Gidrewicz, D., Trivieri, M.G., Zobel, C., Backx, P.H. (2003). Regulation of cardiac excitation-contraction coupling by action potential repolarization: Role of the transient outward potassium current (I(to)). Journal of Physiology, 546, 5–18.

3. Schotten, U., de Haan, S., Verheule, S., Harks, E.G., Frechen, D., Bodewig, E., Greiser, M., Ram, R., Maessen, J., Kelm, M., Allessie, M., Van Wagoner, D.R. (2007). Blockade of atrial-specific K + -currents increases atrial but not ventricular contractility by enhancing reverse mode Na + /Ca2 + -exchange. Cardiovascular Research, 73, 37–47.

4. Sridhar, A. (2007). Regulation of cardiac voltage gated potassium currents in health and disease, Dissertation. The Ohio State University, Columbus, OH.

5. MacKinnon, R. (1991). Determination of the subunit stoichiometry of a voltage-activated potassium channel. Nature, 350, 232–235.

6. MacKinnon, R. (2003). Potassium channels. FEBS Letters, 555, 62–65.

7. Doyle, D.A., Morais, C.J., Pfuetzner, R.A., Kuo, A., Gulbis, J.M., Cohen, S.L., Chait, B.T., MacKinnon, R. (1998). The structure of the potassium channel: molecular basis of K + conduction and selectivity. Science, 280, 69–77.

8. The Superfamily of Voltage-gated channels. (2001). Sinuaer Associates Inc, p. 61–94..

9. Apkon, M., Nerbonne, J.M. (1991). Characterization of two distinct depolarization-activated K + currents in isolated adult rat ventricular myocytes. Journal of General Physiology, 97, 973–1011.

10. Boyle, W.A., Nerbonne, J.M. (1991). A novel type of depolarization-activated K + current in isolated adult rat atrial myocytes. American Journal of Physiology Heart and Circulatory Physiology, 260, H1236–H1247.

11. Xu, H., Guo, W., Nerbonne, J.M. (1999). Four kinetically distinct depolarization-activated K + currents in adult mouse ventricular myocytes. Journal of General Physiology, 113, 661–678.

12. Nerbonne, J.M., Guo, W. (2002). Heterogeneous expression of voltage-gated potassium channels in the heart: Roles in normal excitation and arrhythmias. Journal of Cardiovascular Electrophysiology, 13, 406–409.

13. Guo, W., Li, H., Aimond, F., Johns, D.C., Rhodes, K.J., Trimmer, J.S., Nerbonne, J.M. (2002). Role of heteromultimers in the generation of myocardial transient outward K + currents. Circulation Research, 90, 586–593.

14. Nerbonne, J.M. (2003). Cardiac action potentials and ion channels. In Excitation-Contraction Coupling and Cardiac Contractile Force, Bers, D.M., ed. Kluwer Academic Publishers, New York, pp. 63–100.

15. London, B., Guo, W., Pan, X., Lee, J.S., Shusterman, V., Rocco, C.J., Logothetis, D.A., Nerbonne, J.M., Hill, J.A. (2001). Targeted replacement of KV1.5 in the mouse leads to loss of the 4-aminopyridine-sensitive component of I(K, slow) and resistance to drug-induced qt prolongation. Circulation Research, 88, 940–946.

16. Kodirov, S.A., Brunner, M., Nerbonne, J.M., Buckett, P., Mitchell, G.F., Koren, G. (2004). Attenuation of I(K, slow1) and I(K, slow2) in Kv1/Kv2DN mice prolongs APD and QT intervals but does not suppress spontaneous or inducible arrhythmias. American Journal of Physiology Heart and Circulatory Physiology, 286, H368–H374.

17. Bou-Abboud, E., Li, H., Nerbonne, J.M. (2000). Molecular diversity of the repolarizing voltage-gated K + currents in mouse atrial cells. Journal of Physiology, 529, 345–358.

18. Yue, D.T., Marban, E. (1988). A novel cardiac potassium channel that is active and conductive at depolarized potentials. European Journal of Physiology, 413, 127–133.

19. Fedida, D., Eldstrom, J., Hesketh, J.C., Lamorgese, M., Castel, L., Steele, D.F., Van Wagoner, D.R. (2003). Kv1.5 is an important component of repolarizing K + current in canine atrial myocytes. Circulation Research, 93, 744–751.

20. Brunet, S., Aimond, F., Li, H., Guo, W., Eldstrom, J., Fedida, D., Yamada, K.A., Nerbonne, J.M. (2004). Heterogeneous expression of repolarizing, voltage-gated K + currents in adult mouse ventricles. Journal of Physiology, 559, 103–120.

21. Szuts, V., Ordog, B., Acsai, K., Horvath, Z., Virag, L., Seprenyi, G., Szabad, J., Papa, J.G., Varro, A. (2004). Kv 1.5 channels in ventricular preparations (abstract). Journal of Molecular and Cellular Cardiology, 36, 762.

22. Wettwer, E., Amos, G.J., Posival, H., Ravens, U. (1994). Transient outward current in human ventricular myocytes of subepicardial and subendocardial origin. Circulation Research, 75, 473–482.

23. Christ, T., Wettwer, E., Voigt, N., Hala, O., Radicke, S., Matschke, K., Varro, A., Dobrev, D., Ravens, U. (2008). Pathology-specific effects of the IKur/Ito/IK, ACh blocker AVE0118 on ion channels in human chronic atrial fibrillation. British Journal of Pharmacology, 154, 1619–1630.

24. Sridhar, A., da Cunha, D.N., Lacombe, V.A., Zhou, Q., Fox, J.J., Hamlin, R.L., Carnes, C.A. (2007). The plateau outward current in canine ventricle, sensitive to 4-aminopyridine, is a constitutive contributor to ventricular repolarization. British Journal of Pharmacology, 152, 870–879.

25. Feng, J., Wible, B., Li, G.R., Wang, Z., Nattel, S. (1997). Antisense oligodeoxynucleotides directed against Kv1.5 mRNA specifically inhibit ultrarapid delayed rectifier K + current in cultured adult human atrial myocytes. Circulation Research, 80, 572–579.

26. Volders, P.G., Sipido, K.R., Carmeliet, E., Spatjens, R.L., Wellens, H.J., Vos, M.A. (1999). Repolarizing K + currents ITO1 and IKs are larger in right than left canine ventricular midmyocardium. Circulation, 99, 206–210.

27. Yue, L., Feng, J., Wang, Z., Nattel, S. (1999). Adrenergic control of the ultrarapid delayed rectifier current in canine atrial myocytes. Journal of Physiology, 516, 385–398.

28. Page, R.L., Roden, D.M. (2005). Drug therapy for atrial fibrillation: Where do we go from here?. Nature Reviews Drug Discovery, 4, 899–910.

29. Van Wagoner, D.R., Pond, A.L., McCarthy, P.M., Trimmer, J.S., Nerbonne, J.M. (1997). Outward K + current densities and Kv1.5 expression are reduced in chronic human atrial fibrillation. Circulation Research, 80, 772–781.

30. Li, D., Melnyk, P., Feng, J., Wang, Z., Petrecca, K., Shrier, A., Nattel, S. (2000). Effects of experimental heart failure on atrial cellular and ionic electrophysiology. Circulation, 101, 2631–2638.

31. Nattel, S. (2002). New ideas about atrial fibrillation 50 years on. Nature, 415, 219–226.

32. Sridhar, A., Nishijima, Y., Terentyev, D., Khan, M., Terentyeva, R., Hamlin, R.L., Nakayama, T., Gyorke, S., Cardounel, A.J., Carnes, C.A. (2009). Chronic heart failure and the substrate for atrial fibrillation. Cardiovascular Research, in press.

33. Wettwer, E., Hala, O., Christ, T., Heubach, J.F., Dobrev, D., Knaut, M., Varro, A., Ravens, U. (2004). Role of IKur in controlling action potential shape and contractility in the human atrium: influence of chronic atrial fibrillation. Circulation, 110, 2299–2306.

34. Blaauw, Y., Gogelein, H., Tieleman, R.G., van Hunnick, A., Schotten, U., Allessie, M.A. (2004). "Early" class III drugs for the treatment of atrial fibrillation: Efficacy and atrial selectivity of AVE0118 in remodeled atria of the goat. Circulation, 110, 1717–1724.

35. de Haan, S., Greiser, M., Harks, E., Blaauw, Y., van Hunnick, A., Verheule, S., Allessie, M., Schotten, U. (2006). AVE0118, blocker of the transient outward current (I(to)) and ultrarapid delayed rectifier current (I(Kur)), fully restores atrial contractility after cardioversion of atrial fibrillation in the goat. Circulation, 114, 1234–1242.

36. Gogelein, H., Brendel, J., Steinmeyer, K., Strubing, C., Picard, N., Rampe, D., Kopp, K., Busch, A.E., Bleich, M. (2004). Effects of the atrial antiarrhythmic drug AVE0118 on cardiac ion channels. Naunyn Schmiedebergs Archives of Pharmacology, 370, 183–192.

37. Wirth, K.J., Brendel, J., Steinmeyer, K., Linz, D.K., Rutten, H., Gogelein, H. (2007). In vitro and in vivo effects of the atrial selective antiarrhythmic compound AVE1231. Journal of Cardiovascular Pharmacology, 49, 197–206.

38. Ehrlich, J.R., Ocholla, H., Ziemek, D., Rutten, H., Hohnloser, S.H., Gogelein, H. (2008). Characterization of human cardiac Kv1.5 inhibition by the novel atrial-selective antiarrhythmic compound AVE1231. Journal of Cardiovascular Pharmacology, 51, 380–387.

39. Fedida, D. (2007). Vernakalant (RSD1235): A novel, atrial-selective antifibrillatory agent. Expert Opinions on Investigational Drugs, 16, 519–532.

40. Fedida, D., Orth, P.M., Chen, J.Y., Lin, S., Plouvier, B., Jung, G., Ezrin, A.M., Beatch, G.N. (2005). The mechanism of atrial antiarrhythmic action of RSD1235. Journal of Cardiovascular Electrophysiology, 16, 1227–1238.

41. Eldstrom, J., Wang, Z., Xu, H., Pourrier, M., Ezrin, A., Gibson, K., Fedida, D. (2007). The molecular basis of high-affinity binding of the antiarrhythmic compound vernakalant (RSD1235) to Kv1.5 channels. Molecular Pharmacology, 72, 1522–1534.

42. Orth, P.M., Hesketh, J.C., Mak, C.K., Yang, Y., Lin, S., Beatch, G.N., Ezrin, A.M., Fedida, D. (2006). RSD1235 blocks late INa and suppresses early afterdepolarizations and torsades de pointes induced by class III agents. Cardiovascular Research, 70, 486–496.

43. Jost, N., Virag, L., Bitay, M., Takacs, J., Lengyel, C., Biliczki, P., Nagy, Z., Bogats, G., Lathrop, D.A., Papp, J.G., Varro, A. (2005). Restricting excessive cardiac action potential and QT prolongation: a vital role for IKs in human ventricular muscle. Circulation, 112, 1392–1399.

44. Oros, A., Volders, P.G., Beekman, J.D., van der Nagel, T., Vos, M.A. (2006). Atrial-specific drug AVE0118 is free of torsades de pointes in anesthetized dogs with chronic complete atrioventricular block. Heart Rhythm, 3, 1339–1345.

45. Roy, D., Rowe, B.H., Stiell, I.G., Coutu, B., Ip, J.H., Phaneuf, D., Lee, J., Vidaillet, H., Dickinson, G., Grant, S., Ezrin, A.M., Beatch, G.N. (2004). A randomized, controlled trial of RSD1235, a novel anti-arrhythmic agent, in the treatment of recent onset atrial fibrillation. Journal of the American College of Cardiology, 44, 2355–2361.

46. Roy, D., Pratt, C.M., Torp-Pedersen, C., Wyse, D.G., Toft, E., Juul-Moller, S., Nielsen, T., Rasmussen, S.L., Stiell, I.G., Coutu, B., Ip, J.H., Pritchett, E.L., Camm, A.J. (2008). Vernakalant hydrochloride for rapid conversion of atrial fibrillation: a phase 3, randomized, placebo-controlled trial. Circulation, 117, 1518–1525.

47. Stump, G.L., Wallace, A.A., Regan, C.P., Lynch, J.J. Jr. (2005). In vivo antiarrhythmic and cardiac electrophysiologic effects of a novel diphenylphosphine oxide IKur blocker (2-isopropyl-5-methylcyclohexyl) diphenylphosphine oxide. Journal of Pharmacology and Experimental Therapeutics, 315, 1362–1367.

48. Regan, C.P., Wallace, A.A., Cresswell, H.K., Atkins, C.L., Lynch, J.J. Jr. (2006). In vivo cardiac electrophysiologic effects of a novel diphenylphosphine oxide IKur blocker, (2-Isopropyl-5-methylcyclohexyl) diphenylphosphine oxide, in rat and nonhuman primate. Journal of Pharmacology and Experimental Therapeutics, 316, 727–732.

49. Lagrutta, A., Wang, J., Fermini, B., Salata, J.J. (2006). Novel, potent inhibitors of human Kv1.5 K+ channels and ultrarapidly activating delayed rectifier potassium current. Journal of Pharmacology and Experimental Therapeutics. 317, 1054–1063.

50. Nattel, S., Wang, Z.G., Matthews, C. (1990). Direct electrophysiological actions of pentobarbital at concentrations achieved during general anesthesia. American Jorunal of Physiology Heart and Circulatory Physiology, 259, H1743–H1751.

51. Ford, J.W., Milnes, J.T. (2008). New drugs targeting the cardiac ultra-rapid delayed-rectifier current (I Kur): Rationale, pharmacology and evidence for potential therapeutic value. Journal of Cardiovascular Pharmacology, 52, 105–120.

52. Gaborit, N., Le, B.S., Szuts, V., Varro, A., Escande, D., Nattel, S., Demolombe, S. (2007). Regional and tissue specific transcript signatures of ion channel genes in the non-diseased human heart. Journal of Physiology, 582, 675–693.

CHAPTER 19

Non-Pharmacologic Manipulation of the Autonomic Nervous System in Humans for the Prevention of Life-Threatening Arrhythmias

PETER J. SCHWARTZ

19.1 INTRODUCTION

The evidence indicating that the autonomic nervous system plays a major and critical role in the genesis of life-threatening arrhythmias, especially—but not solely—in the setting of ischemic heart disease, is overwhelming [1–5]. It was progressively realized that whereas sympathetic activation has a profound arrhythmogenic potential, vagal activation has a powerful antifibrillatory effect. Indeed, the findings showing that cardiac electrical stability could be affected in opposite directions by changes in either of the two components of the autonomic nervous system have led to the concept of "autonomic balance." Even though the common perception is that loss of autonomic balance is a potentially dangerous and proarrhythmic condition, this author's view has always been that autonomic imbalance could either become proarrhythmic or antiarrhythmic based on which of the two components was going to prevail. As a matter of fact, this refined concept underlies the therapeutic strategy that aims at modulating the autonomic nervous system with the goal of increasing cardiac electrical stability and of thereby reducing the likelihood of life-threatening cardiac arrhythmias, which constitutes the main objective of this chapter.

Here, the background will be reviewed briefly suggesting that clinically viable approaches to the prevention of sudden cardiac death, with a reduction in overall cardiac mortality, could be derived from experimental investigations that involve manipulation of the autonomic nervous system. Then, the clinical applicability, with specific clinical indications, of these approaches will be discussed. This will be

Novel Therapeutic Targets for Antiarrhythmic Drugs, Edited by George Edward Billman
Copyright © 2010 John Wiley & Sons, Inc.

done sequentially, first for the sympathetic nervous system and then for the parasympathetic nervous system.

19.2 SYMPATHETIC NERVOUS SYSTEM

19.2.1 Experimental Background

A quantitative, but not a qualitative, difference is observed in the arrhythmogenic potential of right and left cardiac sympathetic nerves. The abundant evidence for this has been previously reviewed in detail [4–6]. The much greater likelihood of reproducibly inducing ventricular tachyarrhythmias by stimulation of the left stellate ganglion, particularly during a brief episode of acute myocardial ischemia, has led to the development of a useful animal model in which to assess the efficacy of several different drugs in preventing ventricular tachycardia and fibrillation [7]. The analysis of these responses did show that ventricular tachycardia and fibrillation are favored by the combination of two synergistic effects of sympathetic activation, namely, an increase of the ischemic area and a direct electrophysiologic effect mediated by both α- and β-adrenergic receptors.

The understanding of the neural control of coronary circulation is largely based on the pioneering work by Eric Feigl [8]. Afterward, first we provided clear evidence that, even in conscious animals not pretreated with β-adrenergic receptor blockers, left-sided cardiac sympathetic nerves exert a tonic restraint on the capability of the coronary bed to dilate [9]. Subsequently, we extended this concept by demonstrating that stimulation or ablation of left-sided cardiac sympathetic nerves increases and decreases, respectively, the extent and severity of ischemia produced by a brief coronary occlusion in the same animal, independently of heart rate and blood pressure changes [10].

The relationship between coronary artery occlusion and sympathetic activity was clarified when, 40 years ago, we demonstrated that acute myocardial ischemia elicits a powerful cardio-cardiac sympathetic reflex [11], which directly contributes to the attendant ventricular tachyarrhymias [12]. The group led by Peng Chen has recently amplified these data by showing, by whole nerve recordings in conscious dogs, that ventricular tachyarrhythmias are often preceded by increases in sympathetic activity [13].

The counterpart of the arrhythmogenic effect of left-sided sympathetic activation is represented by the multiple evidence that protective effects result from ablation of the left stellate ganglion with the first thoracic ganglia [14]. This procedure is called "left stellectomy" or "left cardiac sympathetic denervation" according to its being performed in experimental animals or in humans. The effects of left stellectomy, besides those on coronary circulation mentioned above [9, 10], can be summarized as follows: (a) it raises the threshold for ventricular fibrillation, thus making more difficult for a heart to fibrillate [15]; (b) it reduces the arrhythmias associated with acute myocardial ischemia in anesthetized [16] and in conscious animal models [17] for sudden death; (c) it does not produce postdenervation supersensitivity, because it is a preganglionic denervation [18]; and (d) it does not reduce heart rate [19] and does not impair myocardial contractility [19] because the sympathetic control of heart rate on the sinus node is exerted by the right stellate ganglion and because the right-sided sympathetic nerves provide sufficient compensation.

Recently, a series of studies has called attention to the fact that myocardial infarction can lead to nerve sprouting and compensatory reinnervation with a considerable arrhythmogenic potential [20–22]. On the one hand, these findings have raised interest for the potential role of Nerve Growth Factor (NGF) [23], and on the other hand, as the life-threatening arrhythmias were associated with left-sided sympathetic reinnervation, they have supported the concept of sympathetic imbalance [3, 24].

19.2.2   Clinical Evidence

In patients, left cardiac sympathetic denervation (LCSD) has been primarily performed in three clinical conditions: in high-risk patients with a previous myocardial infarction, in patients with the long QT syndrome, and in patients with catecholaminergic polymorphic ventricular tachycardia (CPVT) not protected by β-adrenergic receptor blocker therapy. The results in these three different groups will be summarized briefly here. For more detailed information, the readers are referred to the original publications. LCSD is traditionally performed by a retropleural approach following a small incision in the supraclavicular region. The lower part of the left stellate ganglion is ablated together with the first three to four thoracic ganglia (the fourth is usually cauterized) while leaving intact the upper part of the stellate ganglion: In this way, the Horner syndrome is almost always avoided [25]. Our group had one case only of Horner syndrome in more than 200 surgeries. The time necessary to complete the operation is 35–40 min and the patient is ambulant next day. Some groups are using an approach by video-assisted thoracoscopy [26–28].

19.2.2.1   Post-Myocardial Infarction. Having demonstrated that patients who survive an episode of ventricular fibrillation in the first 24 h after an anterior wall myocardial infarction (MI) are at high risk for sudden death [29], we proceeded with the design of a multicenter clinical trial to assess the efficacy (or lack of it) of LCSD. We enrolled 144 patients whose anterior wall MI had been complicated by ventricular tachycardia or fibrillation. These patients were randomized to either placebo (the efficacy of β-adrenergic receptor blockers had not yet been proven), the β-adrenergic receptor blocker oxprenolol (160 mg), or LCSD. During a mean follow-up of 21 months, the incidence was indeed high in the placebo group (21.3%) and was strikingly reduced by both oxprenolol (2.7%) and LCSD (3.6%), respectively ($P < 0.05$) [30] (Figure 19.1). This study demonstrated that both pharmacological and surgical antiadrenergic interventions can significantly reduce the incidence of sudden cardiac death in high-risk post-MI patients. It also represented an important evidence of the possibility of extrapolating carefully collected experimental data to the clinical setting.

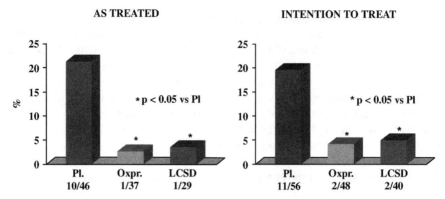

Figure 19.1. Incidence of sudden cardiac death, according to both an "as treated" and "intention to treat" analysis, in a high-risk group of 144 patients who survived a myocardial infarction complicated by either ventricular tachycardia or fibrillation. Pl. = placebo; Oxpr.= oxprenolol (from ref. 30).

19.2.2.2 Long QT Syndrome (LQTS). The definite and major role of LCSD in the management of this leading cause of juvenile sudden death of genetic origin has been widely reported and discussed [25, 28, 31]. The data available in 147 LQTS patients classified as at extremely high risk indicate a reduction in cardiac events greater than 90% [25]. Of special clinical significance is the fact that LCSD has reduced by 95% the number of shocks by the implantable cardioverter defibrillator (ICD) in patients with electrical storms, which have devastating consequences in children [32]. The safety of the procedure, the possibility to performing it in infants below one year of age [25, 28], and its clear efficacy—albeit not 100%—make difficult to justify the choice to implant an ICD in LQTS patients with syncope, but no cardiac arrest, despite β-adrenergic receptor blockers without considering first this once-for-ever simple surgery.

19.2.2.3 Catecholaminergic Polymorphic Ventricular Tachycardia. CPVT is caused by mutations on the ryanodine receptor gene (*RyR2*), which produce an excess release of intracellular calcium and clinically is characterized by life-threatening arrhythmias induced by exercise and stress [33–35]. Although β-adrenergic receptor blockers are the therapy of choice, at least 30% of patients are not protected. ICDs are recommended more and more frequently even though in these patients they often lead to multiple shocks with major psychological consequences and sometimes do not even prevent sudden death [36]. Recently, we have provided the first evidence that LCSD can provide long-term effective prevention of life-threatening arrhythmias in CPVT patients not protected by β-adrenergic receptor blockers and receiving multiple ICD shocks [37] (Figure 19.2). Two groups [27, 28] have just provided additional evidence confirming our data and supporting our concept that CPVT patients not protected by β-adrenergic receptor blockers should not be immediately implanted with an ICD [38] but should first be treated with LCSD. My very personal view is that sooner or later, we will encounter CPVT patients for

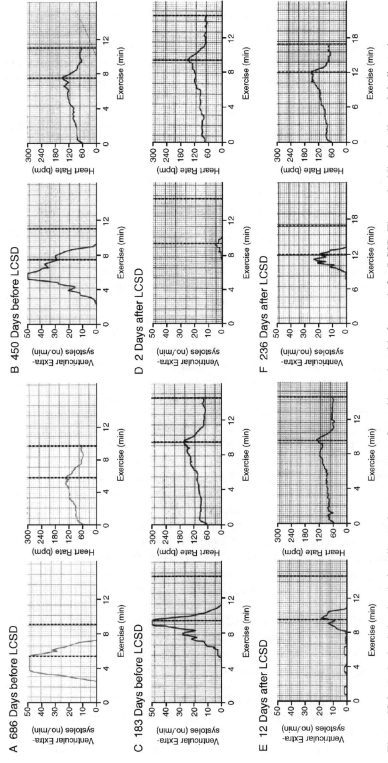

Figure 19.2. Arrhythmia burden during all exercise stress tests performed by patient 2 before and after LCSD. The vertical lines in all panels indicate the end of exercise (left-hand line) and the end of the test (right-hand line). The tests after LCSD were longer than those before LCSD (from ref. 37).

499

whom LCSD will not be sufficient and who will require bilateral cardiac sympathectomy, thus removing also the right stellate ganglion and first three to four thoracic ganglia. For these patients, this approach is likely to be preferable to implanting an ICD. The history of LCSD as clinical therapy has recently been reviewed together with my views on the current approaches and indications [39].

The conclusion of this section is that LCSD is a useful antifibrillatory intervention that prevents sudden death and improves the quality of life for different groups of patients.

19.3 PARASYMPATHETIC NERVOUS SYSTEM

19.3.1 Experimental Background

The turning point was represented by the description of a novel animal model for sudden cardiac death and by the rather amazing host of information that it did produce. This was the result of the partnership of Schwartz, Stone, and Billman [40]. In dogs with a 1-month-old anterior myocardial infarction and with a balloon occluder positioned around the circumflex coronary artery, transient ischemia is produced toward the end of an exercise stress test (exercise and ischemia test). This clinically relevant combination of transient myocardial ischemia at the time of physiologically elevated sympathetic activity results in ventricular fibrillation (VF) in 50% of the animals. Whenever VF occurs, within 10–20 s the animals are defibrillated through steel paddles ligated around the chest, and sinus rhythm is restored. A critical feature of this preparation is that the outcome of the exercise and ischemia test, which is VF or survival without defibrillation, is highly reproducible over several months. On the one hand, this has allowed the evaluation of a large number of antiarrhythmic interventions [41]. On the other hand, it has allowed the identification of markers of either high or low risk for sudden death and cardiac mortality.

In a series of studies [42, 43], we had shown that Baroreceptor Reflex Sensitivity (BRS)—largely a marker of vagal activity—is often depressed after a myocardial infarction and that depressed BRS predicts increased risk for VF during acute myocardial ischemia. We confirmed this experimental finding in a large prospective clinical study conducted in 1284 post-MI patients [44, 45]. These studies together provided the evidence that when vagal activity is reduced, the risk for life-threatening arrhythmias, sudden death, and cardiac mortality increases. They also provided the rationale for exploring the possibility that vagal stimulation might reduce the propensity for VF during acute myocardial ischemia in clinically relevant conditions. Such a possibility had already been demonstrated in anesthetized preparations [5, 46, 47]. We developed chronically implantable electrodes to stimulate the right vagus and then designed a case-control study using our sudden death animal model [48].

From a group of 161 dogs, we identified 59 that survived the exercise ischemia test after having developed VF [48]. They were randomized to repeat the test either in control condition or with vagal stimulation beginning 15 s after onset of coronary occlusion, while the dogs were running. Whereas 92% of the control animals had recurrence of VF, this happened in only 12% of the dogs with vagal stimulation ($P < 0.001$). In addition, we demonstrated that in half of the dogs studied, this antifibrillatory effect was independent of the heart rate reduction. This finding was essential for the subsequent human studies.

In two animal preparations for heart failure, one in rats [49] and one in dogs [50], it was also shown that vagal stimulation reduces mortality and improves cardiac function.

Vagal activity can increase not only with direct electrical stimulation but also in a physiological manner by exercise training. In a model for sudden death, Schwartz et al. [40] demonstrated that exercise training could increase depressed BRS and prevent recurrence of VF in high-risk dogs [51].

Several additional studies were performed in this animal model and have provided significant pathophysiological implications [52, 53]. The interested reader is referred to a comprehensive review by Billman [54].

19.3.2 Clinical Evidence

We always thought that the primary clinical benefit of vagal stimulation was going to be in the prevention of ischemia-related ventricular fibrillation. However, the first attempt to verify whether vagal stimulation could be of value in man has taken place in patients with heart failure [55]. Also among these patients, as in dogs [50], rats [49], and post-MI patients [30], clear evidence has been obtained indicating that when heart failure is accompanied by depressed BRS, there is a higher risk for cardiac mortality [56, 57]. These clinical and experimental studies, taken together, provided a strong rationale for the first study with vagal stimulation in humans [55].

We started with a single-center feasibility and safety study [55] and then moved to a pilot multicenter study [58]. The findings of the latter have been submitted for publication [59]. Vagal stimulation is performed using an implantable neurostimulator system (CardioFit 500; BioControl Medical Ltd.) capable of delivering low current electrical pulses, with adjustable parameters to stimulate the vagus nerve. The stimulator is designed to sense heart rate (via an intracardiac electrode) and deliver stimulation at a fixed delay (70 ms) from the R wave. The stimulator microprocessor responds to the sensed heart rate and can adjust stimulation accordingly (Figure 19.3). In the single-center study, performed in Pavia in 10 patients with advanced heart failure, all procedures were successful. Transient hoarseness in one patient was the sole reported side effect. There were significant improvements in NYHA class, Minnesota quality of life (from 52 ± 14 to 31 ± 18, $P < 0.001$), and left ventricular end-systolic volume (from 208 ± 71 to 190 ± 83 mL, $P = 0.03$). To some surprise, a clear heart rate reduction was observed only in some patients. A good example of the effect of vagal stimulation is shown in Figure 19.4.

We had surmised that, as diabetes often alters vagal responsiveness, the effects of vagal stimulation might have been blunted by analyzing together diabetic and nondiabetic patients. Despite the small number of patients studied so far, clear differences emerge when the data are analyzed separately for the two (small) groups, and the difference is not only quantitative, it is qualitative (Figure 19.5).

This first and limited human experience of chronic vagal stimulation in patients with severe heart failure indicates that this treatment is feasible and suggests that it is also safe, tolerable, and possibly beneficial. This novel approach that modulates the

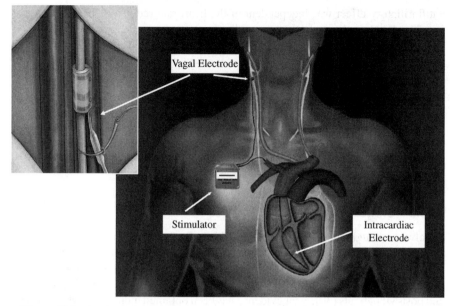

Figure 19.3. A schematic representation of the whole system implanted (from ref. 55).

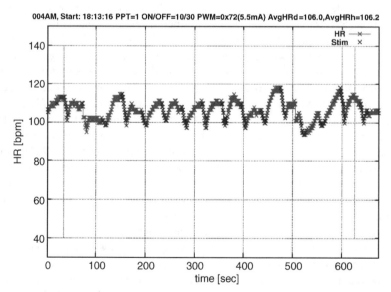

Figure 19.4. Heart rate observed during vagal stimulation (5.5 mAmp, 10 s ON time: red crosses, 30 s OFF time: blue crosses) in patient 4. A reduction of almost 10 b/min, starting from a baseline heart rate of 110 b/min occurs during the 10 s train of pulses (from ref. 55). See color insert.

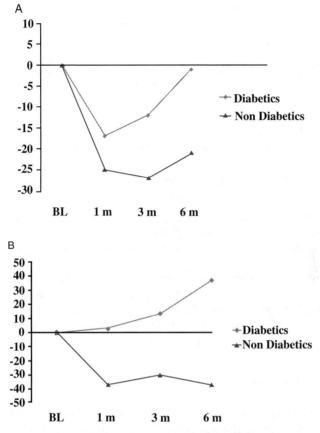

Figure 19.5. Impact of diabetes on the effect of vagal stimulation as for the Minnesota Quality of Life test (**A**) and left ventricular end diastolic volume (**B**).

neural control of the heart seems promising and warrants additional investigation. Indeed, the just completed multicenter study has importantly showed also a marked and significant improvement in left ventricular ejection fraction [59].

The experimental data on the efficacy of exercise training in increasing a depressed BRS in post-MI dogs and in reducing their risk of ventricular fibrillation during acute myocardial ischemia prompted the design and performance of a specific clinical study [60]. Ninety-five consecutive male patients who survived a first and uncomplicated myocardial infarction were randomly allocated to either a 4-week training period or to no training. They were matched for age, left ventricular ejection fraction, site of MI, and BRS. After 4 weeks, BRS improved by 26% among those who trained, whereas it did not change in the group without training. During a 10-year follow-up period, the cardiac mortality among the 16 patients who trained and who had an exercise-induced increase in BRS of at least 3 ms/mm Hg (responders) was strikingly lower compared with that of the trained patients without this increase in BRS (non responders) and of the nontrained patients (0/16 vs 18/79, 23%, $P = 0.04$) (Figure 19.6).

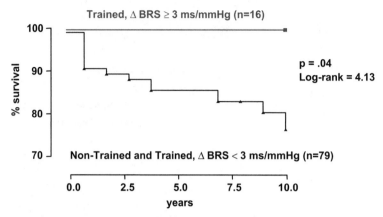

Figure 19.6. Cardiac mortality estimated by the Kaplan-Meier method among the patients with a training-induced increase in (BRS) ≥ 3 ms/mm Hg and the group including patients who trained without the same BRS increase and nontrained patients (from ref. 60).

This prospective randomized study has demonstrated that exercise training can improve long-term cardiovascular mortality in post-MI patients, provided that it shifts autonomic balance toward an increase in vagal activity in quantitatively relevant manner. It also confirms once more the clinical relevance and transferability of the data obtained in our canine model for sudden cardiac death.

19.4 CONCLUSION

These data together provide clear evidence that manipulation of the autonomic nervous system, when performed according to a good understanding of how the system works, can reduce the risk for sudden cardiac death under diverse conditions. Essentially the goals are to either increase cardiac vagal activity or to reduce cardiac sympathetic activity, especially the left-sided one. These goals can be achieved clinically by stimulating directly the right cervical vagus, by exercise training, or by left cardiac sympathetic denervation.

ACKNOWLEDGEMENT

The auther would like to thank Pinuccia De Tomasi, BS, for expert editorial support.

REFERENCES

1. Schwartz, P.J., Brown, A.M., Malliani, A., Zanchetti, A., Eds. Neural Mechanisms in Cardiac Arrhythmias. Raven Press, New York, 1978, p. 442.

2. Schwartz, P.J., Stone, H.L. The role of the autonomic nervous system in sudden coronary death. In: Greenberg, H.M., Dwyer, E.M. (1982). Sudden Coronary Death. Annals of the NY Academy of Sciences, 382, pp. 162–180.

3. Schwartz, P.J. Sympathetic imbalance and cardiac arrhythmias. In: Randall, W.C., Ed. Nervous Control of Cardiovascular Function. Oxford University Press, New York, 1984, pp. 225–251.

4. Schwartz, P.J., Priori, S.G., Sympathetic nervous system and cardiac arrhythmias. In: Zipes, D.P., Jalife, J., Eds. Cardiac Electrophysiology. From Cell to Bedside. WB Saunders Co., Philadelphia, PA, 1990, pp. 330–343.

5. Levy, M.N., Schwartz, P.J., Eds. Vagal Control of the Heart: Experimental Basis and Clinical Implications. Futura Publishing Co., Armonk, NY, 1994, 644.

6. Schwartz, P.J., The autonomic nervous system and life-threatening arrhythmias. In: Shepherd, J.T., Vatner, S.F., Eds. The Nervous Control of the Heart. Harwood Academic Publishers, Amsterdam, The Netherlands, 1996, pp. 329–355.

7. Schwartz, P.J., Vanoli, E., Zaza, A., Zuanetti, G. (1985). The effect of antiarrhythmic drugs on life-threatening arrhythmias induced by the interaction between acute myocardial ischemia and sympathetic hyperactivity. American Heart Journal, 109, 937–948.

8. Feigl, E.O. (1967). Sympathetic control of coronary circulation. Circulation Research, 20, 262–271.

9. Schwartz, P.J., Stone, H.L. (1977). Tonic influence of the sympathetic nervous system on myocardial reactive hyperemia and on coronary blood flow distribution. Circulation Research, 41, 51–58.

10. Janse, M.J., Schwartz, P.J., Wilms-Schopman, F., et al. (1985). Effects of unilateral stellate ganglion stimulation and ablation on electrophysiologic changes induced by acute myocardial ischemia in dogs. Circulation, 72, 585–595.

11. Malliani, A., Schwartz, P.J., Zanchetti, A. (1969). A sympathetic reflex elicited by experimental coronary occlusion. American Journal of Physiology, 217, 703–709.

12. Schwartz, P.J., Foreman, R.D., Stone, H.L., Brown, A.M. (1976). Effect of dorsal root section on the arrhythmias associated with coronary occlusion. American Journal of Physiology, 231, 923–928.

13. Zhou, S., Jung, B.C., Tan, A.Y., et al. (2008). Spontaneous stellate ganglion nerve activity and ventricular arrhythmia in a canine model of sudden death. Heart Rhythm, 5, 131–139.

14. Schwartz, P.J. (1984). The rationale and the role of left stellectomy for the prevention of malignant arrhythmias. Annals of NY Academy of Sciences, 427, 199–221.

15. Schwartz, P.J., Snebold, N.G., Brown, A.M. (1976). Effects of unilateral cardiac sympathetic denervation on the ventricular fibrillation threshold. American Journal of Cardiology, 37, 1034–1040.

16. Schwartz, P.J., Stone, H.L., Brown, A.M. (1976). Effects of unilateral stellate ganglion blockade on the arrhythmias associated with coronary occlusion. American Heart Journal, 92, 589–599.

17. Schwartz, P.J., Stone, H.L. (1980). Left stellectomy in the prevention of ventricular fibrillation due to acute myocardial ischemia in conscious dogs with an anterior myocardial infarction. Circulation, 62, 1256–1265.

18. Schwartz, P.J., Stone, H.L. (1982). Left stellectomy and denervation supersensitivity in conscious dogs. American Journal of Cardiology, 49, 1185–1190.

19. Schwartz, P.J., Stone, H.L. (1979). Effects of unilateral stellectomy upon cardiac performance during exercise in dogs. Circulation Research, 44, 637–645.

20. Zhou, S., Cao, J.-M., Tebb, Z.D., et al. (2001). Modulation of QT interval by cardiac sympathetic nerve sprouting and the mechanisms of ventricular arrhythmia in a canine

model of sudden cardiac death. Journal of Cardiovascular Electrophysiology, 12, 1068–1073.

21. Cao, J.M., Fishbein, M.C., Han, J.B., et al. (2000). Relationship between regional cardiac hyperinnervation and ventricular arrhythmia. Circulation, 101, 1960–1969.

22. Cao, J.M., Chen, L.S., KenKnight, B.H., et al. (2000). Nerve sprouting and sudden cardiac death. Circulation Research, 86, 816–821.

23. Levi Montalcini, R., Booker, B. (1960). Excessive growth of the sympatheticganglia evoked by a protein isolated from mouse salivary glands. Proceedings of the National academy of Sciences USA, 46, 373–384.

24. Schwartz, P.J. (2001). QT prolongation, sudden death, and sympathetic imbalance: The pendulum swings. Journal of Cardiovascular and Electrophysiology, 12, 1074–1077.

25. Schwartz, P.J., Priori, S.G., Cerrone, M., et al. (2004). Left cardiac sympathetic denervation in the management of high-risk patients affected by the long QT syndrome. Circulation, 109, 1826–1833.

26. Li, J., Wang, L., Wang, J. (2003). Video-assisted thoracoscopic sympathectomy for congenital long QT sindrome. Pacing and Clinical Electrophysiology, 26, 870–873.

27. Atallah, J., Fynn-Thompson, F., Cecchin, F., et al. (2008). Video-assisted thoracoscopic cardiac denervation: A potential novel therapeutic option for children with intractable ventricular arrhythmias. Annals of Thoracic Surgery, 86, 1620–1625.

28. Collura, C.A., Johnson, J.N., Moir, C., Ackerman, M.J. (2009). Left Cardiac Sympathetic Denervation for the treatment of long QT syndrome and Catecholaminergic Polymorphic Ventricular Tachycardia using video-assisted thoracic surgery. Heart Rhythm, 6, 752–759.

29. Schwartz, P.J., Zaza, A., Grazi, S., et al. (1985). Effect of ventricular fibrillation complicating acute myocardial infarction on long term prognosis: Importance of the site of infarction. American Journal of Cardiology, 56, 384–389.

30. Schwartz, P.J., Motolese, M., Pollavini, G., et al. (1992). Prevention of sudden cardiac death after a first myocardial infarction by pharmacologic or surgical antiadrenergic interventions. Journal of Cardiovascular Electrophysiology, 3, 2–16.

31. Schwartz, P.J., Crotti, L., Long, Q.T. and short QT syndromes. In: Zipes, D.P., Jalife, J., Eds. Cardiac Electrophysiology. From Cell to Bedside,(5TH Edition.) Elsevier, Philadelphia, PA, 2009.

32. Wolf, M.J., Zeltser, I.J., Salerno, J., et al. (2007). Electrical storm in children with an implantable cardioverter defibrillator: clinical features and outcome. Heart Rhythm, 4, S43.

33. Leenhardt, A., Lucet, V., Denjoy, I., et al. (1995). Catecholaminergic polymorphic ventricular tachycardia in children: a 7-year follow-up of 21 patients. Circulation, 91, 1512–1519.

34. Priori, S.G., Napolitano, C., Memmi, M., et al. (2002). Clinical and molecular characterization of patients with catecholaminergic polymorphic ventricular tachycardia. Circulation, 106, 69–74.

35. Hayashi, M., Denjoy, I., Extramiana, F., et al. (2009). Incidence and risk factors of arrhythmic events in catecholaminergic polymorphic ventricular tachycardia. Circulation, 119, 2426–2434.

36. Mohamed, U., Gollob, M.H., Gow, R.M., Krahn, A.D. (2006). Sudden cardiac death despite an implantable cardioverter-defibrillator in a young female with catecholaminergic ventricular tachycardia. Heart Rhythm, 3, 1486–1489.

37. Wilde, A.A.M., Bhuiyan, Z.A., Crotti, L., et al. (2008). Left cardiac sympathetic denervation for catecholaminergic polymorphic ventricular tachycardia. New England Journal of Medicine, 358, 2024–2029.

38. Napolitano, C., Priori, S.G. (2007). Diagnosis and treatment of catecholaminergic polymorphic ventricular tachycardia. Heart Rhythm, 4, 675–678.

39. Schwartz, P.J., (2009). Cutting nerves and saving lives. Heart Rhythm, 6, 760–763.

40. Schwartz, P.J., Billman, G.E., Stone, H.L. (1984). Autonomic mechanisms in ventricular fibrillation induced by myocardial ischemia during exercise in dogs with healed myocardial infarction. An experimental preparation for sudden cardiac death. Circulation, 69, 790–800.

41. Schwartz, P.J. (1998). Do animal models have clinical value? American Journal of Cardiology, 81, 14D–20D.

42. Billman, G.E., Schwartz, P.J., Stone, H.L. (1982). Baroreceptor reflex control of heart rate: A predictor of sudden cardiac death. Circulation, 66, 874–880.

43. Schwartz, P.J., Vanoli, E., Stramba-Badiale, M., et al. (1988). Autonomic mechanisms and sudden death. New insights from analysis of baroreceptor reflexes in conscious dogs with and without a myocardial infarction. Circulation, 78, 969–979.

44. La Rovere, M.T., Bigger, J.T., Marcus, F., et al. (1998). ATRAMI (Autonomic Tone and Reflexes After Myocardial Infarction). Baroreflex sensitivity and heart-rate variability in prediction of total cardiac mortality after myocardial infarction. Lancet, 351, 478–484.

45. La Rovere, M.T., Pinna, G.D., Hohnloser, S.H., et al. (2001). Baroreflex sensitivity and heart rate variability in the identification of patients at risk for life-threatening arrhythmias. Implications for clinical trials. Circulation, 103, 2072–2077.

46. Myers, R.W., Pearlman, A.S., Hyman, R.M., et al. (1974). Beneficial effect of vagal stimulation and bradycardia during experimental acute myocardial ischemia. Circulation, 49, 943–947.

47. Kolman, B.S., Verrier, R.L., Lown, B. (1975). The effect of vagus nerve stimulation upon vulnerability of the canine ventricle: role of sympathetic-parasympathetic interactions. Circulation, 52, 578–585.

48. Vanoli, E., De Ferrari, G.M., Stramba-Badiale, M. (1991). Vagal stimulation and prevention of sudden death in conscious dogs with a healed myocardial infarction. Circulation Research, 68, 1471–1481.

49. Li, M., Zheng, C., Sato, T., et al. (2004). Vagal nerve stimulation markedly improves long-term survival after chronic heart failure in rats. Circulation, 109, 120–124.

50. Sabbah, H.N., Imai, M., Zaretsky, A., et al. (2007). Therapy with vagus nerve electrical stimulation combined with beta-blockade improves left ventricular systolic function in dogs with heart failure beyond that seen with beta-blockade alone. European Journal of Heart Failure, 6, 114.

51. Billman, G.E., Schwartz, P.J., Stone, H.L. (1984). The effects of daily exercise on susceptibility to sudden cardiac death. Circulation, 69, 1182–1189.

52. Holycross, B.J., Kukielka, M., Nishijima, Y., et al. (2007). Exercise training normalizes beta-adrenoceptor expression in dogs susceptible to ventricular fibrillation. American Journal of Physiology Heart Circulation Physiology, 293, H2702–H2709.

53. Schwartz, P.J., Vanoli, E. (2007). From exercise training to sudden death prevention via adrenergic receptors. American Journal of Physiology Heart Circulation Physiology, 293, H2631–H2633.

54. Billman, G.E. (2006). A comprehensive review and analysis of 25 years of data from an in vivo canine model of sudden cardiac death: Implications for future anti-arrhythmic drug development. Pharmacology and Therapeutics, 111, 808–835.

55. Schwartz, P.J., De Ferrari, G.M., Sanzo, A., et al. (2008). Long term vagal stimulation in patients with advanced heart failure. First experience in man. European Journal of Heart Failure, 10, 884–891.

56. Mortara, A., La Rovere, M.T., Pinna, G.D., et al. (1997). Arterial baroreflex modulation of heart rate in chronic heart failure: clinical and hemodynamic correlates and prognostic implications. Circulation, 96, 3450–3458.

57. La Rovere, M.T., Pinna, G.D., Maestri, R., et al. (2009). Prognostic implications of baroreflex sensitivity in heart failure patients in the beta-blocking era. Journal of the American College of Cardiology, 53, 193–199.

58. De Ferrari, G.M., Sanzo, A., Borggrefe, M., et al. (2008). Chronic vagus nerve stimulation in patients with chronic heart failure is Feasible and appears beneficial. Circulation, 118, S721.

59. De Ferrari, G.M., Crijns, H.J.G.M., Borggrefe, M., et al., for the CardioFit Multicenter Trial Investigators. (2009). Chronic vagus nerve stimulation: a new and promising therapeutic approach for chronic heart failure. Submitted for publication.

60. La Rovere, M.T., Bersano, C., Gnemmi, M., et al. (2002). Exercise-induced increase in baroreflex sensitivity predicts improved prognosis after myocardial infarction. Circulation, 106, 945–949.

CHAPTER 20

Effects of Endurance Exercise Training on Cardiac Autonomic Regulation and Susceptibility to Sudden Cardiac Death: A Nonpharmacological Approach for the Prevention of Ventricular Fibrillation

GEORGE E. BILLMAN

20.1 INTRODUCTION

Given the adverse actions of many antiarrhythmic medications [1–3], as well as the partial protection afforded by even the best agents (e.g., β-adrenergic receptor antagonists [4]) noted in previous chapters, nonpharmacological interventions that could provide a more complete protection from arrhythmias merit consideration. Alterations in cardiac autonomic regulation, particularly during myocardial ischemia, have been shown to play a crucial role in the induction of ventricular fibrillation [5–8]. It is well established that aerobic exercise conditioning can favorably alter cardiac autonomic balance (increase parasympathetic and decrease sympathetic activity) [9–12]. As such, exercise training could thereby provide a safe and effective nonpharmacological therapy for the prevention of lethal ventricular arrhythmias. Therefore, this chapter will evaluate the antiarrhythmic potential of aerobic (endurance) exercise conditioning. First, clinical and experimental evidence that exercise conditioning can reduce the risk for ventricular arrhythmias will be analyzed. Then, the mechanisms that might mediate this with protection will be discussed, with

Novel Therapeutic Targets for Antiarrhythmic Drugs, Edited by George Edward Billman
Copyright © 2010 John Wiley & Sons, Inc.

509

particular emphasis placed on the role of exercise training-induced changes in cardiac autonomic regulation in the prevention of malignant ventricular arrhythmias.

20.2   EXERCISE AND SUSCEPTIBILITY TO SUDDEN DEATH

20.2.1   Clinical Studies

The effects of daily exercise on the incidence of cardiac arrhythmias and sudden death have not been extensively investigated. However, many epidemiological studies indicate that high levels of physical activity may protect against coronary artery disease and reduce cardiac mortality [13–22]. Paffenbarger and Hall [13] found that longshoreman with the highest energy output at work had the lowest incidence of myocardial infarction and other manifestations of ischemic heart disease, including sudden death (Figure 20.1). A meta-analysis of 32 studies confirmed this initial finding, demonstrating that the risk of death from coronary disease was significantly lower in individuals with active compared with sedentary occupations [18]. In a similar manner, both the Harvard Alumni Health Study [20, 21] and the Nurse Health Study [22] found that physical activity was associated with a decreased risk (more than 30% reduction) for coronary heart disease and death [20–22]. Fitness, as measured by the heart rate response at a given level of exercise, has also been linked to cardiac mortality [16]. Ekelund et al. [16], for example, found that individuals with

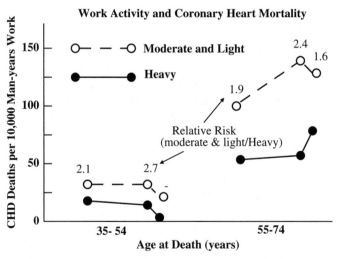

Figure 20.1. The mortality rate from coronary heart disease (CHD) recorded between 1951 and 1972 classified according to physical activity during work and age at death. Note lower the mortality for the men with the higher levels of physical activity in age group. (Reprinted with permission from Paffenbarger and Hall [13], copyright 1975, Massachusetts Medical Society.) A meta-analysis of 32 studies found that the relative risk of death from CHD was significantly lower in individuals with active compared with sedentary occupations [18].

the lowest levels of fitness had a 6.4 to 8.5 greater risk of cardiac disease and death when compared with individuals with the highest levels of fitness. Meyers et al. [23] reported that subjects with cardiovascular disease who had the highest exercise capacity also exhibited the lowest mortality rate during the 14-year follow-up period. Furthermore, Bartels et al. [24] found that the incidence of sudden cardiac death was inversely related to the level of regular physical activity; that is, sedentary individuals had the highest rate of sudden death (4.7 deaths per 10^5 person-years), whereas those in the most active group had the lowest rate (0.9 deaths per 10^5 person-years). It should be emphasized that even modest levels of exercise were associated with significant reductions in mortality. Hakim et al. [25, 26] found that, in elderly men, low-intensity exercise (walking 2 miles or more per day) was associated with a much lower mortality rate (23.8%) during the 12-year follow-up period than was noted in those men that walked less than a mile per day (40.5%) (Figure 20.2). It is interesting to note that walking has also been shown to reduce the incidence of atrial fibrillation in older adults (>65 years old) [27].

The effects of exercise in patients recovering from myocardial infarction strongly suggest that this treatment may reduce mortality in this high-risk group [15, 17, 28–33]. A significant reduction in cardiac death has been reported for patients in multifactorial intervention programs that included daily physical exercise [15]. The decreased cardiovascular mortality resulted primarily from a reduction in the

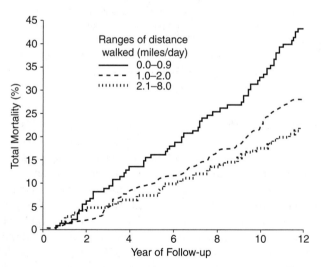

Figure 20.2. Effect of walking on the cumulative mortality reported according to the year of the follow-up in 707 nonsmoking retired men aged 61–81 years enrolled in the Honolulu Heart Program. The distance walked (miles per day) was recorded at the start of the 12-year study. To convert distances walked to kilometers, multiply by 1.609. (Reprinted with permission from Hakim et al. [26], copyright 1998, Massachusetts Medical Society.)

Exercise Training and Mortality Post-Myocardial Infarction

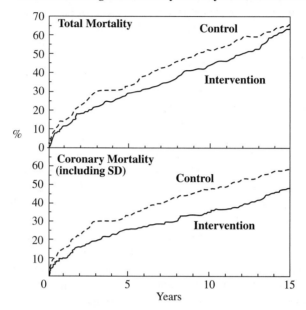

Figure 20.3. The long-term effects of a comprehensive cardiac rehabilitation program on total mortality and death resulting from coronary artery disease. The program consisted of 375 consecutive, nonselected patients under 65 years of age randomly assigned to either the intervention ($n = 188$) or the control group ($n = 187$). After a 15-year follow-up period, the intervention group exhibited a lower incidence of sudden death (16.5% vs. 28.9%, $P = 0.006$) and coronary mortality (47.9 % vs. 58.5 %, $P = 0.04$). (Reprinted with permission from European Society of Cardiology and Oxford University Press, Hamalainen et al. [34]). A meta-analysis of 22 interventional studies found that exercise training produced a 20% reduction in overall mortality. This decrease was from reduced cardiovascular mortality, fatal reinfarction, and sudden death during at least the first 3 years after infarction [17].

incidence of sudden death (5.8% vs 14.4% in the control group); this trend has been maintained for 15 years after the initial study [34] (Figure 20.3). Because exercise was but one factor among many, the effects of the daily exercise program *per se* on sudden death cannot be addressed. A meta-analysis of 22 randomized trials of rehabilitation with exercise after myocardial infarction found that exercise training elicited both significant reductions in the reinfarction rate and in the incidence of sudden death [17]. A 20% overall reduction in cardiac mortality was found (largely based on the reduction in sudden death); this reduction is comparable with the mortality reductions noted for β-adrenergic receptor antagonists [35–37].

Exercise programs have also been shown to improve cardiac autonomic regulation and ventricular function in patients with cardiovascular disease [38–42]. Exercise training improved baroreceptor sensitivity (BRS; the heart rate response to changes in arterial blood pressure that largely reflect cardiac parasympathetic function) in patients recovering from myocardial infarction [32, 38]. Furthermore, the group of

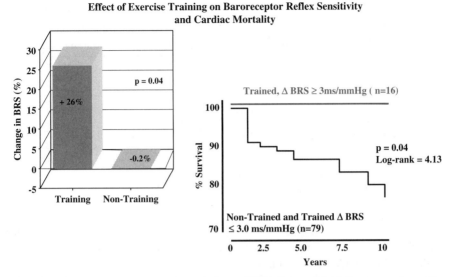

Figure 20.4. A, The effect of exercise training on BRS in myocardial infarction patients. The data are plotted as percent change from pretraining (baseline) after either a 4-week exercise training or equivalent control (nontraining) period. **B**, Cardiac mortality among patients with training-induced increases in BRS ≥ 3 ms/mm Hg compared with nontrained patients and exercise trained individuals with a change in BRS ≤ 3 ms/mm Hg. (Figure made using data reported by La Rovere et al., [32], reprinted with the permission of the American Heart Association).

patients that exhibited the greatest change in BRS (increase ≥ 3.0 ms/mm Hg) exhibited the lowest mortality during a 10-year follow-up period (Figure 20.4). Indeed, no deaths were reported among the patients with a BRS with a change greater than 3.0 ms/mm Hg, whereas more than 20% of the patients with smaller changes in BRS died during the follow-up period [32]. In a similar manner, exercise training improved autonomic balance (i.e., increased heart rate variability) in heart failure patients [43] and may thereby reduce the risk for sudden death. Furthermore, exercise training improved cardiac function and reduced arrhythmia frequency in congestive heart failure patients [43–48]; this patient population has a high risk for sudden death [49, 50]. For example, Hertzeanu et al. [51] found that both the frequency and severity of the arrhythmias were reduced after a 6-month exercise program in post-myocardial infarction patients with ejection fractions less than 30%. Finally, aerobic exercise training reduced the regional difference in ventricular repolarization in patients with heart failure [52], thereby removing the substrate for the formation of reentrant arrhythmias. Thus, the limited clinical data suggest that regular physical exercise may protect against sudden death, as well as improve autonomic balance, in patients with cardiac disease.

It should be noted that strenuous exercise might itself pose a risk for sudden death in high-risk populations, for example, patients recovering from myocardial infarction [24, 53–57]. Numerous anecdotal accounts are available of individuals

Table 20.1. Risk of Sudden Death during Exercise: Effect of Regular Physical Activity

Activity Level	VF death/10^5 person years	Relative Risk fro VF (during exercise)
1 (sedentary)	4.69	389.5
2	4.25	150
3	2.63	-
4 (highest)	0.92	4.0

Data were collected from two districts in Berlin (population = 219,251). During an 18-month period, there were 77 confirmed deaths from ventricular fibrillation. The activity level was determined. The authors concluded that "the protective effects of regular physical exercise for scd" [sudden cardiac death] "by far exceeds the risk increase of the actual strenuous situation" [24].
VF = ventricular fibrillation.

(including trained athletes) who died suddenly during a bout of exercise [58]. Therefore, exercise training may not be completely risk free. However, systematic studies of this paradox have been limited. Bartels et al. [24] demonstrated that the incidence of sudden death increased during a bout of exercise for both sedentary and regular exercisers with the greatest incidence in the sedentary group (Table 20.1). As noted above, the overall incidence of sudden death was much lower in the fit group. Thus, the authors concluded that the protective effect of regular physical activity far exceeded the modestly increased risk for sudden death during exercise. In a similar manner, a large prospective study of male physicians [59] found that, although the incidence of sudden death increased during and shortly after exercise (Table 20.2), the "absolute risk for sudden death during any particular episode of rigorous exertion was extremely low (1 sudden death per 1.51 million episodes of exertion)." These investigators also reported that a history of regular exercise reduced the relative risk for sudden death. In other words, the probability for sudden death, even during exercise, was significantly reduced in those physicians who exercised regularly as compared with their more sedentary colleagues. Corrado et al. [60] found that young athletes had a greater relative risk for death from cardiovascular causes than

Table 20.2. Risk of Sudden Death during Exercise: Effect of Regular Physical Activity (Harvard Physician Study)

Frequency of Habitual Vigorous Exercise	Sudden Deaths (n = 122)	Sudden Deaths Related to Vigorous Exercise (n = 23)	Relative Risk (95% CI)
<1 time/week	32	3	74.1 (22.0–249)
1–4 times/week	67	13	18.9 (10.2–35.1)
≥ 5 times/week	23	7	10.9 (4.5–26.2)

The authors found that the relative risk for sudden death increased during or following vigorous exercise. "However, the absolute risk for sudden death during a particular episode of vigorous exertion was extremely low (1 sudden death per 1.51 million episodes)." They also reported that habitual exercise significantly decreased even this small risk for sudden death [59].
CI = confidence interval.

nonathletes. However, Viskin [61] examined these reports together with others and concluded that arrhythmic death among athletes was rare, with an estimated range from 0.4 to 2.3 per 100,000 person-years. Furthermore, the deaths for truly asymptomatic athletes were even lower, as half of the athletes who died suddenly were found to have a history of syncope. Several authors [24, 54–57, 59], after reviewing the existing literature, concluded that the potential benefits of regular exercise, even in high-risk populations of patients, far exceeded the small risk associated with exercise. Thus, with appropriate monitoring and prudently designed exercise programs, even high-risk patients can benefit from regular physical exercise.

20.2.2 Experimental Studies

Limited experimental evidence indicates that aerobic exercise conditioning may reduce the susceptibility to ventricular fibrillation. A summary of the results of these studies may be found in Tables 20.3 and 20.4. Billman et al. [70] were the first to demonstrate that daily exercise could prevent ventricular fibrillation (VF) induced by acute ischemia in dogs with healed anterior wall myocardial infarctions. A 6-week daily exercise program (treadmill running) prevented ventricular fibrillation in all eight animals previously shown to be susceptible to sudden death. In contrast, sedentary animals (6-week cage rest period) were not protected. If the animals were placed on a cage rest program (n = 2) after the training (i.e., deconditioning), the susceptibility to arrhythmias returned. The heart rate response to an increase in arterial pressure (i.e., BRS) improved in these animals after daily exercise (Figure 20.5), suggesting that the protection may result, in part, from improved cardiac autonomic regulation

Table 20.3. Effect of Exercise Training on Ventricular Arrhythmias: Animal Studies

Study	Model	Results
Noakes et al. [62]	Rat—isolated heart, ischemia	↑ VF threshold
Bakth et al. [63]	Dog—diabetic and normal, without and without epinephrine	↑ VF threshold
Posel et al. [64]	Rat—isolated heart post MI, ischemia	↑ VF threshold
Arad et al. [65]	Rat—isolated heart (swim training)	No Δ VF threshold
Belichard et al. [66]	Rat—ischemia (swim training)	↓ arrhythmias
Hamra and McNeil [67]	Dog—purkinje fibers Ischemia or catechomalines	↓ arrhythmias -ischemia ↑ arrhythmias - catecholamines
Collins et al. [68]	Rat—hypertensive, ischemia	↑ time to arrhythmias
Lujan et al. [69]	Rat—bred for high aerobic capacity, ischemia	↓ arrhythmias

MI = myocardial infarction; VF = ventricular fibrillation.

Table 20.4. Exercise Training and Ventricular Arrhythmias: Canine Model of Sudden Cardiac Death

Study	Results
Billman et al. [70]	↑ baroreflex sensitivity prevented VF
Hull et al. [71]	↑ baroreflex sensitivity ↑ heart rate variability (at rest) ↑ VF threshold prevented VF
Billman and Kukielka [72]	↑ heart rate variability (during exercise or ischemia) prevented VF
Billman et al. [73]	↑ β_2-adrenergic receptor responsiveness prevented VF
Billman and Kukielka [74]	↑ heart rate variability (during recovery from exercise) ↓ heart rate response to exercise onset prevented VF

VF = ventricular fibrillation.

(see below). This initial observation was subsequently confirmed [71–73, 75, 76]. Hull et al. [71] found that a similar 6-week exercise program protected all seven dogs susceptible to ventricular fibrillation that completed the training program, whereas Billman and coworkers found that a 10-week exercise-training program protected eight dogs from tachyarrhythmias induced by ischemia [72, 73, 76]. In contrast, 4 of 11 sedentary susceptible dogs died during the 10-week control period, and the remaining 7 animals still had malignant arrhythmia when tested at the end of this 10-week sedentary period [72, 73, 76]. Representative electrocardiogram (ECG) recordings from the same dog before and at the end of the 10-week exercise training period and from a second animal before and at the end of the 10-week sedentary period are displayed in Figure 20.6, and the composite data from all three canine studies are shown in Figure 20.7. In these studies, heart rate variability (a marker of cardiac parasympathetic regulation) [71, 72, 75] and the electrical current necessary to induce a repetitive ventricular response [71] (i.e., the ventricular fibrillation threshold) also increased after training.

In a similar manner, Opie and co-workers [62, 64] found that exercise training increased the ventricular fibrillation threshold during a coronary occlusion in isolated rat hearts with and without previous myocardial infarction. The amount of electrical current necessary to induce ventricular fibrillation was much greater in hearts obtained from exercise-trained rats as opposed to those obtained from untrained animals. They attributed these differences to reductions in myocardial cyclic adenosine 3′, 5′-monophosphate (cAMP) levels that may reflect a reduction in β-adrenergic receptor activity [62, 64]. Swim training of rats either reduced [66] or did not affect [65] the susceptibility to ventricular fibrillation induced by coronary artery occlusion. More recently, Collins et al. [68] demonstrated that the time to arrhythmia onset induced by myocardial ischemia was significantly increased in exercised (voluntary wheel running) spontaneously hypertensive rats compared with

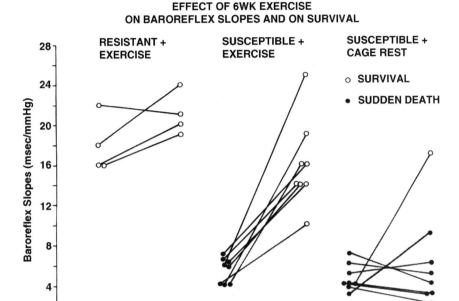

Figure 20.5. Effects of exercise training on BRS and susceptibility to ventricular fibrillation. Baroreceptor slopes (heart rate changes plotted against changes in arterial blood pressure) are shown before and after either a 6-week daily endurance exercise program or an equivalent sedentary (cage rest) period. Ventricular fibrillation is indicated by the closed circles, whereas an incidence of no arrhythmias is indicated by the open circle. Note that exercise training improved BRS (to levels similar to those noted for resistant dogs) and prevented ventricular fibrillation in the eight of eight exercise trained susceptible dogs. In contrast, only one of eight sedentary dogs was protected from sudden death. Interestingly, the sedentary dog that was protected from ventricular fibrillation also exhibited an increase in BRS. (Reprinted with permission from Billman et al. [70]).

sedentary rats. Lujan et al. [69] reported that rats bred for a high aerobic capacity exhibited a lower incidence (3 of 11 rats) of ventricular tachyarrhythmias during myocardial ischemia as compared with low aerobic capacity rats (6 of 7 rats). In the dog, Hamra and McNeil [67] reported that although exercise training reduced the arrhythmias induced by ischemia in isolated purkinje fibers, it enhanced the arrhythmia response to isoproterenol or phenylephrine. In contrast, Bakth et al. [63] demonstrated that exercise conditioning increased ventricular fibrillation threshold in both diabetic and normal dogs. The reduction in ventricular fibrillation threshold induced by epinephrine was attenuated after exercise training; these data once again suggest that exercise alters the autonomic control of the heart [63]. The role that these apparent changes in the autonomic control of the heart play in the exercise conditioning-induced prevention of ventricular fibrillation remains to be determined.

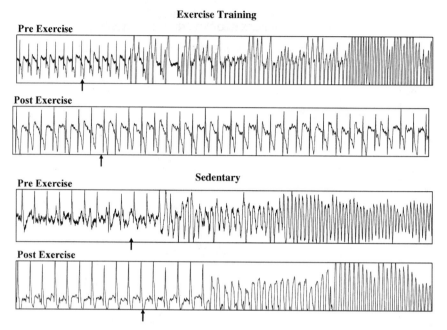

Figure 20.6. Representative ECG recordings from two different susceptible dogs, one dog before and at the end of a 10-week endurance exercise program and one dog before and at the end of a 10-week sedentary period. Note arrhythmias were no longer induced by the exercise plus ischemia test in the exercise-trained animal. The arrow indicates the time at which the treadmill was stopped. (Reprinted with permission from Billman et al. [73]).

20.3 CARDIAC AUTONOMIC NEURAL ACTIVITY AND SUDDEN CARDIAC DEATH

Alterations in cardiac autonomic balance (particularly during myocardial ischemia) contribute significantly to the induction of ventricular fibrillation [5–8]. Several lines of evidence demonstrate that any intervention that elicits an increase in cardiac sympathetic activity also enhances the development of lethal cardiac arrhythmias [6–8]. The direct electrical stimulation of cardiac sympathetic nerves, particularly those originating from the left stellate ganglion, decrease ventricular fibrillation threshold, produce heterogeneities in ventricular refractory period, and induce ventricular arrhythmias [6–8]. Psychological stress or acute bouts of exercise, which are interventions known to increase sympathetic activity, also increase arrhythmia formation during ischemia [18, 54, 59, 60, 77]. Indeed, an excessively large heart rate increase at the onset of exercise (a marker of cardiac sympathetic activation) has been linked to an increased susceptibility to ventricular fibrillation in patients with ischemic heart disease [78]. For example, patients with documented coronary artery disease that exhibited the largest increase in heart rate at exercise onset also had a greater risk for cardiac events (cardiac deaths and nonfatal myocardial infarctions)

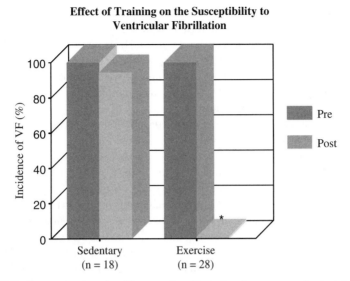

Figure 20.7. Composite data that illustrate the effect of endurance exercise training on the incidence of VF. Exercise training (6 or 10 weeks) prevented VF in 28 of 28 animals susceptible to this malignant arrhythmia. In contrast, the exercise plus ischemia test still induced ventricular fibrillation in all 17 of 18 susceptible animals that completed an equivalent sedentary period. In addition, 4 animals died spontaneously during this sedentary period. *$P < 0.01$ pre vs. post (after 10 weeks). Data used for this figure came from refs 70–73.

than did those subjects with a more modest heart rate increase [78]. Similar results have been obtained in animal studies. Billman [79] found that dogs with healed myocardial infarctions that exhibited the greatest heart rate increases during exercise onset developed ventricular fibrillation during myocardial ischemia more frequently than those animals that proved to be resistant to malignant arrhythmias. The elevated heart rate response to exercise onset was abolished by prior treatment with the β-adrenergic receptor antagonist propranolol. β_2-adrenergic receptor activation may be particularly arrrhythmogenic in these animals (see below). Conversely, interventions that reduce cardiac sympathetic activity have been shown to protect against arrhythmias [6–8, 35–37]. As previously noted, β-adrenergic receptor blockade has been shown to reduce cardiac mortality in patients recovering from myocardial infarction [35–37]. Pooled data from more than 29,000 myocardial infarction patients treated with β-adrenergic receptor antagonists demonstrated that these agents reduced overall mortality by 20% and mortality from sudden death by 30–50% [80–89]. β-adrenergic receptor blockers were most effective in reducing early (1-h to 7-day) cardiac mortality during myocardial infarction [80–83]. Similar results have been reported in animal studies [5, 85].

Alterations in cardiac parasympathetic control also contribute significantly to the risk for sudden death [5–8]. Eckberg et al. [86] were among the first to demonstrate that the patients with the most advanced disease states also exhibited the greatest impairment in parasympathetic activity. Billman and co-workers [87, 88] reported that baroreceptor-mediated reductions in heart rate (baroreceptor reflex sensitivity) were impaired by myocardial infarction, with the greatest impairment noted in animals particularly susceptible to sudden death. Heart rate variability, which is an index of cardiac vagal activity [89–94], was also reduced to a greater extent in animals susceptible to ventricular fibrillation as compared with animals resistant to these malignant arrhythmias [5, 87, 88, 95, 96]. In particular, the susceptible animals exhibited a much greater reduction (withdrawal) of cardiac vagal regulation in response to either submaximal exercise [5, 95, 97, 98] or acute myocardial ischemia [5, 96, 98]. The heart rate recovery following exercise was also depressed (slower reactivation of cardiac parasympathetic regulation) in dogs susceptible to ventricular fibrillation as compared with animals resistant to these malignant arrhythmias [99].

Heart rate variability is reduced in patients recovering from a myocardial infarction, and those patients with the greatest reduction in this variable also have the greatest risk for sudden death [89–94]. Kleiger et al. [100] found that in patients recovering from myocardial infarctions, those with the smallest heart rate variability (standard deviation of R-R interval) had the greatest risk of dying suddenly. The relative risk of mortality was 5.3 times greater in patients with a R-R interval variability less than 50 ms compared with patients with variability greater than 100 ms. This finding has been subsequently confirmed by more recent clinical studies [89–94, 101–105]. To cite just one example, La Rovere et al. [103] reporting for the ATRAMI (Autonomic Tone and Reflexes After Myocardial Infarction) group found that post-myocardial infarction patients with either low heart rate variability or a small heart rate response to an increase in blood pressure (i.e., BRS) had a much greater risk of sudden death than those with well-preserved cardiac vagal tone. The greatest risk for mortality was observed in patients with a large reduction in both markers of cardiac vagal regulation [103]. In a similar manner, heart rate recovery after exercise has been shown to be an independent predictor of mortality across substantial and diverse population groups [106–112]. Cole et al. [107] demonstrated in a multicenter study of 5234 individuals that abnormal heart rate recovery after submaximal exercise predicted death, even after adjustment for various confounding factors; Nishime et al. [112] published similar results from a total of 9454 patients.

When considered together, these clinical and experimental studies clearly suggest that reductions in cardiac parasympathetic regulation play an important role in the development of sudden cardiac death. Thus, one would predict that interventions that alter cardiac parasympathetic control should also alter susceptibility to malignant arrhythmias. Several experimental studies have shown that electrical stimulation of the vagus nerves can reduce ventricular fibrillation threshold, antagonize the effects of sympathetic stimulation, and decrease the incidence of ventricular fibrillation [113–116]. For example, vagal stimulation has been shown to prevent reperfusion arrhythmias in anesthetized cats [116] and ventricular fibrillation in a conscious canine model of sudden death [117]. Cholinergic agonists have also been shown to prevent ischemically induced ventricular fibrillation [117, 118], even when heart rate was held constant by ventricular pacing [118], suggesting an important role for the activation of muscarinic receptors on ventricular cardiomyocytes. Conversely, bilateral vagotomy or the cholinergic antagonist atropine can increase arrhythmia formation [119, 120].

Unfortunately, many cholinergic agonists exert profound gastrointestinal actions, thereby limiting their therapeutic potential. The observation that low doses of cholinergic antagonists paradoxically increased the level of cardiac vagal activity [121] led to the proposal that this treatment could provide an acceptable means of enhancing cardiac parasympathetic activity in patients [122]. Several independent clinical studies [122–125], in fact, demonstrated that low doses of scopolamine augmented markers of cardiac vagal activity in post-myocardial infarction patients. However, Halliwill et al. [97] and Hull et al. [126] both demonstrated that although low doses of cholinergic antagonists increased baseline cardiac vagal activity, as measured by R-R interval variability, this treatment failed to prevent ventricular fibrillation induced by myocardial ischemia. Halliwill et al. [97] demonstrated that the enhanced baseline vagal activity was not maintained when the heart was stressed by either exercise or myocardial ischemia. As such, it is not surprising that this therapy failed to prevent ventricular fibrillation. To be an effective antiarrhythmic therapy, an intervention must not only increases baseline vagal activity but also maintain this enhanced activity when the heart is stressed.

20.4 β_2-ADRENERGIC RECEPTOR ACTIVATION AND SUSCEPTIBILITY TO VF

As previously noted, enhanced sympathetic activation can reduce cardiac electrical stability and induce ventricular fibrillation. Presumably, the activation of myocardial β-adrenergic receptor mediates the arrhythmogenic effects of catecholamines released from the sympathetic nerve terminals. The mammalian myocardium contains both β_1- and β_2 -adrenergic receptors [127]. In the normal heart, the β_1-adrenoceptor is the dominant receptor subtype, and it mediates the inotropic response to the activation of sympathetic nerves. Under certain pathological conditions, however, the activation of β_2-adrenergic receptors may become particularly important [127, 128]. It is now well established that β_1-adrenergic receptor sensitivity decreases substantially during heart failure, whereas β_2-adrenergic receptor number remains relatively constant [127, 128]. As a consequence, the failing heart becomes more dependent on the activation of β_2-adrenergic receptors for inotropic support. The activation of these receptors may help maintain cardiac function in diseased hearts but not without potentially adverse consequences. β_2-adrenergic receptor activation promotes an increase in the calcium current without altering calcium reuptake by the sarcoplasmic reticulum [129]. The resulting elevation in intracellular calcium could provoke oscillations in membrane potential that, in turn, could trigger arrhythmias [130]. Thus, β_2-adrenergic receptor activation would tend to reduce the cardiac electrical stability and increase the propensity for the formation of malignant arrhythmias in the diseased heart.

Recently, Houle et al. [131] demonstrated in dogs with healed myocardial infarctions that the nonselective β-adrenergic receptor agonist isoproterenol provoked significantly larger increases both in heart rate, fractional shortening, and in the velocity of circumferential fiber shortening (Vcf, an index of contractility) in those animals that were susceptible to ventricular fibrillation induced by myocardial ischemia as compared with those animals that were resistant to these malignant arrhythmias [132]. The selective β_2-adrenergic receptor antagonist, ICI 118,551, reduced the isoproterenol response to a much greater extent in the susceptible animals, eliminating any differences noted between the groups [131]. In a similar manner, the calcium transient amplitude and the single-cell isotonic shortening response either to the selective β_2-adrenergic receptor agonist zinterol or to isoproterenol was larger in myocytes obtained from the hearts of susceptible compared with resistant dogs; these differences were also eliminated by the β_2-adrenergic receptor but not by β_1-adrenergic receptor blockade [131, 132]. In the intact dog, β_2-adrenergic receptor blockade also almost completely suppressed VF induced by acute myocardial ischemia, protecting 10 of 11 susceptible animals [131]. In agreement with these findings, zinterol infusion provoked ventricular tachyarrhythmias in rabbits with heart failure induced by myocardial infarction [133]. Furthermore, zinterol elicited aftercontractions and calcium aftertransients in 88% of heart failure compared with 0% of control myocytes [133]. β_2-adrenergic receptor stimulation also induced aftercontractions, aftertransients, increased calcium transient amplitude, and sarcoplasmic reticular calcium load in myocytes from patients with heart failure [133]. When considered together, these data demonstrate that enhanced β_2-adrenergic receptor responsiveness is associated with an increased propensity for ventricular fibrillation because of a calcium-overload-induced spontaneous calcium release from the sarcoplasmic reticulum and resulting afterdepolarizations of the cardiac membrane. One would predict that interventions that restore a more normal β_1- to β_2-adrenergic receptor balance should also protect against ventricular fibrillation.

Clinical studies have not evaluated extensively the contribution of β_2-adrenergic receptor to cardiac mortality. A small clinical trial found that the β_2-adrenergic receptor agonist salbutamol increased episodes of ventricular tachycardia in patients with congestive heart failure [134]. In a similar manner, there are a few case reports in which β_2-adrenergic receptor agonists have precipitated sudden death as a consequence of the cardiac actions of these agents in asthmatic patients [135, 136]. More compelling but indirect evidence in support of the β_2-adrenergic receptor hypothesis is provided by analysis of the numerous β-adrenergic receptor antagonist trials. Overwhelming evidence suggests that β-adrenergic receptor antagonists can protect against arrhythmia formation induced by myocardial ischemia and infarction [35, 36]. Indeed, this marked reduction in cardiac mortality has been verified in at least 32 trials involving approximately 29,000 patients [35, 36]. However, if one carefully examines the clinical studies cited above, it then becomes apparent that not all β-adrenergic receptor antagonists offer the same level of protection, particularly during acute myocardial infarction. Most studies using the β_1-adrenergic receptor antagonist metoprolol failed to report significant reductions in the incidence of ventricular fibrillation during acute myocardial infarction [80, 82]. Furthermore, although atenolol did reduce overall mortality by 15%, the number of patients who died as the result of malignant arrhythmias was not altered [137]. In contrast, propranolol therapy elicited large reductions in both overall mortality (65% decrease) and sudden cardiac death (41% decrease) in post-myocardial infarction patients with persistent

ST-segment depression [84], which is a group of patients known to be at a particularly high risk for subsequent cardiac events [138]. Thus, a better antiarrhythmic protection can be achieved with complete (i.e., β_1- and β_2-adrenergic receptor), rather than selective (i.e., β_1-), β-adrenergic receptor blockade. Exercise training could not only alter cardiac autonomic regulation but also improve β_2- to β_1-adrenergic receptor balance and thereby reduce the risk for malignant ventricular arrhythmias.

20.5   EFFECT OF EXERCISE CONDITIONING ON CARDIAC AUTONOMIC REGULATION

Endurance exercise training is well established to alter autonomic nervous system activity, resulting in an apparent increase in cardiac parasympathetic tone coupled with decreases in sympathetic activity [9–12]. For example, in both humans and animals, the heart rate at submaximal workloads was reduced in trained individuals compared with sedentary controls [9–12, 139–141]. A resting bradycardia is a well-established consequence of exercise training and is, in fact, used as a marker that the exercise trained state has been achieved [9–12, 139–143]. Both acetylcholine content and cholineacetyl transferase were increased in the hearts of trained rats as compared with control animals [144, 145]. In humans, exercise training during recovery from myocardial infarction has been reported to increase heart rate variability [28–32, 39–42]. Thus, these data suggest that endurance exercise training can elicit changes in cardiac autonomic control.

A series of recent studies have comprehensively examined the effects of exercise training both on the parasympathetic [5, 72, 75, 87] and on the β-adrenergic receptor [5, 73, 76] regulation of cardiac function in dogs susceptible or resistant to ventricular fibrillation induced by acute myocardial ischemia. The susceptible ($n = 20$) and resistant ($n = 13$) dogs were randomly assigned to either a 10-week exercise program (susceptible, $n = 9$; resistant $n = 8$) or an equivalent sedentary period (susceptible, $n = 11$; resistant $n = 5$). Heart rate variability was evaluated at rest, during exercise, and during a 2 min occlusion at rest, before and after the 10-week period. As in previous studies [5, 96, 97], pretraining, the coronary occlusion provoked significantly greater increases in heart rate (susceptible 54.9 ± 8.3 vs resistant 25.0 ± 6.1 beats/min) and greater reductions in heart rate variability (susceptible -6.3 ± 0.3 vs. resistant -2.8 ± 0.8 ln ms^2) in the susceptible dogs as compared with the resistant animals. Similar response differences between susceptible and resistant dogs were noted during submaximal exercise. Exercise training significantly reduced the heart rate and heart rate variability response to either submaximal exercise (Figure 20.8) or coronary artery occlusion (Figure 20.9) to a greater extent in the susceptible animals compared with the resistant dogs. In contrast, these variables were not altered in the sedentary susceptible dogs (Figures 20.8 and 20.9). In a similar manner, exercise training attenuated the heart rate response to exercise onset and enhanced (accelerated) the heart rate return toward baseline values (heart rate recovery) following the termination of exercise [74]. Correspondingly, heart rate variability (indices of cardiac vagal regulation) was also enhanced

Effect of Training on the HRV Response to Exercise

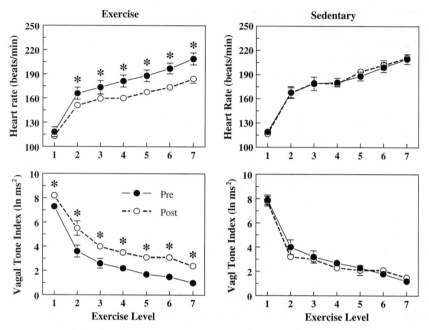

Figure 20.8. The effect of the 10-week exercise training ($n = 9$) or 10-week sedentary period ($n = 7$) on the heart rate and the heart rate variability responses to submaximal exercise in animals susceptible ventricular fibrillation. Exercise elicited significantly smaller increases in heart rate and smaller reductions in the various indices of cardiac vagal activity in the exercise-trained dogs as compared with animals that received a similar sedentary period. The post-training response in the susceptible exercise-trained dogs was no longer different from that noted for the resistant (exercise trained or sedentary) dogs. *$P < 0.01$ exercise-trained versus sedentary, Exercise levels: 1 = 0 kph/0% grade, 2 = 4.8 kph/0% grade, 3 = 6.4 kph/0% grade, 4 = 6.4 kph/4% grade, 5 = 6.4 kph/8% grade, 6 = 6.4 kph 12% grade, 7 = 6.4 kph/16% grade. (Reprinted with permission from Billman and Kukielka, [72])

following exercise training. In marked contrast, neither the heart rate nor the heart rate variability responses to exercise onset or following the termination of exercise were altered in sedentary (time control) animals [74]. Atropine pretreatment eliminated the differences in the indices of cardiac vagal activity and the heart rate response to the termination of exercise noted between the sedentary and exercise-trained dogs [74]. These data suggest that exercise training enhanced cardiac parasympathetic activity.

If enhanced cardiac parasympathetic activity was solely responsible for the antiarrhythmic action of exercise training, then one would predict that inventions that disrupt cardiac parasympathetic actions should also eliminate the beneficial actions of exercise training on cardiac electrical stability (i.e., restore the inducibility of arrhythmias). As previously noted [5, 72, 73, 75, 76, 87], a 10-week exercise-training program completely abolished ventricular fibrillation that was induced by

Effect of Training on the HRV Response to Coronary Occlusion

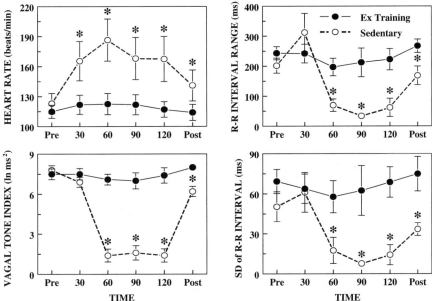

Figure 20.9. The effect of the 10-week exercise training ($n = 9$) or 10-week sedentary ($n = 7$) period on the heart rate and the heart rate variability responses to a 2-min coronary occlusion in animals susceptible to ventricular fibrillation. The coronary occlusion elicited significantly smaller increases in heart rate and smaller reductions in the various indices of cardiac vagal regulation in the exercise-trained dogs as compared with animals that received a similar sedentary period. The posttraining response in the susceptible exercise trained animals was no longer different from that noted for the resistant (either exercise trained or sedentary) dogs. * $P < 0.01$ exercise-trained versus sedentary. Pre = last 30 s before the coronary occlusion, Post = 1 min following coronary occlusion release (i.e., average over 30 s to 60 s post release). (Reprinted with permission from Billman and Kukielka [72]).

acute myocardial ischemia in dogs shown to be susceptible to malignant arrhythmias, whereas a similar 10-week control (sedentary) period failed to protect any animal (Figures 20.6 and 20.7). To evaluate the cardiac parasympathetic contribution to the antiarrhythmic effects of exercise training, studies were repeated after the injection of atropine to abolish any exercise training-induced enhancement of cardiac vagal regulation. This intervention increased heart rate (Figure 20.10A) [72] and provoked reductions in the various indices of heart rate variability but only induced ventricular fibrillation in one of eight trained susceptible dogs (Figure 20.10B) [72]. Thus, exercise training-induced increases in cardiac vagal activity were not solely responsible for the training-induced protection from ventricular fibrillation. Other factors, including alterations in the β-adrenergic receptor regulation of the heart, also contributed to the protection from ventricular fibrillation.

Regular endurance exercise has been shown to improve β-adrenergic receptor responsiveness in normal animals [146, 147], in aged animals [148], and in animals

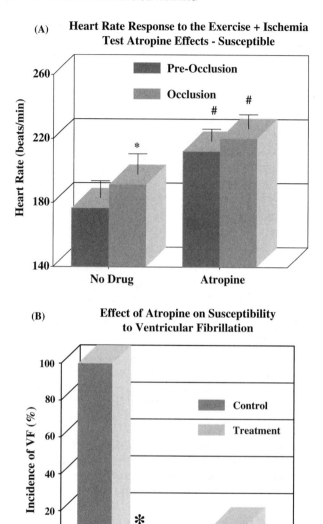

Figure 20.10. **A**. The effect of atropine on the heart rate responses to the exercise plus ischemia in exercise-trained susceptible dogs. Atropine (50 µg/kg, IV given as a bolus 3 min before the coronary occlusion) elicited a large increase in heart rate. * $P < 0.01$ preocclusion versus occlusion, # $P < 0.01$ No drug versus atropine. (Reprinted with Permission of Billman and Kukielka [64].) **B**. The effect of endurance exercise training on the incidence of ventricular fibrillation (VF) before and after atropine treatment. Exercise training (10 weeks) prevented VF in all eight animals that were susceptible to this malignant arrhythmia before training. Despite large increase in heart rate, atropine only reintroduced VF in one exercise-trained dog. Data used for this figure came from ref. 72.

with hypertension [149], despite either a reduction [146] or no change in the β_1-adrenergic receptor density [148, 150]. MacDonnell et al. [149] demonstrated that exercise training could correct the defective inotropic response to β-adrenergic receptor stimulation in spontaneously hypertensive rats. The effects of exercise training on β_2-adrenergic receptor responsiveness in animals with damaged hearts that were susceptible to ventricular fibrillation have been recently evaluated [73]. Before exercise training, the β_2-adrenergic receptor antagonist ICI 118,551 (0.2 mg/kg) significantly reduced the peak contractile (by echocardiography) response to isoproterenol more in the susceptible animals (susceptible $-45.5 \pm 6.5\%$ vs resistant -19.2 6.3%) compared with the resistant dogs. After exercise training, the resistant and the susceptible dogs exhibited similar responses to the β_2-adrenergic receptor antagonist (susceptible $-12.1 \pm 5.7\%$ vs resistant $-16.2 \pm 6.4\%$) (Figure 20.11). In contrast, ICI 118,551 provoked even greater reductions in the isoproterenol response in the sedentary susceptible dogs ($-62.3 \pm 4.6\%$) (Figure 20.11). The β_2-adrenergic receptor agonist zinterol (1 μM) elicited significantly smaller increases in isotonic shortening in ventricular myocytes (Figure 20.12) from susceptible dogs after training ($n = 8$, $7.2 \pm 4.8\%$) than in those from sedentary dogs ($n = 7$, $42.8 \pm 5.8\%$); this response is similar to that noted in the resistant dogs (trained, $n = 6$, $3.0 \pm 1.4\%$; sedentary, $n = 5$, $3.2 \pm 1.8\%$). In a similar manner, exercise training normalized the

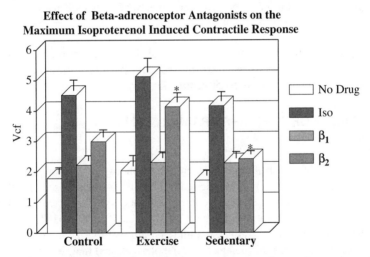

Figure 20.11. Effects of selective β-adrenergic receptor antagonists on the maximum isoproterenol induced Vcf (**A**), fractional shortening (**B**), and heart rate (**C**) responses in susceptible animals before (control $n = 18$) and after either a training ($n = 8$) or a sedentary ($n = 10$) time period. The β_2-adrenoceptor antagonist ICI 118,551 (0.2 mg/kg, IV) elicited a significantly greater reduction in the isoproterenol response in the sedentary animals. In contrast, the β_2-adrenergic receptor r response was significantly reduced in the exercise-trained animals. β_1-adrenergic receptor antagonist = bisoprolol (0.6 mg/kg, IV), isoproterenol = 0.5 μg/kg/min. * $P < 0.01$ control drug treatment response compared with the corresponding drug treatment response for either the 10-week exercise-trained or the 10-week sedentary group. (Reprinted with permission from Billman et al. [73].)

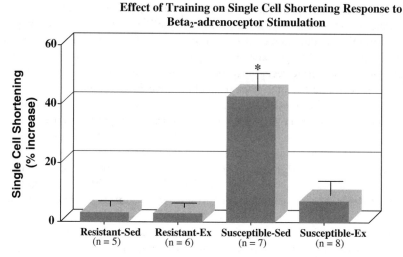

Figure 20.12. The effect of exercise training on the single-cell shortening (% change from control) response to the selective β-adrenergic receptor agonist (zinterol, 1 μM). The responses were compared between ventricular myocytes (6–15 cells per dog) obtained from susceptible (sedentary $n = 7$, trained $n = 8$) and resistant (sedentary $n = 5$, trained $n = 6$) animals. Note the much larger response in the sedentary susceptible animals. * $P < 0.01$ sedentary versus trained. (Reprinted with permission from Billman et al. [73].)

β-adrenergic receptor expression and content [76]. Thus, exercise training can restore cardiac β-adrenergic receptor balance (by reducing $β_2$-adrenergic receptor responsiveness) and could, thereby, prevent ventricular fibrillation.

20.6   EFFECT OF EXERCISE TRAINING ON MYOCYTE CALCIUM REGULATION

The mechanisms by which alterations in cardiac autonomic regulation protect against ventricular fibrillation remain to be elicited fully. It has been proposed that abnormal calcium regulation in diseased hearts contributes not only to contractile dysfunction but also to the development of malignant arrhythmias [8, 130, 151–154]. It is well established that elevated cytosolic calcium (calcium overload) can provoke oscillations in membrane potential (delayed afterdepolarizations) that, if it is of sufficient magnitude to reach threshold, can trigger extrasystoles [8, 130]. These afterdepolarizations have been shown to result primarily from an inward current associated with the activation of the sodium–calcium exchanger current (NCX) in the reverse mode (i.e., 1 Ca^{2+} out of the cell in exchange with 3 Na^+ into the cell) [152–156]. As such, an overexpression of NCX1 (the predominate isoform in the mammalian heart [157–159]), particularly in a setting of elevated cytsolic calcium as could occur during myocardial ischemia [8, 129], would prove to be particularly arrhythmogenic. Several investigators reported both an increased NCX1 expression (protein and/or messenger RNA [mRNA]) and an increase in lethal arrhythmia development (triggered by delayed afterdepolarizations) in animal models of heart failure [153, 160–162]. In a similar manner, heart failure provoked increases in NCX1 expression coupled with decreases in sarcoendoplasmic reticulum Ca^{2+}-ATPase (SERCA) levels in both patients and animals [160–169]. It is well established that patients with the greatest left ventricular function following myocardial infarction also have the greatest risk for sudden death [170]. Thus, changes in calcium regulatory proteins that accompany cardiac disease could provoke abnormalities in myocyte calcium homeostasis that would reduce cardiac electrical stability enhancing the risk for lethal cardiac rhythm disorders.

As noted, exercise training results in a more favorable cardiac autonomic balance (enhanced cardiac vagal and reduced cardiac β_2-adrenergic receptor sensitivity) [5, 72–74]. As changes in intracellular calcium play a critical role in the neural signal transduction process (parasympathetic activation reduces while sympathetic activation increases myocyte calcium), exercise training could also facilitate a more normal myocyte calcium handling. Therefore, exercise-induced changes in calcium regulatory proteins could represent a link between the autonomic nervous system and susceptibility to ventricular fibrillation. In particular, exercise-training-induced changes in NCX1 expression could contribute to an improvement in cardiac myocyte calcium regulation and thereby decrease the risk for arrhythmias.

Only a few studies have examined the effects of exercise training on calcium regulatory proteins, which often yielded conflicting results. For example, both increases [165, 169, 171] and decreases [171, 172] in NCX1 activity have been reported following exercise training in rats with healthy hearts. In contrast, exercise training elicited beneficial changes in NCX1 levels in models of cardiovascular disease. Zhang et al. [173] reported that high-intensity sprint training reduced NCX1 activity and decreased sarcoplasmic reticular calcium content in myocytes obtained from the hearts of rats with a moderate-sized left ventricular infarct. In a similar manner, exercise training reversed the increased expression of NCX1 and decreased SERCA activity (i.e., SERCA and NCX1 protein levels after training were similar to values for the normal hearts) in a canine model of tachycardia-pacing induced heart failure [163]. Sedentary hypertensive rats that were prone to arrhythmia development exhibited an increased NCX1 expression and decreased phospholamban expression compared with normotensive rats [68]. Daily exercise (voluntary wheel running) both reduced arrhythmia formation and normalized phospholamban and NCX1 expression in the hypertensive rats [68]. In contrast, myocardial infarction decreased (rather than increased) NCX1 expression by 30% in infarcted rats compared with sham-treated animals. Interestingly, exercise training elicited beneficial changes even in this study [169]. NCX1 expression increased in trained rats with or without infarction [169] such that, after training, NCX1 levels in the infarcted rats no longer differed from the values observed in the sedentary sham group [169]. After myocardial infarction, NCX1 levels were higher in dogs that were susceptible, as compared with those animals that were resistant, to ventricular fibrillation. In contrast, NCX1 levels were similar in both exercise-trained resistant and susceptible animals (Figure 20.13). Thus, exercise training can restore NCX expression, thereby improving myocyte calcium handling and reducing the risk for malignant arrhythmia.

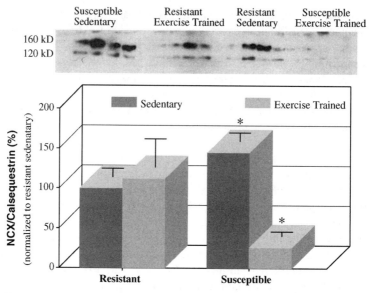

Figure 20.13. Effect of endurance exercise training on NCX protein content. NCX levels were determined by Western blot analysis. Protein content was corrected by calsequesterin levels. The data were then normalized to the resistant sedentary group. * $P < 0.05$ from resistant sedentary group.

20.7   SUMMARY AND CONCLUSIONS

As noted, sudden cardiac death caused by ventricular tachyarrhythmias is the most common cause of death in industrially developed countries [174–176]. Most currently available antiarrhythmic therapies (with the notable exceptions of β-adrenoceptors antagonist [35–37, 175]) have largely proven to be ineffective in preventing untimely deaths. In fact, several initially promising antiarrhythmic compounds were found to induce lethal arrhythmias in some patients, leading to an increase rather than a decrease in overall cardiac mortality [1–3]. Cardiac autonomic balance is altered in patients with cardiac disease, with the patients with the greatest autonomic impairment exhibiting the greatest risk for lethal ventricular tachyarrhythmias [89–94, 100]. It is widely accepted that aerobic exercise training improves cardiac autonomic balance by enhancing cardiac parasympathetic regulation and reducing sympathetic activity perhaps by restoring a more normal β-adrenergic receptor balance (i.e., reducing abnormal $β_2$-adrenoceptor expression and/or sensitivity) [9–12]. A growing body of clinical and epidemiological data clearly indicates that even modest daily physical activity can dramatically reduce cardiac mortality in both healthy individuals and in high-risk patients (patients with heart failure or a previous myocardial infarction) [13–33]. Conversely, the lack of exercise is strongly associated with an increased incidence of many chronic diseases, including coronary artery disease [177]. Exercise training improved cardiac autonomic regulation (enhanced cardiac parasympathetic control and reduced myocardial $β_2$-adrenergic receptor sensitivity) and completely suppressed ventricular fibrillation induced by myocardial ischemia in a canine model for sudden death. In fact, exercise training has proven to be the most effective antiarrhythmic therapy of any of the various treatments evaluated in this canine model of sudden death [5], protecting 100% of the animals (30 of 30 dogs) from ventricular fibrillation after the completion of endurance training (treadmill running) program. As such, aerobic exercise training could prove to be a safe and effective nonpharmacological means of maintaining an optimal cardiac autonomic balance, thereby enhancing cardiac electrical stability and preventing sudden cardiac death.

REFERENCES

1. Echt, D.S., Liebson, P.R., Mitchell, L.B., Peters, R.W., Obiasmanno, D., Barker, A.H., Arensberg, D., Baker, A., Freedman, L., Greene, H.L., Hunter, M.L., Richardson, D.W. (1991). Mortality and morbidity in patients receiving encainide, flecainide, or placebo. New England Journal of Medicine, 324, 782–788.

2. Sager, P.T. (1999). New advances in class III antiarrhythmic drug therapy. Current Opinions in Cardiology, 14, 15–23.

3. Waldo, A.L., Camm, A.J., de Ruyter, H., Friedman, P.L., MacNeil, D.J., Pauls, J.F., Pitt, B., Pratt, C.M., Schwartz, P.J., Veltri, E.P., for the SWORD Investigators (1996). Effect of d-sotalol on mortality in patients with left ventricular dysfunction after recent and remote myocardial infarction. Lancet, 348, 7–12.

4. Buxton, A.E., Lee, K.L., Fisher, J.D., Josephson, M.E., Prystowsky, E.N., Hafley, G. (1999). A randomized study of the prevention of sudden death in patients with coronary artery disease. New England Journal of Medicine, 341, 1882–1890.

5. Billman, G.E. (2006). A comprehensive review and analysis of 25 years of data from an in vivo canine model of sudden cardiac death: implications for future anti-arrhythmic drug development. Pharmacology & Therapeutics, 111, 808–835.

6. Corr, P.B., Yamada, K.A., Witkowski, F.X., Mechanisms controlling cardiac autonomic function and their relationships to arrhythmogenesis. In: Fozzard, H.A., Haber, E., Jennings, R.B., Katz, A.M., Morgan, H.E., Eds. The Heart and Cardiovascular System,. Raven Press, New York, 1986, pp. 1343–1404.

7. Schwartz, P.J., Zipes, D.P., Autonomic modulation of cardiac arrhythmias. In: Zipes, D.P., Jalife, J., Eds. Cardiac Electrophysiology: From Cell to Bedside, 3rd edition) W. B. Saunders Co., Philadelphia, PA, 2000, 300–314.

8. Rubart, M., Zipes, D.P. (2005). Mechanisms of sudden cardiac death. Journal of Clinical Investigation, 115, 2305–2315.

9. Rowell, L.K., Human Circulation: Regulation During Physical Stress. Oxford University Press, New York, 1986, pp. 257–286.

10. Buch, A.N., Coote, J.H., Townsend, J.N. (2002). Morality, cardiac vagal control and physical training—what's the link?. Experimental Physiology, 87, 423–435.

11. Billman, G.E. (2002). Aerobic exercise conditioning: A nonpharmacological antiarrhythmic intervention. Journal of Applied Physiology, 92, 446–454.

12. Bloomquist, C.G., Saltin, B. (1983). Cardiovascular adaptations to physical exercise. Annual Review of Physiology, 45, 169–189.

13. Paffenbarger, R.S., Hall, W.E. (1975). Work activity and coronary heart mortality. New England Journal of Medicine, 292, 545–550.

14. Epstein, L., Miller, G.J., Stitt, F.W., Morris, J.N. (1976). Vigorous exercise in leisure time, coronary risk factors, resting factors, and resting electrocardiograms of middle-aged male civil servants. British Heart Journal, 38, 403–409.

15. Kallio, V., Hamalainen, H., Hakkila, J., Luurila, O.J. (1979). Reduction in sudden deaths by multifactorial intervention programme after myocardial infarction. Lancet, 2, 1091–1094.

16. Ekelund, L.-G., Haskell, W.L., Johnson, J.L., Whaley, F.S., Criqui, M.H., Sheps, D.S. (1988). Physical fitness as a predictor of cardiovascular mortality in asymptomatic North American men: The lipid research clinic mortality follow-up study. New England Journal Medicine, 319, 1379–1384.

17. O'Connor, G.T., Buring, J.E., Yusuf, S., Goldhaber, S.Z., Olmstead, E.M., Paffenbarger, R. S. Jr., Hennekens, C.H. (1989). An overview of randomized trials of rehabilitation with exercise after myocardial infarction. Circulation, 80, 234–244.

18. Berlin, J.A., Colditz, G.A. (1990). A meta-analysis of physical activity in the prevention of coronary heart disease. American Journal of Epidemiology, 132, 612–628.

19. Pekkanen, J., Marti, B., Nissinen, A., Tuomilheto, J., Punsar, S., Karvonen, M.J. (1987). Reduction of premature mortality by high physical activity: A 20-year follow-up of middle-aged Finnish men. Lancet, 1, 1473–1477.

20. Sesso, H.D., Paffenbarger, R.S. Jr., Lee, I.-M. (2000). Physical activity and coronary heart disease in men: The Harvard Alumni Health Study. Circulation, 102, 975–980.

21. Lee, I.-M., Sesso, H., Paffenbarger, R.S. Jr. (2000). Physical activity and coronary heart diesese risk in men: Does the duration of exercise episodes predict risk?. Circulation, 102, 981–986.

22. Manson, J.E., Hu, F.B., Rich-Edwards, J.W., Colditz, G.A., Stampler, M.J., Willet, W.C., Speizer, F.E., Hennekens, C.H. (1999). A prospective study of walking as compared with vigorous exercise in the prevention of coronary heart disease in women. New England Journal of Medicine, 341, 650–658.

23. Meyers, J., Prakash, M., Froechlicher, V., Do, D., Partington, S., Atwood, J.E. (2002). Exercise capacity and mortality among men referred for exercise testing. New England Journal of Medicine, 346, 793–801.

24. Bartels, R., Menges, M., Thimme, W. (1997). Der einfluβ von korperlicher aktivatat auf die inzidenz des plotzlichen herstodes. Medizinische Klinik, 92, 319–325.

25. Hakim, A.A., Curb, J.D., Petrovich, H., Rodriguez, B.L., Yano, K., Ross, G.W., White, L.R., Abbot, R.D. (1999). Effects of walking on coronary heart disease in elderly men—the Honolulu Heart Program. Circulation, 100, 9–13.

26. Hakim, A.A., Petrovich, H., Burchiel, C.M., Ross, G.W., Rodriguez, B.L., White, L.R., Yano, K., Curb, J.D., Abbot, R.D. (1998). Effect of walking on mortality among nonsmoking retired men. New England Journal of Medicine, 338, 94–99.

27. Mozaffarin, D., Furberg, C.D., Psaty, B.M., Siscovick, D. (2008). Physical activity and incidence of atrial fibrillation in older adults. Circulation, 118, 800–807.

28. Malfatto, G., Facchini, M., Bragato, R., Branzi, G., Sala, L., Leonetti, G. (1996). Short and long term effects of exercise training on the tonic autonomic modulation of heart rate variability after myocardial infarction. European Heart Journal, 17, 532–538.

29. Leitch, J.W., Newling, R.P., Basta, M., Inder, K., Dear, K., Fletcher, P.J. (1997). Random-ized trial of hospital-based exercise training after myocardial infarction: Cardiac auto-nomic effects. Journal of the American College of Cardiology, 29, 1263–1268.

30. Oya, M., Itoh, H.Y., Kato, K., Tanabe, K., Murayama, M. (1999). Effects of exercise training on the recovery of the autonomic nervous system and exercise capacity after myocardial infarction. Japanese Circulation Journal, 63, 843–838.

31. La Rovere, M.T., Mortara, A., Sandrone, G., Lombardi, F. (1992). Autonomic nervous system adaptations to short-term exercise training. Chest, 101, 299S–303S.

32. LaRovere, M.T., Bersano, C., Gnemmi, M., Specchia, G., Schwartz, P.J. (2002). Exercise-induced increase in baroreflex sensitivity predicts improved prognosis after myocardial infarction. Circulation, 106, 945–949.

33. Steffen-Batey, L., Nichman, M.Z., Goff, D.C., Frankowski, R.F., Hanis, C.L., Ramsey, D.J., Labarthe, D.R. (2000). Change in level of physical activity and risk of all-cause mortality or reinfarction: The Corpus Christi heart project. Circulation, 102, 2204–2209.

34. Hamalainen, H., Luurila, O.J., Kallio, V., Knuts, L.-R. (1995). Reduction in sudden deaths and coronary mortality in myocardial infarction patients after rehabilitation—15-year follow-up study. European Heart Journal, 16, 1839–1844.

35. Held, P., Yusuf, S. (1989). Early intravenous beta-blockade in acute myocardial infarction. Cardiology, 76, 132–143.

36. Held, P.H., Yusuf, S. (1993). Effects of beta-blockers and Ca^{2+} channel blockers in acute myocardial infarction. European Heart Journal, 14, 18–25.

37. Kendall, M.J., Lynch, K.P., Hjalmarson, A., Kjekshus, J. (1995). β-Blockers and sudden cardiac death. Annals of Internal Medicine, 123, 353–367.

38. Iellamo, F., Legramante, J.M., Massro, M., Raimondo, G., Galante, A. (2000). Effects of a residential exercise training on baroreflex sensitivity and heart rate variability in patients with coronary artery disease. Circulation, 102, 2588–2592.

39. Mazzuero, G., Lanfranchi, P., Colombo, R., Giannuzzi, P., Giordano, A. (1992). Long-term adaptation of 24-h heart rate variability after myocardial infarction. The EAMI Study Group Exercise Training in Anterior Myocardial Infarction. Chest, 101, 304S–308S.

40. Duru, F., Candinas, R., Dziekan, G., Goebbels, U., Myers, J., Dubachi, P. (2000). Effect of exercise training on heart rate variability in patients with new-onset left ventricular dysfunction after myocardial infarction. American Heart Journal, 140, 157–161.

41. Stahle, A., Nordlander, R., Bergfeldt, L. (1999). Aerobic group training improves exercise capacity and heart rate variability in elderly patients with a coronary event. A randomized controlled study. European Heart Journal, 20, 1638–1646.

42. Tygesen, H., Wettervik, C., Wennerblom, B. (2001). Intensive home-based exercise training in cardiac rehabilitation increases exercise capacity and heart rate variability. International Journal of Cardiology, 79, 175–182.

43. Kiilavuori, K., Toivonen, L., Naveri, H., Leinonen, H. (1995). Reversal of autonomic derangement by physical training in chronic heart failure assessed by heart rate variability. European Heart Journal, 16, 490–495.

44. European Heart Failure Training Group. (1998). Experience from controlled trials of physical training in chronic heart failure. European Heart Journal, 19, 466–475.

45. Berlardinelli, R., Georgiou, D., Cianci, G., Purcaro, A. (1999). Randomised, controlled trial of long-term moderate exercise training in chronic heart failure. Circulation, 99, 1173–1182.

46. Coats, A.J., Adamopoulos, S., Radaelli, A., McCance, A., Meyer, T.E., Bernardi, L., Solda, P.L., Davey, P., Ormerod, O., Forfar, C. (1992). Controlled trial of physical training in chronic heart failure. Exercise performance, hemodynamics, ventilation, and autonomic function. Circulation, 85, 2119–2131.

47. Adamopoulos, S., Ponikowski, P., Cerquetani, E., Piepoli, M., Rosano, G., Sleight, P., Coats, A.J. (1995). Circadian pattern of heart rate variability in chronic heart failure patients. Effects of physical training. European Heart Journal, 16, 1308–1310.

48. Radaelli, A., Coats, A.J., Luezzi, S., Piepoli, M., Meyer, T.E., Calciati, A., Finardi, G., Bernardi, L., Slieght, P. (1996). Physical training enhances sympathetic and parasympathetic control of heart rate and peripheral vessels in chronic heart failure. Clinical Sciences, 91, 92–94.

49. Stamler, B.S., Wood, M.A., Ellenbogen, K.A. (1992). Sudden death in patients with congestive heart failure: future directions. PACE—Pacing and Clinical Electrophysiology, 15, 451–470.

50. Ponikowski, P., Anker, S.D., Amadi, A., Chua, T.P., Cerquetani, E., Ondusova, D., O'Sullivan, C., Adamopoulos, S., Piepoli, M., Coats, A.J. (1996). Heart rhythms, ventricular arrhythmias and death in chronic heart failure. Journal of Cardiac Failure, 2, 117–183.

51. Hertzeanu, H.L., Shermesh, J., Aron, L.A. (1993). Ventricular arrhythmias in rehabilitated and non-rehabilitated post-myocardial infarction patients with left ventricular dysfunction. American Journal of Cardiology, 71, 24–27.

52. Ali, A., Mehra, M., Malik, F., Lavie, C.J., Bass, D., Milani, R.V. (1999). Effects of aerobic exercise training on indices of ventricular repolarization in patients with chronic heart failure. Chest, 116, 83–87.

53. Vuori, I., Makarainen, M., Jasskellarnen, A. (1978). Sudden death and physical activity. Cardiology, 63, 287–306.

54. Friedwald, V.E., Spence, D.W. (1990). Sudden death associated with exercise: The risk-benefit issue. American Journal of Cardiology, 66, 183–188.

55. Kohl, H.W., Powell, K.E., Gordon, N.F., Blair, S.N., Paffenbarger, R.S. Jr. (1992). Physical fitness and sudden cardiac death. Epidemiologic Reviews, 14, 37–58.

56. Snell, P.G., Mitchell, J.H. (1999). Physical inactivity an easily modified risk factor?. Circulation, 100, 2–4.

57. Thompson, P.D., Franklin, B.A., Baldy, G.J., Blair, S.N., Corrado, D., Estes, N.A.M., Fulton, J.E., Gordon, N.F., Haskell, W.L., Link, M.S., Maron, B.J., Mittleman, M.A., Pelliccia, A., Wenger, N.K., Willich, S.N., Costa, F. (2007). Exercise and acute cardiovascular events. Placing the risks in perspective. Circulation, 115, 2358–2368.

58. Maron, B.J., Pelliccia, A. (2007). The heart of trained athletes. Cardiac remodeling and the risks of sports, including sudden death. Circulation, 114, 1633–1644.

59. Albert, C., Mittleman, M., Chae, C., Lee, I., Hennekens, C., Manson, J. (2000). Triggering of sudden death from cardiac causes by vigorous exertion. New England Journal of Medicine, 343, 1355–1361.

60. Corrado, D., Basso, C., Rizzoli, G., Schiavon, M., Thiene, G. (2003). Does sports activity enhance the risk of sudden death in adolescent and young adults?. Journal of American College of Cardiology, 42, 1959–1963.

61. Viskin, S. (2007). Antagonist: Routine screening of all athletes prior to participation in competitive sports should be mandatory to prevent sudden cardiac death. Heart Rhythm, 4, 525–528.

62. Noakes, T.N., Higginson, L., Opie, L.H. (1983). Physical training increases VF thresholds of isolated rat hearts during normoxia, hypoxia, and regional ischemia. Circulation, 67, 24–30.

63. Bakth, S., Arena, J., Remy, W.L., Hider, B., Patel, B.C., Lyons, M.M., Regan, T.J. (1986). Arrhythmia susceptibility and myocardial composition in diabetes: Influence of physical conditioning. Journal of Clinical Investigation, 77, 382–395.

64. Posel, D., Noakes, T., Kantor, P., Lambert, M., Opie, L.N. (1989). Exercise training after experimental myocardial infarction increases VF threshold before and after the onset of reinfarction in the isolated rat heart. Circulation, 80, 138–145.

65. Arad, M., Schwalb, H., Mahler, Y., Appelbaum, Y.J., Uretzky, G. (1990). The effect of swimming exercise on spontaneous ventricular defibrillation and VF threshold in the isolated perfused rat heart. Cardiosciences, 1, 295–299.

66. Belichard, P., Pruneau, D., Salzmann, J.L., Rouet, R. (1992). Decreased susceptibility to arrhythmias in hypertrophied hearts of physically trained rats. Basic Research in Cardiology, 87, 344–355.

67. Hamra, M., McNeil, R.S. (1995). Cardiac adrenergic responses and electrophysiology during ischemia: Effect of exercise. Medicine and Science in Sports and Exercise, 27, 993–1002.

68. Collins, H.L., Loka, A.M., DiCarlo, S.E. (2005). Daily exercise-induced cardioprotection is associated with changes in calcium regulatory proteins in hypertensive rats. American Journal of Physiology Heart and Circulatory Physiology, 288, H532–H540.

69. Lujan, H.L., Britton, S.L., Koch, L.G., DiCarlo, S.E. (2006). Reduced susceptibility to ventricular tachyarrhythmias in rats selectively bred for high aerobic capacity. American Journal of Physiology Heart and Circulatory Physiology, 291, H2933–H2941.

70. Billman, G.E., Schwartz, P.J., Stone, H.L. (1984). The effects of daily exercise on susceptibility to sudden cardiac death. Circulation, 69, 1182–1189.

71. Hull, S.S. Jr., Vanoli, E., Adamson, P.B., Verrier, R.L., Foreman, R.D., Schwartz, P.J. (1994). Exercise training confers anticipatory protection from sudden death during acute myocardial ischemia. Circulation, 89, 548–552.

72. Billman, G.E., Kukielka, M. (2006). Effects of endurance exercise training on heart rate variability and susceptibility to sudden cardiac death: Protection is not due to enhanced cardiac vagal regulation. Journal of Applied Physiology, 100, 896–906.

73. Billman, G.E., Kukielka, M., Kelley, R., Moustafa-Bayoumi, M., Altschuld, R.A. (2006). Endurance exercise training attenuates cardiac β_2-adrenoceptor responsiveness and prevents ventricular fibrillation in animals susceptible to sudden death. American Journal of Physiology Heart and Circulatory Physiology, 290, H2590–H2599.

74. Billman, G.E., Kukielka, M. (2007). Effect of endurance exercise training on the heart rate onset and heart rate recovery responses to submaximal exercise in animals susceptible to ventricular fibrillation. Journal of Applied Physiology, 102, 231–240.

75. Kukielka, M., Seals, D.R., Billman, G.E. (2006). Cardiac vagal modulation of heart rate during prolonged submaximal exercise in animals with healed myocardial infarctions: Effects of training. American Journal of Physiology Heart and Circulatory Physiology, 290, H1680–H1685.

76. Holycross, B.J., Kukielka, M., Nishijima, Y., Altschuld, R.A., Carnes, C.A., Billman, G.E. (2007). Exercise training normalizes β-adrenoceptor expression in dogs susceptible to ventricular fibrillation. American Journal of Physiology Heart and Circulatory Physiology, 293, H2702–H2709.

77. Verrier, R.L., Lown, B. (1984). Behavorial stress and cardiac arrhythmias. Annual Review of Physiology, 46, 155–176.

78. Falcone, C., Buzzi, M.P., Klersy, C., Schwartz, P.J. (2005). Rapid heart rate increase at onset of exercise predicts adverse cardiac events in patients with coronary artery disease. Circulation, 112, 1959–1964.

79. Billman, G.E. (2006). Heart rate response to the onset of exercise: Evidence for enhanced cardiac sympathetic activity in animals susceptible to ventricular fibrillation. American Journal of Physiology Heart and Circulatory Physiology, 291, H429–H435.

80. Hjalmarson, A., Armitage, P., Chamberlain, D., Lubsen, J., Yusuf, S., Lubsen, J. (1985). Metoprolol in acute myocardial infarction (MIAMI): A randomised placebo-controlled international trial. European Heart Journal, 6, 199–226.

81. Salathia, K.S., Barber, J.M., McIlmoyle, E.L., Nicholas, J., Evans, A.E., Elwood, J.H., Cran, G., Shanks, R.G., Boyle, D.M. (1985). Very early intervention with metoprolol in suspected acute myocardial infarction. European Heart Journal, 6, 190–198.

82. Hjalmarson, A., Elmfeldt, D., Herlitz, J., Holmberg, S., Malek, I., Nyberg, G., Ryden, L., Swedberg, K., Vedin, A., Waagstein, F., Waldenstrom, A., Waldenstrom, J., Wedel, H., Wilhelmsen, L., Wilhelmsson, C. (1981). Effect on mortality of metoprolol in acute myocardial infarction. A double-blind randomised trial. Lancet, 2, 823–827.

83. Norris, R.M., Barnaby, P.F., Brown, M.A., Geary, G.G., Clarke, E.D., Logan, R.L., Sharpe, D.N. (1984). Prevention of ventricular fibrillation during acute myocardial infarction by intravenous propranolol. Lancet, 2, 883–886.

84. Shivkumar, K., Schultz, L., Goldstein, S., Gheorghiade, M. (1998). Effects of propranolol in patients entered in beta-blocker heart attack trial with their first myocardial infarction and persistent electrocardiographic ST-segment depression. American Heart Journal, 135, 261–267.

85. De Ferrari, G.M., Salvati, P., Grossoni, M., Ukmar, G., Vaga, L., Patrono, C., Schwartz, P.J. (1993). Pharmacologic modulation of the autonomic nervous system in the prevention of sudden cardiac death: a study with propranolol, methacholine and oxotremorine in conscious dogs with a healed myocardial infarction. Journal of the American College of Cardiology, 21, 283–290.

86. Eckberg, D.L., Drabinsky, M., Braunwald, E. (1971). Defective cardiac parasympathetic control in patients with heart disease. New England Journal of Medicine, 285, 877–883.

87. Billman, G.E., Schwartz, P.J., Stone, H.L. (1982). Baroreceptor reflex control of heart rate: A predictor of sudden death. Circulation, 66, 874–880.

88. Schwartz, P.J., Vanoli, E., Stramba-Badiale, M., DeFerrari, G.M., Billman, G.E., Foreman, R.D. (1988). Autonomic mechanisms and sudden death, new insight from the analysis of baroreceptor reflexes in conscious dogs with and without a myocardial infarction. Circulation, 78, 969–979.

89. Bigger, J.T. Jr. (1997). The predictive value of RR variability and baroreflex sensitivity in coronary heart disease. Cardiac Electrophysiology Reviews, 1/2, 198–204.

90. Eckberg, D. (1997). Sympathovagal balance: A critical appraisal. Circulation, 96, 3224–3232.

91. Berntson, G.G., Bigger, J.T., Eckberg, D.L., Grossman, P., Kaufmann, P.G., Malik, M., Nagaraja, H.K., Proges, S.W., Saul, J.P., Stone, P.H., van der Molen, M.W. (1997). Heart rate variability: Origins, methods, and interpretive caveats. Psychophysiology, 34, 623–648.

92. Bigger, J.T., Schwartz, P.J., Markers of vagal activity and the prediction of cardiac death after myocardial infarction. In: Levy, M.N., Schwartz, P.J., Eds. Vagal Control of the Heart: Experimental Basis and Clinical implications. Futura Publishing., Armonk, NY., 1994, pp. 481–508.

93. Task Force of the European society of Cardiology and the North American society of Pacing and Electrophysiology. (1996). Heart rate variability: Standards of measurement, physiological interpretation, and clinical use. Circulation, 93, 1043–1065.

94. Appel, M.L., Berger, R.D., Saul, J.P., Smith, J.M., Cohen, R.J. (1989). Beat to beat variability in cardiovascular variables: Noise or music?. Journal of the American College of Cardiology, 14, 1139–1148.

95. Billman, G.E., Hoskins, R.S. (1989). Time-series analysis of heart rate variability during submaximal exercise. Evidence for reduced cardiac vagal tone in animals susceptible to ventricular fibrillation. Circulation, 80, 146–157.

96. Collins, M.N., Billman, G.E. (1989). Autonomic response to coronary occlusion in animals susceptible to ventricular fibrillation. American Journal of Physiology Heart and Circulatory Physiology, 257, H1886–H1894.

97. Halliwill, J.R., Billman, G.E., Eckberg, D.L. (1998). Effect of a vagomimetic atropine dose on canine cardiac vagal tone and susceptibility to sudden cardiac death. Clinical Autonomic Research, 8, 155–164.

98. Houle, M.S., Billman, G.E. (1999). Low-frequency component of the heart rate variability spectrum: A poor marker of sympathetic activity. American Journal of Physiology Heart and Circulatory Physiology, 267, H215–H223.

99. Smith, L.L., Kukielka, M., Billman, G.E. (2005). Heart rate recovery after exercise: A predictor of ventricular fibrillation susceptibility after myocardial infarction. American Journal of Physiology Heart and Circulatory Physiology, 288, H1763–H1769.

100. Kleiger, R.E., Miller, J.P., Bigger, J.T. Jr., Moss, A.J. (1987). Decreased heart rate variability and its association with increased mortality after acute myocardial infarction. American Journal of Cardiology, 59, 256–262.

101. Bigger, J.T. Jr, Fleiss, J.L., Steinman, R.C., Rolnitzky, L.M., Kleiger, R.E., Rottman, J.N. (1992). Frequency domain measures of heart period variability and mortality after myocardial infarction. Circulation, 85, 164–171.

102. La Rovere, M.T., Specchia, G., Mortara, A., Schwartz, P.J. (1988). Baroreflex sensitivity, clinical correlates and cardiovascular mortality among patients with a first myocardial infarction: A prospective study. Circulation, 78, 816–824.

103. La Rovere, M.T., Bigger, J.T. Jr., Marcus, F.I., Mortara, A., Schwartz, P.J. (1998). Baroreflex sensitivity and heart rate variability in prediction of total cardiac mortality after myocardial infarction. Lancet, 351, 478–484.

104. Hohnloser, S.H., Klingenheben, T., Zabel, M., Li, Y.G. (1997). Heart rate variability used as an arrhythmia risk stratifier after myocardial infarction. PACE—Pacing and Clinical Electrophysiology, 20, 2594–2601.

105. Lanza, G., Guido, V., Galeazzi, M., Mustilli, M., Natali, R., Ierardi, C., Milici, C., Burzotta, F., Pasceri, V., Tomassini, F., Lupi, A., Maseri, A. (1998). Prognostic role of

heart rate variability in patients with recent acute myocardial infarction. American Journal of Cardiology, 82, 1323–1328.

106. Cole, C.R., Blackstone, E.H., Pashikow, F.J., Snader, C.E., Lauer, M.S. (1999). Heart rate recovery immediately after exercise as a predictor of mortality. New England Journal of Medicine, 41, 1351–1357, 1999

107. Cole, C.R., Foody, J.M., Blackstone, E.H., Lauer, M.S. (2000). Heart rate recovery after submaximal exercise testing as a predictor of mortality in a cardiovascularly healthy cohort. Annals of Internal Medicine, 132, 553–555.

108. Jouven, X., Empana, J.P., Schwartz, P.J., Desnosw, M., Courbon, D., Ducimetiere, P. (2005). Heart rate profile during exercise as a predictor of sudden death. New England Journal of Medicine, 352, 1951–1958.

109. Mora, S., Redberg, R.F., Cui, Y., Whiteman, M.K., Flaws, J.A., Sharrett, A.R., Blumenthal, R.S. (2003). Ability of exercise testing to predict cardiovascular and all-cause death in asymptomatic women. JAMA—Journal of the American Medical Association, 290, 1600–1607.

110. Morshedi-Meibodi, A., Larson, M.G., Levy, D., O'Donnel, C.J., Vasan, R.S. (2002). Heart rate recovery after treadmill exercise testing and risk of cardiovascular disease events (the Framingham heart study). American Journal of Cardiology, 90, 848–852.

111. Nissinen, S.I., Makikallio, T.H., Seppanen, T., Tapanainen, J.M., Salo, M., Tulppo, M.P., Huikuri, H.V. (2003). Heart rate recovery after exercise as a predictor of mortality among survivors of acute myocardial infarction. American Journal of Cardiology, 91, 711–714.

112. Nishime, E.O., Cole, C.R., Blackstone, E.H., Pashkow, F.J., Lauer, M.S. (2000). Heart rate recovery and treadmill exercise score as predictors of mortality in patients referred for exercise ECG. JAMA—Journal of the American Medical Association, 284, 1392–1398.

113. Cerati, D., Schwartz, P.J. (1991). Single cardiac vagal activity, acute myocardial ischemia and risk for sudden death. Circulation Research, 69, 1389–1401.

114. Kent, K.M., Smith, E.R., Redwood, D.R., Epstein, S.E. (1973). Electrostability of acutely ischemic myocardium. Influences of heart rate and vagal stimulation. Circulation, 47, 291–298.

115. Kolman, B.S., Verrier, R.L., Lown, B. (1976). The effect of vagus nerve stimulation upon vulnerability of canine ventricle: Role of the sympathetic parasympathetic interaction. Circulation, 52, 578–585.

116. Zuanetti, G., De Ferrari, G.M., Priori, S.G., Schwartz, P.J. (1987). Protective effect of vagal stimulation on reperfusion arrhythmias in cats. Circulation Research, 61, 429–435.

117. Vanoli, E., De Ferrari, G.M., Stramba-Badiale, M., Hull, S.S. Jr., Foreman, R.D., Schwartz, P.J. (1991). Vagal stimulation and prevention of sudden death in conscious dogs with healed myocardial infarction. Circulation Research, 68, 1471–1481.

118. Billman, G.E. (1990). The effect of carbachol and cyclic GMP on susceptibility to ventricular fibrillation. FASEB Journal, 4, 1668–1673.

119. Corr, P.B., Gillis, R.A. (1974). Role of vagus nerves in the cardiovascular changes induced by coronary occlusion. Circulation, 49, 86–97.

120. De Ferrari, G.M., Vanoli, E., Stramba-Badiale, M., Hull, S.S. Jr., Foreman, R.D., Schwartz, P.J. (1991). Vagal reflexes and survival during acute myocardial ischemia in conscious dogs with healed myocardial infarction. American Journal of Physiology Heart and Circulatory Physiology, 261, H63–H69.

121. Kottmeier, C.A., Gravenstein, J.S. (1968). The parasympathomimetic activity of atropine and atropine methylbromide. Anesthesiology, 29, 1125–1133.

122. Casadei, B., Pipillis, A., Sessa, F., Conway, J., Sleight, P. (1993). Low doses of scopolamine increase cardiac vagal tone in the acute phase of myocardial infarction. Circulation, 88, 353–357.

123. Pedretti, R., Columbo, E., Braga, S.S., Caru, B. (1993). Influence of transdermal scopolamine on cardiac sympathovagal interactions after acute myocardial infarction. American Journal of Cardiology, 72, 384–392.

124. De Ferrari, G.M., Mantica, M., Vanoli, E., Hull, S.S. Jr., Schwartz, P.J. (1993). Scopolamine increases vagal tone and vagal reflexes in patients after myocardial infarction. Journal of the American College of Cardiology, 22, 1327–1334.

125. Vybiral, T., Glaeser, D.H., Morris, G., Hess, K.R., Yang, K., Francis, M., Pratt, C.M. (1993). Effects of low-dose transdermal scopolamine on heart rate variability in acute myocardial infarction. Journal of the American College of Cardiology, 22, 1320–1326.

126. Hull, S.S. Jr., Vanoli, E., Adamson, P.B., De Ferrari, G.M., Foreman, R.D., Schwartz, P.J. (1995). Do increases in markers of vagal activity imply protection from sudden death? The case of scopolamine. Circulation, 91, 2516–2519.

127. Altschuld, R.A., Billman, G.E. (2000). β_2-adrenoceptors and ventricular fibrillation. Pharmacology & Therapeutics, 88, 1–14.

128. Bristow, M.R., Ginsburg, R., Umans, V., Fowler, M., Minobe, W., Rasmussen, R., Zera, P., Menlove, R., Shah, P., Jamieson, S., Stinson, E.B. (1986). Beta1- and beta2-adrenergic-receptor subpopulations in nonfailing and failing human ventricular myocardium: Coupling of both receptor subtypes to muscle contraction and selective beta1-receptor down-regulation in heart failure. Circulation Research, 59, 297–309.

129. Altschuld, R.A., Starling, R.C., Hamlin, R.L., Billman, G.E., Hensley, J., Castillo, L., Fertel, R.H., Hohl, C.M., Robitaille, P.M.L., Jones, L.R., Xiao, R.P., Lakatta, E.G. (1995). Response of failing canine and human heart cells to β_2-adrenergic stimulation. Circulation, 92, 1612–1618.

130. Billman, G.E. (1991). The antiarrhythmic and antifibrillatory effects of calcium antagonists. Journal of Cardiovascular Pharmacology, 18, S107–S117.

131. Billman, G.E., Castillo, L.C., Hensley, J., Hohl, C.M., Altschuld, R.A. (1997). β_2-adrenergic receptor antagonists protect against VF: In vivo and in vitro evidence for enhanced sensitivity to β_2- adrenergic stimulation in animals susceptible to sudden death. Circulation, 96, 1914–1922.

132. Houle, M.S., Altshculd, R.A., Billman, G.E. (2001). Enhanced in vivo and in vitro contractile responses in β_2-adreneric receptor stimulation in dogs susceptible to lethal arrhythmias. Journal of Applied Physiology, 91, 1627–1637.

133. DeSantiago, J., Ai, X., Isalm, M., Acuna, G., Ziolo, M.T., Bers, D.M., Pogwizd, S.M. (2008). Arrhythmogenic effects of β_2-adrenergic strimulation in the failing heart are attributable to enhanced sarcoplasmic reticulum Ca load. Circulation Research, 102, 1389–1397.

134. Mettauer, B., Roulou, J.L., Buergess, J.H. (1985). Detriemental arrhtyhmogenic and sustained beneficial hemodynamic effects of oral salbutamol in patients with chronic congestive heart failure. American Heart Journal, 109, 840–847.

135. Robin, R.E., Lewiston, N. (1989). Unexpected, unexplained sudden death in young asthmatic subjects. Chest, 96, 790–793.

136. Robin, R.E., McCauley, R. (1992). Sudden cardiac death in bronchial asthma, and inhaled β-adrenergic agonists. Chest, 101, 1699–1702.

137. ISIS-1 (First International Study of Infarct Survival) Collaborative Group. (1988). Mechanisms for the early mortality reduction produced by beta-blockade started early in acute myocardial infarction: ISIS-1. Lancet, 1, 921–923.

138. Willich, S.N., Stone, P.H., Muller, J.E., Tofler, G.H., Crowder, J., Parker, C., Rutherford, J. D., Turi, Z.G., Robertson, T., Passamani, E., Braunwald, E., the MILIS Group (1987). High-risk subgroups of patients with non-Q wave myocardial infarction based upon direction and severity of ST segment deviation. American Heart Journal, 114, 1110–1119.

139. Smith, M.L., Hudson, D.L., Graitzer, H.M., Raven, P.B. (1989). Exercise training bradycardia: The role of autonomic balance. Medicine and Science in Sports and Exercise, 21, 40–44.

140. Maciel, B., Gallo, L. Jr., Neto, J.A.M., Filho, E.C.L., Filho, J.T., Manco, J.C. (1985). Parasympathetic contribution to bradycardia induced by endurance training in man. Cardiovascular Research, 19, 642–648.

141. Goldsmith, R.L., Bigger, J.T. Jr., Steineman, R.C., Fleiss, J.L. (1992). Comparison of 24-hour parasympathetic activity in endurance trained and untrained young men. Journal of the American College of Cardiology, 20, 552–558.

142. Ordway, G.A., Charles, J.B., Randall, D.C., Billman, G.E., Wekstein, D.R. (1982). Heart rate adaptation to exercise training cardiac-denervated dogs. Journal of Applied Physiology, 56, 1586–1590.

143. DeSchryver, C., Mertens-Strythaggen, J. (1975). Heart tissue acetylcholine in chronically exercised rats. Experientia, 31, 316–318.

144. Ekblom, B., Kilbom, A., Soltysiak, J. (1973). Physical training, bradycardia and autonomic nervous system. Scandinavian Journal of Clinical & Laboratory Investigation, 32, 251–256.

145. Sylvestre-Gervais, L., Nadeau, A., Nguyen, M.H., Tancrede, G., Rousseau-Migneron, S. (1982). Effects of physical training on β-adrenergic receptors in rat myocardial tissue. Cardiovascular Research, 16, 530–535.

146. Barbier, J., Rannou-Bekono, F., Marchais, J., Berthon, P.M., Delamarche, P., Carre, F. (2004). Effect of exercise training on β1, β2, β3, adrenergic and M2 muscarinic receptors in rat heart. Medicine and Science in Sports and Exercise, 36, 949–954.

147. Spina, R.J., Ogawa, T., Coggan, A.R., Holloszy, J.O., Ehsani, A.A. (1992). Exercise training improves left ventricular contractile responses to β-adrenergic agonists. Journal of Applied Physiology, 72, 307–311.

148. Mazzeo, R.S., Podolin, D.A., Henry, V. (1995). Effects of age and endurance training on β-adrenergic receptor characteristics in Fischer 344 rats. Mechanisms of Ageing and Development, 84, 157–169.

149. MacDonnell, S.M., Kubo, H., Crabbe, D.L., Renna, B.F., Reger, P.O., Mohara, J., Smithwick, L.A., Koch, W.J., Houser, S.R., Libonati, J.R. (2005). Improved myocardial β-adrenergic responsiveness and signaling with exercise training in hypertension. Circulation, 111, 3420–3428.

150. Hammond, H.K., White, F.C., Brunton, L.L., Longhurst, J.C. (1987). Association of decreased myocardial β-receptors and chronotropic response to isoproterenol and exercise in pigs following chronic dynamic exercise. Circulation Research, 60, 720–726.

151. Bers, D.M. (2002). Cardiac excitation-contraction coupling. Nature, 415, 198–205.

152. Bers, D.M., Weber, C.R. (2002). Na/Ca exchange function in intact ventricular myocytes. Annals of the New York Academy Sciences, 976, 500–512.

153. Sipido, K.R., Volders, P.G.A., de Groot, S.H., Verdonck, F., Van de Werf, F., Wellens, H.J. J., Vos, M.A. (2000). Enhanced Ca^{2+} release and Na^+-Ca^{2+} exchange activity in hypertrophied canine ventricular myocytes. Potential link between contractile adaption and arrhythmogenesis. Circulation, 102, 2137–2144.

154. Sipido, K.R., Bito, V., Antoons, G., Volder, P.G., Vos, M.A. (2007). Na/Ca exchange and cardiac arrhythmias. Annals of the New York Academy Sciences, 1099, 339–348.

155. Philipson, K.D., Nicoll, D.A. (2000). Sodium-calcium exchange: a molecular prospective. Annual Review of Physiology, 62, 111–133.

156. Satoh, H., Ginsburg, K.S., Qing, K., Terada, H., Hayashi, H., Bers, D.M. (2000). KB-R7943 block of Ca^{2+} influx Na^+/Ca^{2+} exchange does not alter twitches or glycoside Inotropy but prevents Ca^{2+} overload in Rat ventricular myocytes. Circulation, 101, 1441–1446.

157. Nicoll, D.A., Longoni, S., Philipson, K.D. (1990). Molecular cloning and functional expression of the cardiac sarcolemmal Na-Ca exchanger. Science, 250, 562–565.

158. Lee, S.L., Yu, A.S.L., Lytton, J. (1994). Tissue-specific expression of Na^+-Ca^{2+} exchanger isoforms. Journal of Biological Chemistry, 269, 14849–14852.

159. Philipson, K.D., Nicoll, D.A. (2000). Sodium-calcium exchange: A molecular prospective. Annual Review of Physiology, 62, 111–133.

160. Armoundas, A.A., Hobai, I.A., Tomaselli, G.F., Winslow, R.L., O'Rourke, B. (2003). Role of sodium-calcium exchange in modulating the action potential of ventricular myocytes from normal and failing hearts. Circulation Research, 93, 46–53.

161. Pogwizd, S.M., Qi, M., Yuan, W., Samarel, A.M., Bers, D.M. (1999). Upregulation of Na^+-Ca^{2+} exchanger expression and function in an arrhthmogenic rabbit model of heart failure. Circulation Research, 85, 1009–1019.

162. Pogwizd, S.M., Schlotthauer, K., Li, L., Yuan, W., Bers, D.M. (2001). Arrhythmogenesis and contractile dysfunction in heart failure: Roles of sodium-calcium exchange, inward rectifier potassium current, and residual β-adrenergic responsiveness. Circulation Research, 88, 1159–1167.

163. Lu, L., Mei, D.F., Gu, A.G., Wang, S., Lentzer, B., Gutstein, D.E., Zwas, D., Homma, S., Yi, G.H., Wang, J. (2002). Exercise training normalizes altered calcium-handling proteins during development of heart failure. Journal of Applied Physiology, 92, 1524–1530.

164. O'Rourke, B., Kass, D.A., Tomaselli, G.F., Kääb, S., Tunin, R., Marbán, E. (1999). Mechanisms of altered excitation-contraction coupling in canine tachycardia-induced heart failure. Circulation Research, 84, 562–570.

165. Tibbits, G.F., Kashihara, H., O'Reilly, K. (1989). Na^+-Ca^{2+} exchange in cardiac sarcolemma: Modulation of Ca^{2+} affinity by exercise. American Journal of Physiology Heart and Circulatory Physiology, 262, C638–C643.

166. Quinn, F.R., Currie, S., Duncan, A.M., Miller, S., Sayeed, R., Cobbe, S.M., Smith, G.L. (2003). Myocardial infarction causes increased expression but decreased activity of the myocardial Na^+-Ca^{2+} exchanger in the rabbit. Journal of Physiology, 553, 229–242.

167. Schillinger, W., Schneider, H., Minami, K., Ferrari, R., Hasenfuss, G. (2002). Importance of sympathetic activation for the expression of Na^+-Ca^{2+} exchanger in end-stage failing human myocardium. European Heart Journal, 23, 1118–1124.

168. Wei, S.K., Ruknudin, A., Hanlon, S.U., McCurley, J.M., Schulze, D.H., Haigney, M.C. (2003). Protein kinase A hyperphosphorylation increases basal current but decreases beta-adrenergic responsiveness of the sarcolemmal $Na + -Ca2 +$ exchanger in failing pig myocytes. Circulation Research, 92, 897–903.

169. Wisløff, U., Loennechen, J.P., Currie, S., Smith, G.L., Ellingsen, Ø. (2000). Aerobic exercise reduces cardiomyocyte hypertrophy and increases contractility, Ca^{2+} sensitivity and SERCA-2 in rat after myocardial infarction. Cardiovascular Research, 54, 162–174.

170. Bigger, J.T. Jr., Fleiss, J.L., Kleiger, R., Miller, J.P., Rolnitzky, M., The Multicenter Post-Infarction Research Group. (1984). The relationship among ventricular arrhythmias, left ventricular dysfunction, and mortality in the 2 years after myocardial infarction. Circulation, 69, 250–258.

171. Cheung, J.Y., Song, J., Rothblum, L.I., Zhang, X.-Q. (2004). Exercise training improves cardiac function postinfarction: Special emphasis on recent controversies on $Na^{+}-Ca^{2+}$ exchanger. Exercise and Sport Sciences Reviews, 32, 83–89.

172. Palmer, B.M., Lynch, J.M., Synder, S.M., Moore, R.L. (1999). Effects of chronic run training on Na^{+}-dependent Ca^{2+} efflux from rat left ventricular myocytes. Journal of Applied Physiology, 86, 584–591.

173. Zhang, X.-Q., Ng, Y.-C., Musch, T.I., Moore, R.L., Zelis, R., Cheung, J.Y. (1998). Sprint training attenuates myocyte hypertrophy and improves $Ca2 +$ homeostasis in postinfarction myocytes. Journal of Applied Physiology, 84, 544–552.

174. Abildstrom, S.Z., Kobler, L., Torp-Pedersen, C. (1999). Epidemiology of arrhythmic and sudden death in the chronic phase of ischemic heart disease. Cardiac Electrophysiology Reviews, 3, 177–179.

175. Zipes, D.P., Wellens, H.J. (1998). Sudden cardiac death. Circulation, 98, 2334–2351.

176. Zheng, Z.-J., Croft, J.B., Giles, W.H., Mensah, G.A. (2001). Sudden cardiac death in the United States, 1989 to 1998. Circulation, 104, 2158–2163.

177. Booth, F.W., Gordon, S.E., Carlson, C.J., Hamilton, M.T. (2000). Waging war on chronic disease: primary prevention through exercise biology. Journal of Applied Physiology, 88, 774–777.

CHAPTER 21

Dietary Omega-3 Fatty Acids as a Nonpharmacological Antiarrhythmic Intervention

BARRY LONDON and J. MICHAEL FRANGISKAKIS

21.1 INTRODUCTION

Many studies have shown that omega-3 (n-3) polyunsaturated fatty acids (PUFAs) provide protection against heart disease, including both myocardial infarction and arrhythmias [1–4]. The dietary intake of n-3 PUFAs has decreased in developed countries and the ratio of dietary omega-6 (n-6) to n-3 PUFAs has increased, suggesting that a deficiency in n-3 fatty acid intake may contribute to cardiovascular risk [5, 6]. As a result, the American Heart Association recommends that all adults eat fatty fish at least twice each week and that patients with coronary heart disease (CHD) consume approximately 1 g/day of n-3 fatty acids [7, 8].

The mechanisms by which n-3 PUFAs protect against arrhythmias remain uncertain, data from large animal models is lacking, and recent randomized trials have not consistently shown that n-3 PUFAs decrease arrhythmias in high-risk populations [9–12]. In addition, the recommendations for dietary supplementation have been questioned and are not uniformly followed by cardiologists and patients [13]. This result led to a recent workshop sponsored by the National Heart, Lung, and Blood Institute and the Office of Dietary Supplements, which called for additional basic, translational, and clinical research on n-3 PUFAs and arrhythmias [14].

This chapter will review fatty acid biochemistry, the mechanisms by which n-3 PUFAs may affect arrhythmia, animal studies, epidemiological studies, and randomized clinical trials. Areas of uncertainty and recommendations for future research will be emphasized.

Novel Therapeutic Targets for Antiarrhythmic Drugs, Edited by George Edward Billman
Copyright © 2010 John Wiley & Sons, Inc.

21.2 FATTY ACID METABOLISM

21.2.1 Nomenclature

Fatty acids are carboxylic acids made up of a lipophilic carbon backbone and the polar acidic group (R–COOH; Figure 21.1A). The standard nomenclature to describe fatty acids is x:y(n-z), where x is the length of the carbon chain, y is the number of double bonds, and z is the number of the carbon atom relative to the $-CH_3$ or omega (n-) end. The properties of the clinically important fatty acids are largely determined by the length of the carbon chain (long chain, $n = 20$–22; intermediate chain, $n = 18$), the number of double bonds (saturated $= 0$, monounsaturated $= 1$, polyunsaturated ≥ 2), and the location of the first double bond relative to the $-CH_3$ end (n-3, n-6, or n-9) [5, 6].

21.2.2 Dietary Fatty Acids

Long and intermediate chain fatty acids, which are known as essential fatty acids, cannot be synthesized by humans and must be eaten as part of the diet. The most common dietary fatty acids are as follows: omega-6 linoleic acid [18:2(n-6)] found in corn oil, safflower oil, peanuts, and soybeans; omega-3 long chain eicosapentaenoic

Fatty Acid Nomenclature

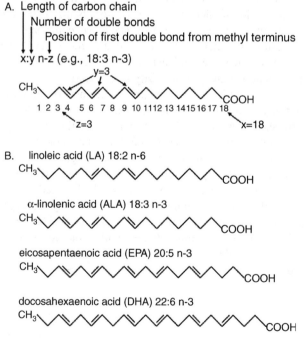

Figure 21.1. Fatty acid nomenclature and examples. **A**, General nomenclature. **B**, Specific examples of dietary intermediate- and long-chain fatty acids.

acid [EPA, 20:5(n-3)] and docosahexaenoic acid [DHA, 22:6(n-3)] found predominantly in fish oils; and omega-3 intermediate chain alpha linolenic acid [ALA, 18:3 (n-3)] found in flaxseed oil, canola oil, and walnuts (Figure 21.1B). Dietary ALA can be partly converted (4–8%) into EPA by the enzyme delta-6 desaturase, although the efficacy seems to vary considerably among individuals [15]. Competition between dietary n-3 and n-6 fatty acids determines the tissue proportions of n-3 and n-6 highly unsaturated fatty acids. These tissue characteristics can be predicted in animals and humans based on diet [16, 17].

21.2.3 Roles of Polyunsaturated Fatty Acids

Fatty acids are important sources of energy for mammalian cells and are the major energy source for the heart under normal conditions [18]. PUFAs are major components of cell membranes and can affect membrane fluidity, enzyme activity, and ion channel activity [19]. PUFAs are also converted into many bioactive substances with autocrine and paracrine properties. EPA is a precursor to the eicosanoids including prostaglandins (platelet aggregation inhibitors), thromboxanes (vasoconstrictors), and leukotrienes (inflammatory mediators). DPA is a precursor to docosanoids and some resolvins (reduce cellular inflammation) [20, 21]. Each of these biological activities could potentially alter arrhythmic risk based on prior works that suggest roles for ischemia and/or inflammation in arrhythmia.

21.3 CELLULAR MECHANISMS

21.3.1 Ion Channel Blockade

N-3 PUFAs have been shown to block cardiac ion channels directly, with evidence derived from studies using heterologous expression systems or cardiac myocytes superfused with n-3 PUFAs as well as from animal models fed diets rich in n-3 PUFAs [22, 23]. Modifications in ion channels can alter arrhythmogenicity by changing action potential duration, intracellular Ca^{2+} release, conduction velocity, and likelihood of afterdepolarizations. The relevance of the individual ion channel effects to clinical arrhythmias has been considerably more difficult to dissect.

21.3.1.1 Sodium Channels. In heterologous expression systems used on either *Xenopus* oocytes or mammalian human embryonic kidney (HEK) cells, the n-3 PUFAs DHA and EPA block the cardiac Na^+ channel SCN5A in a dose-dependent manner [24, 25]. The coexpression of Na^+ channels with its β-1 subunit can modify the effects, and single-point mutations in SCN5A have identified regions of interactions of DHA [25, 26]. Similarly, DHA and EPA block the cardiac Na^+ current (I_{Na}) in neonatal and adult rat ventricular myocytes [27, 28]. Interestingly, the noninactivating component of the I_{Na} may be preferentially altered [27]. Of note, the n-3 PUFA concentrations required for Na^+ channel blockade are similar to plasma concentrations that have been measured in human trials and animal studies that demonstrate protection against arrhythmias and/or sudden death [22, 23].

The changes in I_{Na} may alter arrhythmic risk by several mechanisms. Decreases in I_{Na} may cause arrhythmias as in Brugada syndrome, although selective attenuation of late currents would tend to shorten action potential duration (APD) and the QT interval, prevent afterdepolarizations, and decrease arrhythmias [29]. Decreases in I_{Na} should also decrease conduction velocity, which could selectively depress slow conduction in pathways in the border zone around scars similar to type I antiarrhythmic drugs [30].

21.3.1.2 Potassium Channels.
DHA and EPA inhibit several cardiac K^+ channels at concentrations similar to those that interact with, and block, Na^+ channels. Kv1.5, which is the channel responsible for the human atrial I_{Kur} and the mouse I_{Kslow1} atrial and ventricular delayed rectifier currents, is inhibited by n-3 PUFAs [31, 32]. DHA also inhibits Kv1.2 delayed rectifier channels and Kv4.3 channels responsible for the transient outward current I_{to} [33–35]. Inhibition of the atrial current I_{Kur} could lengthen the effective refractory period and protect against atrial fibrillation [36]. In addition, inhibition of ventricular K^+ channels could both lengthen APD and modify transmembrane Ca^{2+} current and Ca^{2+} transients [3].

N-3 PUFAs inhibit ATP-sensitive K^+ currents (I_{K-ATP}) in neurons from the mammalian hypothalamus [37]. Similar channels are important for glucose regulation in pancreatic β-cells and in protecting cardiac myocytes from ischemic injury [38]. It is not known whether n-3 PUFAs affect cardiac I_{K-ATP}. In addition, it is possible that the redox environment within the myocardium may modulate some electrophysiological effects of n-3 PUFAs on some K^+ channels [39].

21.3.1.3 Calcium Channels and Exchangers.
DHA and EPA reduce the peak inward transmembrane L-type Ca^{2+} current, I_{Ca}, which is responsible for triggering Ca^{2+} release from the sarcoplasmic reticulum (SR) in cardiac myocytes and reduce the efficacy of dihydropyridine agonists and antagonists [40–44]. N-3 PUFAs can also reduce T-type Ca^{2+} currents [45]. This could potentially decrease Ca^{2+} influx into cells, prevent SR Ca^{2+} overload, and decrease arrhythmias under conditions of Ca^{2+} overload, such as digoxin toxicity, ischemia, and/or heart failure [46].

DHA and EPA also seem to affect the properties of the ryanodine receptor (RyR2), which is the channel responsible for Ca^{2+} release from the SR. Increased SR Ca^{2+} release leads to the depolarizing transient inward current (I_{ti}) and to delayed afterdepolarizations through the sodium–calcium exchanger (NCX), and mutations that increase SR leak cause the inherited catecholaminergic polymorphic ventricular tachycardia [47]. Measurements of Ca^{2+} sparks in isolated rodent, rabbit, and human cardiac myocytes; contraction in detergent skinned myocytes; and Ca^{2+} flux in isolated SR vesicles show that n-3 PUFAs decrease Ca^{2+} release and increase SR Ca^{2+} content [41, 44, 48–50]. Although the direct effects of n-3 PUFAs on NCX function is less clear, stabilization of RyR2 would be predicted to suppress triggered activity and arrhythmias.

The electrogenic NCX removes one Ca^{2+} ion in exchange for three Na^+ ions during diastole and may allow Ca^{2+} influx during the action potential. It is responsible for $\sim$30% of cytoplasmic Ca^{2+} removal during each heart beat in the rabbit as opposed to only $\sim$10% in the rat [51]. Dietary supplementation of pigs with a diet rich in n-3 PUFAs resulted in $\sim$60% reduction in NCX current [52]. Consequently, the reduced NCX current may contribute to the antiarrhythmic effects suggested for n-3 PUFAs.

It is clear that n-3 PUFAs can affect multiple ion channels, and the overall effect on myocytes may both be complex and species dependent. Superfusion with EPA and DPA leads to decreased excitability in both rat and guinea pig myocytes, which is consistent with blockade of I_{Na} [53]. At low concentrations in the rat, DHA caused prolongation of APD and increased shortening amplitude, whereas EPA initially increased and then decreased shortening amplitude [44, 53]. In contrast, these same agents only shortened APD and decreased cell shortening in guinea pig myocytes. These differences could be explained, for example, by the absence of the I_{to} K^+ current in guinea pig ventricular myocytes.

Acute superfusion of n-3 PUFAs onto isolated cardiac myocytes, intravenous infusion into animal models, and chronic dietary supplementation may lead to different effects on cardiac ion channels. Unfortunately, relatively little data on ion channel expression and function are available from animal models of arrhythmias following dietary supplementation with n-3 PUFAs. EPA and DHA increase SR Ca^{2+} content in isolated rat cardiac myocytes [41, 44]. In contrast, dietary supplementation with fish oil did not increase SR Ca^{2+} content in rats [54]. Despite these differences, superfusion of n-3 PUFAs onto cells and dietary supplementation both suppress spontaneous Ca^{2+} waves and can reduce dysynchrony in response to isoproterenol [41, 54–57]. Thus, the relationship of findings from superfused isolated cardiac myocytes to arrhythmias *in vivo* remains unclear.

21.3.1.4 Connexins. Connexins, which are formed by hemichannels composed of connexon proteins, mediate intercellular communication for ions and small molecules. Several free fatty acids, including DHA and EPA, uncouple connexin-mediated communication between rat ventricular myocytes [58]. The relevance of these changes to cardiac arrhythmias remains uncertain.

21.3.2 Direct Membrane Effects

Dietary supplementation with n-3 PUFAs leads to increased n-3 fatty acid content in cell membranes that is not observed during acute, intravenous administration of the agents [22, 46, 59–63]. The changes occur rapidly, with dietary supplementation of rats with either fish oil or n-3 PUFAs, both doubling the content of DHA in myocardial membranes after 2 days and reducing arrhythmia susceptibility within 5 days [63, 64]. The n-3 PUFA content of the membrane may affect trafficking of ion channels to the surface membrane as well as localization of channels in subcellular compartments, such as lipid rafts and caveolae [65]. These trafficking changes could alter the number of functional channels in the membrane and affect posttranslational modifications such as phosphorylation and glycosylation.

21.3.3 Phosphorylation

Dietary n-3 PUFA supplementation in animals can reduce β-adrenergic receptor responsiveness, inhibit the activity of protein kinase A (PKA), and inhibit calmodulin kinase II (CaMKII) [66–70]. PKA mediates β-adrenergic receptor signaling and increases I_{Ca} and the K^+ current I_{Ks}. β-adrenergic receptor activation predisposes to arrhythmias and sudden death, whereas β-adrenergic receptor blockers are among the few pharmacological agents that prevent sudden death [71]. CaMKII, similarly, plays an important role in arrhythmia susceptibility in mice and rabbits [72, 73].

21.3.4 Inflammation

Thromboxane A2 and $PGF_{2\alpha}$, which are metabolites of the n-6 fatty acid arachidonic acid, have been implicated in the genesis of tachycardias associated with systemic inflammation [74]. DHA has been shown to reduce inflammatory signaling associated with increased cellular Ca^{2+} and activation of nuclear factor-κB (NF-κB) in neutrophils exposed to pneumococcal toxins [75]. In the setting of ischemia, phospholipase A2 is activated, stimulating the production of additional arachidonate-derived metabolites including platelet activating factor. These mediators have been implicated in ischemia-mediated sudden cardiac death [76]. Dietary n-3 PUFAs are incorporated into myocardial membranes, reduce production of proinflammatory metabolites, and suppress arrhythmias.

21.3.5 Summary

N-3 PUFAs can affect basic arrhythmia mechanisms in several ways. Changes in ion channel function, ion channel surface membrane expression, and Ca^{2+} handling can alter APD, modify triggered activity including afterdepolarizations, and decrease arrhythmia initiation. In addition, changes in excitability, cellular coupling, and inflammation could alter the local substrate that permits reentrant arrhythmias. Little is known about the basic effects of n-3 PUFAs on spatial and temporal dispersion of the electrophysiological properties in the normal myocardium or of their effects on the conduction system. In addition, most arrhythmias occur in the setting of ischemia, prior infarction, and decreased systolic function [77]. Thus, the relative importance of each effect of n-3 PUFAs to arrhythmia susceptibility *in vivo* requires additional study.

21.4 ANIMAL STUDIES

Animal models allow access to physiological measurements and tissues not easily available in human trials and may shed light on antiarrhythmic mechanisms. Studies using short-term intravenous injections and long-term dietary supplementation with n-3 PUFAs have been performed [78, 79].

21.4.1 Acute Intravenous Effects of n-3 PUFAs

Slow intravenous infusion of fish oil extract, DHA, EPA, and α-linolenic acid reduce ventricular fibrillation (VF) in a canine model of exercise-induced adrenergic stress and myocardial ischemia [22, 80, 81]. These findings are analogous to the cellular and molecular studies that have largely focused on immediate responses to these agents. Acute intravenous infusion of n-3 PUFAs also affects electrical remodeling of the dog atrium [82]. The decrease in atrial effective refractory period following rapid atrial pacing was attenuated by n-3 but not n-6 PUFAs.

21.4.2 Dietary Supplementation with n-3 PUFAs

21.4.2.1 Rodents. N-3 fatty acids from fish or plant sources have been shown to decrease arrhythmias and improve survival in rats subjected to surgical myocardial infarctions (MIs), reversible surgical ischemia, and ischemia reperfusion [60–62, 83]. Similarly, dietary n-3 PUFAs improved recovery from ischemic insults, provided resistance to arrhythmias, decreased calcium overload, and prevented changes in Ca^{2+}-handling proteins in isolated hearts, papillary muscles, and isolated cardiac myocytes [54, 59, 64, 84, 85]. In addition, dietary supplementation of aged spontaneously hypertensive rats with n-3 PUFAs suppressed inducible VF without affecting fibrosis, hypertrophy, or abnormal gap junction distribution [86].

Transgenic and gene-targeted mice have helped to elucidate arrhythmia mechanisms related to ion channel mutations and heart failure [87]. To date, they have had little impact regarding the mechanism of action of n-3 PUFAs.

21.4.2.2 Dogs. Dogs treated with EPA (100 mg/kg/day for 8 weeks) showed a reduction in arrhythmias following coronary ligation and treatment with 0.025 mg/kg of digoxin [46]. There was also an increase in the ratio of n-3 PUFAs to n-6 PUFAs in the heart and platelets, along with increased activity of the SR Ca^{2+} ATPase (SERCA2a.)

21.4.2.3 Pigs. Cardiac myocytes isolated from pigs fed a diet rich in fish oil for 8 weeks had shorter action potentials, less E-4031–induced APD prolongation, and fewer E-4031–induced early afterdepolarizations (EADs) than myocytes isolated from pigs fed sunflower oil [88]. Surprisingly, hearts isolated from pigs fed a diet rich in fish oil or sunflower oil and perfused had more episodes of spontaneous ventricular tachycardia following left anterior descending coronary artery ligation than hearts from pigs fed a control diet [89]. This finding seems to be caused by an increase in excitable myocardium early after coronary ligation.

21.4.2.4 Marmoset Monkeys. Programmed electrical stimulation of the hearts of Marmoset monkeys fed either tuna fish oil or sunflower seed oil for 30 months triggered fewer arrhythmias than in monkeys fed saturated fat diets [90]. The diets rich in PUFAs decreased inducible arrhythmias at baseline, during intravenous isoproterenol infusion, and in the setting of reversible surgical ischemia. Mortality was also reduced.

21.4.2.5 Summary. On the whole, the findings from animal models seem to support the benefits of n-3 fatty acids and their potential role in arrhythmia prevention. Additional well-controlled studies of sudden cardiac death in large animal models are needed, however.

21.5 CLINICAL STUDIES

21.5.1 Observational Studies

Consumption of fish rich in n-3 PUFAs seems to lower the risk of dying from coronary heart disease [3, 7]. Populations with diets high in seafood (e.g., 400 g/day), such as the Greenland Inuits and Japanese living on Okinawa, were shown to have a low incidence of death from heart disease [91, 92]. These findings catalyzed several studies to test whether n-3 PUFAs prevent arrhythmias and sudden cardiac death.

21.5.1.1 Total Cardiovascular Mortality. Many, large prospective cardio-vascular cohort studies compared the dietary history of fish intake with the risk of all-cause cardiovascular mortality [93–98]. Some of these studies showed that higher dietary fish intake was associated with lower cardiovascular mortality [97, 98]. Others did not, possibly because of the absence of a significant proportion of the population with little or no fish intake [93–96]. A meta-analysis combined these studies and reported a statistically significant 7% lower risk of cardiac mortality for each 20 g/day of fish intake [99]. Of note, the meta-analysis of these and additional studies failed to show any association between similar levels of dietary n-3 PUFA intake and nonfatal myocardial infarction [99–103]. The presence of an effect on mortality without an effect on nonfatal myocardial infarction raises the possibility that n-3 PUFAs selectively decrease fatal arrhythmic events.

The intermediate chain n-3 PUFA ALA is present in nuts; if beneficial in arrhythmia prevention, it could be useful to populations where fish is not readily available or palatable and would circumvent concerns regarding toxin accumulation in fish oil [104]. The evidence for a direct benefit of ALA on arrhythmia risk in humans is less well developed than for the long chain n-3 PUFAs EPA and DHA, however [3]. Inverse associations between the dietary intake of ALA and risk of fatal CHD have been observed in most but not all prospective cohort studies [98, 105–108].

21.5.1.2 Sudden Cardiac Death. Several studies examined the effect of dietary n-3 PUFA consumption equivalent to one fatty fish meal per week on sudden death. In a population-based, case-control study of patients suffering sudden cardiac arrest in Seattle, a dietary intake of n-3 fatty acids was associated with a 50% decreased risk of cardiac arrest, whereas high blood levels of PUFAs were associated with a 70% decreased risk [109]. A prospective examination of subjects in the male U.S. Physicians' Health Study showed a 52% decrease in sudden cardiac death for similar levels of n-3 PUFA dietary intake and an even greater decrease associated with blood n-3 PUFA levels [100, 110]. Another prospective study of >45,000 healthy men showed a 42% decrease in sudden cardiac death risk associated with n-3 PUFA intake independent of n-6 PUFA intake [111]. Finally, a study conducted among individuals over age 65 showed higher serum n-3 PUFA levels and similar protection against sudden cardiac death following consumption of baked, but not fried fish [103].

Two studies have examined the association between ALA intake and sudden cardiac death. In the Health Professional Follow-Up Study, ALA intake was not significantly related to risk of sudden cardiac death [111]. In contrast, high levels of ALA intake were associated with an ~40% decreased risk of sudden cardiac death in the Nurses' Health Study [112]. Similar to the data reported for EPA and DHA, the protective effects of ALA were specific for sudden cardiac death and not related to coronary artery disease.

Ventricular tachyarrhythmias underlie approximately 80–90% of sudden cardiac deaths [113]. Thus, while subject to some limitations, these studies suggest that n-3 PUFA consumption and high levels of n-3 PUFAs in the blood may protect against ventricular arrhythmias.

21.5.1.3 Atrial Fibrillation.
The association between n-3 PUFA intake and atrial arrhythmias is uncertain. In one study composed of 4815 indsividuals over age 65, subjects who consumed the most fish had a 31% reduction in risk of new-onset atrial fibrillation during 12 years of follow-up [114]. In contrast, the Danish Diet, Cancer, and Health Study of 47,949 younger individuals found that increased fish consumption was associated with up to a 34% increased incidence of atrial fibrillation over 5.7 years of follow-up [115]. In the Rotterdam Study of 5184 subjects, dietary intake of DHA/EPA and fish were not associated with the risk of developing atrial fibrillation [116].

21.5.2 Randomized Trials

To test directly whether there was a causal relationship between n-3 PUFA dietary intake, arrhythmias, and sudden cardiac death, trials randomizing subjects to either diets rich in fish or fish oil supplements were undertaken.

21.5.2.1 Dietary Modifications.
Randomized treatment trials were conducted among patients with known preexisting cardiac disease. The Diet and Reinfarction Trial (DART) randomized 2033 men after myocardial infarction to either get or not get advice to eat at least two portions of fatty fish per week [117]. The fish advice arm had a 29% reduction in 2-year all-cause mortality, largely related to cardiac mortality, without any decrease in nonfatal MIs. The DART-2 trial subsequently randomized 3114 men with chronic angina to (1) no dietary advice or (2) fatty fish or to n-3 PUFA supplementation with fish oil capsules [118]. Surprisingly, the investigators found a 26% higher risk of cardiac death and a 54% increased risk of sudden death among men randomly assigned to the fish advice group. This second trial, while suffering from significant technical difficulties, is difficult to reconcile with the observational studies on dietary fish intake.

In the Lyon Diet Heart Study, a Mediterranean diet rich in ALA after a myocardial infarction was associated with higher levels of ALA and a 47–72% reduction in combined cardiovascular endpoints that was sustained for up to 4 years [119, 120]. Unfortunately, differences between the treatment and control groups in this non-placebo-controlled study make the findings difficult to interpret.

21.5.2.2 N-3 PUFA Supplementation. Many trials have tested the efficacy of n-3 fatty acid supplements [121–127]. The largest by far, the GISSI (Gruppo Italiano per la Sperimentazione della Streptochinasi nell'Infarto miocardico) Prevenzione trial, randomized 11,324 patients with recent myocardial infarction to a combination of low-dose n-3 PUFAs (850 mg EPA and DHA daily) in an open-label fashion [121]. The patients assigned to n-3 PUFA had a significant reduction in death and nonfatal myocardial infarction, largely because of a 45% reduction in sudden cardiac death that was evident within several months; there was no benefit on nonfatal myocardial infarction or stroke [128]. Subgroup analyses suggested that the benefit may be greatest among patients with systolic dysfunction left ventricular ejection fraction ([LVEF] $\leq 40\%$) [129]. Thus, the GISSI-Prevenzione trial supports a benefit to n-3 PUFA supplementation and was a major factor driving the American Heart Association recommendations for consumption of 1 g/day of EPA plus DHA in subjects with heart disease [8]. The findings of this and the other smaller studies are limited, however, by the lack of a placebo control group.

The Japan EPA Lipid Intervention Study (JELIS), randomized 18,645 participants with hypercholesterolemia, to a statin plus high dose EPA (1.8 grams/day) versus a statin alone in an open-label fashion [130]. Treatment with EPA decreased a combined end point of major coronary events by 19%, driven by unstable angina and nonfatal myocardial infarction. Similar results were present in subgroup analysis based on the presence or absence of a history of coronary artery disease, although only the secondary prevention subgroup reached statistical significance. There was no difference in total cardiac death or sudden death between the treatment groups, possibly because of the high baseline fish intake and low cardiac death rate in the Japanese population [131].

As a follow-up to the GISSI-Prevenzione trial, the GISSI-HF trial randomized, in a double-blinded 2×2 factorial design, with a heterogeneous group of 6,975 patients with class-II-IV heart failure ($\sim$50% ischemic) to receive either 1 g of EPA/DHA, rosuvastatin, both active drugs, or placebos for a mean of 3.9 years [132]. Treatment with n-3 PUFAs led to a statistically significant but small (9%) decrease in total mortality but no change in sudden cardiac death.

The Norwegian vegetable oil experiment of 1965–1966 randomized over 13,000 participants to an ALA supplement (linseed oil 10 mL/day; ALA 5.25 g/d) or placebo [133]. Unfortunately, insufficient events occurred in the primary prevention population in 1 year to support any conclusions.

The Omega Trial is an ongoing randomized, double-blind trial that seeks to randomize 3800 patients within 1 year of an myocardial infarction to 1 g of long-chain n-3 fatty acids or placebo, with sudden cardiac death as the primary end point [134]. The Alpha Omega Trial is an ongoing randomized, double-blind trial in 4800 Dutch men with an myocardial infarction during the last 10 years [135]. Participants are being randomized in a 2×2 design to 40 months of low dose EPA + DHA (400 mg), ALA (2 g), both agents, or placebos with coronary mortality as the primary end point and sudden cardiac death as a secondary end points.

Two other large-scale, randomized, placebo-controlled trials are also planned in diabetic patients. The ASCEND (A Study of Cardiovascular Events in Diabetes) Trial plans to randomize 10,000 diabetic patients in a 2×2 factorial design to 100 mg aspirin, 1 g n-3 PUFAs, both, or placebo [136]. The ORIGIN (Outcome Reduction with Initial Glargine InterventioN) Trial plans to enroll 12,500 diabetic patients with a history of cardiovascular disease in a 2×2 factorial design comparing insulin glargine, 1 g n-3 fatty PUFA supplementation, both, or placebo [137]. The primary end points for both trials will be composite end points involving serious cardiovascular events.

21.5.2.3 *Implantable Cardioverter-Defibrillator (ICD) Trials.* The reduction in sudden cardiac death risk reported in observational studies and some clinical trials, along with the basic science data, has led to the hypothesis that n-3 PUFAs are antiarrhythmic in humans. ICDs have created the potential to test directly whether long-chain n-3 PUFAs reduce ventricular arrhythmias. In one small study, acute infusion of n-3 PUFAs was shown to decrease arrhythmias in subjects with ICDs during acute electrophysiology testing by programmed stimulation [138]. To test more clinically relevant uses of n-3 PUFAs, three double-blind, randomized trials of n-3 PUFA supplementation have been performed using patients who had an ICD in place for a life-threatening arrhythmia [9–11].

Raitt et al. [11] reported that 1.8 g of fish oil tended to increase the risk of ventricular tachycardia (VT) or VF in patients with ICDs, with 51% of patients assigned to fish oil having received ICD therapies compared with 41% of patients assigned to placebo at 1 year ($p = 0.19$) [11]. In the subgroup of patients whose prior arrhythmia was VT, 66% of patients assigned to fish oil received ICD therapies compared with 43% of patients assigned to placebo ($P < 0.01$). Conversely, the Fatty Acid Arrhythmia Trial (FAAT) reported that 4 g of fish oil per day tended to decrease the risk of VT/VF, with a 28% event rate at 1 year in those assigned to fish oil compared with 39% of patients assigned to placebo ($P = 0.057$) [10]. If therapies for episodes of probable VT/VF were included, or if noncompliant patients were excluded, the risk reduction became significant ($P < 0.04$). Finally, the Study on Omega-3 Fatty acids and Ventricular Arrhythmia (SOFA) showed no difference following treatment with 2 g of fish oil, with a 30% event rate at 1 year in those assigned to fish oil compared with 33% of patients assigned to placebo ($P = 0.33$) [9]. In the subgroup of patients who previously had a myocardial infarction, there was a trend toward a beneficial effect of fish oil ($P = 0.13$).

Possible explanations for the differing results in these trials include the dosage of EPA/DHA and the amount of fish the patients were allowed to eat (Table 21.1) [9–11]. Consistent with this, baseline n-3 fatty acid levels in red blood cells were higher in the Raitt trial (4.7%) as compared with the FAAT trial (3.4%), and it is possible that patients in the Raitt and SOFA trials were already eating sufficient dietary n-3 PUFAs

Table 21.1. Implantable Cardioverter-Defibrillator Trial Comparison

Study	Number of Subjects	Enrollment Criteria	Therapy	Placebo	Red Cell Membrane n-3 PUFA	Follow-up Duration	Primary End Point Results at 1 Year
Raitt [11]	200	• 6 United States centers • 02/99-07/03 • Hx: VT/VF within 3 months • Excl: >1 fatty fish/week or fish supplements in prior month	1.8 g fish oil/day (1.3 g EPA + DHA)	1.8 g olive oil/day (0 g EPA + DHA)	~8.3% Rx ~4.7% Plac (P < 0.05)	24 Months	51% Rx 41% Plac (n = 104; P = 0.19)
FAAT [10]	402	• 18 United States centers • 04/99-09/01 • Hx: cardiac arrest, VT/VF, syncope with positive EPS within 12 months • Excl: N/A	4 g fish oil/day (2.6 g EPA + DHA)	1.8 g olive oil/day (0 g EPA + DHA)	7.6% Rx 3.5% Plac (P < 0.0001)	12 Months	28% Rx 39% Plac (n = 135; P = 0.057)
SOFA [9]	546	• 26 European centers • 10/01-08/04 • Hx: VT/VF within 12 months • Excl: supplemental n-3 PUFAs in prior 3 months or >8 gm n-3 PUFAs from seafood/month	2 g fish oil/day (0.8 g EPA + DHA)	2 g sunflower oil/day	N/A	12 Months	30% Rx 33% Plac (n = 171; P = 0.33)

Abbreviations: Hx = history; Excl = exclusion criteria; EPS = electrical programmed stimulation; Rx = therapy arm; Plac = placebo arm.

to obtain the maximum antiarrhythmic benefit [100]. In addition, limiting patients enrollment to those who have already experienced an episode of sustained VT/VF increases the event rate, but it may not be representative of subjects shown to benefit from n-3 PUFAs in prior observational and randomized trials. Similarly, inclusion of antitachycardia pacing as an end point in all of the trials likely led to the inclusion of some clinically insignificant arrhythmias [139].

21.5.2.4 Atrial Fibrillation. AFib is common after coronary artery bypass surgery CABG. In one study evaluating the utility of fish oil in limiting the onset of atrial fibrillation after CABG, 160 patients scheduled for CABG were randomized to 2 g/day of fish oil beginning 5 days prior to surgery and continuing until hospital discharge [140]. Postoperative atrial fibrillation was reduced in subjects randomized to n-3 fatty acids (15.2%) as compared with those in the control group (33.3%, $P = 0.013$).

21.5.3 Surrogate Markers for Arrhythmias

Noninvasive markers are used to estimate the risk of cardiac events including sudden death. Several studies have examined the impact of n-3 PUFAs on these intermediate end points.

21.5.3.1 Heart Rate and Heart Rate Variability. Both resting heart rate and heart rate during exercise have been associated with the risk of sudden cardiac death [141]. A meta-analysis of 30 randomized trials demonstrated that fish oil decreased resting heart rate by 2.5 beats/min in subjects with baseline heart rates $\geq$69 beats/min [142]. Decreased heart rate variability reflects changes in the autonomic nervous system and is characteristic of patients with severe heart disease and an increased risk of sudden death. A 12-week regimen of dietary supplementation with either 2.0 or 6.6 g/day n-3 PUFAs resulted in increased heart rate variability in men [143, 144].

21.5.3.2 QTc Prolongation. Prolongation of the corrected QT interval (QTc) on the surface electrocardiogram (ECG) is associated with increased risk of arrhythmias in patients with inherited ion channel mutations (long QT syndrome) and in patients with heart failure [145, 146]. In the ATTICA study of 3042 healthy Greek men and women, subjects who consumed at least 300 g per week of fish had a mean QTc that was 13.6% ($\sim$60 ms) lower than those with no fish intake [147].

21.5.4 Summary

In summary, considerable epidemiological evidence supports a role for n-3 PUFAs in arrhythmia prevention. Randomized trials have not shown n-3 PUFA supplementation to be antiarrhythmic in all clinical settings, however. Several complexities in the trial designs, patient populations, and therapeutic regimens may explain the complexities. Additional studies will be needed to define the clinical settings where n-3 PUFAs are most beneficial.

21.6 FUTURE DIRECTIONS

Cardiac electrical activity is extremely complex. Ion channels, exchangers, and pumps have spatial and temporal gradients of expression, undergo posttranslational modifications such as phosphorylation and glycosylation, and exist in macromolecular complexes. In addition, the metabolic state of the myocyte, mechanical forces, autonomic tone, extracellular matrix, geometry, fibrosis, and scar all interact to modulate arrhythmic risk.

Ongoing efforts to understand the links between diet and cardiac rhythm more accurately have the potential to improve public health and welfare. n-3 PUFAs clearly have an impact on the fundamental elements (ion channels, exchangers, and modulators) of cardiac electrical activity. However, the translation of this understanding into evidence-based policy guidelines that can decrease the incidence of arrhythmias and sudden cardiac death requires additional basic work on cellular mechanisms, new animal models, and human trials targeted to identify both the populations that would benefit from n-3 PUFAs and the mechanisms underlying the benefit.

REFERENCES

1. Balk, E., Chung, M., Lichtenstein, A., Chew, P., Kupelnick, B., Lawrence, A., DeVine, D., Lau, J. (2004). Effects of omega-3 fatty acids on cardiovascular risk factors and intermediate markers of cardiovascular disease. Evidence Report—Technology Assessment, 2004, 1–6.

2. Wang, C., Chung, M., Lichtenstein, A., Balk, E., Kupelnick, B., DeVine, D., Lawrence, A., Lau, J. (2004). Effects of omega-3 fatty acids on cardiovascular disease. Evidence Report - Technology Assessment, 1–8.

3. Wang, C., Harris, W.S., Chung, M., Lichtenstein, A.H., Balk, E.M., Kupelnick, B., Jordan, H.S., Lau, J. (2006). n-3 Fatty acids from fish or fish-oil supplements, but not alpha-linolenic acid, benefit cardiovascular disease outcomes in primary- and secondary-prevention studies: A systematic review. American Journal of Clinical Nutrition, 84, 5–17.

4. Harris, W.S., Miller, M., Tighe, A.P., Davidson, M.H., Schaefer, E.J. (2008). Omega-3 fatty acids and coronary heart disease risk: Clinical and mechanistic perspectives. Atherosclerosis, 197, 12–24.

5. DeFilippis, A.P., Sperling, L.S. (2006). Understanding omega-3's. American Heart Journal, 151, 564–570.

6. Lands, W.E. (1992). Biochemistry and physiology of n-3 fatty acids. The Journal of the Federation of American Societies for Experimental Biology, 6, 2530–2536.

7. Kris-Etherton, P.M., Harris, W.S., Appel, L.J. (2002). Fish consumption, fish oil, omega-3 fatty acids, and cardiovascular disease. Circulation, 106, 2747–2757.

8. Kris-Etherton, P.M., Harris, W.S., Appel, L.J. (2003). Omega-3 fatty acids and cardiovascular disease: new recommendations from the American Heart Association. Arteriosclerosis, Thrombosis, and Vascular Biology. 23, 151–152.

9. Brouwer, I.A., Zock, P.L., Camm, A.J., Bocker, D., Hauer, R.N., Wever, E.F., Dullemeijer, C., Ronden, J.E., Katan, M.B., Lubinski, A., Buschler, H., Schouten, E.G. (2006). Effect

of fish oil on ventricular tachyarrhythmia and death in patients with implantable cardioverter defibrillators: The Study on Omega-3 Fatty Acids and Ventricular Arrhythmia (SOFA) randomized trial. Journal of the American Medical Association, 295, 2613–2619.

10. Leaf, A., Albert, C.M., Josephson, M., Steinhaus, D., Kluger, J., Kang, J.X., Cox, B., Zhang, H., Schoenfeld, D. (2005). Prevention of fatal arrhythmias in high-risk subjects by fish oil n-3 fatty acid intake. Circulation, 112, 2762–2768.

11. Raitt, M.H., Connor, W.E., Morris, C., Kron, J., Halperin, B., Chugh, S.S., McClelland, J., Cook, J., MacMurdy, K., Swenson, R., Connor, S.L., Gerhard, G., Kraemer, D.F., Oseran, D., Marchant, C., Calhoun, D., Shnider, R., McAnulty, J. (2005). Fish oil supplementation and risk of ventricular tachycardia and ventricular fibrillation in patients with implantable defibrillators: A randomized controlled trial. Journal of the American Medical Association, 293, 2884–2891.

12. Jenkins, D.J., Josse, A.R., Dorian, P., Burr, M.L., LaBelle Trangmar, R., Kendall, C.W., Cunnane, S.C. (2008). Heterogeneity in randomized controlled trials of long chain (fish) omega-3 fatty acids in restenosis, secondary prevention and ventricular arrhythmias. Journal of the American College of Nutrition, 27, 367–378.

13. Fish Oil Supplements. (2006). The Medical Letter, 48, 59–60.

14. London, B., Albert, C., Anderson, M.E., Giles, W.R., Van Wagoner, D.R., Balk, E., Billman, G.E., Chung, M., Lands, W., Leaf, A., McAnulty, J., Martens, J.R., Costello, R. B., Lathrop, D.A. (2007). Omega-3 fatty acids and cardiac arrhythmias: Prior studies and recommendations for future research: A report from the National Heart, Lung, and Blood Institute and Office Of Dietary Supplements Omega-3 Fatty Acids and their Role in Cardiac Arrhythmogenesis Workshop. Circulation, 116, e320–335.

15. Burdge, G. (2004). Alpha-linolenic acid metabolism in men and women: nutritional and biological implications. Current Opinion in Clinical Nutrition and Metabolic Care, 7, 137–144.

16. Lands, W.E., Libelt, B., Morris, A., Kramer, N.C., Prewitt, T.E., Bowen, P., Schmeisser, D., Davidson, M.H., Burns, J.H. (1992). Maintenance of lower proportions of (n - 6) eicosanoid precursors in phospholipids of human plasma in response to added dietary (n - 3) fatty acids. Biochimica et Biophysica Acta, 1180, 147–162.

17. Essential Fatty Acids: Relating Diets and Tissue HUFA. http://efaeducation.nih.gov/sig/hufacalc.html. Accessed January 23, 2009.

18. Park, T.S., Yamashita, H., Blaner, W.S., Goldberg, I.J. (2007). Lipids in the heart: A source of fuel and a source of toxins. Current Opinion in Lipidology, 18, 277–282.

19. Youdim, K.A., Martin, A., Joseph, J.A. (2000). Essential fatty acids and the brain: Possible health implications. International Journal of Developmental Neuroscience, 18, 383–399.

20. Serhan, C.N. (2005). Novel eicosanoid and docosanoid mediators: Resolvins, docosatrienes, and neuroprotectins. Current Opinion in Clinical Nutrition and Metabolic Care, 8, 115–121.

21. Serhan, C.N., Hong, S., Gronert, K., Colgan, S.P., Devchand, P.R., Mirick, G., Moussignac, R.L. (2002). Resolvins: A family of bioactive products of omega-3 fatty acid transformation circuits initiated by aspirin treatment that counter proinflammation signals. Journal of Experimental Medicine, 196, 1025–1037.

22. Billman, G.E., Kang, J.X., Leaf, A. (1999). Prevention of sudden cardiac death by dietary pure omega-3 polyunsaturated fatty acids in dogs. Circulation, 99, 2452–2457.

23. Leaf, A., Kang, J.X., Xiao, Y.F., Billman, G.E. (2003). Clinical prevention of sudden cardiac death by n-3 polyunsaturated fatty acids and mechanism of prevention of arrhythmias by n-3 fish oils. Circulation, 107, 2646–2652.

24. Xiao, Y.F., Wright, S.N., Wang, G.K., Morgan, J.P., Leaf, A. (1998). Fatty acids suppress voltage-gated Na + currents in HEK293t cells transfected with the alpha-subunit of the human cardiac Na + channel. Proceedings of the National Academy of Sciences USA, 95, 2680–2685.

25. Xiao, Y.F., Wright, S.N., Wang, G.K., Morgan, J.P., Leaf, A. (2000). Coexpression with beta(1)-subunit modifies the kinetics and fatty acid block of hH1(alpha) Na(+) channels. American Journal of Physiology—Heart and Circulatory Physiology, 279, H35–46.

26. Xiao, Y.F., Ke, Q., Wang, S.Y., Auktor, K., Yang, Y., Wang, G.K., Morgan, J.P., Leaf, A. (2001). Single point mutations affect fatty acid block of human myocardial sodium channel alpha subunit Na + channels. Proceedings of the National Academy of Sciences USA, 98, 3606–3611.

27. Leifert, W.R., McMurchie, E.J., Saint, D.A. (1999). Inhibition of cardiac sodium currents in adult rat myocytes by n-3 polyunsaturated fatty acids. Journal of Physiology, 520, 671–679.

28. Xiao, Y.F., Kang, J.X., Morgan, J.P., Leaf, A. (1995). Blocking effects of polyunsaturated fatty acids on Na + channels of neonatal rat ventricular myocytes. Proceedings of the National Academy of Sciences USA, 92, 11000–11004.

29. Saint, D.A. (2008). The cardiac persistent sodium current: An appealing therapeutic target?. British Journal of Pharmacology, 153, 1133–1142.

30. Pu, J., Balser, J.R., Boyden, P.A. (1998). Lidocaine action on Na + currents in ventricular myocytes from the epicardial border zone of the infarcted heart. Circulation Research, 83, 431–440.

31. Nerbonne, J.M., Nichols, C.G., Schwarz, T.L., Escande, D. (2001). Genetic manipulation of cardiac K(+) channel function in mice: What have we learned, and where do we go from here? Circulation Research, 89, 944–956.

32. Honore, E., Barhanin, J., Attali, B., Lesage, F., Lazdunski, M. (1994). External blockade of the major cardiac delayed-rectifier K + channel (Kv1.5) by polyunsaturated fatty acids. Proceedings of the National Academy of Sciences USA, 91, 1937–1941.

33. Garratt, J.C., McEvoy, M.P., Owen, D.G. (1996). Blockade of two voltage-dependent potassium channels, mKv1.1 and mKv1.2, by docosahexaenoic acid. European Journal of Pharmacology, 314, 393–396.

34. Poling, J.S., Karanian, J.W., Salem, N. Jr., Vicini, S. (1995). Time- and voltage-dependent block of delayed rectifier potassium channels by docosahexaenoic acid. Molecular Pharmacology, 47, 381–390.

35. Singleton, C.B., Valenzuela, S.M., Walker, B.D., Tie, H., Wyse, K.R., Bursill, J.A., Qiu, M.R., Breit, S.N., Campbell, T.J. (1999). Blockade by N-3 polyunsaturated fatty acid of the Kv4.3 current stably expressed in Chinese hamster ovary cells. British Journal of Pharmacology, 127, 941–948.

36. Van Wagoner, D.R. (2003). Electrophysiological remodeling in human atrial fibrillation. Pacing and Clinical Electrophysiology, 26, 1572–1575.

37. Lam, T.K., Pocai, A., Gutierrez-Juarez, R., Obici, S., Bryan, J., Aguilar-Bryan, L., Schwartz, G.J., Rossetti, L. (2005). Hypothalamic sensing of circulating fatty acids is required for glucose homeostasis. Nature Medicine, 11, 320–327.

38. Negroni, J.A., Lascano, E.C., del Valle, H.F. (2007). Glibenclamide action on myocardial function and arrhythmia incidence in the healthy and diabetic heart. Cardiovascular and Hematological Agents in Medicinal Chemistry, 5, 43–53.

39. Jude, S., Bedut, S., Roger, S., Pinault, M., Champeroux, P., White, E., Le Guennec, J.Y. (2003). Peroxidation of docosahexaenoic acid is responsible for its effects on I TO and I SS in rat ventricular myocytes. British Journal of Pharmacology, 139, 816–822.

40. Hallaq, H., Smith, T.W., Leaf, A. (1992). Modulation of dihydropyridine-sensitive calcium channels in heart cells by fish oil fatty acids. Proceedings of the National Academy of Sciences USA, 89, 1760–1764.

41. Negretti, N., Perez, M.R., Walker, D., O'Neill, S.C. (2000). Inhibition of sarcoplasmic reticulum function by polyunsaturated fatty acids in intact, isolated myocytes from rat ventricular muscle. Journal of Physiology, 523, 367–375.

42. O'Neill, S.C., Perez, M.R., Hammond, K.E., Sheader, E.A., Negretti, N. (2002). Direct and indirect modulation of rat cardiac sarcoplasmic reticulum function by n-3 polyunsaturated fatty acids. Journal of Physiology, 538, 179–184.

43. Pepe, S., Bogdanov, K., Hallaq, H., Spurgeon, H., Leaf, A., Lakatta, E. (1994). Omega 3 polyunsaturated fatty acid modulates dihydropyridine effects on L-type Ca2 + channels, cytosolic Ca2 +, and contraction in adult rat cardiac myocytes. Proceedings of the National Academy of Sciences USA, 91, 8832–8836.

44. Rodrigo, G.C., Dhanapala, S., Macknight, A.D. (1999). Effects of eicosapentaenoic acid on the contraction of intact, and spontaneous contraction of chemically permeabilized mammalian ventricular myocytes. Journal of Molecular and Cellular Cardiology, 31, 733–743.

45. Danthi, S.J., Enyeart, J.A., Enyeart, J.J. (2005). Modulation of native T-type calcium channels by omega-3 fatty acids. Biochemical and Biophysical Research Communications, 327, 485–493.

46. Kinoshita, I., Itoh, K., Nishida-Nakai, M., Hirota, H., Otsuji, S., Shibata, N. (1994). Antiarrhythmic effects of eicosapentaenoic acid during myocardial infarction–enhanced cardiac microsomal (Ca(2 +)-Mg2 +)-ATPase activity. Japanese Circulation Journal, 58, 903–912.

47. Priori, S.G., Napolitano, C., Memmi, M., Colombi, B., Drago, F., Gasparini, M., DeSimone, L., Coltorti, F., Bloise, R., Keegan, R., Cruz Filho, F.E., Vignati, G., Benatar, A., DeLogu, A. (2002). Clinical and molecular characterization of patients with catecholaminergic polymorphic ventricular tachycardia. Circulation, 106, 69–74.

48. Honen, B.N., Saint, D.A., Laver, D.R. (2003). Suppression of calcium sparks in rat ventricular myocytes and direct inhibition of sheep cardiac RyR channels by EPA, DHA and oleic acid. Journal of Membrane Biology, 196, 95–103.

49. Swan, J.S., Dibb, K., Negretti, N., O'Neill, S.C., Sitsapesan, R. (2003). Effects of eicosapentaenoic acid on cardiac SR Ca(2 +)-release and ryanodine receptor function. Cardiovascular Research, 60, 337–346.

50. Den Ruijter, H.M., Berecki, G., Verkerk, A.O., Bakker, D., Baartscheer, A., Schumacher, C.A., Belterman, C.N., de Jonge, N., Fiolet, J.W., Brouwer, I.A., Coronel, R. (2008). Acute administration of fish oil inhibits triggered activity in isolated myocytes from rabbits and patients with heart failure. Circulation, 117, 536–544.

51. Despa, S., Islam, M.A., Pogwizd, S.M., Bers, D.M. (2002). Intracellular [Na +] and Na + pump rate in rat and rabbit ventricular myocytes. Journal of Physiology, 539, 133–143.

52. Verkerk, A.O., van Ginneken, A.C., Berecki, G., den Ruijter, H.M., Schumacher, C.A., Veldkamp, M.W., Baartscheer, A., Casini, S., Opthof, T., Hovenier, R., Fiolet, J.W., Zock, P.L., Coronel, R. (2006). Incorporated sarcolemmal fish oil fatty acids shorten pig ventricular action potentials. Cardiovascular Research, 70, 509–520.

53. Macleod, J.C., Macknight, A.D., Rodrigo, G.C. (1998). The electrical and mechanical response of adult guinea pig and rat ventricular myocytes to omega3 polyunsaturated fatty acids. European Journal of Pharmacology, 356, 261–270.

54. Leifert, W.R., Dorian, C.L., Jahangiri, A., McMurchie, E.J. (2001). Dietary fish oil prevents asynchronous contractility and alters Ca(2 +) handling in adult rat cardiomyocytes. Journal of Nutritional Biochemistry, 12, 365–376.

55. Jahangiri, A., Leifert, W.R., Patten, G.S., McMurchie, E.J. (2000). Termination of asynchronous contractile activity in rat atrial myocytes by n-3 polyunsaturated fatty acids. Molecular and Cellular Biochemistry., 206, 33–41.

56. Leaf, A., Xiao, Y.F., Kang, J.X. (2002). Interactions of n-3 fatty acids with ion channels in excitable tissues. Prostaglandins, Leukotrienes and Essential Fatty Acids, 67, 113–120.

57. Rinaldi, B., Di Pierro, P., Vitelli, M.R., D'Amico, M., Berrino, L., Rossi, F., Filippelli, A. (2002). Effects of docosahexaenoic acid on calcium pathway in adult rat cardiomyocytes. Life Sciences, 71, 993–1004.

58. Burt, J.M., Massey, K.D., Minnich, B.N. (1991). Uncoupling of cardiac cells by fatty acids: Structure-activity relationships. American Journal of Physiology, 260, C439–448.

59. Anderson, K.E., Du, X.J., Sinclair, A.J., Woodcock, E.A., Dart, A.M. (1996). Dietary fish oil prevents reperfusion Ins(1,4,5)P3 release in rat heart: possible antiarrhythmic mechanism. American Journal of Physiology, 271, H1483–1490.

60. Lepran, I., Nemecz, G., Koltai, M., Szekeres, L. (1981). Effect of a linoleic acid-rich diet on the acute phase of coronary occlusion in conscious rats: influence of indomethacin and aspirin. Journal of Cardiovascular Pharmacology, 3, 847–853.

61. Hock, C.E., Beck, L.D., Bodine, R.C., Reibel, D.K. (1990). Influence of dietary n-3 fatty acids on myocardial ischemia and reperfusion. American Journal of Physiology, 259, H1518–1526.

62. McLennan, P.L. (1993). Relative effects of dietary saturated, monounsaturated, and polyunsaturated fatty acids on cardiac arrhythmias in rats. American Journal of Clinical Nutrition, 57, 207–212.

63. Owen, A.J., Peter-Przyborowska, B.A., Hoy, A.J., McLennan, P.L. (2004). Dietary fish oil dose- and time-response effects on cardiac phospholipid fatty acid composition. Lipids, 39, 955–961.

64. Yang, B., Saldeen, T.G., Nichols, W.W., Mehta, J.L. (1993). Dietary fish oil supplementation attenuates myocardial dysfunction and injury caused by global ischemia and reperfusion in isolated rat hearts. Journal of Nutrition, 123, 2067–2074.

65. Ma, D.W., Seo, J., Switzer, K.C., Fan, Y.Y., McMurray, D.N., Lupton, J.R., Chapkin, R.S. (2004). n-3 PUFA and membrane microdomains: A new frontier in bioactive lipid research. Journal of Nutritional Biochemistry, 15, 700–706.

66. Reibel, D.K., Holahan, M.A., Hock, C.E. (1988). Effects of dietary fish oil on cardiac responsiveness to adrenoceptor stimulation. American Journal of Physiology, 254, H494–499.

67. Reithmann, C., Scheininger, C., Bulgan, T., Werdan, K. (1996). Exposure to the n-3 polyunsaturated fatty acid docosahexaenoic acid impairs alpha 1-adrenoceptor-mediated

contractile responses and inositol phosphate formation in rat cardiomyocytes. Naunyn-Schmiedeberg's Archives of Pharmacology, 354, 109–119.

68. Wince, L.C., Hugman, L.E., Chen, W.Y., Robbins, R.K., Brenner, G.M. (1987). Effect of dietary lipids on inotropic responses of isolated rat left atrium: Attenuation of maximal responses by an unsaturated fat diet. Journal of Pharmacology and Experimental Therapeutics, 241, 838–845.

69. Mirnikjoo, B., Brown, S.E., Kim, H.F., Marangell, L.B., Sweatt, J.D., Weeber, E.J. (2001). Protein kinase inhibition by omega-3 fatty acids. Journal of Biological Chemistry, 276, 10888–10896.

70. Speizer, L.A., Watson, M.J., Brunton, L.L. (1991). Differential effects of omega-3 fish oils on protein kinase activities in vitro. American Journal of Physiology, 261, E109–114.

71. Pogwizd, S.M., Bers, D.M. (2004). Cellular basis of triggered arrhythmias in heart failure. Trends in Cardiovascular Medicine, 14, 61–66.

72. Anderson, M.E., Braun, A.P., Wu, Y., Lu, T., Wu, Y., Schulman, H., Sung, R.J. (1998). KN-93, an inhibitor of multifunctional Ca + + /calmodulin-dependent protein kinase, decreases early afterdepolarizations in rabbit heart. Journal of Pharmacology and Experimental Therapeutics, 287, 996–1006.

73. Zhang, R., Khoo, M.S., Wu, Y., Yang, Y., Grueter, C.E., Ni, G., Price, E.E. Jr., Thiel, W., Guatimosim, S., Song, L.S., Madu, E.C., Shah, A.N., Vishnivetskaya, T.A., Atkinson, J.B., Gurevich, V.V., Salama, G., Lederer, W.J., Colbran, R.J., Anderson, M.E. (2005). Calmodulin kinase II inhibition protects against structural heart disease. Nature Medicine, 11, 409–417.

74. Takayama, K., Yuhki, K., Ono, K., Fujino, T., Hara, A., Yamada, T., Kuriyama, S., Karibe, H., Okada, Y., Takahata, O., Taniguchi, T., Iijima, T., Iwasaki, H., Narumiya, S., Ushikubi, F. (2005). Thromboxane A2 and prostaglandin F2alpha mediate inflammatory tachycardia. Nature Medicine, 11, 562–566.

75. Fickl, H., Cockeran, R., Steel, H.C., Feldman, C., Cowan, G., Mitchell, T.J., Anderson, R. (2005). Pneumolysin-mediated activation of NFkappaB in human neutrophils is antagonized by docosahexaenoic acid. Clinical and Experimental Immunology, 140, 274–281.

76. Henry, P.D., Pacifico, A. (1998). Altering molecular mechanisms to prevent sudden arrhythmic death. Lancet, 351, 1276–1278.

77. Huang, B., El-Sherif, T., Gidh-Jain, M., Qin, D., El-Sherif, N. (2001). Alterations of sodium channel kinetics and gene expression in the postinfarction remodeled myocardium. Journal of Cardiovascular Electrophysiology, 12, 218–225.

78. Jordan, H., Matthan, N., Chung, M., Balk, E., Chew, P., Kupelnick, B., DeVine, D., Lawrence, A., Lichtenstein, A., Lau, J. (2004). Effects of omega-3 fatty acids on arrhythmogenic mechanisms in animal and isolated organ/cell culture studies. Evidence Report—Technology Assessment, 1–8.

79. Matthan, N.R., Jordan, H., Chung, M., Lichtenstein, A.H., Lathrop, D.A., Lau, J. (2005). A systematic review and meta-analysis of the impact of omega-3 fatty acids on selected arrhythmia outcomes in animal models. Metabolism, 54, 1557–1565.

80. Billman, G.E., Hallaq, H., Leaf, A. (1994). Prevention of ischemia-induced ventricular fibrillation by omega 3 fatty acids. Proceedings of the National Academy of Sciences USA, 91, 4427–4430.

81. Billman, G.E. (2006). A comprehensive review and analysis of 25 years of data from an in vivo canine model of sudden cardiac death: Implications for future anti-arrhythmic drug development. Pharmacology and Therapeutics, 111, 808–835.

82. da Cunha, D.N., Hamlin, R.L., Billman, G.E., Carnes, C.A. (2007). n-3 (omega-3) polyunsaturated fatty acids prevent acute atrial electrophysiological remodeling. British Journal of Pharmacology, 150, 281–285.

83. McLennan, P.L., Abeywardena, M.Y., Charnock, J.S. (1985). Influence of dietary lipids on arrhythmias and infarction after coronary artery ligation in rats. Canadian Journal of Physiology and Pharmacology, 63, 1411–1417.

84. Charnock, J.S., McLennan, P.L., Abeywardena, M.Y., Dryden, W.F. (1985). Diet and cardiac arrhythmia: Effects of lipids on age-related changes in myocardial function in the rat. Annals of Nutrition and Metabolism, 29, 306–318.

85. Pepe, S., McLennan, P.L. (2002). Cardiac membrane fatty acid composition modulates myocardial oxygen consumption and postischemic recovery of contractile function. Circulation, 105, 2303–2308.

86. Mitasikova, M., Smidova, S., Macsaliova, A., Knezl, V., Dlugosova, K., Okruhlicova, L., Weismann, P., Tribulova, N. (2008). Aged male and female spontaneously hypertensive rats benefit from n-3 polyunsaturated fatty acids supplementation. Physiological Research, 57, S39–48.

87. Salama, G., London, B. (2007). Mouse models of long QT syndrome. Journal of Physiology, 578, 43–53.

88. Den Ruijter, H.M., Verkerk, A.O., Berecki, G., Bakker, D., van Ginneken, A.C., Coronel, R. (2006). Dietary fish oil reduces the occurrence of early afterdepolarizations in pig ventricular myocytes. Journal of Molecular and Cellular Cardiology, 41, 914–917.

89. Coronel, R., Wilms-Schopman, F.J., Den Ruijter, H.M., Belterman, C.N., Schumacher, C.A., Opthof, T., Hovenier, R., Lemmens, A.G., Terpstra, A.H., Katan, M.B., Zock, P. (2007). Dietary n-3 fatty acids promote arrhythmias during acute regional myocardial ischemia in isolated pig hearts. Cardiovascular Research, 73, 386–394.

90. McLennan, P.L., Bridle, T.M., Abeywardena, M.Y., Charnock, J.S. (1992). Dietary lipid modulation of ventricular fibrillation threshold in the marmoset monkey. American Heart Journal, 123, 1555–1561.

91. Bang, H.O., Dyerbert, J. (1980). Lipid metabolism and ischemic heart disease in Greenland Eskimos. In: Draper, H., ed. Advances in Nutrition Research. Plenum Press, New York, 1–22.

92. Kagawa, Y., Nishizawa, M., Suzuki, M., Miyatake, T., Hamamoto, T., Goto, K., Motonaga, E., Izumikawa, H., Hirata, H., Ebihara, A. (1982). Eicosapolyenoic acids of serum lipids of Japanese islanders with low incidence of cardiovascular diseases. Journal of Nutritional Science and Vitaminology, 28, 441–453.

93. Ascherio, A., Rimm, E.B., Stampfer, M.J., Giovannucci, E.L., Willett, W.C. (1995). Dietary intake of marine n-3 fatty acids, fish intake, and the risk of coronary disease among men. New England Journal of Medicine, 332, 977–982.

94. Curb, J.D., Reed, D.M. (1985). Fish consumption and mortality from coronary heart disease. New England Journal of Medicine, 313, 821–822.

95. Morris, M.C., Manson, J.E., Rosner, B., Buring, J.E., Willett, W.C., Hennekens, C.H. (1995). Fish consumption and cardiovascular disease in the physicians' health study: A prospective study. American Journal of Epidemiology, 142, 166–175.

96. Vollset, S.E., Heuch, I., Bjelke, E. (1985). Fish consumption and mortality from coronary heart disease. New England Journal of Medicine, 313, 820–821.

97. Daviglus, M.L., Stamler, J., Orencia, A.J., Dyer, A.R., Liu, K., Greenland, P., Walsh, M.K., Morris, D., Shekelle, R.B. (1997). Fish consumption and the 30-year risk of fatal myocardial infarction. New England Journal of Medicine, 336, 1046–1053.

98. Dolecek, T.A. (1992). Epidemiological evidence of relationships between dietary polyunsaturated fatty acids and mortality in the multiple risk factor intervention trial. Proceedings of the Society for Experimental Biology and Medicine, 200, 177–182.

99. He, K., Song, Y., Daviglus, M.L., Liu, K., Van Horn, L., Dyer, A.R., Greenland, P. (2004). Accumulated evidence on fish consumption and coronary heart disease mortality: A meta-analysis of cohort studies. Circulation, 109, 2705–2711.

100. Albert, C.M., Hennekens, C.H., O'Donnell, C.J., Ajani, U.A., Carey, V.J., Willett, W.C., Ruskin, J.N., Manson, J.E. (1998). Fish consumption and risk of sudden cardiac death. Journal of the American Medical Association, 279, 23–28.

101. Hu, F.B., Bronner, L., Willett, W.C., Stampfer, M.J., Rexrode, K.M., Albert, C.M., Hunter, D., Manson, J.E. (2002). Fish and omega-3 fatty acid intake and risk of coronary heart disease in women. Journal of the American Medical Association, 287, 1815–1821.

102. Iso, H., Kobayashi, M., Ishihara, J., Sasaki, S., Okada, K., Kita, Y., Kokubo, Y., Tsugane, S. (2006). Intake of fish and n3 fatty acids and risk of coronary heart disease among Japanese: The Japan Public Health Center-Based (JPHC) Study Cohort I. Circulation, 113, 195–202.

103. Mozaffarian, D., Lemaitre, R.N., Kuller, L.H., Burke, G.L., Tracy, R.P., Siscovick, D.S. (2003). Cardiac benefits of fish consumption may depend on the type of fish meal consumed: the Cardiovascular Health Study. Circulation, 107, 1372–1377.

104. Bolger, P.M., Schwetz, B.A. (2002). Mercury and health. New England Journal of Medicine, 347, 1735–1736.

105. Ascherio, A., Rimm, E.B., Giovannucci, E.L., Spiegelman, D., Stampfer, M., Willett, W.C. (1996). Dietary fat and risk of coronary heart disease in men: cohort follow up study in the United States. British Medical Journal, 313, 84–90.

106. Hu, F.B., Stampfer, M.J., Manson, J.E., Rimm, E.B., Wolk, A., Colditz, G.A., Hennekens, C.H., Willett, W.C. (1999). Dietary intake of alpha-linolenic acid and risk of fatal ischemic heart disease among women. American Journal of Clinical Nutrition, 69, 890–897.

107. Pietinen, P., Ascherio, A., Korhonen, P., Hartman, A.M., Willett, W.C., Albanes, D., Virtamo, J. (1997). Intake of fatty acids and risk of coronary heart disease in a cohort of Finnish men. The Alpha-Tocopherol, Beta-Carotene Cancer Prevention Study. American Journal of Epidemiology, 145, 876–887.

108. Oomen, C.M., Ocke, M.C., Feskens, E.J., Kok, F.J., Kromhout, D. (2001). alpha-Linolenic acid intake is not beneficially associated with 10-y risk of coronary artery disease incidence: The Zutphen Elderly Study. American Journal of Clinical Nutrition, 74, 457–463.

109. Siscovick, D.S., Raghunathan, T.E., King, I., Weinmann, S., Wicklund, K.G., Albright, J., Bovbjerg, V., Arbogast, P., Smith, H., Kushi, L.H., et al. (1995). Dietary intake and cell membrane levels of long-chain n-3 polyunsaturated fatty acids and the risk of primary cardiac arrest. Journal of the American Medical Association, 274, 1363–1367.

110. Albert, C.M., Campos, H., Stampfer, M.J., Ridker, P.M., Manson, J.E., Willett, W.C., Ma, J. (2002). Blood levels of long-chain n-3 fatty acids and the risk of sudden death. New England Journal of Medicine, 346, 1113–1118.

111. Mozaffarian, D., Ascherio, A., Hu, F.B., Stampfer, M.J., Willett, W.C., Siscovick, D.S., Rimm, E.B. (2005). Interplay between different polyunsaturated fatty acids and risk of coronary heart disease in men. Circulation, 111, 157–164.

112. Albert, C.M., Oh, K., Whang, W., Manson, J.E., Chae, C.U., Stampfer, M.J., Willett, W.C., Hu, F.B. (2005). Dietary alpha-linolenic acid intake and risk of sudden cardiac death and coronary heart disease. Circulation, 112, 3232–3238.

113. Greene, H.L. (1990). Sudden arrhythmic cardiac death--mechanisms, resuscitation and classification: The Seattle perspective. American Journal of Cardiology, 65, 4B–12B.

114. Mozaffarian, D., Psaty, B.M., Rimm, E.B., Lemaitre, R.N., Burke, G.L., Lyles, M.F., Lefkowitz, D., Siscovick, D.S. (2004). Fish intake and risk of incident atrial fibrillation. Circulation, 110, 368–373.

115. Frost, L., Vestergaard, P. (2005). n-3 Fatty acids consumed from fish and risk of atrial fibrillation or flutter: the Danish Diet, Cancer, and Health Study. American Journal of Clinical Nutrition, 81, 50–54.

116. Brouwer, I.A., Heeringa, J., Geleijnse, J.M., Zock, P.L., Witteman, J.C. (2006). Intake of very long-chain n-3 fatty acids from fish and incidence of atrial fibrillation. The Rotterdam Study. American Heart Journal, 151, 857–862.

117. Burr, M.L., Fehily, A.M., Gilbert, J.F., Rogers, S., Holliday, R.M., Sweetnam, P.M., Elwood, P.C., Deadman, N.M. (1989). Effects of changes in fat, fish, and fibre intakes on death and myocardial reinfarction: Diet and reinfarction trial (DART). Lancet, 2, 757–761.

118. Burr, M.L., Ashfield-Watt, P.A., Dunstan, F.D., Fehily, A.M., Breay, P., Ashton, T., Zotos, P.C., Haboubi, N.A., Elwood, P.C. (2003). Lack of benefit of dietary advice to men with angina: results of a controlled trial. European Journal of Clinical Nutrition, 57, 193–200.

119. de Lorgeril, M., Renaud, S., Mamelle, N., Salen, P., Martin, J.L., Monjaud, I., Guidollet, J., Touboul, P., Delaye, J. (1994). Mediterranean alpha-linolenic acid-rich diet in secondary prevention of coronary heart disease. Lancet, 343, 1454–1459.

120. de Lorgeril, M., Salen, P., Martin, J.L., Monjaud, I., Delaye, J., Mamelle, N. (1999). Mediterranean diet, traditional risk factors, and the rate of cardiovascular complications after myocardial infarction: Final report of the Lyon Diet Heart Study. Circulation, 99, 779–785.

121. Dietary supplementation with n-3 polyunsaturated fatty acids and vitamin E after myocardial infarction: Results of the GISSI-Prevenzione trial. Gruppo Italiano per lo Studio della Sopravvivenza nell'Infarto miocardico. (1999). Lancet, 354, 447–455.

122. Leng, G.C. , Lee, A.J., Fowkes, F.G., Jepson, R.G., Lowe, G.D., Skinner, E.R., Mowat, B.F. (1998). Randomized controlled trial of gamma-linolenic acid and eicosapentaenoic acid in peripheral arterial disease. Clinical Nutrition, 17, 265–271.

123. Nilsen, D.W., Albrektsen, G., Landmark, K., Moen, S., Aarsland, T., Woie, L. (2001). Effects of a high-dose concentrate of n-3 fatty acids or corn oil introduced early after an acute myocardial infarction on serum triacylglycerol and HDL cholesterol. American Journal of Clinical Nutrition, 74, 50–56.

124. Sacks, F.M., Stone, P.H., Gibson, C.M., Silverman, D.I., Rosner, B., Pasternak, R.C. (1995). HARP Research Group. Controlled trial of fish oil for regression of human coronary atherosclerosis. Journal of the American College of Cardiology, 25, 1492–1498.

125. Singh, R.B., Niaz, M.A., Sharma, J.P., Kumar, R., Rastogi, V., Moshiri, M. (1997). Randomized, double-blind, placebo-controlled trial of fish oil and mustard oil in patients with suspected acute myocardial infarction: The Indian experiment of infarct survival–4. Cardiovascular Drugs and Therapy, 11, 485–491.

126. von Schacky, C., Angerer, P., Kothny, W., Theisen, K., Mudra, H. (1999). The effect of dietary omega-3 fatty acids on coronary atherosclerosis. A randomized, double-blind, placebo-controlled trial. Annals of Internal Medicine, 130, 554–562.

127. Harper, C.R., Jacobson, T.A. (2005). Usefulness of omega-3 fatty acids and the prevention of coronary heart disease. The American Journal of Cardiology, 96, 1521–1529.

128. Marchioli, R., Barzi, F., Bomba, E., Chieffo, C., Di Gregorio, D., Di Mascio, R., Franzosi, M.G., Geraci, E., Levantesi, G., Maggioni, A.P., Mantini, L., Marfisi, R.M., Mastrogiuseppe, G., Mininni, N., Nicolosi, G.L., Santini, M., Schweiger, C., Tavazzi, L., Tognoni, G., Tucci, C., Valagussa, F. (2002). Early protection against sudden death by n-3 polyunsaturated fatty acids after myocardial infarction: time-course analysis of the results of the Gruppo Italiano per lo Studio della Sopravvivenza nell'Infarto Miocardico (GISSI)-Prevenzione. Circulation, 105, 1897–1903.

129. Macchia, A., Levantesi, G., Franzosi, M.G., Geraci, E., Maggioni, A.P., Marfisi, R., Nicolosi, G.L., Schweiger, C., Tavazzi, L., Tognoni, G., Valagussa, F., Marchioli, R. (2005). Left ventricular systolic dysfunction, total mortality, and sudden death in patients with myocardial infarction treated with n-3 polyunsaturated fatty acids. European Journal of Heart Failure, 7, 904–909.

130. Yokoyama, M., Origasa, H., Matsuzaki, M., Matsuzawa, Y., Saito, Y., Ishikawa, Y., Oikawa, S., Sasaki, J., Hishida, H., Itakura, H., Kita, T., Kitabatake, A., Nakaya, N., Sakata, T., Shimada, K., Shirato, K. (2007). Effects of eicosapentaenoic acid on major coronary events in hypercholesterolaemic patients (JELIS): A randomised open-label, blinded endpoint analysis. Lancet, 369, 1090–1098.

131. Mozaffarian, D. (2007). JELIS, fish oil, and cardiac events. Lancet, 369, 1062–1063.

132. Tavazzi, L., Maggioni, A.P., Marchioli, R., Barlera, S., Franzosi, M.G., Latini, R., Lucci, D., Nicolosi, G.L., Porcu, M., Tognoni, G. (2008). Effect of n-3 polyunsaturated fatty acids in patients with chronic heart failure (the GISSI-HF trial): A randomised, double-blind, placebo-controlled trial. Lancet, 372, 1223–1230.

133. Natvig, H., Borchgrevink, C.F., Dedichen, J., Owren, P.A., Schiotz, E.H., Westlund, K. (1968). A controlled trial of the effect of linolenic acid on incidence of coronary heart disease. The Norwegian vegetable oil experiment of 1965–66. Scandinavian Journal of Clinical and Laboratory Investigation Supplementum, 105, 1–20.

134. Rauch, B., Schiele, R., Schneider, S., Gohlke, H., Diller, F., Gottwik, M., Steinbeck, G., Heer, T., Katus, H., Zimmer, R., Erdogan, A., Pfafferott, C., Senges, J. (2006). Highly purified omega-3 fatty acids for secondary prevention of sudden cardiac death after myocardial infarction-aims and methods of the OMEGA-study. Cardiovascular Drugs and Therapy, 20, 365–375.

135. Alpha Omega Trial. http://clinicaltrials.gov/ct2/show/NCT00139464. Accessed January 23, 2009.

136. ASCEND (A Study of Cardiovascular Events iN Diabetes) Trial. http://clinicaltrials.gov/ct2/show/NCT00135226. Accessed January 23, 2009.

137. ORIGIN (Outcome Reduction with Initial Glargine InterventioN) Trial. http://www.clinicaltrials.gov/ct/show/NCT00069784. Accessed March 13, 2009.

138. Schrepf, R., Limmert, T., Claus Weber, P., Theisen, K., Sellmayer, A. (2004). Immediate effects of n-3 fatty acid infusion on the induction of sustained ventricular tachycardia. Lancet, 363, 1441–1442.

139. Ellenbogen, K.A., Levine, J.H., Berger, R.D., Daubert, J.P., Winters, S.L., Greenstein, E., Shalaby, A., Schaechter, A., Subacius, H., Kadish, A. (2006). Are implantable cardio-verter defibrillator shocks a surrogate for sudden cardiac death in patients with non-ischemic cardiomyopathy? Circulation, 113, 776–782.

140. Calo, L., Bianconi, L., Colivicchi, F., Lamberti, F., Loricchio, M.L., de Ruvo, E., Meo, A., Pandozi, C., Staibano, M., Santini, M. (2005). N-3 Fatty acids for the prevention of atrial fibrillation after coronary artery bypass surgery: A randomized, controlled trial. Journal of the American College of Cardiology, 45, 1723–1728.

141. Jouven, X., Zureik, M., Desnos, M., Guerot, C., Ducimetiere, P. (2001). Resting heart rate as a predictive risk factor for sudden death in middle-aged men. Cardiovascular Research, 50, 373–378.

142. Mozaffarian, D., Geelen, A., Brouwer, I.A., Geleijnse, J.M., Zock, P.L., Katan, M.B. (2005). Effect of fish oil on heart rate in humans: A meta-analysis of randomized controlled trials. Circulation, 112, 1945–1952.

143. Christensen, J.H., Schmidt, E.B. (2007). Autonomic nervous system, heart rate variability and n-3 fatty acids. Journal of Cardiovascular Medicine, S19–22.

144. Christensen, J.H., Gustenhoff, P., Korup, E., Aaroe, J., Toft, E., Moller, J., Rasmussen, K., Dyerberg, J., Schmidt, E.B. (1996). Effect of fish oil on heart rate variability in survivors of myocardial infarction: A double blind randomised controlled trial. British Medical Journal, 312, 677–678.

145. Algra, A., Tijssen, J.G., Roelandt, J.R., Pool, J., Lubsen, J. (1991). QTc prolongation measured by standard 12-lead electrocardiography is an independent risk factor for sudden death due to cardiac arrest. Circulation, 83, 1888–1894.

146. Vrtovec, B., Delgado, R., Zewail, A., Thomas, C.D., Richartz, B.M., Radovancevic, B. (2003). Prolonged QTc interval and high B-type natriuretic peptide levels together predict mortality in patients with advanced heart failure. Circulation, 107, 1764–1769.

147. Chrysohoou, C., Panagiotakos, D.B., Pitsavos, C., Skoumas, J., Krinos, X., Chloptsios, Y., Nikolaou, V., Stefanadis, C. (2007). Long-term fish consumption is associated with protection against arrhythmia in healthy persons in a Mediterranean region--the ATTICA study. American Journal of Clinical Nutrition, 85, 1385–1391.

■ GENERAL INDEX

Ablation: 135, 155, 165, 237, 431, 461
Acetylation: 157
Acidosis: 28, 104, 110, 346–348, 439, 446
Action potential:
  Dispersion: 317, 416, 431–433, 439
  Prolongation: 10, 23, 74, 131, 132, 156,
    161, 175, 177, 215, 254, 355, 316, 317,
    369, 370, 372, 467, 486, 488, 549
  Restitution: 416
  Shortening: 8–12, 21, 25, 26, 158, 183, 188,
    193, 273, 285, 316, 326, 353, 355, 373,
    374, 383, 384, 393, 396, 416, 417, 421,
    422, 432, 546, 547, 549
  Upstroke velocity (Vmax): 110, 111, 115,
    116, 120–122, 348, 395, 416, 421, 436,
    450
Activation recovery interval: 106, 434,
  435, 445
Adrenergic receptors
  α-adrenergic receptors: 157, 284, 285,
    485, 496
  β-adrenergic receptors: 21, 63, 72, 83, 161,
    210, 302, 350, 352, 433, 485, 496, 516,
    521–523, 525, 527–529, 548
  β_1-adrenergic receptors: 70, 164, 280, 284,
    285, 521–523, 527
  β_2-adrenergic receptors: 136, 235, 316,
    344, 355, 516, 519, 521–523, 527
Afterdepolarizations: 136, 235, 316,
  344, 355, 522, 528, 529, 545,
  546, 548
  Delayed afterdepolarizations (DADs):
    116, 179, 276, 277, 279, 280, 301–304,
    314, 316–318, 321, 322, 324, 326, 328,
    339, 348, 350, 354, 355, 415, 470, 528,
    529, 546

Early afterdepolarizations (EADs): 158,
  215, 216, 235, 272, 274, 275, 282, 283,
  316–318, 321, 324, 326, 327, 339, 350,
  354, 355, 370, 415, 467, 549
Alternans: 251, 301, 302, 304–306, 324, 418,
  439, 443
Andersen (Andresen-Tawil) syndrome: 23,
  180
Angina pectoris: 72, 74, 76, 102, 112, 203,
  215, 216, 400, 551, 552
Anoxia: 107–109, 323
Anisotrophy: 127–129, 431, 432, 450
Antianginal: 76, 161, 206, 208, 213, 215, 255
Antiischemic: 76
Antioxidant: 305, 307, 418–420, 422,
  423, 469
Apoptosis: 136, 284, 285, 342
Arrhythmia Phase (or type) 1a: 103, 104,
  107–113, 417, 418
  Phase (or type) 1b: 103, 111, 113–115, 418
Athletes: 188, 514, 515
Atrial Fibrillation: 1, 18, 20, 22, 26, 64, 80, 81,
  165, 201, 205–208, 212, 213, 216–221,
  236, 237, 242, 244, 248–251, 254, 255,
  313, 324, 326, 327, 346, 353, 371,
  444–446, 453, 485–488, 511, 546, 551,
  555, see chapter 17
Atrial flutter: 208, 212, 219, 220, 242, 488,
  489
Atroventricular node (AV node): 5, 6, 8, 64,
  81, 157, 158, 162–165, 175, 193, 202,
  204, 211, 214, 235, 314, 322, 367, 414,
  432, 488
Autoinhibitory: 341
Automaticity: 20, 59, 116, 163, 202, 386, 414,
  415, 444

Novel Therapeutic Targets for Antiarrhythmic Drugs, Edited by George Edward Billman
Copyright © 2010 John Wiley & Sons, Inc.

INDEX OF DRUG AND CHEMICAL NAMES

Novel Therapeutic Targets for Antiarrhythmic Drugs, Edited by George Edward Billman
Copyright © 2010 John Wiley & Sons, Inc.